Diabetes

Novel Insights and Therapies

Diabetes

Novel Insights and Therapies

Anas Islam, MPharm
Badruddeen, PhD
Editors

AAP | APPLE ACADEMIC PRESS

First edition published 2027

Apple Academic Press Inc.
1265 Goldenrod Circle, NE,
Palm Bay, FL 32905 USA

760 Laurentian Drive, Unit 19,
Burlington, ON L7N 0A4, Canada

CRC Press
2385 NW Executive Center Drive,
Suite 320, Boca Raton FL 33431

4 Park Square, Milton Park,
Abingdon, Oxon, OX14 4RN, UK

Apple Academic Press exclusively co-publishes with CRC Press, an imprint of Taylor & Francis Group, LLC

Library and Archives Canada Cataloguing in Publication

CIP data on file with Canada Library and Archives

Library of Congress Cataloging-in-Publication Data

CIP data on file with US Library of Congress

ISBN: 978-1-77964-458-9 (hbk)
ISBN: 978-1-77964-459-6 (ebk)

DOI: 10.1201/9781779644596

About the Editors

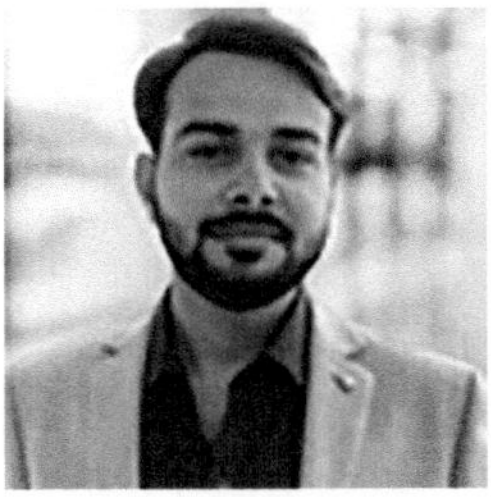

Anas Islam, MPharm
Researcher and Lecturer, Faculty of Pharmacy, Integral University, Lucknow, India

Anas Islam is a distinguished professional in the field of pharmacology, with a keen focus on the evaluation of therapeutic agents and their impact on various health conditions. Possessing a master's degree in pharmacology and currently pursuing a PhD in pharmacy, Mr. Islam has established himself as a dedicated and knowledgeable researcher with a profound understanding of pharmaceutical sciences. His commitment to advancing therapeutic solutions is evident through his significant contributions to academia and research. Mr. Islam has published several book chapters and served as an editor for a comprehensive volume in the field. His research findings have been featured in reputable journals, showcasing the depth of his contributions to the scientific community.

In addition to his research pursuits, Mr. Islam serves as a lecturer in the Faculty of Pharmacy at Integral University, Lucknow, where he imparts knowledge in subjects such as pharmacology, toxicology, and pharmacotherapeutics. His role as an educator underscores his dedication to nurturing the next generation of professionals in the pharmaceutical field. With a strong educational background, an extensive research portfolio, and a commitment to excellence, Mr. Anas Islam is a respected figure in the field, contributing significantly to the advancement of pharmaceutical sciences. As he continues his doctoral studies and engages in cutting-edge research, Mr. Islam remains at the forefront of shaping the future of pharmacological research and education.

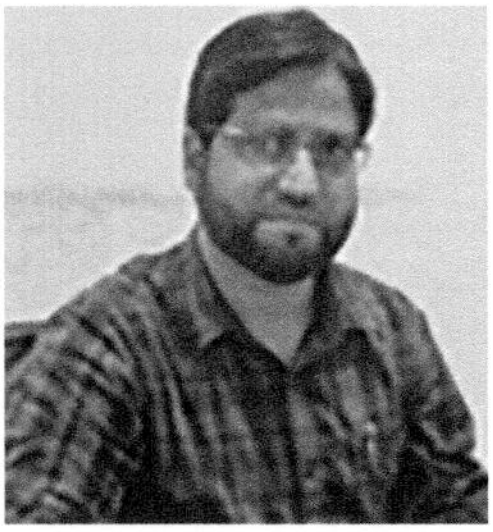

Badruddeen, PhD
Professor, Faculty of Pharmacy, Integral University Lucknow, Uttar Pradesh, India

Badruddeen, PhD, stands as a distinguished figure in the field of pharmacology, holding a PhD in pharmacology from Integral University, Lucknow, India, awarded in 2014. With a robust academic background that includes both BPharm and MPharm degrees from Jamia Hamdard, New Delhi, India, he has emerged as a leading expert in the assessment of safety, toxicity, and clinical efficacy of both herbal and allopathic drugs. His scholarly contributions are underscored by an impressive citation count of more than 1,000 and an h-index of 16—figures that reflect the substantial impact of his work in the field.

Dr. Badruddeen's expertise spans cardiovascular, neurodegenerative, and endocrine diseases, reflecting his comprehensive understanding of diverse therapeutic areas. A prolific author, he has published numerous original articles in esteemed journals, showcasing his dedication to advancing scientific knowledge in pharmacology. As an academic book editor and a member of the editorial boards of prestigious journals, he actively contributes to shaping the discourse in his field. Beyond his research endeavors, Dr. Badruddeen is deeply involved in academic leadership and ethical oversight. He has successfully supervised a dozen research scholars, demonstrating his commitment to mentorship and knowledge dissemination. His affiliations include memberships in esteemed organizations such as the Indian Science Congress Association, where he actively engages with the broader scholarly community. Dr. Badruddeen holds key positions in various committees and centers, further emphasizing his commitment to ethical and responsible research practices. He serves as the member secretary of the Institutional Animal Ethics Committee (IAEC), coordinator of the Adverse Drug Monitoring Center (AMC), chair of the Causality Assessment Committee (CAC), and a member of the Animal House Facility at Integral University. In these roles, he plays a vital part in upholding the highest standards of research ethics and animal welfare.

Contents

Contributors .... *ix*

Abbreviations .... *xiii*

Preface .... *xix*

PART I: Understanding Diabetes 1

1. Definition, Classification, and Epidemiological Perspectives 3
Sara Khan, Anas Islam, Badruddeen, and Yusuf Asad

2. Etiological Insights and Pathophysiological Mechanisms of Diabetes 33
Ayeza Sarwar Kalam, Sahil Hussain, Mohammad Irfan Khan, and Alina Khan

PART II: Diagnosis and Management 61

3. Diagnostic Modalities and Holistic Management Strategies for Diabetes 63
Mohd. Mursal, Mohammad Ahmad, Deeba Shamim Jairajpuri, and Asad Ahmad

4. Navigating Diabetes Complications and Comorbidities 83
Mohsin Vahid Khan, Mohammad Rumman, Gulam Rabbani, Mohd Kamil Hussain, and Nafees Ahmad

PART III: Natural and Innovative Therapies 127

5. Harnessing Nature: Exploring Natural Products in Diabetes Management 129
Tahreen Taj, Swastik Verma, Ashwin Kotnis, Prashul Sethi, Himanshu Sharma, and Sumel Ashique

6. Revolutionizing Diabetes Care with Nanotechnology Innovations 205
Purba Mandal, Aditya Singh, Juber Akhtar, and Perwez Alam

7. Decoding the Genomic Foundations of Diabetes 247
Raja Chakraverty, Iryna Vlasenko, and Shambo Samrat Samajdar

PART IV: Advanced Scientific Insights 271

8. Proteomics in Diabetes: Unveiling the Complexities of the Proteomic Landscape 273
Muhammad Muzammal, Sana Fatima, Hamna Batool Hashmi, Maria Shafiq, and Arshad Farid

9. Immunomodulation in Diabetes: The Dynamic Role of the Immune System 309
Amit Anand, Akshansh Kumar, S. N. Manjula, Neeraj Kumar Fuloria, and Kenganora Mruthunjaya

10. Synthetic Innovations: Engineering Solutions in Diabetes 345
Wan Nurhidayah Wan Hanaffi, Nazish Naseem, Usama Ahmad, Anas Islam, and Mohd. Muazzam Khan

PART V: Personalized and Regenerative Medicine 381

11. Personalized Medicine Strategies Tailored to Diabetes Management 383
Farogh Ahsan, Shahzadi Bano, Tarique Mahmood, Abdul Rahman Khan, and Mohd. Masih Uzzaman Khan

12. Stem Cell Therapy: A Paradigm Shift in Diabetes Treatment............427
Arshi Waseem, Miroslaw Janowski, and Syed Shadab Raza

Index 447

Contributors

Asad Ahmad
Faculty of Pharmacy, Integral University, Lucknow, Uttar Pradesh, India

Mohammad Ahmad
Faculty of Pharmacy, Integral University, Lucknow, Uttar Pradesh, India

Nafees Ahmad
Department of Chemistry, Integral University, Lucknow, Uttar Pradesh, India

Usama Ahmad
Faculty of Pharmacy, Integral University, Lucknow, Uttar Pradesh, India

Farogh Ahsan
Department of Pharmacy, Integral University, Dasauli, Lucknow, Uttar Pradesh, India

Juber Akhtar
Faculty of Pharmacy, Integral University, Dasauli, Lucknow, Uttar Pradesh, India

Perwez Alam
Department of Pharmacognosy, College of Pharmacy, King Saud University, Riyadh, Kingdom of Saudi Arabia

Amit Anand
Department of Pharmacognosy, JSS College of Pharmacy, JSS Academy of Higher Education and Research, Mysuru, Karnataka, India

Yusuf Asad
Department of Biomedical Engineering, Rowan University, Glassboro, New Jersey, United States

Sumel Ashique
Department of Pharmaceutical Technology, School of Health and Medical Sciences, Adamas University, Kolkata, West Bengal, India

Badruddeen
Faculty of Pharmacy, Integral University, Lucknow, Uttar Pradesh, India

Shahzadi Bano
Department of Applied Sciences, Jahangirabad Institute of Technology, Jahangirabad Fort, Barabanki, Uttar Pradesh, India

Raja Chakraverty
Department of Critical Care Medicine, Institute of Post Graduate Medical Education and Research, Kolkata, West Bengal, India

Arshad Farid
Gomal Center of Biochemistry and Biotechnology, Gomal University, Dera Ismail Khan, Khyber Pakhtunkhwa, Pakistan

Sana Fatima
Gomal Center of Biochemistry and Biotechnology, Gomal University, Dera Ismail Khan, Khyber Pakhtunkhwa, Pakistan

Neeraj Kumar Fuloria
Department of Pharmaceutical Chemistry, Faculty of Pharmacy, AIMST University, Semeling Campus, Bedong, Kedah, Malaysia

Wan Nurhidayah Wan Hanaffi
Laboratoire de Chimie Physique Macromoléculaire, Université de Lorraine, CNRS, Nancy, France; Department of Immunology, School of Medical Sciences, Universiti Sains Malaysia, Kelantan, Malaysia

Hamna Batool Hashmi
Gomal Center of Biochemistry and Biotechnology, Gomal University, Dera Ismail Khan, Khyber Pakhtunkhwa, Pakistan

Mohd Kamil Hussain
Department of Chemistry, Government Raza Postgraduate College, Rampur, Uttar Pradesh, India

Sahil Hussain
Faculty of Pharmacy, Integral University, Lucknow, Uttar Pradesh, India;
College of Health and Life Sciences, Hamad Bin Khalifa University, Doha, Qatar

Anas Islam
Faculty of Pharmacy, Integral University, Lucknow, Uttar Pradesh, India

Deeba Shamim Jairajpuri
Department of Biochemistry, Arabian Gulf University, Manama, Bahrain

Miroslaw Janowski
Department of Diagnostic Radiology and Nuclear Medicine, University of Maryland, Baltimore, Maryland, United States

Ayeza Sarwar Kalam
Faculty of Pharmacy, Integral University, Lucknow, Uttar Pradesh, India

Abdul Rahman Khan
Department of Chemistry, Integral University, Dasauli, Lucknow, Uttar Pradesh, India

Alina Khan
Department of Toxicology and Medical Elementology, Jamia Hamdard, New Delhi, Delhi, India

Mohammad Irfan Khan
Faculty of Pharmacy, Integral University, Lucknow, Uttar Pradesh, India

Mohd. Masih Uzzaman Khan
Department of Pharmaceutical Chemistry and Pharmacognosy, Unaizah College of Pharmacy, Qassim University, Unaizah, Al-Qassim, Saudi Arabia

Mohd. Muazzam Khan
Faculty of Pharmacy, Integral University, Lucknow, Uttar Pradesh, India

Mohsin Vahid Khan
Department of Biosciences, Integral University, Lucknow, Uttar Pradesh, India

Sara Khan
Faculty of Pharmacy, Integral University, Lucknow, Uttar Pradesh, India

Ashwin Kotnis
All India Institute of Medical Sciences, Bhopal, Madhya Pradesh, India

Akshansh Kumar
Department of Pharmaceutical Biotechnology, JSS College of Pharmacy, JSS Academy of Higher Education and Research, Mysuru, Karnataka, India

Tarique Mahmood
Department of Pharmacy, Integral University, Dasauli, Lucknow, Uttar Pradesh, India

Purba Mandal
Faculty of Pharmacy, Integral University, Dasauli, Lucknow, Uttar Pradesh, India

S. N. Manjula
Department of Pharmacology, JSS College of Pharmacy, JSS Academy of Higher Education and Research, Mysuru, Karnataka, India

Kenganora Mruthunjaya
Department of Pharmacognosy, JSS College of Pharmacy, JSS Academy of Higher Education and Research, Mysuru, Karnataka, India

Mohd. Mursal
Faculty of Pharmacy, Integral University, Lucknow, Uttar Pradesh, India

Muhammad Muzammal
Gomal Center of Biochemistry and Biotechnology, Gomal University, Dera Ismail Khan, Khyber Pakhtunkhwa, Pakistan

Nazish Naseem
Faculty of Pharmacy, Integral University, Lucknow, Uttar Pradesh, India

Gulam Rabbani
School of Chemical Engineering, Yeungnam University, Gyeongsan, Gyeongbuk, Republic of Korea

Syed Shadab Raza
Department of Biotechnology, Laboratory for Stem Cell and Restorative Neurology, Era's Lucknow Medical College and Hospital, Era University, Sarfarazganj, Lucknow, Uttar Pradesh, India; Department of Stem Cell Biology and Regenerative Medicine, Era's Lucknow Medical College and Hospital, Era University, Sarfarazganj, Lucknow, Uttar Pradesh, India

Mohammad Rumman
Department of Biosciences, Integral University, Lucknow, Uttar Pradesh, India

Shambo Samrat Samajdar
Diabetes and Allergy-Asthma Therapeutics Speciality Clinic, Kolkata, West Bengal, India

Prashul Sethi
Department of Pharmacology, College of Pharmacy, Shri Venkateswara University, Gajraula, Uttar Pradesh, India

Maria Shafiq
Gomal Medical College, Dera Ismail Khan, Khyber Pakhtunkhwa, Pakistan

Himanshu Sharma
Department of Pharmacology, NIMS Institute of Pharmacy, NIMS University Rajasthan, Jaipur, Rajasthan, India

Aditya Singh
Faculty of Pharmacy, Integral University, Dasauli, Lucknow, Uttar Pradesh, India

Tahreen Taj
Department of Pharmacology, Yenepoya Pharmacy College and Research Center, Yenepoya (Deemed to Be) University, Mangalore, Karnataka, India

Swastik Verma
All India Institute of Medical Sciences, Bhopal, Madhya Pradesh, India

Iryna Vlasenko
International Diabetes Federation, Brussels, Belgium

Arshi Waseem
Department of Biotechnology, Laboratory for Stem Cell and Restorative Neurology, Era's Lucknow Medical College and Hospital, Era University, Sarfarazganj, Lucknow, Uttar Pradesh, India

Abbreviations

2D	two-dimensional
2DGE	two-dimensional gel electrophoresis
3D	three-dimensional
4-HNE	4-hydroxy-2-nonenal
ACTH	adrenocorticotropic hormone
AD	Alzheimer's disease
AGE	advanced glycation end-product
AI	artificial intelligence
AINS	arginine–insulin complexes
AMP	adenosine monophosphate
AMPK	AMP-activated protein kinase
Ang-II	angiotensin-II
ANS	autonomic nervous systems
APC	antigen-presenting cell
ApoB	apolipoprotein B
ApoH	apolipoprotein H
AT	adipose tissue
BB	bio-breeding
BGL	blood glucose level
BMI	body mass index
BSL	blood sugar level
CAD	coronary artery disease
CAM	complementary and alternative medicine
CAT	catalase
CAT	computed axial tomography
CBG	capillary blood glucose
CBT	cognitive behavioral therapy
CEPC	cell-engineered pancreatic construct
CGM	continuous glucose monitoring
CHF	congestive heart failure
ChIP	chromatin immunoprecipitation
CKD	chronic kidney disease
CNT	carbon nanotube
CoA	certificate of analysis
COPD	chronic obstructive pulmonary disease
CPAP	continuous positive airway pressure

CPP	cell-penetrating peptide
CS	chitosan
CT	computed tomography
CVD	cardiovascular disease
DC	dendritic cell
DFI	diabetic foot infections
DFU	diabetic foot ulcers
DI	disposition index
DIAGRAM	diabetes genetics replication and meta-analysis
DKA	diabetic ketoacidosis
DM	diabetes mellitus
DME	diabetic macular edema
dPCR	digital PCR
DPP	diabetes prevention program
DPP-4	dipeptidyl peptidase-4
DRN	diabetic retinal neurodegeneration
DSME	diabetes self-management education
EBFC	enzyme biofuel cell
EBs	embryoid bodies
ECM	enhancing extracellular matrix
ED	erectile dysfunction
EGCG	epigallocatechin gallate
EGF	epidermal growth factor
EHR	electronic health records
EIR	early insulin response
ELSI	ethical, legal, and societal implications
EPIC	European Prospective Investigation into Cancer and Nutrition
ER	endoplasmic reticulum
ESC	embryonic stem cell
ESRD	end-stage renal disease
ETC	electron transport chain
FAD	flavin adenine dinucleotide
FFA	free fatty acids
FHD	family history of diabetes
FPG	fasting plasma glucose
FSD	female sexual dysfunction
FUS	focused ultrasound system
GA	Golgi apparatus
GAD	glutamic acid decarboxylase
GDM	gestational diabetes mellitus
GFR	glomerular filtration rate
GLP-1	glucagon-like peptide-1

GMP	good manufacturing practices
GOx	glucose oxidase
GPx	glutathione peroxidase
GRI	glucose-responsive insulins
GRP	glucose-regulated protein
GSIS	glucose-stimulated insulin secretion
GWAS	genome-wide association studies
HbA1C	hemoglobin A1C
HCLF	high-carbohydrate, low-fat
HCS	high-content screening
HDL	high-density lipoprotein
HEMA	hydroxyethyl methacrylate
hESC	human embryonic stem cells
hIAPP	human islet amyloid polypeptide
HIPAA	Health Insurance Portability and Accountability Act
HLA	human leucocytes antigen
HNF	hepatocyte nuclear transcription factor
HNF-4α	hepatocyte nuclear factor 4α
hPSC	human pluripotent stem cells
HSC	hematopoietic stem cells
HSL	hormone-sensitive lipase
IAA	insulin autoantibody
IAPP	islet amyloid polypeptide
ICA	islet cell antibodies
IDDM	insulin-dependent diabetes mellitus
IDF	International Diabetes Federation
IDL	intermediate-density lipoprotein
IFG	impaired fasting glucose
IFN	interferons
IGT	impaired glucose tolerance
IL	interleukin
IPC	insulin-producing cell
IPF-1	insulin promoter factor 1
iPSC	induced pluripotent stem cell
IR	insulin resistance
IRS	insulin receptor substrate
KATP	potassium ATP
LDL	low-density lipoprotein
LMICs	low- and middle-income countries
LPL	less lipoprotein lipase
LSF	lisofylline
LTBI	latent tuberculosis infection

MAF	minor allele frequency
MEMS	micro-electromechanical systems
MFGM	milk's fat globule membrane
MGC	metagenomic cluster
MHC	major histocompatibility complex
MIP	macrophage inflammatory protein
miRNA	microRNA
ML	machine learning
MMP2	matrix metalloproteinase 2
MN	microneedle
MODY	maturity-onset diabetes of the young
MRI	magnetic resonance imaging
MS	mass spectrometry
MSC	mesenchymal stem cell
NAD	nicotinamide adenine dinucleotide
NAFLD	nonalcoholic fatty liver disease
NCBI	National Center for Biotechnology Information
NDDG	National Diabetes Data Group
NEMS	nanoelectromechanical systems
NGS	next-generation sequencing
NGT	normal glucose tolerance
NIDDM	non-insulin-dependent diabetes mellitus
NK	natural killer
NMR	nuclear magnetic resonance
NOD	non-obese diabetic
NP	nanoparticle
NPDR	non-proliferative diabetic retinopathy
NPH	neutral protamine Hagedorn
nTreg	natural Treg
OCT	optical coherence tomography
OGTT	oral glucose tolerance test
OPTN	organ procurement and transplantation network
OSA	obstructive sleep apnea
PAD	peripheral artery disease
PAI-1	plasminogen activator inhibitor-1
PAni-NP	polyaniline nanoparticles
PBA	phenylboronic acid
PCPMs	pH-responsive cationic polymeric micelles
PCSK9	proprotein convertase subtilisin/Kexin type 9
PDI	protein disulfide isomerase
PDR	proliferative diabetic retinopathy
PET	positron emission tomography

PG	plasma glucose
PHI	personal health information
PKC	protein kinase C
PLGA	poly(lactic-co-glycolic acid)
PLP	pyridoxal phosphate
PNDM	permanent neonatal diabetes mellitus
PRS	polygenic risk scores
PTP1B	protein tyrosine phosphatase 1 B
RBCM	red blood cell membrane
REG1	regenerating protein 1
ROS	reactive oxygen species
RWD	real-world data
SCFA	short-chain fatty acid
SC-β	stem cell-derived β
SELDI TOF-MS	surface-enhanced laser desorption/ionization time-of-flight spectrometry
SFA	saturated fatty acids
SGDC	sodium-glycodeoxycholate
SGLT2	sodium-dependent glucose-linked co-transporter 2
SLN	solid lipid nanoparticle
SMR	standardized mortality rate
SNP	single nucleotide polymorphism
SNS	sympathetic nervous system
SOD1	superoxide dismutase 1
SOI	silicon-on-insulator
STZ	streptozotocin
T1D	type 1 diabetes
T1DM	type 1 diabetes mellitus
T2D	type 2 diabetes
T2DM	type 2 diabetes mellitus
TCM	traditional Chinese medicine
TGs	triglycerides
TiO2	titanium dioxide
TLA	transmucosal adhesive
TNDM	transient neonatal diabetes mellitus
TNF	tumor necrosis factor
TXN	thioredoxin
UNOS	United Network for Organ Sharing
UPR	unfolded protein response
VEGF	vascular endothelial growth factor
VLDL	very-low-density cholesterol
WC	waist circumference

WHO	World Health Organization
ZDF	Zucker diabetic fatty
ZF	Zucker fatty

Preface

In the ever-evolving field of medical science, diabetes remains one of the most challenging chronic diseases to manage and fully understand. With its increasing global prevalence, the urgency for innovative therapeutic strategies and deeper insights into its complex pathophysiology has never been more acute. *Diabetes: Novel Insights and Therapies* is designed to meet this need, providing a comprehensive exploration of cutting-edge developments in diabetes research and care. This book aims to bridge the gap between traditional approaches and modern innovations, offering readers a detailed overview of the latest advancements shaping the future of diabetes management.

This book is crafted for a diverse audience, encompassing healthcare professionals, researchers, academics, and students in the medical sciences. Each chapter is meticulously structured to provide both foundational knowledge and advanced insights into various aspects of diabetes—from epidemiology and pathophysiology to groundbreaking therapeutic techniques such as stem cell therapy and nanotechnology. By integrating these diverse themes, the book offers a holistic view of diabetes that highlights the interdisciplinary nature of contemporary medical research and practice.

One of the unique features of this volume is its emphasis on both established and emerging therapeutic strategies. It explores the traditional use of natural products in diabetes management, re-evaluating their roles through the lens of modern science and integrating them with innovative treatment approaches. This blend of old and new encapsulates the spirit of the book—acknowledging the roots of traditional medicine while forging ahead into the uncharted territories of genomic medicine, proteomics, and synthetic biology.

Diabetes: Novel Insights and Therapies also addresses the critical role of personalized medicine in diabetes care, highlighting the importance of tailoring treatments to individual genetic profiles. This approach not only enhances the efficacy of therapeutic interventions but also mitigates the risks and side effects associated with generalized treatment protocols. The book's comprehensive discussion of the dynamic role of the immune system in diabetes provides profound insights that are crucial for the development of immunomodulatory therapies.

In preparing this manuscript, contributions from leading experts in various fields of diabetes research have been meticulously compiled and edited to ensure clarity, depth, and accessibility. Each chapter is supported by the latest research findings, offering readers evidence-based perspectives and practical insights that can be applied in both clinical and research settings. The inclusion of advanced scientific research techniques and results aims to foster a deeper understanding of diabetes at the molecular level, empowering healthcare professionals and researchers to develop more effective diagnostics and therapies.

The benefits of reading *Diabetes: Novel Insights and Therapies* are manifold. Clinicians will find practical guidance for daily practice, enriched by the latest research outcomes. Academics and students will appreciate the detailed scientific discussions that can enhance their studies and foster new research initiatives. Industry professionals in pharmaceuticals and biotechnology will gain insights into the emerging market trends and innovations that are driving the future of diabetes care. Lastly, general readers with an interest in diabetes or chronic disease management will discover valuable information on prevention strategies and holistic management approaches that go beyond conventional medical advice.

As the landscape of diabetes care continues to expand and evolve, *Diabetes: Novel Insights and Therapies* serves as a crucial resource, offering readers not just information but a comprehensive perspective on where diabetes treatment is headed in the 21st century. It is our hope that this book will not only inform but also inspire new thinking and innovation in the fight against diabetes.

We are excited to present this book to you, confident that it will make a significant contribution to your professional libraries and enhance your understanding of one of the most pressing health challenges of our time.

PART I
Understanding Diabetes

CHAPTER 1

Definition, Classification, and Epidemiological Perspectives

SARA KHAN,[1] ANAS ISLAM,[1] BADRUDDEEN,[1,*] and YUSUF ASAD[2]

[1]*Faculty of Pharmacy, Integral University, Lucknow, Uttar Pradesh, India*

[2]*Department of Biomedical Engineering, Rowan University, Glassboro, New Jersey, United States*

*Corresponding author

ABSTRACT

Diabetes mellitus (DM) is a chronic endocrine condition characterized by increased blood glucose levels (BGLs) due to inadequate insulin synthesis, insulin resistance, or both. Diabetes is categorized into three primary types: type 1 diabetes mellitus (T1DM), type 2 diabetes mellitus (T2DM), and gestational diabetes mellitus (GDM). T1DM is an autoimmune disorder causing pancreatic beta cell death, while T2DM involves insulin resistance and relative insulin deficit. Gestational diabetes occurs during pregnancy and may lead to T2DM after childbirth. Diagnosis relies on blood glucose measurements, HbA1c levels, oral glucose tolerance tests (OGTTs), and random blood sugar assessment. The worldwide incidence of diabetes is increasing, with 537 million cases in 2021 and projections of 783 million by 2045. T2DM constitutes over 90% of cases and is influenced by weight and lifestyle factors. Diabetes is associated with comorbidities like cardiovascular disease (CVD), neuropathy, nephropathy, and retinopathy, affecting morbidity, mortality, and quality of life. Environmental contaminants and metabolic syndrome contribute to diabetes etiology. Advances in data collection, analysis, and technology

Diabetes: Novel Insights and Therapies. Anas Islam and Badruddeen (Eds)

DOI: 10.1201/9781779644596-2

have improved diabetes management, enabling personalized treatment strategies. Future research should focus on patient-centered approaches, prevention, and complication management. Public health policies must address rising prevalence, economic burden, and the need for tailored interventions to combat the global diabetes epidemic.

1.1 INTRODUCTION

Diabetes mellitus (DM) is a common endocrine condition that disrupts the body's capacity to create or effectively use insulin. This leads to increased blood glucose levels (BGLs), either from inadequate insulin secretion by the pancreas or from the inability of cells to react to the existing insulin (Shivashankar and Mani, 2011). The disorder is classified into three main groups (Mukhtar et al., 2020). Type 1 diabetes mellitus (T1DM), also known as insulin-dependent diabetes or juvenile diabetes, arises when the body cannot synthesize insulin and requires insulin injections or the use of an insulin pump for treatment (Quattrin et al., 2023). Type 2 diabetes mellitus (T2DM), sometimes referred to as non-insulin-dependent diabetes or adult-onset diabetes, is defined by insulin resistance, whereby cells fail to effectively use insulin. This disease may manifest with or without total insulin insufficiency (Tokhirovna, 2024). The third form of gestational diabetes occurs during pregnancy in women with no history of diabetes and may sometimes result in type 2 diabetes after pregnancy (Sweeting et al., 2024). Diabetes mellitus management often includes insulin and oral hypoglycemic agents (Mohajan and Mohajan, 2024).

Diabetes is a complex and diverse condition that is diagnosed by measuring blood glucose levels (BGLs) regardless of its underlying causes (Hughes et al., 2023). Although this method is practical, it oversimplifies the nature of the disease, which can hinder research and patient care. Recent approaches, such as palette, threshold, and gradient models, aim to better understand and manage diabetes by recognizing its variability and the different factors that influence disease progression and complications (Leslie et al., 2023). Understanding this heterogeneity through precision medicine could lead to better prevention, treatment, and personalized care; improve health outcomes; and guide the development of new therapies. Given its widespread impact and potential for severe complications, understanding diabetes is crucial for enhancing patient health and reducing the healthcare burden (Misra et al., 2023).

1.2 DEFINITION OF DIABETES

1.2.1 HISTORICAL PERSPECTIVE

Diabetes mellitus has a long history, with references appearing as early as 3000 years ago in ancient Egyptian texts. In 1675, Thomas Willis appended "mellitus" to the term, reflecting the sweet taste of patients' urine and blood, a feature that was also observed by ancient Indian doctors. The 19th century saw significant advancements in our understanding of diabetes. Claude Bernard's research in 1857 highlighted the role of the liver in glucose production, whereas Mering and Minkowski's 1889 discovery of the pancreas's role paved the way for Banting and Best's successful insulin isolation in 1921, which transformed diabetes treatment (Ahmed, 2002). Ancient Indian scholars, including Sushruta and Charaka, had already recognized two forms of diabetes, corresponding to what we now call type 1 and type 2 diabetes. The Persian physician Avicenna also made key observations regarding symptoms and treatments. These historical contributions reflect a persistent global effort to understand and treat diabetes throughout the ages (Lakhtakia, 2013).

1.2.2 MODERN DEFINITION

Historical accounts of diabetes are based on noticeable symptoms such as extreme thirst and frequent urination (McAulay, 2001). In contrast, contemporary definitions of diabetes mellitus are based on a thorough understanding of its metabolic and physiological processes. Diabetes is now recognized as a chronic condition characterized by persistently elevated blood sugar levels (BSLs) caused by problems with insulin production, insulin action, or a combination of both (Ramachandran et al., 2024).

1.2.3 PATHOPHYSIOLOGICAL BASIS

The pathophysiology of diabetes is characterized by impaired glucose regulation caused by insulin production, function, or a combination of both. In type 1 diabetes, the immune system obliterates pancreatic beta cells that produce insulin, resulting in diminished insulin levels and increased BGLs. Type 2 diabetes is defined by insulin resistance, whereby cells react inadequately to insulin, along with diminished insulin secretion from the pancreas (Tesauro et al., 2020). Hormonal alterations during pregnancy can induce insulin resistance and insufficient insulin synthesis, leading to gestational diabetes. Monogenic diabetes caused by genetic mutations and secondary diabetes caused by other health issues or drugs are two distinct types of diabetes. These disturbances cause persistent high BGLs and issues with glucose metabolism that must be addressed (Avagimyan et al., 2022).

1.2.4 DIAGNOSTIC CRITERIA

Based on extensive research and evidence, the WHO and ADA have established various diagnostic criteria for identifying diabetes and prediabetes (Kumar et al., 2016).

1.2.4.1 BLOOD GLUCOSE LEVELS

These are key indicators for diagnosing and managing diabetes. Normal fasting BGLs typically range from 70 to 99 mg/dL. The following criteria are generally used (Karter et al., 2001):

1.2.4.1.1 HbA1c levels

The hemoglobin A1C (HbA1C) assay has been a crucial tool for monitoring chronic glycemia for the past two decades (Greci et al., 2003). Traditionally regarded as a measure of average BGLs over the last 10–12 weeks, the current findings reveal that it more accurately reflects glucose management in the previous weeks. The average glycemia in the month before the test accounted for 50% of the HbA1C result, while the 30–60 days previously contributed 25%, and the 60–120 days before the test accounted for the remaining 25%. Both fasting and postprandial glucose levels influence HbA1C values. Post-meal glucose had a more significant impact when HbA1C was below 7.5%, whereas fasting glucose was more influential when HbA1C exceeded 7.5% (Beach, 1979; Curt et al., 2002). The relationship between HbA1C levels and the risk of diabetes complications, as demonstrated by studies such as the DCCT and UKPDS, has led to its adoption as a key metric in diabetes care. In 2010, the ADA recommended using HbA1C to diagnose diabetes, setting a cut-off of 6.5%, based on studies linking HbA1C levels to the risk of developing retinopathy, a common complication of diabetes (Pathmanatham and Somasundaram, 2014).

1.2.4.1.2 Oral glucose tolerance test (OGTT)

It is widely used in both clinical practice and research to diagnose T2DM and impaired glucose tolerance (IGT) (Kuo et al., 2021). It is also a key research tool for the study of glucose metabolism and insulin sensitivity. While the specific aims and procedures may vary between clinical and research settings, the standard 2-hour post-glucose blood glucose measurement is commonly used, following guidelines from the American Diabetes Association (ADA) (Jagannathan et al., 2020). In this test, the patient was required to fast for at least 8 h before a baseline blood glucose measurement was obtained. Subsequently, the patient consumed a drink containing approximately 75 g of glucose. Blood samples were drawn at various time points, typically 30 min, 1 h, and 2 h, to track blood glucose changes. The main focus was on the 2-hour glucose level to evaluate how efficiently the body manages glucose. Elevated glucose levels at this stage suggest IGT or diabetes (Mari et al., 2001). The OGTT is also used to identify gestational diabetes and assess insulin resistance and other metabolic disorders (McDonald et al., 1965).

1.2.4.1.3 Random blood sugar test

It is a diagnostic method used to measure BGLs at any given time (Rashed et al., 2020). Unlike fasting blood sugar tests, which require the patient to fast for several hours, random blood sugar tests can be performed without any prior preparation (Aliyu et al., 2020). It is often used in situations where quick results are needed, or when symptoms of diabetes are present. A random blood sugar test revealed a glucose level of 200 mg/dL or above, accompanied by diabetic symptoms, often signifying diabetes, and may need further testing for verification. This test is especially useful in emergency settings or during routine checkups to quickly identify potential blood sugar issues (Hariyono and Leo, 2018).

1.3 CLASSIFICATION OF DIABETES

1.3.1 TYPE 1 DIABETES MELLITUS (T1DM)

It is a chronic condition caused by autoimmune destruction of pancreatic β-cells (Thrower and Bingley et al., 2014). This destruction, mediated by

T cells, leads to the presence of autoantibodies against β cell antigens. T1DM typically presents with a sudden onset of symptoms such as weight loss, excessive urination, and excessive thirst, which are linked to insulin deficiency and can also increase the risk of ketoacidosis (Lambert and Bingle, 2002). T1DM can occur at any age, with more than half of the cases emerging after 20 years of age. The disease has a complex origin, and autoimmune attack on β-cells can begin in early childhood, with the speed of cell destruction varying among individuals. The protracted preclinical period of T1DM indicates potential prospects for early therapies to postpone or avert the manifestation of symptoms (Syed, 2022). It is mostly an autoimmune condition characterized by the obliteration of pancreatic beta cells, leading to complete insulin insufficiency. The condition progresses over time, eventually leading to significant beta cell loss and clinical symptoms of hyperglycemia when approximately 80–90% of beta cells are destroyed (Van Belle et al., 2011).

T1DM has a strong genetic component. The HLA region on chromosome 6, particularly the HLA-DR3 and HLA-DR4 haplotypes, significantly increases susceptibility to T1DM. Other genetic loci associated with an increased risk include the insulin (*INS*) gene, PTPN22, and CTLA-4, which are involved in immune regulation (Todd, 2010). Environmental triggers are believed to initiate autoimmune responses in genetically predisposed individuals. Viral infections, dietary factors, and environmental toxins are potential triggers. Changes in the gut microbiome and vitamin D deficiency have also been implicated in T1DM pathogenesis (Knip et al., 2005; Norris et al., 2003). Patients with T1DM typically present symptoms of hyperglycemia, including polyuria, polydipsia, polyphagia, and unintentional weight loss. Diabetic ketoacidosis (DKA) may occur in severe cases and is characterized by nausea, vomiting, abdominal pain, and confusion. Chronic complications include retinopathy, nephropathy, neuropathy, and cardiovascular disease (CVD) (Atkinson et al., 2014).

1.3.2 TYPE 2 DIABETES MELLITUS (T2DM)

It is characterized by insulin resistance and a relative shortage of insulin. Initially, the body adjusts to insulin resistance by increasing insulin secretion. Over time, beta cells fail to maintain sufficient insulin production, leading to hyperglycemia. Insulin resistance mainly affects the muscle, liver, and adipose tissue, leading to reduced glucose uptake and utilization (Defronzo et al., 2015). T2DM has a strong genetic basis, with multiple genes influencing insulin secretion, insulin action, and beta cell function. Family history is a significant risk factor, and numerous loci associated with T2DM have been identified through Genome-Wide Association Studies (GWAS) (Florez, 2008). Obesity, sedentary behavior, and poor dietary habits are significant risk factors for T2DM. A marked visceral fat build-up leads to insulin resistance. Additional considerations include age, ethnicity, and history of gestational diabetes or polycystic ovary syndrome (Hu et al., 2001). T2DM often manifests gradually, with individuals remaining asymptomatic for an extended period. The typical symptoms include polyuria, polydipsia, visual impairment, and fatigue. Chronic complications are similar to those of T1DM and include microvascular and macrovascular complications (ADA, 2014).

1.3.3 GESTATIONAL DIABETES MELLITUS (GDM)

Glucose intolerance is defined as glucose intolerance that begins or is first recognized during pregnancy. It is often identified during the second or third trimester using the oral glucose tolerance test (OGTT). If inadequately managed, GDM may pose health hazards for both the mother and the baby (Metzger et al., 2008).

Risk factors for GDM include obesity, advanced maternal age, familial diabetes history, prior GDM occurrence, and certain ethnicities (Ferrara, 2007). GDM is caused by increased insulin resistance and insufficient insulin production during gestation. Hormones from the placenta, including human placental lactogens, progesterone, and cortisol, play a role in insulin resistance. In GDM, pancreatic β cells are inadequately adjusted for heightened demand (Catalano et al., 1999). This may result in preeclampsia, cesarean section, and an elevated risk of developing T2DM. Fetuses face hazards such as macrosomia, newborn hypoglycemia, jaundice, respiratory distress syndrome, and an increased likelihood of developing obesity and T2DM later in life (Hod et al., 2015).

1.3.4 OTHER SPECIFIC TYPES

1.3.4.1 MONOGENIC DIABETES SYNDROMES

Monogenic diabetes arises from mutations in a single gene that affect beta cell functionality, including MODY and neonatal diabetes. These forms are distinct from T1DM and T2DM, and often present with early onset diabetes with a strong family history (Ellard et al., 2013).

1.3.4.2 SECONDARY DIABETES

Secondary diabetes can arise from conditions that damage the pancreas, such as pancreatitis, cystic fibrosis, hemochromatosis, or hormonal disturbances, such as Cushing's syndrome or acromegaly. It may also result from certain autoimmune conditions and infections that affect the pancreatic function (ADA, 2014).

1.3.4.3 DRUG OR CHEMICAL-INDUCED DIABETES

Certain medications can induce diabetes by impairing insulin action or beta cell function. Common culprits include glucocorticoids, thiazide diuretics, atypical antipsychotics, and immunosuppressants. Chemical exposure to certain pesticides has also been linked to an increased risk (Piccinini et al., 2016).

1.4 EPIDEMIOLOGICAL PERSPECTIVES

1.4.1 GLOBAL PREVALENCE AND INCIDENCE

In 2000, the global prevalence of diabetes among adults aged $\geq$ 20 years was estimated to be approximately 171 million cases, representing an 11% increase over the previous estimate of 154 million cases. This increase is not due to changes in demographic data, such as the proportion of older adults, but rather reflects updated survey data and the more inclusive reporting criteria used by the International Diabetes Federation (IDF) *Diabetes Atlas* (2000). The IDF *Diabetes Atlas* (2000) reported 151 million cases in individuals aged 20–79 years, which closely aligns with the current estimate of 147 million cases in this age group.

The IDF's future projections suggest a significant rise in diabetes cases; estimates for 2003 were 194 million, with forecasts predicting 334 million cases by 2025 (IDF, 2003). This expected increase is largely attributed to factors such as population aging, urbanization, and rising obesity rates. Even if obesity rates remain stable, the number of diabetes cases is projected to double by 2030. Given the observed increase in obesity and its role as a major risk factor for diabetes, the actual future prevalence may be even higher than the current estimates.

Interventions to combat diabetes, including dietary changes, increased physical activity, and pharmacological treatments, are essential and should be implemented more widely to reduce the prevalence of diabetes. Additionally, improved survival rates, especially in developed countries, may contribute to the increasing number of diabetes cases (IDF, 2003).

Current estimates face limitations such as a lack of comprehensive data, especially from Eastern Europe and Southeast Asia. Previous estimates used different statistical models, which may have affected the accuracy. For example, earlier methods used logistic regression models for age-specific prevalence, whereas more recent approaches incorporated quadratic models that can alter prevalence estimates for older age groups (IDF, 2000).

Given that many surveys used in these estimates are over a decade old, the current prevalence may have been underestimated. Future updates are anticipated as new data becomes available. This ongoing epidemic of diabetes poses significant human and economic challenges, particularly as other health issues in less developed countries decline. Addressing this growing public health crisis requires concerted global efforts (IDF, 2003).

1.4.1.1 TRENDS OVER TIME

In 2000, there were approximately 171 million cases globally, and by 2023, this number had risen to approximately 537 million cases (IDF, 2023). This increase is driven by rising obesity rates, aging populations, and urbanization. The IDF (2023) projects that the number of people with diabetes will exceed 640 million by 2030 and could reach approximately 780 million by 2045. This projection underscores a continuing and accelerating trend in the global prevalence of diabetes.

It has been rising steadily owing to lifestyle changes, including increased sedentary behavior and poor dietary habits. Research indicates that the incidence of type 2 diabetes is increasing at an alarming rate in many countries, particularly among younger populations (Zheng et al., 2018).

Advances in diabetes management, including better medications, technology (such as continuous glucose monitors), and educational programs, have improved disease management and patient outcomes. However, these advancements have not kept pace with the increasing prevalence (ADA, 2020). There is a growing focus on prevention, with greater emphasis on lifestyle interventions. These measures have shown effectiveness in reducing the incidence of type 2 diabetes when implemented widely (Diabetes Prevention Program Research Group, 2002).

1.4.1.2 REGIONAL VARIATIONS

Regional variations in high-income countries and low- and middle-income countries (LMICs) are summarized in Tables 1.1 and 1.2.

TABLE 1.1 Regional Variations in High-Income Countries

North America and Europe	Western Europe
Diabetes prevalence is high in North America and Europe, with significant increases over recent decades. In the United States, the prevalence of diabetes among adults has been rising, with about 11% of the adult population affected as of 2021 (Centers for Disease Control and Prevention [CDC], 2022). This increase is partly due to higher rates of obesity and an aging population.	The United Kingdom and Germany have also reported high diabetes prevalence, with increasing rates of T2DM linked to rising obesity levels and sedentary lifestyles (*European Journal of Public Health*, 2020)

TABLE 1.2 Regional Variations in Low- and Middle-Income Countries

Asia	Africa
In China and India, the prevalence of diabetes has surged dramatically. China, for instance, has one of the highest numbers of diabetes cases globally, with over 116 million people living with diabetes as of 2021 (IDF, 2023). Rapid urbanization, dietary changes, and increasing obesity rates contribute to this trend.	Diabetes prevalence is also rising in Africa, although the rates are lower compared to more developed regions. However, the number of cases is growing rapidly due to urbanization and lifestyle changes. For example, Nigeria has seen a significant increase in diabetes cases over recent years (IDF Africa Region, 2021).

1.4.2 RISK FACTORS

1.4.2.1 GENETIC PREDISPOSITION

Genetic predisposition is a concept that describes an individual's increased likelihood of developing certain diseases due to an inherited genetic makeup. In the case of type 1 diabetes, genetic predisposition plays a significant role (Corder et al., 1993; King et al., 2003; Miki et al., 1994;

Shoji et al., 1998). This condition is strongly associated with the HLA complex on chromosome 6. HLA-DR3 and HLA-DR4 are associated with an increased risk of IDDM, particularly in Caucasian populations. Individuals carrying both the DR3 and DR4 antigens face an even higher risk, suggesting that multiple genetic factors influence susceptibility. Advancements in recombinant DNA technology have allowed researchers to more precisely identify specific susceptibility genes within the HLA class II region. The focus has shifted from HLA-DR antigens to DQ determinants, which are now believed to be critical in IDDM susceptibility. Specific variations in the DQA and DQB genes have been linked to an increased risk of IDDM. These include the absence of aspartic acid at position 57 on the DQβ chain and the presence of arginine at position 52 on the DQα chain (Deschamps et al., 1991). The concept of susceptibility molecules, formed by different combinations of DQα and DQβ chains, helps explain why certain individuals are at a higher risk for IDDM (Radah and Mohan, 2007; Sirdah and Reading, 2020).

1.4.2.2 LIFESTYLE AND BEHAVIORAL FACTORS

Lifestyle and behavioral variables include everyday behaviors and activities that may affect health outcomes (National Cancer Institute, 2019). Physical inactivity and inadequate nutrition are associated with chronic illnesses, including CVDs and type 2 diabetes. The American Heart Association (2015) indicated that sedentary activity and poor eating habits contribute substantially to the incidence of CVD. Furthermore, high alcohol use is correlated with a heightened risk of liver disease (Rehm et al., 2009).

1.4.2.3 SOCIOECONOMIC AND ENVIRONMENTAL FACTORS

These factors significantly influence health outcomes. Low socioeconomic status is often associated with worse health outcomes, owing to restricted access to healthcare services and increased exposure to environmental risks. Individuals in lower socioeconomic strata are more prone to reside in regions with elevated pollution levels, which have been associated with respiratory and cardiovascular ailments (Pope et al., 2002). Environmental variables, including exposure to hazardous chemicals, substandard living conditions, and insufficient access to clean water, may intensify health inequities. Research indicates that air pollution exposure correlates with an increased prevalence of chronic respiratory disorders such as asthma and chronic obstructive pulmonary disease (COPD) (Brook et al., 2010). Moreover, socioeconomic status affects dietary choices because lower-income groups often have limited access to nutritional foods, resulting in elevated obesity rates and associated health issues (Drewnowski and Almiron-Roig, 2010).

1.4.3 AGE AND GENDER DISTRIBUTION

1.4.3.1 AGE-SPECIFIC TRENDS

The prevalence of diabetes is age-specific across various populations. Research indicates that older adults, particularly men, show a marked increase in diabetes prevalence, whereas trends differ for younger demographics and women. In Japan, the prevalence of diabetes among men aged $\geq$ 70 years has significantly increased, with projections suggesting a rise from 9.9% in 2010 to 13.1% by 2030 (Charvat et al., 2015). In Korea, the prevalence among the elderly also rose, while young women showed stable rates, indicating that age-related risk factors, such as obesity and sarcopenia, play crucial roles (Koo and Moon, 2016).

1.4.3.2 GENDER DIFFERENCES IN PREVALENCE

A study in Taiwan revealed that the prevalence of diabetes increased from 4.6% to 9.3% in men and slightly decreased in women from 7.9% to 6.4% between 1993 and 2008 (Chang et al., 2010). The LEAD study found that men had a higher prevalence of diabetes (7.3%) than women (3.7%), with notable differences in comorbidities (Breyer et al., 2020). While these findings highlight the increasing burden of diabetes, particularly among older men, they also underscore the need for targeted public health strategies to effectively address these disparities.

1.4.4 COMPLICATIONS AND COMORBIDITIES

1.4.4.1 MICROVASCULAR COMPLICATIONS

1. **Diabetic Retinopathy:** It is a primary cause of blindness and is heavily influenced by both the length and intensity of high BSLs (Fong et al., 2004; Gabbay et al., 1975; Keenan et al., 2007; UK Prospective Diabetes Study Group, 1998). It can begin developing

years before a diabetes diagnosis is made, advancing from early-stage retinopathy, characterized by microaneurysms and retinal swelling, to more severe proliferative retinopathy, marked by the growth of abnormal blood vessels and a high risk of blindness (Gabbay et al., 2004; Kunisaki et al., 1995). Interventions, such as laser photocoagulation, are crucial to prevent severe progression (Aiello et al., 1995; Watkins, 1995).

2. **Diabetic Nephropathy:** As the foremost cause of kidney failure in the United States, diabetic nephropathy begins with minor protein leaks in the urine (microalbuminuria) and can escalate to significant proteinuria and severe kidney damage (Chaturvedi et al., 2001; Gross et al., 2005). Early detection and aggressive management using ACE inhibitors or ARBs, coupled with rigorous blood sugar and blood pressure control, are vital for slowing the progression of kidney damage and safeguarding renal function (Alder et al., 2003; Heart Outcomes Prevention Evaluation Study Investigators, 2000; Rossing et al., 2003; The DCCT Research Group, 1993).

3. **Diabetic Neuropathy:** Characterized by nerve damage due to prolonged high BSLs, diabetic neuropathy presents as sensory, focal, or autonomic nerve dysfunction. The symptoms range from burning pain and tingling to complete numbness, significantly increasing the risk of foot ulcers and amputation (ADA, 2007; Boulton et al., 2005). Management centers on strict blood sugar regulation and targeted treatment for pain relief using drugs, such as duloxetine and pregabalin, although no treatment is universally effective (Abbott et al., 2002; Maser et al., 2003).

1.4.4.2 MACROVASCULAR COMPLICATIONS

Diabetes significantly increases the risk of macrovascular complications, predominantly through the progression of atherosclerosis, which leads to narrowing and hardening of arteries (Beckaman et al., 2002; Laing et al., 2003; Paterson et al., 2007). This condition begins with ongoing inflammation and damage to the endothelium, resulting in the accumulation of oxidized low-density lipoprotein (LDL) particles in arterial walls (Buse et al., 2007; Haffner et al., 1998; Hogan et al., 1971). These particles attract monocytes, which transform into macrophages and form foam cells (Almdal et al., 2004; Avogaro et al., 2007; Lehto et al., 1996). The presence of foam cells then promotes the recruitment of T-lymphocytes and proliferation of smooth muscle cells, culminating in the formation of atherosclerotic plaques with a fibrous cap (Laing et al., 2003; Nathan et al., 2005). The rupture of these plaques can result in serious events such as heart attacks or strokes (UKPDS, 1998a, b).

In addition to atherosclerosis, diabetes increases the likelihood of thrombosis due to heightened platelet activity and a pro-coagulant state (Colhoun et al., 2004; Lindholm et al., 2002). Elevated BGLs lead to decreased NO production and increased oxidative stress, which enhances platelet aggregation (Collins et al., 2003). Additionally, elevated levels of plasminogen activator inhibitor-1 (PAI-1) impair the body's ability to break down clots. CVD remains the primary cause of death in individuals with diabetes, particularly in those with type 2 diabetes (Frick et al., 2007). Therefore, comprehensive management, including strict control of blood pressure, lipid levels, and blood sugar, is essential to reduce these macrovascular risks and enhance cardiovascular health in patients (Koskinen et al., 1992; Manninen et al., 1988).

1.4.4.3 COMMON COMORBID CONDITIONS

Diabetes mellitus (DM) is frequently associated with various comorbid conditions that exacerbate its severity and complicate its management. Understanding these comorbidities is crucial for effective treatment and improved patient outcome (Sasako, 2024) (Table 1.3).

TABLE 1.3 Various Comorbid Conditions in Diabetes

Common Comorbid Conditions in Diabetes	Description	References
Hypertension	A prevalent comorbidity, with incidence rates twice as high in diabetic patients compared to non-diabetics; often linked to insulin resistance.	Bodke et al. (2023)
Dyslipidemia	Commonly coexists with diabetes, contributing to cardiovascular risks.	Rathi et al. (2017)
Neuropathy	A significant complication affecting diabetic patients, leading to increased morbidity.	Rathi et al. (2017)
Cognitive impairment	Macrovascular complications and depressive symptoms mediate cognitive decline in individuals with type 2 diabetes.	Whitelock et al. (2021)
Infections	UTIs are notably frequent among diabetic patients, particularly in females.	Bodke et al. (2023)

While these comorbidities significantly affect diabetes management, some studies suggest that lifestyle interventions and targeted treatments can mitigate their effects, emphasizing the importance of comprehensive care strategies (Teck, 2022).

1.4.5 MORTALITY AND MORBIDITY

1.4.5.1 MORTALITY RATES

Diabetes substantially impacts worldwide mortality, with rates differing according to variables such as diabetes type, age, sex, and geographic region. Research has demonstrated that type 2 diabetes is correlated with elevated death rates relative to those of type 1 diabetes. A study in the Netherlands reported mortality rates of 67.7 per 10,000 person-years for type 1 diabetes and 324.2 per 10,000 person-years for type 2 diabetes, with cancer identified as a significant cause of death (Bak et al., 2024). A multi-country analysis in the Americas highlighted a stable diabetes mortality rate from 2000 to 2019 but identified a 1.5% annual increase in deaths from diabetic kidney disease, particularly among men (Antini et al., 2024). Gender disparities are evident, as seen in England, where women with type 2 diabetes had a higher standardized mortality rate (SMR) of 1.72 compared to 1.46 for men, pointing to significant differences in outcomes (Heald, 2023). The causes of death among diabetic patients also vary. In Mongolia, sepsis is the leading cause of death, followed by renal failure, accounting for 65% of cases (Sankhuu et al., 2023). Additionally, young individuals are not spared, with diabetes causing approximately 16,300 deaths in those under 25 years of age globally in 2019, predominantly due to type 1 diabetes, emphasizing the need for improved healthcare access for younger populations (Cousin et al., 2022). Despite advances in diabetes management, the persistently high mortality rates, especially among specific demographics, underline the urgent need for targeted interventions and improved health care services.

1.4.5.2 MORBIDITY BURDEN

Diabetes imposes a substantial morbidity burden due to its chronic nature. Patients with diabetes are at a higher risk of developing CVD, kidney failure, neuropathy, and retinopathy. These complications not only increase hospitalizations and healthcare costs but also contribute to long-term disability among diabetic individuals (IDF, 2021). For instance, the risk of CVD is significantly elevated in patients with diabetes, making them more susceptible to heart attacks and strokes. Moreover, diabetes is a leading cause of end-stage renal disease (ESRD), which requires costly and intensive treatments, such as dialysis or kidney transplantation (Centers for Disease Control and Prevention, 2022). The combination of these factors results in a considerable morbidity burden that affects both individuals and healthcare systems worldwide.

1.4.5.3 IMPACT ON QUALITY OF LIFE

Managing diabetes requires constant monitoring of BGLs and lifestyle modifications, which can be both time-consuming and stressful. This continuous management can lead to psychological distress, including anxiety and depression, further diminishing the quality of life (Peyrot et al., 2019). Complications, such as neuropathy, can cause chronic pain and disability, limiting mobility and independence. Moreover, diabetic retinopathy can lead to vision loss, severely affecting an individual's ability to perform daily activities. These physical and psychological challenges associated with diabetes significantly impair overall quality of life, making effective management and support crucial (Rubin and Peyrot, 2020).

1.5 CURRENT TRENDS AND FUTURE DIRECTIONS

1.5.1 ADVANCES IN UNDERSTANDING DIABETES EPIDEMIOLOGY

Advancements in diabetes epidemiology have significantly enhanced our understanding of the prevalence, risk factors, and molecular underpinnings of diabetes. Recent research highlights the integration of omics technologies, which have provided insights into genetic, epigenetic, and metabolic markers associated with diabetes, paving the way for precision medicine (Yu et al., 2024).

The global prevalence of diabetes reached 537 million adults in 2021 and is projected to rise to 783 million by 2045, with a disproportionate burden in LMICs (Forouhi and Wareham, 2022). Type 2 diabetes accounts for over 90% of all cases and is driven by obesity and lifestyle factors (Forouhi and Wareham, 2022). Advances in molecular genetics have identified numerous mutations linked to diabetes, thereby enhancing our understanding of its pathogenesis (Kharroubi and Darwish, 2015). Omics research has illustrated the heterogeneity of diabetes, emphasizing the need for tailored epidemiological studies (Yu et al., 2024).

The evolving diagnostic thresholds for diabetes, influenced by various studies, highlight the need for standardized criteria across populations (Balkau and Holt, 2019). While these advancements provide a clearer picture of diabetes epidemiology, challenges remain in fully understanding the complexities of the disease and ensuring equitable healthcare access globally.

1.5.2 EMERGING RISK FACTORS

Emerging risk factors for diabetes mellitus are increasingly being recognized, particularly in relation to environmental contaminants and metabolic syndrome. Recent studies have highlighted the complex interplay between these factors and the development of diabetes, necessitating further investigation.

1.5.2.1 ENVIRONMENTAL CONTAMINANTS

Substances such as endocrine disruptors, perfluorinated compounds, and bisphenols (e.g., BPS and BPF) have been linked to glycemic dysregulation. These contaminants may interfere with glucose metabolism and contribute to diabetes risk (Moreno-Gómez-Toledano et al., 2024; Niu et al., 2024). A systematic review indicated a significant association between bisphenol exposure and diabetes, particularly BPS (Moreno-Gómez-Toledano et al., 2024).

1.5.2.2 METABOLIC SYNDROME

Obesity, hyperlipidemia, and hypertension are associated with insulin resistance and an increased risk (Hayden, 2024). New insights suggest that factors such as leptin resistance, mitochondrial stress, and vascular inflammation also play critical roles in the development (Hayden, 2024). While these emerging factors present significant concerns, it is essential to consider that traditional lifestyle factors such as diet and physical activity continue to be fundamental in diabetes prevention and management.

1.5.3 INNOVATIONS IN DATA COLLECTION AND ANALYSIS

Innovations in data collection and analysis for diabetes management have transformed patient care and treatment strategies significantly. Recent advancements in technology, machine learning (ML), and real-world data (RWD) to enhance diabetes care have led to more personalized and effective management approaches.

1.5.3.1 TECHNOLOGICAL ADVANCEMENTS

CGMs and automated insulin delivery systems have revolutionized real-time monitoring and management of diabetes (Kang, 2024). Health management applications for smartphones and wearables facilitate the integration of patient-generated health data with electronic health records (EHRs), thereby enhancing clinical decision-making (Kang, 2024).

1.5.3.2 MACHINE LEARNING APPLICATIONS

ML techniques analyze vast datasets from EHRs and wearable devices, providing insights into blood glucose patterns and treatment outcomes (Khanam et al., 2024). These algorithms improve the predictive capabilities (Khanam et al., 2024).

1.5.3.3 REAL-WORLD DATA UTILIZATION

The use of RWD has expanded research opportunities, allowing examination of diverse populations and interventions (Gregg et al., 2023). Datasets such as DiaTrend, which include extensive longitudinal data from wearable devices, support the development of novel analytical solutions to improve diabetes management (Prioleau et al., 2023). Although these innovations promise enhanced diabetes care, challenges such as data quality and potential biases in RWD must be addressed to ensure reliable outcomes.

1.5.4 FUTURE RESEARCH PRIORITIES

Future research on diabetes is increasingly focused on patient-centered priorities, technological advancements, and the management of complications. The following key areas have emerged as critical for future research:

1. **Patient-Centered Research Priorities:** One study identified that individuals with diabetes prioritize research on improving

diabetes technology and understanding the causes of diabetes, with specific interests varying by diabetes type (Hendrieckx et al., 2024). The James Lind Alliance emphasizes the importance of involving patients in research to align studies with their needs, highlighting priorities such as lifestyle interventions and psychosocial support (Oliver and Holt, 2019).

2. **Complications and Management:** Research on diabetic foot disease has revealed significant priorities in prevention and management strategies, including understanding healing factors and improving treatment outcomes (Collings et al., 2022). The need for better management of diabetes-related complications such as neuropathy is underscored, with calls for more effective diagnostic and treatment approaches (Oliver and Holt, 2020).
3. **Technological Innovations:** Continuous glucose monitoring (CGM) and automated insulin delivery systems are highlighted as areas that require further research to enhance diabetes management (Oliver and Holt, 2020). While these priorities reflect a consensus on the need for innovative and patient-focused research, some argue that the complexity of diabetes necessitates a broader approach that includes basic science and public health strategies to address the multifaceted nature of the disease (Franceschi, 2024).

1.5.5 IMPLICATIONS FOR PUBLIC HEALTH POLICY

They are multifaceted and address prevention, management, and economic impacts. Effective policies must consider the rising prevalence of diabetes, the economic burden it imposes, and the need for tailored interventions across contexts. Diabetes, particularly type 2 diabetes, is largely preventable and increasingly prevalent owing to obesity and lifestyle factors (Watkins, 2023). Countries are urged to develop specific action plans to halt this rise, as seen in Iran's establishment of a diabetes subcommittee to create a national service framework (Peykari et al., 2022).

Public health programs for diabetes management can significantly affect the economy. For instance, a policy that reduces complications by 0.42% could yield substantial tax revenue and decrease productivity losses in Italy (Di et al., 2022). Telemedicine and innovative treatments are recommended to enhance patient care and improve economic outcomes (Di et al., 2022).

Addressing barriers to early diagnosis, such as insurance gaps and symptom normalization, is crucial for effective diabetes management (Chard et al., 2022). Policymakers must consider diverse healthcare contexts and risk factors when designing interventions (Peykari et al., 2022). While these strategies highlight the importance of targeted public health policies, challenges remain in ensuring equitable access to care and addressing the social determinants of health that contribute to the prevalence of diabetes.

1.6 CONCLUSION

In conclusion, diabetes mellitus is a significant and complex global health challenge, characterized by its chronic nature and widespread prevalence. With over 537 million cases worldwide in 2021, the disease demands urgent attention, particularly type 2 diabetes, which constitutes the majority of diagnoses owing to its strong correlation with obesity and lifestyle factors. Beyond its direct impact, diabetes is closely linked to a range of comorbidities and complications, underscoring its substantial burden on morbidity and mortality. Emerging insights into risk factors, including environmental contaminants and metabolic syndrome, have further highlighted the evolving dimensions of this condition. Advancements in technology, data analytics, and innovative research methodologies have opened up new pathways for understanding, managing, and mitigating diabetes. As the field progresses, these tools will be pivotal in shaping effective interventions and fostering better outcomes for individuals with diabetes worldwide.

KEYWORDS

- **data analytics**
- **diabetes mellitus**
- **end-stage renal disease**
- **insulin resistance**
- **machine learning**
- **metabolic syndrome**
- **public health interventions**
- **real-world data**

REFERENCES

Abbott, C. A., Carrington, A. L., Ashe, H., Bath, S., Every, L. C., Griffiths, J., et al. (2002). The North-West Diabetes Foot Care Study: Incidence of, and risk factors for, new diabetic foot ulceration in a community-based patient cohort. *Diabetes Med, 19*, 377–384.

Adler, A. I., Stevens, R. J., Manley, S. E., Bilous, R. W., Cull, C. A., & Holman, R. R. (2003). Development and progression of nephropathy in type 2 diabetes: The United Kingdom Prospective Diabetes Study (UKPDS 64). *Kidney Int, 63*, 225–232.

Ahmed, A. M. (2002). History of diabetes mellitus. *Saudi Medical Journal, 23*(4), 373–378.

Aiello, L. P., Pierce, E. A., Foley, E. D., Takagi, H., Chen, H., Riddle, L., et al. (1995). Suppression of retinal neovascularization *in vivo* by inhibition of vascular endothelial growth factor (VEGF) using soluble VEGF-receptor chimeric proteins. *Proc Natl Acad Sci U S A, 92*, 10457–10461.

Aliyu, I. S., Aliyu, T. M., Bakari, A. G., Hassan, S. S., Onyemelukwe, G. C., & Sani, B. G. (2006). Relationship between random blood sugar and body mass index in an African population. *International Journal of Diabetes and Metabolism, 14*(3), 144–145.

Almdal, T., Scharling, H., Jensen, J. S., & Vestergaard, H. (2004). The independent effect of type 2 diabetes mellitus on ischemic heart disease, stroke, and death: A population-based study of 13,000 men and women with 20 years of follow-up. *Arch Intern Med, 164*, 1422–1426.

American Diabetes Association (ADA). (2014). Standards of medical care in diabetes—2014. *Diabetes Care, 37*(Supplement 1), S14–S80.

American Diabetes Association. (2007). Standards of medical care in diabetes—2007 [Position Statement]. *Diabetes Care, 30*, S4–S41.

American Diabetes Association. (2020). Standards of medical care in diabetes—2020. *Diabetes Care, 43*(Supplement 1), S1–S212. https://doi.org/10.2337/dc20-S001 (accessed on 2nd February 2026).

American Heart Association. (2015). Physical activity and cardiovascular health. *Circulation, 131*(6), e1–e10.

Antini, C., Caixeta, R., Luciani, S., & Hennis, A. J. (2024). Diabetes mortality: Trends and multi-country analysis of the Americas from 2000 to 2019. *International Journal of Epidemiology, 53*(1), dyad182.

Atkinson, M. A., Eisenbarth, G. S., & Michels, A. W. (2014). Type 1 diabetes. *The Lancet, 383*(9911), 69–82.

Avagimyan, A., Popov, S., & Shalnova, S. (2022). The pathophysiological basis of diabetic cardiomyopathy development. *Current Problems in Cardiology, 47*(9), 101156.

Avogaro, A., Giorda, C., Maggini, M., Mannucci, E., Raschetti, R., Lombardo, F., et al. (2007). Incidence of coronary heart disease in type 2 diabetic men and women: Impact of microvascular complications, treatment, and geographic location. *Diabetes Care, 30*, 1241–1247.

Bak, J. C., de Vries, S. A., Serné, E. H., Groenwold, R. H., de Valk, H. W., Mul, D., et al. (2024). Mortality patterns in Dutch diabetes outpatients. *Diabetes, Obesity and Metabolism. 26(10), 4213–4224.*

Balkau, B., & Holt, R. I. G. (2019). Learning about diabetes through epidemiology. *Diabetic Medicine, 36*(10), 1195–1198.

Bartoli, E., Fra, G. P., & Schianca, G. C. (2011). The oral glucose tolerance test (OGTT) revisited. *European Journal of Internal Medicine, 22*(1), 8–12.

Beach, K. W. (1979). A theoretical model to predict the behavior of glycosylated hemoglobin levels. *Journal of Theoretical Biology, 81*, 547–561.

Beckman, J. A., Creager, M. A., & Libby, P. (2002). Diabetes and atherosclerosis: Epidemiology, pathophysiology, and management. *JAMA, 287*, 2570–2581.

Bodke, H., Wagh, V., & Kakar, G. (2023). Diabetes mellitus and prevalence of other comorbid conditions: A systematic review. *Cureus, 15*(11), e49374.

Boulton, A. J., Vinik, A. I., Arezzo, J. C., Bril, V., Feldman, E. L., Freeman, R., et al. (2005). Diabetic neuropathies: A statement by the American Diabetes Association. *Diabetes Care, 28*, 956–962.

Breyer, M. K., Ofenheimer, A., Altziebler, J., Hartl, S., Burghuber, O. C., Studnicka, M., et al. (2020). Marked differences in prediabetes- and diabetes-associated comorbidities between men and women—Epidemiological results from a general population-based cohort aged 6–80 years—The LEAD (Lung, hEart, sociAl, boDy) study. *European Journal of Clinical Investigation, 50*(3), e13207.

Brook, R. D., Franklin, B., Cascio, W., Hong, Y. L., Howard, G., Lipsett, M., et al. (2010). Air pollution and cardiovascular outcomes: A review. *Circulation, 121*(21), 2331–2378.

Buse, J. B., Ginsberg, H. N., Bakris, G. L., Clark, N. G., Costa, F., Eckel, R., et al. (2007). Primary prevention of cardiovascular diseases in people with diabetes mellitus: A scientific statement from the American Heart Association and the American Diabetes Association. *Diabetes Care, 30*, 162–172.

Catalano, P. M., & Tyzbir, E. D. (1999). Insulin resistance and carbohydrate metabolism in pregnancy. *Baillière's Clinical Endocrinology and Metabolism, 13*(1), 73–92.

Centers for Disease Control and Prevention (CDC). (2022). *National Diabetes Statistics Report, 2022.* Centers for Disease Control and Prevention. https://www.cdc.gov/diabetes/pdfs/data/statistics/national-diabetes-statistics-report.pdf (accessed on 2nd February 2026).

Chang, H. Y., Hsu, C. C., Pan, W. H., Liu, W. L., Cheng, J. Y. C., Tseng, C. H., et al. (2010). Gender differences in trends in diabetes prevalence from 1993 to 2008 in Taiwan. *Diabetes Research and Clinical Practice, 90*(3), 358–364.

Chard, S., Girling, L., Harris-Wallace, B., Henderson, L., Roth, E. G., & Eckert, J. K. (2022). "Here it was waiting for me:" Diabetes diagnosis pathways and implications for health policy. *Journal of Elder Policy, 2*(2), 111–140.

Charvat, H., Goto, A., Goto, M., Inoue, M., Heianza, Y., Arase, Y., et al. (2015). Impact of population aging on trends in diabetes prevalence: A meta-regression analysis of 160,000 Japanese adults. *Journal of Diabetes Investigation, 6*(5), 533–542.

Chaturvedi, N., Bandinelli, S., Mangili, R., Penno, G., Rottiers, R. E., & Fuller, J. H. (2001). Microalbuminuria in type 1 diabetes: Rates, risk factors and glycemic threshold. *Kidney Int, 60*, 219–227.

Colhoun, H. M., Betteridge, D. J., Durrington, P. N., Hitman, G. A., Neil, H. A., Livingstone, S. J., et al. (2004). Primary prevention of cardiovascular disease with atorvastatin in type 2 diabetes in the Collaborative Atorvastatin Diabetes Study (CARDS): Multicenter randomized placebo-controlled trial. *Lancet, 364*, 685–696.

Collings, R., Shalhoub, J., Atkin, L., Game, F., Hitchman, L., & Long, L. (2022). Research priorities in diabetic foot disease. *J Vasc Soc GB Irel, 1*(4), 124–129.

Collins, R., Armitage, J., Parish, S., Sleigh, P., & Peto, R. (2003). MRC/BHF Heart Protection Study of cholesterol-lowering with simvastatin in 5963 people with diabetes: A randomized placebo-controlled trial. *Lancet, 361*, 2005–2016.

Corder, E. H., Saunders, A. M., Risch, N., Strittmatter, W. J., Schmechel, D., Gaskell, P. C., et al. (1993). Protective effect of apolipoprotein E type 2 allele for late onset Alzheimer disease. *Nature Genetics, 7*(2), 180–184.

Cousin, E., Duncan, B. B., Stein, C., Ong, K. L., Vos, T., Abbafati, C., et al. (2022). Diabetes mortality and trends before 25 years of age: An analysis of the Global Burden of Disease Study 2019. *The Lancet Diabetes & Endocrinology, 10*(3), 177–192.

DeFronzo, R. A., Ferrannini, E., Groop, L., et al. (2015). Type 2 diabetes mellitus. *Nature Reviews Disease Primers, 1*(1), 1–22.

Deschamps, I., Beressi, J. P., Khalil, I., Robert, J. J., & Hors, J. (1991). The role of genetic predisposition to type I (insulin-dependent) diabetes mellitus. *Annals of Medicine, 23*(4), 427–435.

Di Brino, E., Basile, M., Rumi, F., Calabrò, G. E., & Cicchetti, A. (2022). PP153 The economic and fiscal impact of public health programs for diabetic patients in Italy. *International Journal of Technology Assessment in Health Care, 38*(S1), S90–S90.

Diabetes Prevention Program Research Group. (2002). Reduction in the incidence of type 2 diabetes with lifestyle intervention or metformin. *New England Journal of Medicine, 346*(6), 393–403. https://doi.org/10.1056/NEJMoa012512 (accessed on 2nd February 2026).

Drewnowski, A., & Almiron-Roig, E. (2010). Human perceptions of food and the implications for dietary choices. *Appetite, 55*(1), 13–20.

Ellard, S., & Hattersley, A. T. (2013). Genetic basis of monogenic diabetes. *Pediatric Diabetes, 14*(3), 167–173.

Ferrara, A. (2007). Increasing prevalence of gestational diabetes mellitus: A public health perspective. *Diabetes Care, 30*(Supplement 2), S141–S146.

Florez, J. C. (2008). Newly identified loci highlight beta cell dysfunction as a key cause of type 2 diabetes: Where are the insulin resistance genes? *Diabetology, 51*(7), 1100–1110.

Fong, D. S., Aiello, L. P., Ferris, F. L. III, & Klein, R. (2004). Diabetic retinopathy. *Diabetes Care, 27*, 2540–2553.

Forouhi, N. G., & Wareham, N. J. (2022). Epidemiology of diabetes. *Medicine, 50*(10), 638–643.

Franceschi, R. (2024). Special issue—Diabetes mellitus: Current research and future perspectives. *J. Pers. Med, 14*, 308.

Frick, M. H., Elo, O., Haapa, K., Heinonen, O. P., Heinsalmi, P., Helo, P., et al. (1987). Helsinki Heart Study: Primary-prevention trial with gemfibrozil in middle-aged men with dyslipidemia: Safety of treatment, changes in risk factors, and incidence of coronary heart disease. *N Engl J Med, 317*, 1237–1245.

Gabbay, K. H. (1975). Hyperglycemia, polyol metabolism, and complications of diabetes mellitus. *Annu Rev Med, 26*, 521–536.

Gabbay, K. H. (2004). Aldose reductase inhibition in the treatment of diabetic neuropathy: Where are we in 2004? *Curr Diab Rep, 4*, 405–408.

Greci, L. S., Kailasam, M., Malkani, S., Katz, D. L., Hulinsky, I., Ahmadi, R., et al. (2003). Utility of HbA1c levels for diabetes case finding in hospitalized patients with hyperglycemia. *Diabetes Care, 26*(4), 1064–1068.

Gregg, E. W., Patorno, E., Karter, A. J., Mehta, R., Huang, E. S., White, M., et al. (2023). Use of real-world data in population science to improve the prevention and care of diabetes-related outcomes. *Diabetes Care, 46*(7), 1316–1326.

Gross, J. L., de Azevedo, M. J., Silveiro, S. P., Canani, L. H., Caramori, M. L., & Zelmanovitz, T. (2005). Diabetic nephropathy: Diagnosis, prevention, and treatment. *Diabetes Care, 28*, 164–176.

Haffner, S. M., Lehto, S., Ronnemaa, T., Pyorala, K., & Laakso, M. (1998). Mortality from coronary heart disease in subjects with type 2 diabetes and in nondiabetic subjects with and without prior myocardial infarction. *N Engl J Med, 339*, 229–234.

Hariyono, H., & Leo Yosdimyati, R. (2018). The relationship of emotional response with random blood sugar levels in type 2 diabetes mellitus. *Journal of Applied Science and Research, 6*(6), 7–11.

Hayden, M. R. (2024). A closer look at the perivascular unit in the development of enlarged perivascular spaces in obesity, metabolic syndrome, and type 2 diabetes mellitus. *Biomedicines, 12*(1), 96.

Heald, A. H., Stedman, M., Laing, I., Gibson, M., & Whyte, M. (2023). Type 2 diabetes and mortality in females versus males in England: The Salford diabetes cohort. *Cardiovascular Endocrinology & Metabolism, 12*(1), e0276.

Heart Outcomes Prevention Evaluation Study Investigators. (2000). Effects of ramipril on cardiovascular and microvascular outcomes in people with diabetes mellitus: Results of the HOPE study and MICRO-HOPE substudy. *Lancet, 355*, 253–259.

Hendrieckx, C., Russell-Green, S., Skinner, T., Ng, A. H., Lee, C., Barlow, S., et al. (2024). Diabetes research matters: A three-round priority-setting survey consultation with adults living with diabetes and family members in Australia. *The Patient-Patient-Centered Outcomes Research, 17*(4), 441–455.

Hod, M., Kapur, A., Sacks, D. A., et al. (2015). The International Federation of Gynecology and Obstetrics (FIGO) initiative on gestational diabetes mellitus: A pragmatic guide for diagnosis, management, and care. *International Journal of Gynecology & Obstetrics, 131*(S3), S173–S211.

Hogan, P., Dall, T., & Nikolov, P. (2003). Economic costs of diabetes in the US in 2002. *Diabetes Care, 26*, 917–932.

Hu, F. B., Manson, J. E., Stampfer, M. J., et al. (2001). Diet, lifestyle, and the risk of type 2 diabetes mellitus in women. *New England Journal of Medicine, 345*(11), 790–797.

Hughes, M. S., Addala, A., & Buckingham, B. (2023). Digital technology for diabetes. *New England Journal of Medicine, 389*(22), 2076–2086.

IDF Africa Region. (2021). *Diabetes Atlas: Africa.* International Diabetes Federation. https://www.idf.org/our-network/regions-members/africa.html (accessed on 2nd February 2026).

International Diabetes Federation. (2000). *IDF Diabetes Atlas 2000.* International Diabetes Federation.

International Diabetes Federation. (2003). *IDF Diabetes Atlas 2003.* International Diabetes Federation.

International Diabetes Federation. (2021). *IDF Diabetes Atlas, 10th edition.*

International Diabetes Federation. (2023). *IDF Diabetes Atlas 2023.* International Diabetes Federation. https://doi.org/10.1038/s41591-020-1060-3 (accessed on 2nd February 2026).

Jagannathan, R., Neves, J. S., Dorcely, B., Chung, S. T., Tamura, K., Rhee, M., et al. (2020). The oral glucose tolerance test: 100 years later. *Diabetes, Metabolic Syndrome and Obesity*, 3787–3805.

Kang, S. (2024). Technological innovations transforming diabetes care in practice. *The Journal of Korean Diabetes, 25*(2), 57–61.

Kannel, W. B., & McGee, D. L. (1979). Diabetes and cardiovascular disease: The Framingham study. *JAMA, 241*, 2035–2038.

Karter, A. J., Ackerson, L. M., Darbinian, J. A., D'Agostino, R. B., Ferrara, A., Liu, J., et al. (2001). Self-monitoring of blood glucose levels and glycemic control: The Northern California Kaiser Permanente Diabetes Registry. *The American Journal of Medicine, 111*(1), 1–9.

Keenan, H. A., Costacou, T., Sun, J. K., Doria, A., Cavellerano, J., Coney, J., et al. (2007). Clinical factors associated with resistance to microvascular complications in diabetic patients of extreme disease duration: The 50-year medalist study. *Diabetes Care, 30*, 1995–1997.

Khanam, A., Masoodi, F. S., & Bamhdi, A. (2024). From data to insights: Leveraging machine learning for diabetes management. In *A Biologist's Guide to Artificial Intelligence* (pp. 97–123). Academic Press.

Kharroubi, A. T., & Darwish, H. M. (2015). Diabetes mellitus: The epidemic of the century. *World Journal of Diabetes, 6*(6), 850.

King, M. C., Marks, J. H., & Mandell, J. B. (2003). Breast and ovarian cancer risks due to inherited mutations in BRCA1 and BRCA2. *Science, 302*(5645), 643–646.

Knip, M., Veijola, R., Virtanen, S. M., et al. (2005). Environmental triggers and determinants of type 1 diabetes. *Diabetes, 54*(Supplement 2), S125–S136.

Koo, B. K., & Moon, M. K. (2016). Are we in the same risk of diabetes mellitus? Gender- and age-specific epidemiology of diabetes in 2001 to 2014 in the Korean population. *Diabetes & Metabolism Journal, 40*(3), 175–181.

Koskinen, P., Manttari, M., Manninen, V., Huttunen, J. K., Heinonen, O. P., & Frick, M. H. (1992). Coronary heart disease incidence in NIDDM patients in the Helsinki Heart Study. *Diabetes Care, 15*, 820–825.

Kumar, R., Nandhini, L. P., Kamalanathan, S., Sahoo, J., & Vivekanadan, M. (2016). Evidence for current diagnostic criteria of diabetes mellitus. *World Journal of Diabetes, 7*(17), 396.

Kunisaki, M., Bursell, S. E., Clermont, A. C., Ishii, H., Ballas, L. M., Jirousek, M. R., et al. (1995). Vitamin E prevents diabetes-induced abnormal retinal blood flow via the diacylglycerol–protein kinase C pathway. *Am J Physiol, 269*, E239–E246.

Kuo, F. Y., Cheng, K. C., Li, Y., & Cheng, J. T. (2021). Oral glucose tolerance test in diabetes, the old method revisited. *World Journal of Diabetes, 12*(6), 786.

Laing, S. P., Swerdlow, A. J., Carpenter, L. M., Slater, S. D., Burden, A. C., Botha, J. L., et al. (2003). Mortality from cerebrovascular disease in a cohort of 23,000 patients with insulin-treated diabetes. *Stroke, 34*, 418–421.

Laing, S. P., Swerdlow, A. J., Slater, S. D., Burden, A. C., Morris, A., Waugh, N. R., et al. (2003). Mortality from heart disease in a cohort of 23,000 patients with insulin-treated diabetes. *Diabetology, 46*, 760–765.

Lakhtakia, R. (2013). The history of diabetes mellitus. *Sultan Qaboos University Medical Journal, 13*(3), 368.

Lambert, P., & Bingley, P. J. (2002). What is type 1 diabetes? *Medicine, 30*(1), 1–5.

Lehto, S., Ronnemaa, T., Pyorala, K., & Laakso, M. (1996). Predictors of stroke in middle-aged patients with non-insulin-dependent diabetes. *Stroke, 27*, 63–68.

Leslie, R. D., Ma, R. C. W., Franks, P. W., Nadeau, K. J., Pearson, E. R., & Redondo, M. J. (2023). Understanding diabetes heterogeneity: Key steps towards precision medicine in diabetes. *The Lancet Diabetes & Endocrinology, 11*(11), 848–860.

Lindholm, L. H., Ibsen, H., Dahlof, B., Devereux, R. B., Beevers, G., de Faire, U., et al. (2002). Cardiovascular morbidity and mortality in patients with diabetes in the Losartan Intervention for Endpoint reduction in hypertension study (LIFE): A randomized trial against atenolol. *Lancet, 359*, 1004–1010.

Manninen, V., Elo, M. O., Frick, M. H., Haapa, K., Heinonen, O. P., Heinsalmi, P., et al. (1988). Lipid alterations and decline in the incidence of coronary heart disease in the Helsinki Heart Study. *JAMA, 260*, 641–651.

Mari, A., Pacini, G., Murphy, E., Ludvik, B., & Nolan, J. J. (2001). A model-based method for assessing insulin sensitivity from the oral glucose tolerance test. *Diabetes Care, 24*(3), 539–548.

Maser, R. E., Mitchell, B. D., Vinik, A. I., & Freeman, R. (2003). The association between cardiovascular autonomic neuropathy and mortality in individuals with diabetes: A meta-analysis. *Diabetes Care, 26*, 1895–1901.

McAulay, V., Deary, I. J., & Frier, B. M. (2001). Symptoms of hypoglycemia in people with diabetes. *Diabetic Medicine, 18*(9), 690–705.

McDonald, G. W., Fisher, G. F., & Burnham, C. (1965). Reproducibility of the oral glucose tolerance test. *Diabetes, 14*(8), 473–480.

Meier, N. W., Böhm, R., Korn, L., & Betsch, C. (2020). Individual preferences for voluntary vs. mandatory vaccination policies: An experimental analysis. *European Journal of Public Health, 30*(1), 50–55. https://doi.org/10.1093/eurpub/ckz181 (accessed on 2nd February 2026).

Metzger, B. E., Gabbe, S. G., Persson, B., et al. (2008). International Association of Diabetes and Pregnancy Study Groups recommendations on the diagnosis and classification of hyperglycemia in pregnancy. *Diabetes Care, 33*(3), 676–682.

Miki, Y., Swensen, J., Shattuck-Eidens, D., et al. (1994). A strong candidate for the breast and ovarian cancer susceptibility gene BRCA1. *Science, 266*(5182), 66–71.

Misra, S., Wagner, R., Ozkan, B., Schön, M., Sevilla-Gonzalez, M., Prystupa, K., et al. (2023). Precision subclassification of type 2 diabetes: A systematic review. *Communications Medicine, 3*(1), 138.

Mohajan, D., & Mohajan, H. K. (2024). Oral hypoglycemic agents: Non-insulin medications for type 2 diabetes patients. *Innovation in Science and Technology, 3*(1), 23–31.

Moreno-Gómez-Toledano, R. (2024). *Environmental Health Literacy Update—New Evidence, Methodologies and Perspectives: New Evidence, Methodologies and Perspectives.* BoD–Books on Demand.

Mukhtar, Y., Galalain, A., & Yunusa, U. (2020). A modern overview on diabetes mellitus: A chronic endocrine disorder. *European Journal of Biology, 5*(2), 1–14.

Nathan, D. M., Cleary, P. A., Backlund, J. Y., Genuth, S. M., Lachin, J. M., Orchard, T. J., et al. (2005). Intensive diabetes treatment and cardiovascular disease in patients with type 1 diabetes. *N Engl J Med, 353*, 2643–2653.

National Cancer Institute. (2019). *Harms of smoking and health benefits of quitting.* Smoking and Tobacco Control. https://www.cancer.gov/about-cancer/causes-prevention/risk/tobacco (accessed on 2nd February 2026).

Niu, H., Xu, M., Tu, P., Xu, Y., Li, X., Xing, M., et al. (2024). Emerging contaminants: An emerging risk factor for diabetes mellitus. *Toxics, 12*(1), 47.

Norris, J. M., Barriga, K., Klingensmith, G., et al. (2003). Timing of initial cereal exposure in infancy and risk of islet autoimmunity. *JAMA, 290*(13), 1713–1720.

Oliver, N., & Holt, R. I. G. (2019). The James Lind Alliance research priorities for diabetes. *Diabetic Medicine, 36*(3), 267–268.

Paterson, A. D., Rutledge, B. N., Cleary, P. A., Lachin, J. M., & Crow, R. S. (2007). The effect of intensive diabetes treatment on resting heart rate in type 1 diabetes: The Diabetes Control and Complications Trial/Epidemiology of Diabetes Interventions and Complications study. *Diabetes Care, 30*, 2107–2112.

Pathmanathan, S., & Somasundaram, N. P. (2014). HbA1c and diabetes–An overview. *Sri Lanka Journal of Diabetes Endocrinology and Metabolism, 3*(2).

Peykari, N., Ghaemi, F., Nasli, E., Hazaveh, A. R. M., Yousefi, E., Monji, H., et al. (2022). Policy implications for diabetes prevention and control: An experience from Iran. *Medical Journal of the Islamic Republic of Iran, 36.*

Peyrot, M., Burns, K., Davies, M., Forbes, A., Hermanns, N., Holt, R., et al. (2019). Diabetes Attitudes, Wishes and Needs 2 (DAWN2): A multinational, multistakeholder study of psychosocial issues in diabetes and person-centered diabetes care. *Diabetes Research and Clinical Practice, 156*, 107839.

Piccinini, F., & Bergman, M. (2016). A mechanistic approach to the etiology of type 2 diabetes. *Diabetes Care, 39*(7), 1131–1139.

Pope, C. A., Dockery, D. W., & Schwartz, J. (2002). Review of epidemiological studies on short-term exposure to air pollution: Epidemiological evidence of a relationship between short-term exposure and mortality. *Environmental Health Perspectives, 110*(8), 103–109.

Prioleau, T., Bartolome, A., Comi, R., & Stanger, C. (2023). DiaTrend: A dataset from advanced diabetes technology to enable development of novel analytic solutions. *Scientific Data, 10*(1), 556.

Quattrin, T., Mastrandrea, L. D., & Walker, L. S. (2023). Type 1 diabetes. *The Lancet, 401*(10394), 2149–2162.

Radha, V., & Mohan, V. (2007). Genetic predisposition to type 2 diabetes among Asian Indians. *Indian Journal of Medical Research, 125*(3), 259–274.

Ramachandran, A., Snehalatha, C., Raghavan, A., & Nanditha, A. (2024). Classification and diagnosis of diabetes. In *Textbook of Diabetes* (pp. 22–27).

Rashed, E., Alkout, T., Eltomy, S., Etekbali, O. R., & Alkout, A. M. (2020). The effects of red blood cells parameters on HbA1c and random blood sugar levels in diabetics diagnosis. *International Journal of Diabetes and Clinical Research, 7*, 1–7.

Rathi, A., Bansal, R., & Saha, K. (2017). Presence of co-morbidities in patients suffering from diabetes mellitus type 2 attending two clinics in Delhi. *MOJ Immunology, 5*(3), 00160.

Rehm, J., Samokhvalov, A. V., & Shield, K. D. (2009). Global burden of alcoholic liver diseases. *Alcohol Research & Health, 33*(4), 259–268.

Rohlfing, C. L., England, J. D., Weidmeyer, H. M., et al. (2002). Defining the relationship between plasma glucose and HbA1c. *Diabetes Care, 25*, 275–278.

Rossing, K., Jacobsen, P., Pietraszek, L., & Parving, H. H. (2003). Reno protective effects of adding angiotensin II receptor blocker to maximal recommended doses of ACE inhibitor in diabetic nephropathy: A randomized double-blind crossover trial. *Diabetes Care, 26*, 2268–2274.

Rubin, R. R., & Peyrot, M. (2020). Quality of life and diabetes. *Diabetes/Metabolism Research and Reviews, 15*(3), 205–218.

Sankhuu, Y., Altaisaikhan, O., Battsogt, M. O., Byambasukh, O., & Khasag, A. (2023). Diabetes-related mortality in a developing country: An exploration of tertiary hospital data. *Journal of Clinical Medicine, 12*(20), 6687.

Sasako, T. (2024). Exploring mechanisms underlying diabetes comorbidities and strategies to prevent vascular complications. *Diabetology International, 15*(1), 34–40.

Shivashankar, M., & Mani, D. (2011). A brief overview of diabetes. *International Journal of Pharmacy and Pharmaceutical Sciences, 3*(4), 22–27.

Shoji, M., Kanekiyo, M., & Murakami, M. (1998). Apolipoprotein E and Alzheimer's disease. *Journal of Clinical Neuroscience, 5*(2), 120–124.

Sirdah, M. M., & Reading, N. S. (2020). Genetic predisposition in type 2 diabetes: A promising approach toward a personalized management of diabetes. *Clinical Genetics, 98*(6), 525–547.

Sweeting, A., Hannah, W., Backman, H., Catalano, P., Feghali, M., Herman, W. H., et al. (2024). Epidemiology and management of gestational diabetes. *The Lancet, 404*(10448), 175–192.

Syed, F. Z. (2022). Type 1 diabetes mellitus. *Annals of Internal Medicine, 175*(3), ITC33–ITC48.

Teck, J. (2022). Diabetes-associated comorbidities. *Primary Care: Clinics in Office Practice, 49*(2), 275–286.

Tesauro, M., & Mazzotta, F. A. (2020). Pathophysiology of diabetes. In *Transplantation, Bioengineering, and Regeneration of the Endocrine Pancreas* (pp. 37–47). Academic Press.

The DCCT Research Group. (1993). The effect of intensive treatment of diabetes on the development and progression of long-term complications in insulin-dependent diabetes mellitus. *N Engl J Med, 329*, 977–986.

Thrower, S. L., & Bingley, P. J. (2014). What is type 1 diabetes? *Medicine, 42*(12), 682–686.

Tokhirovna, E. G. (2024). Risk factors for developing type 2 diabetes mellitus. *Education, Science and Innovative Ideas in the World, 36*(5), 64–69.

U.K. Prospective Diabetes Study Group. (1998a). Efficacy of atenolol and captopril in reducing risk of macrovascular and microvascular complications in type 2 diabetes: UKPDS 39. *BMJ, 317*, 713–720.

U.K. Prospective Diabetes Study Group. (1998b). Tight blood pressure control and risk of macrovascular and microvascular complications in type 2 diabetes: UKPDS 38. *BMJ, 317*, 703–713.

UK Prospective Diabetes Study Group. (1998c). Intensive blood glucose control with sulphonylureas or insulin compared with conventional treatment and risk of complications in patients with type 2 diabetes (UKPDS 33). *Lancet, 352*, 837–853.

Watkins, D. A., & Ali, M. K. (2023). Measuring the global burden of diabetes: Implications for health policy, practice, and research. *The Lancet, 402*(10397), 163–165.

Watkins, P. J. (2003). Retinopathy. *BMJ, 326*, 924–926.

Whitelock, V., Rutters, F., Rijnhart, J. J., Nouwen, A., & Higgs, S. (2021). The mediating role of comorbid conditions in the association between type 2 diabetes and cognition: A cross-sectional observational study using the UK Biobank cohort. *Psych Neuroendocrinology, 123*, 104902.

Yu, G., Tam, H. C., Huang, C., Shi, M., Lim, C. K., Chan, J. C., et al. (2024). Lessons and applications of omics research in diabetes epidemiology. *Current Diabetes Reports, 24*(3), 27–44.

Zheng, Y., Ley, S. H., & Hu, F. B. (2018). Global etiology and epidemiology of type 2 diabetes mellitus and its cardiovascular implications. *Nature Reviews Endocrinology, 14*(2), 88–98. https://doi.org/10.1038/nrendo.2017.151 (accessed on 2nd February 2026).

CHAPTER 2

Etiological Insights and Pathophysiological Mechanisms of Diabetes

AYEZA SARWAR KALAM,[1] SAHIL HUSSAIN,[1,2] MOHAMMAD IRFAN KHAN,[1,*] and ALINA KHAN[3]

[1]*Faculty of Pharmacy, Integral University, Lucknow, Uttar Pradesh, India*

[2]*College of Health and Life Sciences, Hamad Bin Khalifa University, Doha, Qatar*

[3]*Department of Toxicology and Medical Elementology, Jamia Hamdard, New Delhi, Delhi, India*

*Corresponding author

ABSTRACT

Hyperglycemia, an ongoing metabolic condition caused by deficiencies in the release of insulin, production, or both, is a hallmark of diabetes mellitus. This chapter explores etiological insights and pathophysiological mechanisms underlying diabetes, aiming to provide a comprehensive understanding of its complex nature. The section delineates the interaction between predisposition due to genes, circumstances, and lifestyle variables as the key etiological factors that contribute to the emergence and advancement of diabetes. Insights into the roles of insulin resistance, pancreatic β-cell dysfunction, and aberrant glucagon secretion are discussed, shedding light on the mechanisms involved in glucose homeostasis and dysregulation. Additionally, the impact of inflammatory pathways, oxidative stress, and adipose

Diabetes: Novel Insights and Therapies. Anas Islam and Badruddeen (Eds)

DOI: 10.1201/9781779644596-3

tissue dysfunction on the pathophysiology of diabetes was examined, highlighting their contribution to insulin resistance and β-cell failure. Furthermore, emerging concepts such as gut microbiota-host interaction and epigenetic modifications have been explored for their potential implications in diabetes etiology and pathogenesis. Through the synthesis of current research findings, this chapter offers valuable perspectives on the underlying mechanisms driving diabetes onset and progression, paving the way for innovative therapeutic approaches and preventive strategies.

2.1 INTRODUCTION

The initial population to develop chronic diabetes, marked by dropping pounds and polyuria, was Egyptian. Nevertheless, Aertaeus, a Greek physician, was the first to employ the term DM. Mellitus is a Latin word for honey (sugar), and diabetes is the Greek term meaning "to pass through." As a significant cause of both prolonged disease and untimely death, diabetes claims the lives of about one person every 10 seconds in terms of annual fatalities. Insulin has become an epidemic on an international level due to the rise in overweight individuals and the advent of global urbanization. Despite the challenges in obtaining an accurate estimate of prevalence owing to variations in data collection standards and methodologies across different regions, current surveys predict that, by 2025, the proportion of people with diabetes will increase from 4% in 1995 to 6.4% (King et al., 1998).

Moreover, it is projected to undergo rapid changes, with a 42% surge from 51 to 72 million in developed nations and a 170% increase from 84 to 228 million in developing regions. Globally, the number of adults affected by diabetes is anticipated to increase from 194 million in 2003 to almost 380 million by 2025. By 2025, the nations most affected by this outbreak will include India, China, and the United States. Another concern is the substantial proportion (nearly 50%) of patients who remain undiagnosed even today. Consequently, there is an increasing trend in diabetes, particularly in urban settings. Hence, nations worldwide will confront a considerable increase in the healthcare burden, given that diabetic patients are susceptible to both immediate and long-term complications, leading to premature mortality (Kaul et al., 2012).

2.1.1 CLASSIFICATION OF DIABETES MELLITUS

2.1.1.1 TYPE 1 DIABETES MELLITUS (T1DM)

T1DM, also known as juvenile-onset diabetes or insulin-dependent diabetes, is an autoimmune disease that causes the death of pancreatic islet cells and is composed of activated CD^{4+} and CD^{8+} T cells as well as macrophages that infiltrate the system (Phillips et al., 2009). The initiation of T1DM typically manifests during childhood and early adulthood, specifically before the age of 35. Both genetic and environmental factors influence predisposition to this form of diabetes. Studies focusing on genetics have revealed a close correlation between the human leukocyte antigen (HLA) gene found on chromosome 6 and T1DM. Furthermore, HLA-DR, which is located next to HLA, is important for T1DM (Gorodezky et al., 2006). Existing evidence suggests that specific viruses may contribute to the onset of T1DM (Jun and Yoon, 2004). Idiopathic diabetes, known as T1DM, is a variant that lacks autoimmune involvement, with a lower occurrence rate compared to autoimmune T1DM, predominantly observed in African and Asian populations. The underlying causes and mechanisms remain unclear and are characterized by deficient insulin production and susceptibility to ketoacidosis without antibodies to β-cells (Harris et al., 1998). Fulminant T1DM, a subtype of T1DM, is characterized by rapid or extensive damage to β-cells (Shibasaki et al., 2013).

2.1.1.2 TYPE 2 DIABETES MELLITUS(T2DM)

Insulin resistance causes insufficient production and secretion of insulin, which is a symptom of type 2 diabetes typically diagnosed after the fourth decade of life and constitutes approximately 90% of global diabetes cases. The prevalence and incidence of T2DM increases with age (Masharani, 2005). T2DM subgroups are distinguished by the presence or absence of obesity. Obese T2DM patients encounter insulin resistance due to altered cell receptors, particularly in abdominal fat distribution. Non-obese T2DM individuals exhibit post-receptor insulin resistance and insufficient insulin production and release. Obesity and metabolic abnormalities can cause diabetes in emerging countries. The high prevalence of diabetes in these areas is caused by changes in diet and lifestyle (Galicia-Garcia et al., 2020).

2.1.1.3 GESTATIONAL DIABETES MELLITUS (GDM)

Pregnancy causes GDM to develop, and temporary insulin resistance is caused by glucose swings and increased insulin production in the placenta. Although GDM usually resolves post-pregnancy, complications such as maternal and fetal mortality risks, teratogenic effects, and diabetic nephropathy-related preeclampsia can arise (de Souza Rugolo et al., 2011).

2.1.1.4 MATURITY-ONSET DIABETES OF THE YOUNG (MODY)

A small proportion of individuals with diabetes are affected by MODY, a monogenic form of the disease. This condition typically manifests in the subsequent phases of life. The pathogenesis of the six MODY variants has been associated with mutations in several genes, including hepatocyte nuclear factor 4α (HNF-4α), glucokinase (MODY 2), HNF-1α, insulin promoter factor 1 (IPF-1), HNF-1β, and NEUROD1. Predominantly, changes in the HNF-1α gene are most prevalent, being responsible for over 70% of instances of MODY. Among the MODY subtypes, MODY 2 and MODY 3 are the most frequently encountered, with MODY 3 being characterized by a significant impairment in insulin secretion. Despite its rarity, an accurate diagnosis of MODY is crucial to ascertain the underlying cause of diabetes and to determine the most suitable therapeutic approach. Various secondary forms of diabetes can be triggered by conditions such as pancreatitis, Cushing syndrome, Klinefelter syndrome, and hyperthyroidism (Fajans et al., 2001).

2.2 ETIOLOGICAL FACTORS

2.2.1 GENETIC PREDISPOSITION

Genetics are a major factor in the onset of DM. T1DM is a complex illness with a significant hereditary component that arises from an inflammatory mechanism which destroys the cells of the pancreas preferentially and irrevocably (European Consortium for IDDM Genome Studies, 2001). The etiology of this condition involves a combination of ecological and biological elements. The genetic factors contributing to the etiology of T1DM are intricate. The disease prevalence in first-degree relatives of T1DM patients (5 to 6%) is increased compared to the general population (0.3 to 0.5%) (Degnbol and Green, 1978; Tillil and

Köbberling, 1987; Wagener et al., 1982). In the case of identical twins, the rate of concordance for T1DM is approximately 34% (Mier and van den Hurk, 1975).

When taken in conjunction with studies carried out on experimental animals, including the non-obese diabetic (NOD) mouse and the bio-breeding (BB) rat, they indicate that many genes contribute to the genetic basis of the illness, while other variables are equally important in its course. Analyses spanning over 15 years on major histocompatibility complex (MHC) antigens have gathered substantial evidence indicating that the primary vulnerability factors are located in the MHC region of chromosome 6 (Svejgaard et al., 1977; Svejgaard and Ryder, 1989).

T2DM is also known to cause multifaceted disarray, which is influenced by multiple genes found on various chromosomes, thereby enhancing its vulnerability. MODY is an example of a single-gene defect that causes only a minority of type 2 diabetes cases. T2DM represents a diverse and intricate cluster of conditions that cause elevated plasma glucose dose in the blood, stemming from impairments in both insulin secretion and action. The global increase in T2DM cases underscores the significance of environmental factors, including rapid lifestyle changes and escalating physical inactivity, as triggers for the condition. Nevertheless, compelling evidence from twin studies, family studies, and epidemiological investigations substantiates the etiology of the function of the genomic component in T2DM (Radha and Mohan, 2007). Evidence suggests that hereditary factors play a major role in the onset of type 2 diabetes.

- Disease recurrence differs significantly across ethnicities, and some ethnic variance is attributed to environmental factors rather than to inherited traits. Nonetheless, noteworthy variations in the frequency of illness between ethnically similar groups sharing common environments suggest that genetic predisposition is a contributing factor to the disease (Diamond, 2003).
- The monozygotic twins' high correlation rate (over 80%) and the significant drop in concordance among dizygotic twins by 50% provide compelling evidence for genetic involvement in the etiology of T2DM (Poulsen et al., 1999; Vaag et al., 1995).
- Evidence from various studies supports a genetic foundation for metrics related to both insulin sensitivity and insulin secretion (Elbein et al., 1999; Gerich, 1998).

2.2.2 ENVIRONMENTAL INFLUENCES

2.2.2.1 ENVIRONMENTAL FACTORS AND T1DM

Environmental factors are related to the etiology and prognosis of T1DM and T2DM. There are significant regional and racial disparities in T1DM frequency and severity (Karovonen et al., 1993). The highest documented occurrences of T1DM are observed in Nordic nations, with Finland exhibiting the highest incidence rate (35/100,000/year) among the population of children aged 0–14 years. Conversely, the least frequent are reported in Asia (0.5–1.3/100,000/year). Additionally, reduced incidences have been noted in regions of Africa and Latin America (Rewers et al., 1988). Changes in the environment and genetics may be responsible for notable variations in T1DM incidence ("Childhood Diabetes, Epidemics, and Epidemiology," 1992; LaPorte et al., 1985).

Several studies have shown that there is significant variance in the incidence and medical characteristics of diabetes (Meigs, 2010). This heterogeneity between ethnic groups may be influenced by both context-modifying variables and genetic predispositions. Moreover, this could imply that different ethnic groups have different genetic makeup. Overeating and the incidence of diabetes appear to be positively correlated. Following their immigration to Israel, several populations, such as the Yemenite and Kurdish Jews, have experienced a notable improvement in the overall prevalence of diabetes, along with major modifications to their dietary habits (Cohen and Marom, 1993).

Thus, environmental factors contribute to the ethnic variance observed in the onset of DM. Nonetheless, such distinctions regarding the clinical manifestations of diabetes across various ethnic groups suggest a genetic component (Meigs, 2010). Between 1988 and 1995, France had a yearly prevalence of children with T1DM which was comparable with the rates in Nordic nations. The annual prevalence of adolescent T1DM is comparable, although the total adolescent incidence in France is still lower. This means that environmental variables have a significant impact on the pathophysiology of type 1 diabetes (Charkaluk et al., 2002).

2.2.2.2 ENVIRONMENTAL FACTORS AND T2DM

The incidence of T2DM is markedly elevated (8.9%) among South African Indians, in contrast to South African blacks (4.2%). Variations in the occurrence throughout Asia of T2DM across people of different ethnic origins have also been reported. The aggregate occurrence of T2DM within Aborigines and Malays living in identical circumstances locality is found to be 4.4% and 11.3%, respectively. This observation further substantiates the notion that ethnicity, alongside other factors, may play a vital role in the heightened prevalence of DM (Ali et al., 1993).

Pregnancy has been demonstrated to correlate with diminished glucose tolerance attributed to insulin resistance, particularly during later stages of gestation. In some women, cellular dysfunction exacerbates glucose resistance, which results in the development of diabetes mellitus (Geronooz et al., 1999). Several studies have reported pronounced variance in the ethnic distribution of GDM (Hughes et al., 1995). The prevalence of T2DM is very high (>50%) among the Pima Indians of Arizona (Pettitt et al., 1980) and the urbanized Pacific Islanders of Nauru (King and Rewers, 1993) and Fiji (Hoskins et al., 1987), therefore suggesting that the pathophysiology of diabetes may be influenced by hereditary (ethnic) factors (Adeghate et al., 2006).

2.2.2.3 LOCATION

The geographic location has also been associated with the pathogenesis of DM. In a study examining the prevalence of childhood-onset T1DM between Caribbean communities of Black African descent, notable differences were observed in the prevalence of T1DM. The prevalence of T1DM was recorded as the highest (2.57/100,000) in Barbados and the lowest (0.09/100,000) in St. Croix (Tull et al., 1997). Al-Nuaim's research in Saudi Arabia (Al-Nuaim, 1997) revealed that the frequency, corrected for age, of diabetes mellitus (DM) was notably higher in urban areas, with rates of 12% in males and 14% in females, compared to rural areas, where the prevalence was 7% in males and 7.7% for females. El Mugamer and colleagues in the United Arab Emirates obtained comparable outcomes (El Mugamer et al., 1995). In Asia, it has additionally been shown that the incidence of type T2DM varies amongst urban and rural populations. The frequency of T2DM differed significantly between the two distinct groups in a study on the incidence of DM in adults residing in suburban and rural regions. Within a traditional hamlet, the incidence of type 2 diabetes is 2.8%, whereas in an urban area, it is 8.2% (Ali et al., 1993). Given that Japanese Americans and native Japanese have identical DNA, external factors, such as geographic location, could contribute to the genesis of type 2 diabetes. There may be two causes for the disparity in diabetes prevalence between urban and rural areas. In particular, compared to those in the countryside, people in metropolitan areas could be wealthier or consume more processed foods. Second, relative to their metropolitan parallels, people in rural areas were more inclined to engage in aerobic exercise, which lowered the risk of developing type 2 diabetes.

2.2.3 CULTURAL ASPECTS

2.2.3.1 OBESITY

Obesity serves as a robust indicator of the onset of T2DM, a condition that has recently exhibited an increase in prevalence across numerous nations. Diabetes develops due to a complex interplay between inherited and extrinsic variables, which include regular energy intake compared to expenditure, nutrient balance of eating habits, and physiological characteristics, and is correlated with a heightened frequency of T2DM cases, with research indicating that weight accumulation during adolescence contributes to obesity in adulthood. The increase in overweight and obesity during adulthood is linked to increased susceptibility to T2DM.

Low educational attainment has been identified as a significant predictor of overweight and obesity in Iranian women. Given the connection between obesity and diabetes prevalence, various studies have established specific age and sex criteria. Individuals with a higher body mass index (BMI) develop T2DM earlier in life, while those with a lower BMI tend to experience an increased incidence as they age. According to some studies, waist circumference (WC) and the waist-to-hip ratio could serve as more accurate measures of the frequency of diabetes and cardiovascular risk factors than BMI in certain age categories, and visceral fat, particularly abdominal obesity, is considered a strong indicator of these risks.

One study found that intra-abdominal fat, as determined by computed axial tomography (CAT), is a reliable anthropometric predictor of diabetes onset in Japanese American men. As central adiposity significantly contributes to the development of diabetes, it is important to recognize the normal BMI range of 18.5–24.9 kg/m^2 for various populations. Several studies have linked a BMI of 21 kg/m^2 with an increased risk of diabetes. However, a higher BMI threshold may be more suitable for Pacific Islander populations because of their greater muscle mass compared with European populations. As recommended by the WHO, adhere to the BMI range of 18.5–24.9 kg/m^2 and an average mean of 21 kg/m^2 due to conflicting data about the diameter of the waist and waist-to-hip ratio (Rahati et al., 2014).

2.2.3.2 PHYSICAL INACTIVITY

It is defined as a succession of organized and repetitive movements of the skeletal muscles and is intricately linked to energy expenditure (Polikandrioti and Dokoutsidou, 2009). Multiple studies have established a correlation between physical inactivity and the development of T2DM (Polikandrioti and Dokoutsidou, 2009; Steyn et al., 2004). Exercise plays a pivotal role in controlling blood sugar levels (BSLs) and protein and fat metabolism, enhancing insulin sensitivity, averting diabetes complications, improving muscle function, and fostering cardiovascular health, thereby extending life expectancy. Furthermore, physical activity confers mental health benefits by boosting energy levels, enhancing self-esteem, and reducing depressive symptoms (Sato et al., 2003). The key components of a successful exercise are length, magnitude, and frequency. The workouts should start with a 30-minute time limit, with a warm-up period ranging from 5 to 10 minutes and ending with recuperation exercises every time. The minimum suggested regularity was three times per week. Low-intensity, long-duration exercise regimes are generally considered the safest and ideal for patients with diabetes (Polikandrioti and Dokoutsidou, 2009).

2.2.3.3 EXCESSIVE AND EXTENDED STRESS

Stress that is both intense and prolonged—a feature of modern life—may be additionally connected to glucose intolerance, which increases the chance of developing diabetes. Diabetes that develops after extended periods of intense stress may be caused by adrenal hormone activation, particularly glucocorticoids, which are associated with glucose resistance (Huang et al., 1997).

2.2.3.4 ABNORMAL INSULIN SECRETION AND ACTION

The majority of individuals diagnosed with T2DM exhibit diminished insulin secretion relative to plasma glucose concentrations. This phenomenon occurs alongside a progressive loss of pancreatic cells, albeit not to the degree observed in T1DM. Islet amyloid constitutes a defining characteristic of pancreatic pathology in patients with T2DM. Amyloid originating from islet amyloid polypeptide (IAPP) may contribute to the etiology (Ferrannini, 1998).

2.2.3.5 BODY MASS AND LOCATION OF FAT

One significant risk factor associated with the emergence of type 2 diabetes is adiposity (Dowse et al., 1990; Haffner et al., 1986; Ohlson et al., 1988). BMI is directly associated with an elevated risk of T2DM across ethnic cohorts (Trevisan et al., 1998). The prominence of intra-abdominal adiposity, as opposed to subcutaneous fat, is critical for the pathogenesis of DM (Bray, 1987; Kissebah et al., 1982; Kissebah and Peiris, 1989). Numerous studies have documented a robust correlation between obesity and T2DM. A survey of 3229 individuals with diabetes mellitus revealed that 57.7% of diabetic women were considered fat and 30.2% to be obese (Abdella et al., 1995).

2.2.3.6 DIETARY COMPONENTS AND OBESITY

Obesity is prevalent in approximately 80% of individuals afflicted with T2DM. A strong associative link exists between obesity and the incidence of T2DM (Bray, 1987; James, 1998; Kissebah et al., 1982). The proliferation of energy-dense foods, characterized by high levels of saturated fats, refined and simple sugars, and a deficiency of complex carbohydrates (such as fibers), might encourage the development of obesity and T2DM. Diets that are heavy in fat, moderate in carbohydrates, and lacking in fiber are associated with a higher incidence of diabetes, according to a new study examining the incidence of diabetes in the Mexican population (Lerman et al., 1998).

2.3 PATHOPHYSIOLOGICAL MECHANISMS

Diabetes is mostly caused by insulin resistance, and several studies have examined the environmental and genetic variables that lead to type 2 diabetes (Kosasih and Bonavida, 2021).

2.3.1 *INSULIN RESISTANCE (IR)*

The ability of the human body to use insulin is influenced by accessibility. For those with T1DM, insulin is absent, although peripheral tissues develop resistance to its actions in T2DM. The brain, which requires stable blood glucose levels (BGLs) for optimal function, relies on the secretion of insulin by pancreatic β-cells in response to increased blood glucose. Medications, such as oral antihyperglycemic agents and insulin, are used to counteract hyperglycemia (Moini, 2019; Zahoor et al., 2022). The central nervous system responds to plasma glucose levels by triggering the release of energy substrates. Reduced BGLs lead to an increase in autonomic activity. Hypoglycemia serves as an indication of lower BGLs and aids in the diagnosis of diabetes. Various reactions occur in response to hypoglycemia, including decreased insulin release, increased glucagon and epinephrine secretion, exacerbated sympathoadrenal symptoms, and in severe cases, cognitive impairment, seizures, stroke, fainting, or coma. Intravenous or oral glucose administration is a rapid intervention to rectify hypoglycemia and restore normal BGLs (Moini, 2019).

In type 1 diabetes mellitus (T1DM), disease progression is determined by the rate at which autoimmune destruction of pancreatic β cells occurs. Diabetic ketoacidosis (DKA) is a severe complication in individuals with diabetes. Rapid fat breakdown results in the conversion of fat to ketones, leading to blood acidification. Because β-cells are destroyed, DKA is increasingly common in young people and children and frequently presents as an initial sign of illness. The gradual increase in fasting plasma glucose (FPG) levels reflects slow progression of the condition. However, patients become more dependent on insulin as their insulin insufficiency progresses, which also causes severe hyperglycemia and ketoacidosis. Eventually, patients depend solely on insulin treatment because of the seriousness and development of T1DM (Banday et al., 2020). The pathogenesis of type 2 diabetes is defined by insulin resistance and insufficiency, which are linked to increased amounts of fatty acids and cytokines that cause inflammation in the circulatory system. This leads to higher glucose synthesis in the liver, enhanced fat failure, and decreased glucose delivery into target cells (Khardori, 2017).

Excessive glucagon secretion and deficient insulin release from α- and β-cells, respectively, contribute to hyperglycemia, and the failure of individuals to adjust for insulin resistance by boosting insulin production, which results in increased glucose levels, is the basis for the recognition of type 2 diabetes. The slow and often asymptomatic progression of T2DM may delay its early detection, sometimes presenting with mild hyperglycemia. Symptoms such as polydipsia, weight loss, vision disturbances, and growth abnormalities typically manifest in advanced stages of the disease. The etiology of this particular type of diabetes involves a combination of genetic and environmental factors. The disorder is frequently associated with a variety of lifestyle factors, including suboptimal dietary patterns, advancing age, sedentary behavior, familial predisposition to diabetes, high BMI, antecedent GDM in females, and pathophysiological conditions such as atherosclerosis, dyslipidemia, and hypertension. GDM is defined as the onset of diabetes or impaired glucose tolerance (IGT) in the second or third trimester of pregnancy. Early in pregnancy, fasting and random BGLs are typically below the normal reference range. However, a significant increase in the third trimester glucose level indicates the diagnosis of GDM (Banday et al., 2020).

2.3.2 PANCREATIC B-CELL DYSREGULATION

The primary cause of the two common types of diabetes mellitus (DM), T1DM and T2DM, is a reduction in functional β-cell density. Preventing or reversing this condition requires in-depth knowledge of the fundamental pathways that lead to β-cell malfunction. Fundamental pathogenic distinctions are present between the two DM types: T1DM is characterized by immune-mediated processes, whereas T2DM is primarily influenced by metabolic pathways. These distinct mechanisms exert differential effects on the initial β-cell impairment and ultimate consequences. Over the last 10 years, a great deal of development has been made in this area, mainly because of studies on β-cells in relation to human diseases. Such advancements encompass analyses of islet architecture and human β-cell gene expression pertaining to T1DM and T2DM, as well as the identification and characterization of the roles played by candidate genes associated with T1DM and T2DM at the β-cell level, along with the endoplasmic reticulum (ER) stress signaling pathways that lead to β-cell dysfunction in T1DM (predominantly driven by inositol-requiring enzyme 1 (IRE1)) and T2DM (mostly reliant on RNA-like endoplasmic reticulum kinase (PERK), a protein kinase/eIF2α mechanisms) (Eizirik et al., 2020).

β-cell dysfunction has been linked to the death of β-cells (Christensen and Gannon, 2019). According to a recent study, the essential molecular pathways or external variables of cellular biology could collaborate in greater detail in T2DM, resulting in β-cell malfunction (Halban et al., 2014). In conditions of nutritional excess, similar to what is seen in obesity, the occurrence of hyperglycemia and hyperlipidemia often leads to insulin resistance (IR) and chronic inflammation. In such cases, β-cells, particularly those with a genetic predisposition, are subjected to harmful stressors such as inflammation, ER stress, metabolic/oxidative stress, and amyloid stress, which may compromise island integrity (Christensen and Gannon, 2019).

Both hyperglycemia and a buildup of free fatty acids (FFAs) cause ER stress by activating pathways that lead to apoptosis and the unfolded protein response (UPR), which in turn causes β-cell malfunction (Yamamoto et al., 2019). Physiological and oxidative stress are induced by lipotoxicity, glucose toxicity, and glucolipotoxicity linked to obesity, which damages β-cells (Halban et al., 2014).

Stress from elevated levels of saturated fat and protein can activate the UPR through various mechanisms. These include direct disruption of ER homeostasis, stimulation of inositol trisphosphate (IP3) receptors, or inhibition of Sarco/endoplasmic Reticulum Ca^{2+} ATPase (SERCA), which is essential for ER Ca^{2+} mobilization. Additionally, sustained high glucose levels enhance the production of islet amyloid polypeptides (IAPP) and proinsulin in β-cells. Owing to oxidative stress in protein folding, this buildup of misfolded insulin and IAAP causes a rise in the production of reactive oxygen species (ROS) (Yamamoto et al., 2019).

Such occurrences interfere with the regular physiologic mobilization of ER Ca^{2+} and stimulate pro-apoptotic signals, pro-insulin mRNA degradation, and the production of interleukin (IL)-1β, which increases the swelling of local islets and attracts monocytes (Yamamoto et al., 2019). To meet the metabolic demands, insulin secretion must be precisely regulated. Therefore, maintaining the integrity of islets is essential for the reaction of β-cells to metabolic demands. The previously discussed mechanisms may eventually lead to the breakdown of islet integrity and structure in various diseases. This hinders the best possible interaction between cells within pancreatic islets, which will ultimately exacerbate hyperglycemia by contributing to irregular glucagon and insulin secretion. Inadequate production of glucose or its precursors, together with malfunctions in the secretion pathways, may cause insulin secretory dysfunction, which is the main cause of β-cell failure and a central feature of type 2 diabetes. GLUT-2 expression reduction, for instance, has been shown to have a negative impact on the subsequent signaling cascade (Hoang Do and Thorn, 2015), and mistakes in proinsulin synthesis are other frequently observed occurrences associated with insufficient insulin synthesis or the onset of diabetes (Liu et al., 2018).

2.3.3 GLUCAGON SECRETION ABERRATIONS

As glucagon and insulin have different effects on glucose metabolism, pancreatic islet β- and α-cells are thought to be functional antagonists. In previous studies, the intra-islet hypothesis, which holds that insulin inhibits glucagon release, has been the most widely accepted explanation for the processes behind glucagon production. In contrast, glucagon is used in tests of β-cell activity and is a strong promoter of insulin release. Glucagon functions as an enhancer of insulin secretion and is used to assess β-cell functionality. In recent years, α-cells have garnered increased scholarly interest owing to their capacity to promote insulin release from adjacent β-cells, with the interplay between α- and β-cells emerging as pivotal for the maintenance of glucose homeostasis *in vivo*. In the context of carbohydrate breakdown, glucagon not only functions as the opposite of diabetes in terms of its regulation, yet its release is also more sensitive to changes in the bloodstream level of certain amino acids than it is for changes in BGLs. Glucagon plays an important role in both the breakdown of amino acids and burning of hepatocellular lipids (Hædersdal et al., 2023; Unger, 1978).

2.3.4 OXIDATIVE STRESS

The production of ROS in pancreatic β-cells is significantly influenced by hyperglycemia, hyperlipidemia, and inflammation. Basal levels of ROS play a crucial role in insulin secretion. Llanos et al. (2015) illustrated that the activation of RyR channels, which are necessary for insulin secretion, is dependent on ROS generation and a moderate influx of Ca^{2+} following glucose stimulation. This increase in intracellular Ca^{2+} levels is facilitated by the activation of RyR channels (Llanos et al., 2015).

Exposing islet cells to H_2O_2 for basic glucose results in enhanced insulin secretion, highlighting the crucial role of ROS in this process. However, in pathological states, excessive ROS accumulation leads to oxidative stress, primarily arising from the mitochondrial electron transport chain (ETC). When glucose and lipid levels are high, the concentrations of nicotinamide adenine dinucleotide (NAD) and flavin adenine dinucleotide (FAD) increase, which results in the overproduction of ROS due to ETC overload and electron leakage from complexes I and III (El-Azzouny et al., 2014; Newsholme et al., 2019).

Electrons react with oxygen molecules to produce O_2, which is quickly converted into H_2O_2. If not neutralized, H_2O_2 can react with transition metals, such as Cu^{2+} and Fe^{2+}, to generate highly reactive hydroxyl radicals and OH^- through the Fenton reaction. Despite the presence of antioxidant defenses, such as catalase (CAT), glutathione peroxidase (GPx), thioredoxin (TXN), and peroxiredoxins in β-cells, reduced levels of CAT and GPx1 make these cells more susceptible to ROS-induced damage. ROS production in β-cells under hyperglycemic conditions involves several mitochondrial pathways, including protein kinase C (PKC) activation, advanced glycation end-product (AGE) formation, hexosamine and polyol pathway activation, and oxidative phosphorylation. Additionally, hyperlipidemia worsens ROS production by activating NOX, inducing matrix metalloproteinase 2 (MMP2), and increasing macrophage infiltration. Both hyperglycemia and hyperlipidemia exacerbate oxidative stress by impairing antioxidant defenses, as shown by the decreased reduced-to-oxidized glutathione ratio in hyperglycemia and lower levels of superoxide dismutase 1 (SOD1) and SOD2 in hyperlipidemia in β cells. However, according to a study by Dai et al., hyperglycemia does not affect superoxide or antioxidant enzyme levels in human islets, whereas hyperlipidemia increases superoxide levels and decreases antioxidant enzyme levels, suggesting that hyperlipidemia is a primary driver of ROS production (Eguchi et al., 2021).

2.3.5 ADIPOSE TISSUE DYSFUNCTION

In the past few decades, the conventional understanding of fatty tissue as the only location for preserving fat has changed to acknowledge its critical function in the cellular breakdown of fat and carbohydrates. Adipose tissue produces many hormones and cytokines, including IL-6, adiponectin, leptin, PAI-1, tumor necrosis factor-α (TNF-α), and IL-6. Insulin resistance is mostly influenced by two substances released in high amounts by larger adipocytes: free fatty acids (FFAs) and TNF-α (IR) (Hotamisligil et al., 1995).

The detrimental effect of FFAs on insulin sensitivity results in elevated lipolysis within adipocytes, as insulin plays a crucial role in regulating hormone-sensitive lipase (HSL), which governs triglyceride breakdown. TNF-α further intensifies this effect by promoting triglyceride hydrolysis in fatty tissues. TNF-α also contributes to insulin resistance (IR) by down-regulating key genes involved in insulin signaling and adipocyte differentiation, such as CCAAT-enhancer-binding protein-α, PPAR-γ, glucose transporter type 4, insulin receptor substrate-1 (IRS-1), adiponectin, and long-chain fatty acid acyl-coenzyme A synthase. This adds another layer to the molecular mechanisms underlying IR development. By decreasing the synthesis of glucose within the liver and increasing the oxidation of fatty acids within the liver and muscle tissues, adiponectin increases insulin sensitivity, an effect mediated by the increased activity of 5' adenosine monophosphate (AMP)-activated protein kinase (Goldstein and Scalia, 2004).

Single-nucleotide polymorphisms (SNPs) in the promoter region of the leptin gene may be involved in the development of IR, obesity, and type 2 diabetes mellitus (T2DM). SNPs in the adiponectin promoter were connected to a two-fold increase in the occurrence of type 2 diabetes in an investigation of people who were very obese individuals. Adipose tissue malfunction increases the incidence of nonalcoholic fatty liver disease (NAFLD) in people who are obese, insulin-resistant, and diabetic. More lipids build up in the liver as a result of the portal circulation's enhanced influx of fatty acids and IL-6. In animal models of chronic liver injury, leptin has been implicated as a possible contributor to liver cirrhosis; however, in leptin-resistant individuals, its significance may diminish (Amrita et al., 2021; Hajer et al., 2008; Melistas et al., 2009; Vasseur et al., 2005).

2.4 EMERGING INSIGHTS

2.4.1 GUT MICROBIOTA-HOST INTERACTION

The complex interactions between the essential elements of the stomach, including the gut microbiota, affect numerous gut activities. These microbes are essential for controlling the porosity of gastrointestinal mucosa. It oversees the digestion and absorption of nutritional polysaccharides to yield short-chain fatty acids (SCFAs), helping to elucidate the importance of modulating the build-up of fat and the consequent emergence of obesity-associated disorders. This highlights their pivotal role as the primary cause of corpulence and its aftermath. Additionally, gut microbes are essential for human transcription, immune system modulation, the regulation of inflammatory processes, and energy extraction from food. Alteration of the human colonic microbiota via nutrition may benefit the host in several ways. Simple treatment interventions that aim to slow down the progression of low-level chronic inflammation and IR must be used (Blandino et al., 2016).

There can be significant variations in the gut microbiota composition of patients with diabetes. Significant correlations between certain gut microbial populations, bacterial genetic components, and chemical reactions have been found in an extensive human metagenome-wide association analysis among T2DM patients (Larsen et al., 2010). These individuals exhibited elevated concentrations of *Lactobacillus* spp. compared to those who did not have diabetes (Lê et al., 2013).

While *Clostridium* spp. exhibited a negative association with fasting glucose, HbA1c, insulin, C-peptide, and plasma triglyceride levels, *Lactobacillus* spp. showed a favorable correlation with both parameters. In contrast, there was a positive correlation between *Clostridium* species and both adiponectin and high-density lipoprotein (HDL) cholesterol. Gene-predisposed obese and diet-induced leptin-resistant mouse models were shown to have 26 different metagenomic clusters (MGCs) compared to animals with normal glucose tolerance (NGT) and diabetes. Studies conducted on diverse populations have also demonstrated that the gut microbiota of people with diabetes generally contain reduced quantities of bacteria that produce butyrate, such as *Faecalibacterium prausnitzii* and *Roseburia intestinalis*, in conjunction with a higher percentage of *Lactobacillus gasseri*, *Streptococcus mutans*, and bacteria belonging to the order *Clostridiales* (Lau et al., 2011).

Similarly, the ratios of Bacteroidetes to Firmicutes and *Bacteroides/Prevotella* groups to *C. coccoides/Eubacterium rectale* groups were positively correlated with plasma glucose concentrations. Furthermore, it was shown that the Betaproteobacteria class showed a positive connection with plasma glucose levels and was significantly enriched in diabetic participants compared to non-diabetic subjects. Additionally, the gut microbiota has been reported to have an inflammatory impact that triggers autoimmune diabetes (Wen et al., 2008).

An essential element for the pathophysiology of autoimmune T1DM is a pathogenic cascade that compromises the gut immune system. The similarity in lymphocyte-homing receptors between the stomach and inflammation-ridden pancreatic tissues explains the association between gut microbiota and autoimmune diabetes (Cani et al., 2007).

2.4.2 EPIGENETIC MODIFICATIONS

Although external variables, such as psychological and ecological effects, are just as significant in relation to wellness and disease, genes play a substantial role in the genesis of illnesses and medical conditions, indicating that the DNA sequence alone does not solely dictate the clinical phenotype (Fraga and Esteller, 2005; Moosavi and Motevalizadeh, 2016). Genetic alterations influence the synthesis of specific proteins, whereas epigenetic modifications can activate or deactivate genes; these epigenetic alterations do not alter the fundamentals. DNA sequences are thought to be important modulators of gene activity in a variety of clinical conditions. The field of epigenetics explores how behavioral and environmental factors can induce alterations that modulate gene functionality, with the notable advantage that these modifications may either be retained within the genome and transmitted to subsequent generations or, conversely, be reversible (Tammen et al., 2013). The predominant epigenetic alterations include DNA methylation, histone modifications, and non-coding RNAs, whereas modifications to DNA and histones can either condense or relax the chromatin structure to regulate the accessibility of transcription factors, and non-coding RNAs exert control over gene expression at the RNA level (Handy et al., 2011; Kowluru and Mohammad, 2022).

2.5 IMPLICATIONS FOR THERAPY AND PREVENTION

The three main tenets of diabetes care are improving general health, preventing related issues, and controlling BSLs. Changes in daily life can include eating a healthy diet and performing regular exercise, which are integral to the effective management of DM. Pharmacological treatments include a diverse array of medications such as insulin, oral hypoglycemic agents, glucagon-like peptide-1 (GLP-1) receptor agonists, and sodium-dependent glucose cotransporter-2 (SGLT-2) inhibitors. The formulation of individualized treatment strategies, which consider the duration of the disease, its severity, and the preferences of the patient, is vital for attaining optimal glycemic regulation.

Novel treatment methods are being investigated at a faster pace owing to the developments in diabetes research. The individualized healthcare paradigm provides an opportunity to tailor therapies to individual patients by focusing on certain hereditary and molecular characteristics. Additionally, studies have investigated the potential of therapies targeted at modifying immune responses, inflammatory conditions, and the gut microbiome to improve glucose management and minimize complications (Blaslov et al., 2019; Sprague et al., 2006; Venerando et al., 2002; Zhou et al., 2018).

The complexity of diabetes is highlighted by the division of the illness into several subtypes, discovery of atypical symptoms, and diagnosis of GDM. This difference is essential for modifying therapeutic methods and tactics (Nadhiya et al., 2024).

2.6 CONCLUSION

Diabetes mellitus is a multifaceted metabolic illness that results from a complex interplay of factors related to genes, environment, and lifestyle. This chapter discusses the pathophysiological processes and etiological concepts that underlie diabetes, offering a thorough summary of the variables that influence the development and course of the disease.

Genetic predisposition is a major factor in the development of type 1 and 2 diabetes. Certain genetic indicators, such as differences in the HLA region and correlations with certain autoimmune responses, have been shown to be important contributors to T1DM. In contrast, insulin resistance and decreased insulin production in T2DM are the result of interactions between many genes on separate chromosomes. The genetic variety among diabetes diseases is further highlighted by monogenic types, such as maturity-onset diabetes of the young (MODY).

The genetic predisposition to diabetes is strongly influenced by environmental and lifestyle variables. Owing to its link to insulin resistance, obesity, especially central adiposity, has been identified as a significant risk factor for type 2 diabetes. Physical inactivity and dietary habits of simple carbohydrates and saturated fats increase this risk by causing metabolic disruption. Chronic stress and exposure to certain pharmaceutical compounds have also been linked to disruption of glucose homeostasis. This is related to the onset of diabetes.

Insulin resistance is a key pathophysiological mechanism in T2DM in which peripheral tissues are unable to react to insulin as required, resulting in persistent hyperglycemia. β-cell dysfunction, a condition in which the pancreatic β-cells are unable to adjust to increasing insulin demand, leading to decreased insulin production, exacerbates this disease. Oxidative stress and inflammatory pathways are also important because they cause cellular damage and exacerbate insulin resistance. The gradual nature of β-cell degeneration in diabetes is highlighted by the formation of IAPP in the pancreatic tissues.

It is necessary to understand these pathophysiological and etiological elements to develop therapeutic and preventative measures. The occurrence of type 2 diabetes may be considerably decreased by addressing modifiable risk factors, including obesity, via lifestyle treatments, such as dietary changes and increased physical activity. Timely interventions and customized treatment techniques are made possible by the early identification of genetic markers and at-risk individuals. Furthermore, investigating the molecular pathways underlying insulin resistance and β-cell malfunction provides opportunities for the creation of innovative pharmaceuticals targeted at re-establishing appropriate glucose metabolism.

KEYWORDS

- **diabetes mellitus**
- **genetic predisposition**
- **insulin resistance**
- **metabolism**
- **oxidative stress**
- **pancreatic tissues**
- **pharmaceuticals**
- **β-cell dysfunction**

REFERENCES

Abdella, N. A., Khogali, M. M., Salman, A. D., Ghuneimi, S. A., & Bajaj, J. S. (1995). Pattern of non-insulin dependent diabetes mellitus in Kuwait. *Diabetes Research and Clinical Practice, 29*(2), 129–136. https://doi.org/10.1016/0168-8227(95)01128-5 (accessed on 2nd February 2026).

Adeghate, E., Schattner, P., & Dunn, E. (2006). An update on the etiology and epidemiology of diabetes mellitus. *Annals of the New York Academy of Sciences, 1084*(1), 1–29. https://doi.org/10.1196/annals.1372.029 (accessed on 2nd February 2026).

Ali, O., Tan, T. T., Sakinah, O., Khalid, B. A. K., Wu, L. L., & Ng, M. L. (1993). Prevalence of NIDDM and impaired glucose tolerance in Aborigines and Malays in Malaysia and their relationship to sociodemographic, health, and nutritional factors. *Diabetes Care, 16*(1), 68–75. https://doi.org/10.2337/diacare.16.1.68 (accessed on 2nd February 2026).

Al-Nuaim, A. R. (1997). Prevalence of glucose intolerance in urban and rural communities in Saudi Arabia. *Diabetic Medicine: A Journal of the British Diabetic Association, 14*(7), 595–602. https://doi.org/10.1002/(SICI)1096-9136(199707)14:7<595::AID-DIA377>3.0.CO;2-C (accessed on 2nd February 2026).

Amrita, J., Mahajan, M., Bhanwer, A. J. S., & Matharoo, K. (2021). Association of *AdipoQ* gene variation (rs1501299) and oxidative stress with cardiovascular disease in North West Indian population of Punjabi women. *Journal of Medical Biochemistry, 40*(1), 49–59. https://doi.org/10.5937/jomb0-24704 (accessed on 2nd February 2026).

Banday, M. Z., Sameer, A. S., & Nissar, S. (2020). Pathophysiology of diabetes: An overview. *Avicenna Journal of Medicine, 10*(04), 174–188. https://doi.org/10.4103/ajm.ajm_53_20 (accessed on 2nd February 2026).

Blandino, G., Inturri, R., Lazzara, F., Di Rosa, M., & Malaguarnera, L. (2016). Impact of gut microbiota on diabetes mellitus. *Diabetes & Metabolism, 42*(5), 303–315. https://doi.org/10.1016/j.diabet.2016.04.004 (accessed on 2nd February 2026).

Blaslov, K., Kruljac, I., Mirošević, G., Gaćina, P., Kolonić, S. O., & Vrkljan, M. (2019). The prognostic value of red blood cell characteristics on diabetic retinopathy development and progression in type 2 diabetes mellitus. *Clinical Hemorheology and Microcirculation, 71*(4), 475–481. https://doi.org/10.3233/CH-180422 (accessed on 2nd February 2026).

Bray, G. A. (1987). Overweight is risking fate: Definition, classification, prevalence, and risks. *Annals of the New York Academy of Sciences, 499*, 14–28. https://doi.org/10.1111/j.1749-6632.1987.tb36194.x (accessed on 2nd February 2026).

Cani, P. D., Amar, J., Iglesias, M. A., Poggi, M., Knauf, C., Bastelica, D., et al. (2007). Metabolic endotoxemia initiates obesity and insulin resistance. *Diabetes, 56*(7), 1761–1772. https://doi.org/10.2337/db06-1491 (accessed on 2nd February 2026).

Charkaluk, M. L., Czernichow, P., & Lévy-Marchal, C. (2002). Incidence data of childhood-onset type I diabetes in France during 1988–1997: The case for a shift toward younger age at onset. *Pediatric Research, 52*(6), 859–862. https://doi.org/10.1203/00006450-200212000-00008 (accessed on 2nd February 2026).

Cohen, A. M., & Marom, L. (1993). Diabetes and accompanying obesity, hypertension and ECG abnormalities in Yemenite Jews 40 years after immigration to Israel. *Diabetes Research (Edinburgh, Scotland), 23*(2), 65–74.

de Souza Rugolo, L. M. S., Bentlin, M. R., & Trindade, C. E. P. (2011). Preeclampsia: Effect on the fetus and newborn. *Neo Reviews, 12*(4), e198–e206.

Degnbol, B., & Green, A. (1978). Diabetes mellitus among first- and second-degree relatives of early onset diabetics. *Annals of Human Genetics, 42*(1), 25–47. https://doi.org/10.1111/j.1469-1809.1978.tb00929.x (accessed on 2nd February 2026).

Diamond, J. (2003). The double puzzle of diabetes. *Nature, 423*(6940), 599–602. https://doi.org/10.1038/423599a (accessed on 2nd February 2026).

Dowse, G. K., Gareeboo, H., Zimmet, P. Z., Alberti, K. G., Tuomilehto, J., Fareed, D., et al. (1990). High prevalence of NIDDM and impaired glucose tolerance in Indian, Creole, and Chinese Mauritians. Mauritius Noncommunicable Disease Study Group. *Diabetes, 39*(3), 390–396. https://doi.org/10.2337/diab.39.3.390 (accessed on 2nd February 2026).

Eguchi, N., Vaziri, N. D., Dafoe, D. C., & Ichii, H. (2021). The role of oxidative stress in pancreatic β cell dysfunction in diabetes. *International Journal of Molecular Sciences, 22*(4), Article 4. https://doi.org/10.3390/ijms22041509 (accessed on 2nd February 2026).

Eizirik, D. L., Pasquali, L., & Cnop, M. (2020). Pancreatic β-cells in type 1 and type 2 diabetes mellitus: Different pathways to failure. *Nature Reviews Endocrinology, 16*(7), 349–362. https://doi.org/10.1038/s41574-020-0355-7 (accessed on 2nd February 2026).

el Mugamer, I. T., Ali Zayat, A. S., Hossain, M. M., & Pugh, R. N. (1995). Diabetes, obesity and hypertension in urban and rural people of Bedouin origin in the United Arab Emirates. *The Journal of Tropical Medicine and Hygiene, 98*(6), 407–415.

El-Azzouny, M., Evans, C. R., Treutelaar, M. K., Kennedy, R. T., & Burant, C. F. (2014). Increased glucose metabolism and glycolipid formation by fatty acids and GPR40 receptor signaling underlies the fatty acid potentiation of insulin secretion. *The Journal of Biological Chemistry, 289*(19), 13575–13588. https://doi.org/10.1074/jbc.M113.531970 (accessed on 2nd February 2026).

Elbein, S. C., Hasstedt, S. J., Wegner, K., & Kahn, S. E. (1999). Heritability of pancreatic β-cell function among nondiabetic members of Caucasian familial type 2 diabetic kindreds. *The Journal of Clinical Endocrinology & Metabolism, 84*(4), 1398–1403. https://doi.org/10.1210/jcem.84.4.5604 (accessed on 2nd February 2026).

European Consortium for IDDM Genome Studies. (2001). A genome wide scan for type 1–diabetes susceptibility in Scandinavian families: Identification of new loci with evidence of interactions. *The American Journal of Human Genetics, 69*(6), 1301–1313.

Fajans, S. S., Bell, G. I., & Polonsky, K. S. (2001). Molecular mechanisms and clinical pathophysiology of maturity-onset diabetes of the young. *New England Journal of Medicine, 345*(13), 971–980. https://doi.org/10.1056/NEJMra002168 (accessed on 2nd February 2026).

Ferrannini, E. (1998). Insulin resistance versus insulin deficiency in non-insulin-dependent diabetes mellitus: Problems and prospects. *Endocrine Reviews, 19*(4), 477–490. https://doi.org/10.1210/edrv.19.4.0336 (accessed on 2nd February 2026).

Fraga, M. F., & Esteller, M. (2005). Towards the human cancer epigenome: A first draft of histone modifications. *Cell Cycle (Georgetown, Tex.), 4*(10), 1377–1381. https://doi.org/10.4161/cc.4.10.2113 (accessed on 2nd February 2026).

Galicia-Garcia, U., Benito-Vicente, A., Jebari, S., Larrea-Sebal, A., Siddiqi, H., Uribe, K. B., et al. (2020). Pathophysiology of type 2 diabetes mellitus. *International Journal of Molecular Sciences, 21*(17), 6275. https://doi.org/10.3390/ijms21176275 (accessed on 2nd February 2026).

Gerich, J. E. (1998). The genetic basis of type 2 diabetes mellitus: Impaired insulin secretion versus impaired insulin sensitivity. *Endocrine Reviews, 19*(4), 491–503. https://doi.org/10.1210/edrv.19.4.0338 (accessed on 2nd February 2026).

Geronooz, I., Scheen, A. J., & Foidart, J. M. (1999). [Gestational diabetes: Definition, screening and management]. *Revue Medicale de Liege, 54*(5), 429–433.

Goldstein, B. J., & Scalia, R. (2004). Adiponectin: A novel adipokine linking adipocytes and vascular function. *The Journal of Clinical Endocrinology and Metabolism, 89*(6), 2563–2568. https://doi.org/10.1210/jc.2004-0518 (accessed on 2nd February 2026).

Gorodezky, C., Alaez, C., Murguía, A., Rodríguez, A., Balladares, S., Vazquez, M., et al. (2006). HLA and autoimmune diseases: Type 1 diabetes (T1D) as an example. *Autoimmunity Reviews, 5*(3), 187–194. https://doi.org/10.1016/j.autrev.2005.06.002 (accessed on 2nd February 2026).

Hædersdal, S., Andersen, A., Knop, F. K., & Vilsbøll, T. (2023). Revisiting the role of glucagon in health, diabetes mellitus and other metabolic diseases. *Nature Reviews. Endocrinology, 19*(6), 321–335. https://doi.org/10.1038/s41574-023-00817-4 (accessed on 2nd February 2026).

Haffner, S. M., Stern, M. P., Hazuda, H. P., Rosenthal, M., Knapp, J. A., & Malina, R. M. (1986). Role of obesity and fat distribution in non-insulin-dependent diabetes mellitus in Mexican Americans and non-Hispanic whites. *Diabetes Care, 9*(2), 153–161. https://doi.org/10.2337/diacare.9.2.153 (accessed on 2nd February 2026).

Hajer, G. R., Van Haeften, T. W., & Visseren, F. L. J. (2008). Adipose tissue dysfunction in obesity, diabetes, and vascular diseases. *European Heart Journal, 29*(24), 2959–2971. https://doi.org/10.1093/eurheartj/ehn387 (accessed on 2nd February 2026).

Halban, P. A., Polonsky, K. S., Bowden, D. W., Hawkins, M. A., Ling, C., Mather, K. J., et al. (2014). β-cell failure in type 2 diabetes: Postulated mechanisms and prospects for prevention and treatment. *Diabetes Care, 37*(6), 1751–1758. https://doi.org/10.2337/dc14-0396 (accessed on 2nd February 2026).

Handy, D. E., Castro, R., & Loscalzo, J. (2011). Epigenetic modifications: Basic mechanisms and role in cardiovascular disease. *Circulation, 123*(19), 2145–2156. https://doi.org/10.1161/CIRCULATIONAHA.110.956839 (accessed on 2nd February 2026).

Harris, M. I., Flegal, K. M., Cowie, C. C., Eberhardt, M. S., Goldstein, D. E., Little, R. R., et al. (1998). Prevalence of diabetes, impaired fasting glucose, and impaired glucose tolerance in US adults: The Third National Health and Nutrition Examination Survey, 1988–1994. *Diabetes Care, 21*(4), 518–524.

Hoang Do, O., & Thorn, P. (2015). Insulin secretion from beta cells within intact islets: Location matters. *Clinical and Experimental Pharmacology and Physiology, 42*(4), 406–414. https://doi.org/10.1111/1440-1681.12368 (accessed on 2nd February 2026).

Hoskins, P. L., Handelsman, D. J., Hannelly, T., Silink, M., Yue, D. K., & Turtle, J. R. (1987). Diabetes in the Melanesian and Indian peoples of Fiji: A study of risk factors. *Diabetes Research and Clinical Practice, 3*(5), 269–276. https://doi.org/10.1016/S0168-8227(87)80050-5 (accessed on 2nd February 2026).

Hotamisligil, G. S., Arner, P., Caro, J. F., Atkinson, R. L., & Spiegelman, B. M. (1995). Increased adipose tissue expression of tumor necrosis factor-α in human obesity and insulin resistance. *The Journal of Clinical Investigation, 95*(5), 2409–2415. https://doi.org/10.1172/JCI117936 (accessed on 2nd February 2026).

Huang, Z., Cabanela, V., & Howell, T. (1997). Stress, bottle-feeding, and diabetes. *The Lancet, 350*(9081), 889. https://doi.org/10.1016/S0140-6736(05)62075-2 (accessed on 2nd February 2026).

Hughes, P. F., Agarwal, M., Newman, P., & Morrison, J. (1995). Screening for gestational diabetes in a multi-ethnic population. *Diabetes Research and Clinical Practice, 28*(1), 73–78. https://doi.org/10.1016/0168-8227(95)01051-E (accessed on 2nd February 2026).

James, W. P. (1998). What are the health risks? The medical consequences of obesity and its health risks. *Experimental and Clinical Endocrinology & Diabetes: Official Journal, German Society of Endocrinology [and] German Diabetes Association, 106*(Suppl 2), 1–6. https://doi.org/10.1055/s-0029-1212028 (accessed on 2nd February 2026).

Jun, H. S., & Yoon, J. W. (2004). A new look at viruses in type 1 diabetes. *ILAR Journal, 45*(3), 349–374.

Kaul, K., Tarr, J. M., Kohner, E. M., & Chibber, R. (2012). Introduction to diabetes mellitus. *Advances in Experimental Medicine and Biology, 771*, 1–11.

Khardori, R. (2017). Type 2 diabetes mellitus: Practice essentials, background, pathophysiology. *Medscape*.

King, H., & Rewers, M. (1993). Global estimates for prevalence of diabetes mellitus and impaired glucose tolerance in adults. WHO Ad Hoc Diabetes Reporting Group. *Diabetes Care, 16*(1), 157–177. https://doi.org/10.2337/diacare.16.1.157 (accessed on 2nd February 2026).

King, H., Aubert, R. E., & Herman, W. H. (1998). Global burden of diabetes, 1995–2025: Prevalence, numerical estimates, and projections. *Diabetes Care, 21*(9), 1414–1431. https://doi.org/10.2337/diacare.21.9.1414 (accessed on 2nd February 2026).

Kissebah, A. H., & Peiris, A. N. (1989). Biology of regional body fat distribution: Relationship to non-insulin-dependent diabetes mellitus. *Diabetes/Metabolism Reviews, 5*(2), 83–109. https://doi.org/10.1002/dmr.5610050202 (accessed on 2nd February 2026).

Kissebah, A. H., Vydelingum, N., Murray, R., Evans, D. J., Hartz, A. J., Kalkhoff, R. K., & Adams, P. W. (1982). Relation of body fat distribution to metabolic complications of obesity. *The Journal of Clinical Endocrinology and Metabolism, 54*(2), 254–260. https://doi.org/10.1210/jcem-54-2-254 (accessed on 2nd February 2026).

Kosasih, F. R., & Bonavida, B. (2021). Chapter 16—YY1-mediated regulation of type 2 diabetes via insulin. In B. Bonavida (Ed.), *YY1 in the Control of the Pathogenesis and Drug Resistance of Cancer* (pp. 271–287). Academic Press. https://doi.org/10.1016/B978-0-12-821909-6.00005-5 (accessed on 2nd February 2026).

Kowluru, R. A., & Mohammad, G. (2022). Epigenetic modifications in diabetes. *Metabolism, 126*, 154920. https://doi.org/10.1016/j.metabol.2021.154920 (accessed on 2nd February 2026).

LaPorte, R. E., Tajima, N., Akerblom, H. K., Berlin, N., Brosseau, J., Christy, M., et al. (1985). Geographic differences in the risk of insulin-dependent diabetes mellitus: The importance of registries. *Diabetes Care, 8*(Suppl 1), 101–107. https://doi.org/10.2337/diacare.8.1.s101 (accessed on 2nd February 2026).

Larsen, N., Vogensen, F. K., Van Den Berg, F. W. J., Nielsen, D. S., Andreasen, A. S., Pedersen, B. K., et al. (2010). Gut microbiota in human adults with type 2 diabetes differs from non-diabetic adults. *PLoS ONE, 5*(2), e9085. https://doi.org/10.1371/journal.pone.0009085 (accessed on 2nd February 2026).

Lau, K., Benitez, P., Ardissone, A., Wilson, T. D., Collins, E. L., Lorca, G., et al. (2011). Inhibition of type 1 diabetes correlated to a *Lactobacillus johnsonii* N6.2-mediated Th17 bias. *The Journal of Immunology, 186*(6), 3538–3546. https://doi.org/10.4049/jimmunol.1001864 (accessed on 2nd February 2026).

Lê, K. A., Li, Y., Xu, X., Yang, W., Liu, T., Zhao, X., et al. (2013). Alterations in fecal *Lactobacillus* and *Bifidobacterium* species in type 2 diabetic patients in Southern China population. *Frontiers in Physiology, 3*, Article 496. https://doi.org/10.3389/fphys.2012.00496 (accessed on 2nd February 2026).

Lerman, I. G., Villa, A. R., Martinez, C. L., Cervantes Turrubiatez, L., Aguilar Salinas, C. A., Wong, B., et al. (1998). The prevalence of diabetes and associated coronary risk factors in urban and rural older Mexican populations. *Journal of the American Geriatrics Society, 46*(11), 1387–1395. https://doi.org/10.1111/j.1532-5415.1998.tb06005.x (accessed on 2nd February 2026).

Liu, M., Weiss, M. A., Arunagiri, A., Yong, J., Rege, N., Sun, J., et al. (2018). Biosynthesis, structure, and folding of the insulin precursor protein. *Diabetes, Obesity and Metabolism, 20*(S2), 28–50. https://doi.org/10.1111/dom.13378 (accessed on 2nd February 2026).

Llanos, P., Contreras-Ferrat, A., Barrientos, G., Valencia, M., Mears, D., & Hidalgo, C. (2015). Glucose-dependent insulin secretion in pancreatic β-cell islets from male rats requires Ca^{2+} release via ROS-stimulated ryanodine receptors. *PLoS ONE, 10*(6), e0129238. https://doi.org/10.1371/journal.pone.0129238 (accessed on 2nd February 2026).

Masharani, U. (2005). Diabetes mellitus and hypoglycemia. In *Current Medical Diagnosis and Treatment* (pp. 1157–1201).

Meigs, J. B. (2010). Epidemiology of type 2 diabetes and cardiovascular disease: Translation from population to prevention. *Diabetes Care, 33*(8), 1865–1871. https://doi.org/10.2337/dc10-0641 (accessed on 2nd February 2026).

Melistas, L., Mantzoros, C. S., Kontogianni, M., Antonopoulou, S., Ordovas, J. M., & Yiannakouris, N. (2009). Association of the +45T>G and +276G>T polymorphisms in the adiponectin gene with insulin resistance in nondiabetic Greek women. *European Journal of Endocrinology, 161*(6), 845–852. https://doi.org/10.1530/EJE-09-0492 (accessed on 2nd February 2026).

Mier, P. D., & van den Hurk, J. J. (1975). Lysosomal hydrolases of the epidermis. 2. Ester hydrolases. *The British Journal of Dermatology, 93*(4), 391–398. https://doi.org/10.1111/j.1365-2133.1975.tb06512.x (accessed on 2nd February 2026).

Moini, J. (2019). Pathophysiology of diabetes. In *Epidemiology of Diabetes* (pp. 25–43). Elsevier. https://doi.org/10.1016/B978-0-12-816864-6.00003-1 (accessed on 2nd February 2026).

Moosavi, A., & Motevalizadeh Ardekani, A. (2016). Role of epigenetics in biology and human diseases. *Iranian Biomedical Journal, 5*, 246–258. https://doi.org/10.22045/ibj.2016.01 (accessed on 2nd February 2026).

N/A. (1992). Childhood diabetes, epidemics, and epidemiology: An approach for controlling diabetes. World Health Organization DIAMOND Project Group on Epidemics. *American Journal of Epidemiology, 135*(7), 803–816.

Nadhiya, J., Vijayalakshmi, M. K., & Showbharnikhaa, S. (2024). A brief review on diabetes mellitus: Short communication. *Journal of Pharma Insights and Research, 2*(1), Article 1.

Newsholme, P., Keane, K. N., Carlessi, R., & Cruzat, V. (2019). Oxidative stress pathways in pancreatic β-cells and insulin-sensitive cells and tissues: Importance to cell metabolism, function, and dysfunction. *American Journal of Physiology-Cell Physiology, 317*(3), C420–C433. https://doi.org/10.1152/ajpcell.00141.2019 (accessed on 2nd February 2026).

Ohlson, L. O., Larsson, B., Björntorp, P., Eriksson, H., Svärdsudd, K., Welin, L., et al. (1988). Risk factors for type 2 (non-insulin-dependent) diabetes mellitus. Thirteen and one-half years of follow-up of the participants in a study of Swedish men born in 1913. *Diabetology, 31*(11), 798–805. https://doi.org/10.1007/BF00277480 (accessed on 2nd February 2026).

Pettitt, D. J., Knowler, W. C., Baird, H. R., & Bennett, P. H. (1980). Gestational diabetes: Infant and maternal complications of pregnancy in relation to third-trimester glucose tolerance in the Pima Indians. *Diabetes Care, 3*(3), 458–464. https://doi.org/10.2337/diacare.3.3.458 (accessed on 2nd February 2026).

Phillips, J. M., Parish, N. M., Bland, C., Sawyer, Y., De La Peña, H., & Cooke, A. (2009). Type 1 diabetes development requires both CD4+ and CD8+ T cells and can be reversed by non-depleting antibodies targeting both T cell populations. *The Review of Diabetic Studies, 6*(2), 97–103. https://doi.org/10.1900/RDS.2009.6.97 (accessed on 2nd February 2026).

Polikandrioti, M., & Dokoutsidou, H. (2009). The role of exercise and nutrition in type II diabetes mellitus management. *Health Science Journal, 3*(4).

Poulsen, P., Ohm Kyvik, K., Vaag, A., & Beck-Nielsen, H. (1999). Heritability of type II (non-insulin-dependent) diabetes mellitus and abnormal glucose tolerance—A population-based twin study. *Diabetology, 42*(2), 139–145. https://doi.org/10.1007/s001250051131 (accessed on 2nd February 2026).

Radha, V., & Mohan, V. (2007). Genetic predisposition to type 2 diabetes among Asian Indians. *The Indian Journal of Medical Research, 125*(3), 259–274.

Rahati, S., Shahraki, M., Arjomand, G., & Shahraki, T. (2014). Food pattern, lifestyle and diabetes mellitus. *International Journal of High-Risk Behaviors and Addiction, 3*(1). https://doi.org/10.5812/ijhrba.8725 (accessed on 2nd February 2026).

Sakai, K., Matsumoto, K., Nishikawa, T., Suefuji, M., Nakamaru, K., Hirashima, Y., et al. (2003). Mitochondrial reactive oxygen species reduce insulin secretion by pancreatic β-cells. *Biochemical and Biophysical Research Communications, 300*(1), 216–222. https://doi.org/10.1016/S0006-291X(02)02832-2 (accessed on 13th August 2024).

Sato, Y., Nagasaki, M., Nakai, N., & Fushimi, T. (2003). Physical exercise improves glucose metabolism in lifestyle-related diseases. *Experimental Biology and Medicine, 228*(10), 1208–1212. https://doi.org/10.1177/153537020322801017 (accessed on 2nd February 2026).

Shibasaki, S., Imagawa, A., & Hanafusa, T. (2013). Fulminant type 1 diabetes mellitus: A new class of type 1 diabetes. In S. I. Ahmad (Ed.), *Diabetes* (Vol. 771, pp. 20–23). Springer New York. https://doi.org/10.1007/978-1-4614-5441-0_3 (accessed on 2nd February 2026).

Sprague, R. S., Stephenson, A. H., Bowles, E. A., Stumpf, M. S., & Lonigro, A. J. (2006). Reduced expression of G(i) in erythrocytes of humans with type 2 diabetes is associated with impairment of both cAMP generation and ATP release. *Diabetes, 55*(12), 3588–3593. https://doi.org/10.2337/db06-0555 (accessed on 2nd February 2026).

Steyn, N., Mann, J., Bennett, P., Temple, N., Zimmet, P., Tuomilehto, J., et al. (2004). Diet, nutrition and the prevention of type 2 diabetes. *Public Health Nutrition, 7*(1a), 147–165. https://doi.org/10.1079/PHN2003586 (accessed on 2nd February 2026).

Svejgaard, A., & Ryder, L. P. (1989). HLA and insulin-dependent diabetes: An overview. *Genetic Epidemiology, 6*(1), 1–14. https://doi.org/10.1002/gepi.1370060104 (accessed on 2nd February 2026).

Svejgaard, A., Platz, P., & Ryder, L. P. (1977). Associations between HLA and some non-rheumatic diseases and possible explanations. *Clinics in Rheumatic Diseases, 3*(2), 239–253. https://doi.org/10.1016/S0307-742X(21)00019-9 (accessed on 2nd February 2026).

Tammen, S. A., Friso, S., & Choi, S. W. (2013). Epigenetics: The link between nature and nurture. *Molecular Aspects of Medicine, 34*(4), 753–764. https://doi.org/10.1016/j.mam.2012.07.018 (accessed on 2nd February 2026).

Tillil, H., & Köbberling, J. (1987). Age-corrected empirical genetic risk estimates for first-degree relatives of IDDM patients. *Diabetes, 36*(1), 93–99. https://doi.org/10.2337/diab.36.1.93 (accessed on 2nd February 2026).

Trevisan, R., Vedovato, M., & Tiengo, A. (1998). The epidemiology of diabetes mellitus. *Nephrology, Dialysis, Transplantation, 13*(Suppl 8), 2–5. https://doi.org/10.1093/ndt/13.suppl_8.2 (accessed on 2nd February 2026).

Tull, E. S., Jordan, O. W., Simon, L., Laws, M., Smith, D. O., Vanterpool, H., et al. (1997). Incidence of childhood-onset IDDM in Black African-heritage populations in the Caribbean. *Diabetes Care, 20*(3), 309–310. https://doi.org/10.2337/diacare.20.3.309 (accessed on 2nd February 2026).

Unger, R. H. (1978). Role of glucagon in the pathogenesis of diabetes: The status of the controversy. *Metabolism, 27*(11), 1691–1709. https://doi.org/10.1016/0026-0495(78)90291-3 (accessed on 2nd February 2026).

Vaag, A., Henriksen, J. E., Madsbad, S., Holm, N., & Beck-Nielsen, H. (1995). Insulin secretion, insulin action, and hepatic glucose production in identical twins discordant for non-insulin-dependent diabetes mellitus. *Journal of Clinical Investigation, 95*(2), 690–698. https://doi.org/10.1172/JCI117715 (accessed on 2nd February 2026).

Vasseur, F., Helbecque, N., Lobbens, S., Vasseur-Delannoy, V., Dina, C., Clément, K., et al. (2005). Hypoadiponectinemia and high risk of type 2 diabetes are associated with adiponectin-encoding (ACDC) gene promoter variants in morbid obesity: Evidence for a role of ACDC in diabesity. *Diabetology, 48*(5), 892–899. https://doi.org/10.1007/s00125-005-1729-z (accessed on 2nd February 2026).

Venerando, B., Fiorilli, A., Croci, G., Tringali, C., Goi, G., Mazzanti, L., et al. (2002). Acidic and neutral sialidase in the erythrocyte membrane of type 2 diabetic patients. *Blood, 99*(3), 1064–1070. https://doi.org/10.1182/blood.v99.3.1064 (accessed on 2nd February 2026).

Wagener, D. K., Sacks, J. M., LaPorte, R. E., & MaCgregor, J. M. (1982). The Pittsburgh Study of Insulin-Dependent Diabetes Mellitus: Risk for diabetes among relatives of

IDDM. *Diabetes, 31*(2), 136–144. https://doi.org/10.2337/diab.31.2.136 (accessed on 2nd February 2026).

Wen, L., Ley, R. E., Volchkov, P. Y., Stranges, P. B., Avanesyan, L., Stonebraker, A. C., et al. (2008). Innate immunity and intestinal microbiota in the development of type 1 diabetes. *Nature, 455*(7216), 1109–1113. https://doi.org/10.1038/nature07336 (accessed on 2nd February 2026).

Zahoor, I., Singh, S., Behl, T., Sharma, N., Naved, T., Subramaniyan, V., et al. (2022). Emergence of microneedles as potential therapeutics in diabetes mellitus. *Environmental Science and Pollution Research, 29*(3), 3302–3322. https://doi.org/10.1007/s11356-021-17346-0 (accessed on 2nd February 2026).

Zhou, Z., Mahdi, A., Tratsiakovich, Y., Zahorán, S., Kövamees, O., Nordin, F., et al. (2018). Erythrocytes from patients with type 2 diabetes induce endothelial dysfunction via arginase I. *Journal of the American College of Cardiology, 72*(7), 769–780. https://doi.org/10.1016/j.jacc.2018.05.052 (accessed on 2nd February 2026).

PART II
Diagnosis and Management

CHAPTER 3

Diagnostic Modalities and Holistic Management Strategies for Diabetes

MOHD. MURSAL,[1] MOHAMMAD AHMAD,[1,*]
DEEBA SHAMIM JAIRAJPURI,[2] and ASAD AHMAD[1]

[1]*Faculty of Pharmacy, Integral University, Lucknow, Uttar Pradesh, India*

[2]*Department of Biochemistry, Arabian Gulf University, Manama, Bahrain*

*Corresponding author

ABSTRACT

Diabetes mellitus (DM) is a chronic metabolic disorder marked by elevated blood glucose levels (BGLs) due to defects in insulin secretion, action, or both. Early diagnosis and holistic management are crucial for preventing complications, improving quality of life, and reducing healthcare costs. Diagnostic modalities for diabetes have evolved, offering methods for accurately detecting and monitoring conditions, such as fasting plasma glucose (FPG), oral glucose tolerance tests (OGTTs), hemoglobin A1c, and continuous glucose monitoring (CGM) systems. Holistic management strategies include lifestyle modification, pharmacotherapy, and complementary therapies. A balanced diet, regular physical activity, and weight management are essential lifestyle interventions. Pharmacotherapy, including oral hypoglycemic agents and insulin therapy, is critical for glycemic control. Complementary therapies such as acupuncture, yoga, and herbal supplements may provide benefits for stress reduction and well-being. Patient-centered care emphasizes tailoring treatment plans to individual preferences, values, and goals. Technology such as CGM and

Diabetes: Novel Insights and Therapies. Anas Islam and Badruddeen (Eds)

DOI: 10.1201/9781779644596-5

insulin pumps enables real-time data monitoring and personalized treatment adjustments. Challenges remain in coordination, healthcare system constraints, patient engagement, and technological barriers. Future directions should focus on enhancing interdisciplinary training, advocating for policy reforms, improving patient education, and advancing technology to optimize diabetes management outcomes and improve the quality of life for individuals with diabetes.

3.1 INTRODUCTION

Diabetes mellitus (DM) is a chronic metabolic disease that has become a global health concern. Diabetes is characterized by elevated blood glucose levels (BGLs), or hyperglycemia, which can be caused by abnormalities in insulin secretion, action, or both. The two primary types of diabetes are type 1 diabetes, which is often diagnosed in childhood and involves the autoimmune destruction of insulin-producing beta cells in the pancreas, and type 2 diabetes, which is more common and usually occurs in adulthood and is characterized by insulin resistance and relative insulin deficiency (Figure 3.1). Gestational diabetes, which occurs during pregnancy, is another condition that highlights the diverse manifestations of the disease.

Globally, the prevalence of diabetes is increasing at a steady rate. The IDF estimates that 463 million adults worldwide had diabetes in 2019, and by 2045, there will be more than 700 million people. This increasing frequency is caused by a number of variables, such as urbanization and aging populations, dietary changes, sedentary lifestyles, and increasing obesity rates. Additionally, genetic predispositions and socioeconomic factors contribute to the growing burden of diabetes.

Owing to consequences such as cardiovascular disease (CVD), renal failure, neuropathy, and retinopathy, diabetes is linked to significant morbidity and death that affect not only individuals but also healthcare systems and economies. With direct medical costs such as hospital stays, prescription drugs, and medical supplies, as well as indirect costs such as missed work and disability, the economic impact is significant. This combined cost burden highlights the need for efficient management and preventive techniques.

To effectively manage diabetes, comprehensive treatment plans that are individualized for each patient must be made after an early and correct diagnosis. Maintaining BGLs within a target range, reducing the chance of complications, and improving the quality of life for those with diabetes are the three main goals of this dual strategy. Diagnostic modalities for diabetes have evolved over the years, offering various methods for accurately detecting and monitoring conditions (Ojo et al., 2023).

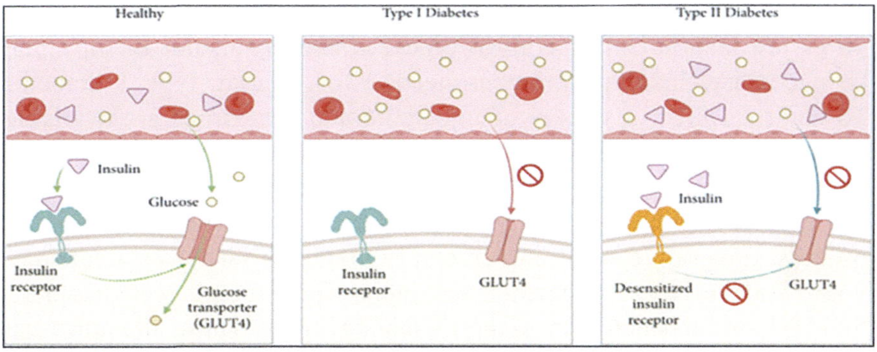

FIGURE 3.1 Difference between type I and II diabetes.

Source: Reprinted from Cheng et al. (2022). http://creativecommons.org/licenses/by/4.0/

Blood glucose testing remains the cornerstone for diabetes diagnosis. Many tests are used to diagnose and track diabetes, including hemoglobin A1c (HbA1c) test, random plasma glucose test, oral glucose tolerance test (OGTT), and fasting plasma glucose (FPG) tests. While the OGTT evaluates BGLs both before and after ingestion of a glucose-rich beverage, the FPG test checks BGLs after an overnight fast. The HbA1c test provides an average BGL over the previous two–three months, providing insights into long-term glucose control, while the random plasma glucose test can be performed at any time, regardless of when a meal is eaten. In addition to traditional blood glucose tests, continuous glucose monitoring (CGM) systems have emerged as valuable tools for the management of diabetes. CGM devices measure glucose levels in real time using a sensor inserted under the skin, providing continuous data that helps individuals and healthcare providers make informed decisions about treatment adjustments. These advancements in diagnostic technologies have significantly improved the ability to effectively monitor and manage diabetes (Abdoli et al., 2018).

Holistic management strategies for diabetes encompass a broad spectrum of approaches, including lifestyle modifications, pharmacotherapy, and complementary therapies. The core elements of diabetes management include lifestyle treatments, such as dietary adjustments, physical exercise, weight control, and smoking cessation. Improved insulin sensitivity and stable BGLs can be achieved with a well-balanced diet high in fiber, whole grains, lean proteins, and healthy fats, as well as frequent exercise. In particular, pharmacotherapy is essential for the management of type 1 diabetes and severe type 2 diabetes. When oral drugs are insufficient to control type 2 diabetes, insulin therapy may be necessary. Insulin therapy is needed for treating type 1 diabetes. To control BGLs, a variety of injectable and oral drugs are available, including SGLT2 inhibitors, DPP-4 inhibitors, metformin, sulfonylureas, and GLP-1 receptor agonists. The patient's health situation, preferences, and response to therapy play a role in the customized medicine selection process. Integrative and complementary therapies, such as acupuncture, yoga, and herbal supplements, are increasingly being recognized for their potential benefits in diabetes management. These therapies can complement conventional treatments and contribute to overall well-being, stress reduction, and improved glycemic control (Westman, 2021). Integrative and complementary therapies, such as acupuncture, yoga, and herbal supplements, are increasingly being recognized for their potential benefits in diabetes management. These therapies can complement conventional treatments and contribute to overall well-being, stress reduction, and improved glycemic control (Westman, 2021). Moreover, patient education and psychological support are critical for fostering adherence to treatment regimens and enhancing the quality of life of individuals with diabetes. Education empowers patients with knowledge of their condition, enabling them to make informed decisions and adopt healthier lifestyles.

3.2 IMPORTANCE OF EARLY DIAGNOSIS AND HOLISTIC MANAGEMENT IN DIABETES

Diabetes mellitus is a chronic disease with potentially severe complications that cannot be effectively managed. Early diagnosis and holistic management of diabetes are critical for preventing complications, reducing healthcare costs, and improving the quality of life of those affected. This section explores the significance of early diagnosis and comprehensive integrative approaches for managing diabetes. Early diagnosis of diabetes is essential for several reasons. One of the primary benefits is the prevention of or delay in diabetes-related complications. Chronic hyperglycemia can lead to damage to various organs, resulting in complications, such as CVD, retinal degeneration, nephropathy, and neuropathy. Early identification of diabetes allows for timely intervention, which can mitigate the risk of these complications. Early diagnosis also provides an opportunity for improved glycemic control. Initiating treatment and lifestyle modifications at an early stage can help maintain BGLs within a target range, thereby preventing the adverse effects of prolonged hyperglycemia (Goetsch and Wiebe, 1995).

Similarly, diabetes control and early identification can greatly enhance a person's quality of life. People can prevent the symptoms of uncontrolled diabetes, such as weariness, frequent urination, and excessive thirst, by maintaining appropriate BGLs, which will improve their general health. Additionally, early diagnosis and management of diabetes can reduce long-term healthcare costs. By averting these problems, people and healthcare systems can save a great deal of money by avoiding the need for expensive hospital stays and treatments. Moreover, prompt diagnosis gives patients the ability to manage their health. Better outcomes and a sense of agency in controlling one's illness can result from people making educated decisions about their lifestyles and treatment with the right information and assistance.

The holistic management of diabetes involves a comprehensive approach that integrates various strategies to address the physical, emotional, and psychological aspects of the disease. A balanced diet, frequent exercise, and weight control are examples of lifestyle changes that are essential for managing diabetes. Nutritional therapy involves consuming various foods that provide essential nutrients while maintaining BGLs. Glycemic control can be enhanced by placing an emphasis on whole grains, lean proteins, healthy fats, fruits, and vegetables that are high in fiber. Frequent exercise improves insulin sensitivity and aids blood glucose control. Activities, such as walking, swimming, and strength training, are also beneficial. It is critical to reach and stay at a healthy weight, particularly in patients with type 2 diabetes. Weight loss can enhance glycemic control and insulin sensitivity, thereby lowering the requirement for medication (Vijan and Hayward, 2004).

Pharmacotherapy plays a critical role in diabetes management. Insulin therapy is crucial for patients with type 1 diabetes and some patients with type 2 diabetes. Insulin treatment aids in controlling blood sugar levels (BSLs) and averting issues. Several oral medicines are available for the treatment of type 2 diabetes, such as SGLT2 inhibitors, DPP-4 inhibitors, sulfonylureas, and metformin. However, the methods by which these drugs reduce BGLs vary. Other injectable drugs, such as GLP-1 receptor agonists, can assist in controlling diabetes in addition to insulin by increasing insulin secretion and encouraging fullness.

Monitoring and self-management of diabetes are crucial aspects of diabetes care. Individuals who regularly check their BGLs are better able to manage their BSLs and make educated choices regarding their medicine, diet, and exercise regimen. CGM systems provide a more complete view of glycemic control by providing real-time data on the glucose levels. These systems can alert individuals to hyperglycemia and hypoglycemia and facilitate timely interventions. Education is the cornerstone of diabetes management. Being aware of the illness, its side effects, and its management techniques gives people the ability to take charge of their health. Programs for diabetes self-management education (DSME) offer important knowledge and abilities for successful diabetes management. Diabetes management can be difficult. Therefore, emotional support is essential. The stress and emotional strain of diabetes can be managed by people using support groups, counseling, and mental health services. Tai chi, yoga, and meditation are examples of complementary and integrative therapies that can help to lower stress and enhance general well-being. Stress management is crucial because chronic stress can adversely affect BGLs. Some individuals find benefits from complementary therapies such as acupuncture and certain herbal supplements. Although these should not replace conventional treatments, they can complement a holistic management plan (Petersen et al., 2021).

The importance of early diagnosis and holistic management of diabetes cannot be overstated. Early diagnosis helps prevent complications, improves glycemic control, enhances the quality of life, reduces healthcare costs, and empowers patients. Holistic management, incorporating lifestyle modifications, pharmacotherapy, monitoring, education, support, and complementary therapies, provides a comprehensive approach for managing diabetes. By addressing the multifaceted nature of diabetes, healthcare providers can offer more effective and personalized care, ultimately leading to better outcomes for individuals living with diabetes.

3.3 OVERVIEW OF DIABETES AS A GLOBAL HEALTH CONCERN

Diabetes mellitus is not only a serious personal health issue, but also a worldwide health issue with broad ramifications. Globally, the prevalence of diabetes has been increasing at an alarming rate, posing a serious threat to public health systems, economies, and the well-being of millions of people. This section provides an overview of diabetes as a global health issue, examining its prevalence, impact, and the urgent need for coordinated global action.

3.3.1 RISING PREVALENCE OF DIABETES

Over the past few decades, the prevalence of diabetes has significantly increased. The IDF estimated that 463 million people worldwide had diabetes in 2019, and by 2045, there will be 700 million more. Many factors, such as population aging, urbanization, dietary changes, sedentary lifestyles, and the worldwide obesity pandemic, are contributing to this spike. While type 1 diabetes is less common and is typically diagnosed in childhood or adolescence, type 2 diabetes accounts for the majority of cases and is increasingly being diagnosed in younger age groups, including children and adolescents.

3.3.2 IMPACT ON HEALTH AND WELL-BEING

Diabetes has a profound impact on an individual's health and well-being. It is linked to a host of issues affecting almost all organ systems. CVD, which includes heart attack and stroke, is the primary cause of morbidity and mortality. Retinopathy, diabetic neuropathy, and nephropathy are additional common consequences that substantially lower the quality of life. Diabetic nephropathy is the primary cause of kidney failure; however, diabetic neuropathy can cause excruciating pain and incapacity. Untreated diabetic retinopathy can result in blindness (Ogurtsova et al., n.d.).

The chronic nature of diabetes requires ongoing medical care and self-management, which can be physically and emotionally demanding. A daily regimen of blood glucose monitoring, medication, and lifestyle modifications requires a high level of commitment and can lead to burnout and psychological distress. Moreover, the social and economic burdens of diabetes are substantial. The direct medical costs associated with diabetes are high owing to the need for medications, regular monitoring, and treatment of complications. Indirect costs such as loss of productivity and disability further exacerbate the economic impact of the disease (Widyahening et al., 2022).

3.3.3 GLOBAL DISPARITIES AND CHALLENGES

The burden of diabetes is not evenly distributed across the world. Low- and middle-income countries (LMICs) are experiencing the greatest increase in the prevalence of diabetes and face significant challenges in managing the disease. These regions often lack the healthcare infrastructure, resources, and trained healthcare professionals required to provide adequate diabetes care. Access to essential medications, including insulin, is limited in many LMICs, which makes effective diabetes management difficult. Additionally, public awareness of diabetes and its complications is often low, hindering early diagnosis and timely intervention (Owen et al., 2022).

High-income countries are not immune to the diabetes epidemic but generally have more resources to address the disease. However, even in these countries, disparities exist among socioeconomic and ethnic groups. Minority populations and individuals from lower socioeconomic backgrounds often have higher rates of diabetes and face barriers in accessing quality healthcare (Liakos et al., 2023).

3.3.4 THE NEED FOR GLOBAL ACTION

Addressing diabetes as a global health concern requires coordinated effort at multiple levels. Public health strategies should focus on prevention, early diagnosis, and effective management. Prevention efforts should target risk factors that can be altered, including diet, physical inactivity, and obesity. The incidence of type 2 diabetes can be decreased, and healthy lifestyles can be promoted with the aid of community-based interventions, public health campaigns, and legislative reforms. Early diagnosis is crucial for preventing complications and improving patient outcomes. Strengthening primary healthcare systems to ensure the timely screening and diagnosis of diabetes is essential. Integrating diabetes care into primary health care can help make services more accessible and affordable, particularly in LMICs. Effective management of diabetes requires a multifaceted approach, including medication, lifestyle changes, and patient education.

Ensuring access to affordable medication and medical supplies is critical. Additionally, educating patients about self-management and providing psychosocial support can empower them to take control of their health and improve their quality of life (Bae et al., 2022).

3.4 DIAGNOSTIC MODALITIES FOR DIABETES

Accurate diagnosis and monitoring of its progression are critical components of effective diabetes management. Several diagnostic modalities have been used to detect diabetes and monitor conditions over time. These include blood glucose monitoring, various laboratory tests, and diagnostic imaging techniques, each of which plays a unique role in providing a comprehensive assessment of a patient's glycemic status and associated complications.

3.4.1 BLOOD GLUCOSE MONITORING

Monitoring BGLs is crucial for the diagnosis and treatment of diabetes. The OGTT, random plasma glucose test, and FPG test are the main techniques used for tracking BGLs. The FPG test checks BGLs following a minimum 8-hour overnight fast. Diabetes is diagnosed when BGLs are 126 mg/dL (7.0 mmol/L) or greater on two different occasions. This simple examination is frequently used for preliminary screening.

The OGTT is a more comprehensive test that evaluates how the body processes glucose levels. It entails taking blood glucose readings both before and two hours after ingestion of a beverage high in glucose. Diabetes is confirmed by a two-hour plasma glucose level of 200 mg/dL (11.1 mmol/L) or greater. This test is particularly useful for diagnosing gestational diabetes and can reveal issues with glucose metabolism that might not be apparent with fasting glucose alone (Holt Ma et al., 1991).

Regardless of when you last had a meal, you can perform a random plasma glucose test at any time of the day. Diabetes is suggested by a result of 200 mg/dL (11.1 mmol/L) or greater combined with hyperglycemia symptoms, such as excessive thirst, frequent urination, and unexplained weight loss. When fasting is not an option, this test is useful for the diagnosis of diabetes.

CGM systems have become vital tools in diabetes management, especially for patients with type 1 diabetes and those requiring intensive insulin therapy. CGM devices continually measure the interstitial fluid's glucose levels using a sensor implanted beneath the skin. They provide real-time data and trend analysis, alerting users to hypo- or hyperglycemic events, thus enabling more precise and timely adjustments to insulin therapy and lifestyle modifications (Mookiah et al., 2015a).

3.4.2 LABORATORY TESTS

Laboratory tests are indispensable for diagnosing diabetes and assessing long-term glycemic control. An important diagnostic tool is the hemoglobin A1c (HbA1c) test, which calculates the proportion of glycated hemoglobin in the blood and represents the average BGLs over the previous two–three months. Diabetes was indicated by an HbA1c score of 6.5% or greater on two different tests. This test is useful for both initial diagnosis and continuing care, because it provides information on the degree of blood glucose control that has been maintained over time.

C-peptide levels and autoantibody tests are important laboratory tests. C-peptide, a by-product of insulin production, helps differentiate between type 1 and type 2 diabetes by indicating the level of endogenous insulin production. Low levels suggest type 1 diabetes, whereas high levels suggest type 2 diabetes. Autoantibody tests detect the presence of specific antibodies associated with type 1 diabetes, aiding the diagnosis of autoimmune diabetes (Kumar et al., n.d.; Owen et al., 2022).

Urine tests, such as those for detecting microalbuminuria, are used to identify the early signs of kidney damage, a common complication of diabetes. Microalbuminuria indicates the presence of small amounts of albumin in the urine, which can be an early marker of diabetic nephropathy. Timely detection allows for early intervention to prevent the progression to more severe kidney diseases (Ortiz-Martínez et al., 2022).

3.4.3 DIAGNOSTIC IMAGING TECHNIQUES

Diagnostic imaging techniques are crucial to identify and manage diabetes-related complications. Ultrasound and Doppler studies are commonly used to assess blood flow and detect peripheral artery disease (PAD), which is prevalent among patients with diabetes. PAD can lead to severe complications, including non-healing ulcers and amputations, making its early detection and management vital. Optical coherence tomography (OCT) and fundus photography are two forms of retinal imaging that are crucial for identifying diabetic retinopathy, which is one of the main causes of vision loss. By taking precise pictures of the retina, fundus photography makes it possible to identify retinal abnormalities such as hemorrhages and microaneurysms. OCT enables the identification of structural problems such as macular edema by providing cross-sectional images of the retina. For individuals with diabetes to maintain their vision, early detection and treatment of retinal impairment is essential (Noguerol et al., 2017).

Magnetic resonance imaging (MRI) and computed tomography (CT) are used to evaluate complications affecting the internal organs. For instance, MRI can be used to assess the extent of fatty liver disease, which is common in individuals with type 2 diabetes. CT can identify pancreatic abnormalities, such as cysts or tumors, that may affect insulin production. These advanced imaging techniques provide detailed insights into the extent and severity of organ involvement and guide appropriate therapeutic interventions (Anwar et al., 2020).

3.5 HOLISTIC MANAGEMENT STRATEGIES FOR DIABETES

Diabetes mellitus demands a comprehensive management approach that extends beyond glycemic control to encompass holistic strategies addressing lifestyle, pharmacology, psychological well-being, and complementary therapies; every element is essential to reach the best possible health results and improve the quality of life for people with diabetes.

3.5.1 LIFESTYLE MODIFICATIONS

Lifestyle modifications are fundamental in diabetes management, focusing on improving glycemic control and reducing cardiovascular risk factors. A well-balanced diet that prioritizes fruits, vegetables, whole grains, lean meat, and healthy fats helps to control BSLs and improves general health. Dietary strategies may include carbohydrate counting or glycemic index considerations to manage postprandial glucose spikes. Increasing insulin sensitivity, reducing BGLs, and strengthening cardiovascular fitness require regular physical activity. Resistance training should be performed in addition to 150 min/week of moderate-intensity exercise to increase muscle mass and enhance glucose metabolism. Weight management through calorie control and healthy eating habits is crucial, especially for individuals with type 2 diabetes, as excess weight contributes to insulin resistance and complicates glycemic control (Patel et al., 2024).

3.5.2 PHARMACOLOGICAL INTERVENTIONS

Pharmacological interventions are essential when lifestyle modifications alone are insufficient to achieve the target glycemic goals. Oral hypoglycemic agents, such as SGLT2 inhibitors, metformin, sulfonylureas, DPP-4 inhibitors, and GLP-1 receptor agonists, are frequently administered to reduce BGLs via different mechanisms (Sharma et al., n.d.). Metformin, a first-line treatment for type 2 diabetes, improves insulin sensitivity and lowers glucose synthesis in the liver. While DPP-4 and SGLT2 inhibitors enhance glycemic control through various processes, including glucose metabolism and renal glucose reabsorption, sulfonylureas promote insulin production from pancreatic beta cells. GLP-1 receptor agonists help to control weight by increasing satiety and inhibiting glucagon release by stimulating insulin production. Insulin therapy is still essential for people with type 1 diabetes and might be required for patients with type 2 diabetes who need strict glycemic control (Ortiz-Martínez et al., 2022).

3.5.3 PSYCHOLOGICAL SUPPORT AND BEHAVIORAL INTERVENTIONS

Psychological support and behavioral interventions are integral to managing the emotional and mental health aspects of diabetes. Living with a chronic condition, such as diabetes, can be stressful and overwhelming, impacting adherence to treatment plans and overall well-being (Syed, 2022). Counseling, support groups, and cognitive behavioral therapy (CBT) can help individuals cope with diabetes-related stress, depression, and anxiety. Behavioral interventions focus on promoting healthy behaviors, enhancing self-management skills, and improving adherence to treatment regimens. Empowering patients with education on diabetes self-care and providing ongoing support are essential for promoting psychological resilience and improving treatment outcomes (Chew et al., 2018).

3.5.4 COMPLEMENTARY AND ALTERNATIVE THERAPIES

Complementary and alternative therapies offer additional avenues for managing diabetes and improving overall health outcomes. Acupuncture, yoga, meditation, and herbal supplements are among the practices with potential advantages in lowering stress, promoting better glycemic management, and boosting general well-being, as have been investigated (Holt Ma et al., 2024). Acupuncture may help alleviate neuropathic pain associated with diabetes, whereas yoga and meditation can reduce stress levels and promote relaxation, potentially lowering blood pressure and improving sleep quality. Herbal supplements, such as cinnamon and fenugreek, have shown promising results in lowering BGLs, although their efficacy and safety require further research and monitoring. It is imperative that people who are thinking about including alternative therapies in their diabetes management strategy speak with healthcare professionals to ensure safe and seamless integration (Mookiah et al., 2015b).

3.6 INTEGRATIVE APPROACHES TO DIABETES MANAGEMENT

Diabetes management is increasingly embracing integrative approaches that leverage multidisciplinary care teams, prioritize patient-centered care, and integrate technology to optimize outcomes. This shift recognizes that diabetes is a complex, chronic condition that requires more than just medical treatment; it demands a comprehensive strategy that addresses the medical, psychological, and lifestyle aspects of the disease.

3.6.1 MULTIDISCIPLINARY CARE TEAMS

To provide comprehensive and coordinated care, multidisciplinary care teams that bring together medical specialists from several specialties play a critical role in diabetes management. Endocrinologists, primary care doctors, nurses, nutritionists, pharmacists, and behavioral health specialists are frequently involved in these teams. Each team member contributes specialized knowledge and skills to address various aspects of diabetes care, such as medical management, dietary counseling, mental health support, and patient education. Collaborative decision making and regular team meetings ensure holistic assessment, personalized treatment plans, and continuity of care (Zhang et al., 2017). By working together, multidisciplinary teams can effectively manage complex cases, promptly address diabetes-related complications, and improve patient outcomes through coordinated intervention. For instance, an endocrinologist can adjust medication regimens based on the latest glucose readings, while a dietitian can provide personalized nutritional advice to support these adjustments. Behavioral health specialists can help patients manage psychological stress associated with diabetes, which can be a significant barrier to effective self-management. Pharmacists play a critical role in the management of medication adherence and can identify potential drug interactions and side effects. Regular communication among team members helps monitor progress and make necessary adjustments to the care plan. This collaborative approach not only improves clinical outcomes, but also enhances patient satisfaction by providing a more comprehensive and supportive healthcare experience (Cianciosi et al., 2024).

3.6.2 PATIENT-CENTERED CARE

Patient-centered care is fundamental in diabetes management, emphasizing the importance of tailoring treatment plans to individual preferences, values, and goals. This approach recognizes that each patient's experience with diabetes is unique and influenced by factors such as lifestyle, cultural background, socioeconomic status, and personal health beliefs. Healthcare providers engage in shared decision making with patients, involving them in treatment decisions and goal setting. Patient education is integral to promoting self-management skills, enhancing health literacy, and empowering patients to play an active role in their health (Klein et al., 2022).

By prioritizing patients' perspectives and preferences, healthcare providers can build trust, improve treatment adherence, and achieve better long-term health outcomes for individuals with diabetes. For example, a patient who values natural remedies may be more compliant with a treatment plan that includes dietary changes and physical activity alongside conventional medicine. Incorporating cultural sensitivity into education and communication can help bridge gaps and ensure that advice is relevant and respectful (Skinner et al., 2020). Additionally, socioeconomic factors, such as access to healthy foods or safe places to exercise, allow for a more realistic and attainable goal setting. By fostering a collaborative and respectful relationship, healthcare providers can support patients in navigating their diabetes management journey more effectively, leading to improved overall well-being and disease management (Tomic et al., n.d.).

3.6.3 TECHNOLOGY INTEGRATION

Technology integration is revolutionizing diabetes care by offering advanced tools and solutions to monitor glucose levels, track health metrics, and enhance communication between patients and healthcare providers. With the help of real-time data on glucose trends provided by CGM devices, patients can make timely modifications to their insulin therapy and lifestyle choices. Insulin pumps optimize glycemic control and lower the risk of hypoglycemia by automating insulin delivery based on CGM readings. The use of digital platforms and mobile applications, remote monitoring, online consultations, and individualized coaching can enhance treatment adherence and expand access to care. Utilizing machine learning (ML) techniques and artificial intelligence (AI), data are analyzed to forecast glucose patterns and customize treatment suggestions (Magliano and Boyko, 2022).

By leveraging technology, healthcare providers can deliver more personalized, proactive, and effective diabetes management, empowering patients to achieve better health outcomes and quality of life. For instance, a CGM system can alert a patient to impending hyperglycemia or hypoglycemia, allowing immediate corrective action (Matoori, 2022). Patients in underserved or rural locations can receive professional advice and treatment plans without having to travel owing to telemedicine systems. Furthermore, AI-driven insights can help identify patterns and trends that might be missed during routine checkups, leading to earlier interventions and more precise adjustments to treatment. These technological advancements make it easier for patients to remain engaged with their health management and for providers to offer continuous, comprehensive support. By embracing these tools, diabetes care can become more dynamic, responsive, and tailored to individual needs, ultimately improving outcomes and enhancing the quality of life of those living with diabetes (Pectasides and Kalva, 2011).

3.7 CHALLENGES AND FUTURE DIRECTION

Despite significant advancements in diabetes management through integrative approaches, several challenges remain, and addressing these issues is crucial for future progress. One major challenge is ensuring effective coordination and communication among the diverse members of multidisciplinary care teams. Successful collaboration among endocrinologists, primary care physicians, nurses, dietitians, pharmacists, and behavioral health specialists requires overcoming differences in schedules, communication methods, and practice settings, which can delay information sharing and decision making. Another challenge lies in healthcare system constraints (Harrison et al., 2022). Issues such as limited resources, rigid structural frameworks, and insufficient reimbursement models can hinder the establishment and maintenance of effective multidisciplinary teams as well as limit the adoption of patient-centered care practices and advanced technologies. In addition, patient engagement and adherence to treatment plans pose significant difficulties (Elsayed et al., 2022). Patients may struggle with health literacy, cultural barriers, or psychological resistance to lifestyle changes, all of which can undermine the effectiveness of patient-centered approaches. The integration of technology into diabetes care also presents challenges, including the high cost of devices, such as continuous glucose monitors and insulin pumps, the need for technological literacy, and concerns about data privacy and security. Future studies for improving diabetes management should focus on several key areas to overcome these challenges. Enhanced interdisciplinary training programs should be developed to equip healthcare professionals with the skills needed for effective team-based care and collaborative practice. Policy and reimbursement reforms are necessary to support an integrative approach by promoting coordinated care, advanced technologies, and patient-centered practices. To improve patient engagement, future efforts should emphasize comprehensive, culturally sensitive educational programs and personalized coaching that addresses individual needs and barriers. Technological advancements should continue to aim for more affordable, user-friendly devices and sophisticated AI-driven solutions for personalized care, with a focus on equitable access for all patients (Pop-Busui et al., 2022). Finally, ongoing research and innovation are essential to explore the effectiveness of multidisciplinary teams, patient-centered interventions, and emerging technologies, ensuring that new strategies are developed and tested to optimize diabetes management outcomes for diverse patient populations. By addressing these challenges and pursuing future directions, the field of diabetes management can continue to evolve, offering more effective, inclusive, and patient-focused care.

3.8 CONCLUSION

In conclusion, integrative approaches to diabetes management—combining multidisciplinary care teams, patient-centered care, and advanced technology—represent a significant advancement in diabetes care. By leveraging the expertise of diverse healthcare professionals, focusing on individual patient needs, and utilizing cutting-edge tools, we can offer more effective and personalized management for this complex condition. However, challenges, such as coordination among team members, system constraints, patient engagement, and technological barriers, must be addressed. Looking forward, enhancing interdisciplinary training, advocating policy reforms, improving patient education, and advancing technology will be crucial for overcoming these obstacles. Embracing these future directions will help to achieve better health outcomes and improve the quality of life of those living with diabetes.

KEYWORDS

- **artificial intelligence**
- **continuous glucose monitoring**
- **diabetes mellitus**
- **lifestyle modification**
- **machine learning**
- **patient-centered care**
- **pharmacotherapy**

REFERENCES

Abdoli, S., Doosti Irani, M., Hardy, L. R., & Funnell, M. (2018). A discussion paper on stigmatizing features of diabetes. *Nursing Open, 5*(2), 113–119. https://doi.org/10.1002/NOP2.112 (accessed on 2nd February 2026).

Anwar, F., Qurat-Ul-Ain, Ejaz, M. Y., & Mosavi, A. (2020). A comparative analysis on diagnosis of diabetes mellitus using different approaches–A survey. *Informatics in Medicine Unlocked, 21*, 100482. https://doi.org/10.1016/j.imu.2020.100482 (accessed on 2nd February 2026).

Bae, J., Han, K., Ko, S., Yoon, Y., et al. (2022). Diabetes fact sheet in Korea 2021. *Diabetes & Metabolism Journal, 46*(3), 417–426. https://doi.org/10.4093/dmj.2022.0106 (accessed on 2nd February 2026).

Cheng, P., Wang, L., & Gong, W. (2022). Cellular immunity of patients with tuberculosis combined with diabetes. *Journal of Immunology Research, 2022*(1), 6837745. https://doi.org/10.1155/2022/6837745 (accessed on 2nd February 2026).

Chew, B. H., Fernandez, A., & Shariff-Ghazali, S. (2018). Psychological interventions for behavioral adjustments in diabetes care–A value-based approach to disease control.

Psychology Research and Behavior Management, 11, 145–155. https://doi.org/10.2147/PRBM.S117224 (accessed on 2nd February 2026).

Cianciosi, D., Armas Diaz, Y., Grosso, G., Quiles, J. L., Giampieri, F., & Battino, M. (2024). Association between diagnostic imaging and biochemical markers: A possible tool for monitoring metabolic disorders. *Current Opinion in Food Science, 55*, 101109. https://doi.org/10.1016/j.cofs.2023.101109 (accessed on 2nd February 2026).

Elsayed, N. A., Aleppo, G., Aroda, V. R., Bannuru, R. R., Brown, F. M., Bruemmer, D., et al (2022). Summary of revisions: Standards of care in diabetes—2023. *American Diabetes Association*. https://doi.org/10.2337/dc23-SREV (accessed on 2nd February 2026).

Goetsch, V. L., & Wiebe, D. J. (1995). Diabetes mellitus. In *Handbook of Health Behavior Research II* (pp. 513–533). https://doi.org/10.1007/978-1-4899-1028-8_25 (accessed on 2nd February 2026).

Harrison, A. V., Lorenzo, F. R., & McClain, D. A. (2022). Iron and the pathophysiology of diabetes. *Annual Review of Physiology*. https://doi.org/10.1146/annurev-physiol-022522 (accessed on 2nd February 2026).

Holt, M. A. R. I., Flyvbjerg, A., & Goldstein, B. J. (1991). Characteristics of types of diabetes mellitus II in regional general hospital Than Rondahaim, Simalungun District. *Medalion Journal*. http://medalionjournal.com/index.php/go/article/view/64 (accessed on 2nd February 2026).

Holt, R. I. G., Flyvbjerg, A., & Goldstein, B. J. (2024). *Textbook of Diabetes*. https://books.google.com/books?hl=en&lr=&id=OrvtEAAAQBAJ&oi=fnd&pg=PP17&dq=diabetes&ots=UiaIMJ2Zit&sig=aagXAIGxNevT8wPQ8fneYVHj1cM (accessed on 2nd February 2026).

Klein, S., Gastaldelli, A., Yki-Järvinen, H., & Smith, P. S. (2022). Why does obesity cause diabetes? *Cell Metabolism, 34*, 11–20. https://doi.org/10.1016/j.cmet.2021.12.012.

Kumar, A., Gangwar, R., & Zaidi, A. A. (2024). Prevalence of diabetes in India: A review of IDF diabetes atlas 10th edition. *Current Diabetes Reviews, 20*(1), 105–114. https://www.ingentaconnect.com/content/ben/cdr/2024/00000020/00000001/art00013 (accessed on 2nd February 2026).

Liakos, A., Karagiannis, T., Avgerinos, I., Malandris, K., Tsapas, A., & Bekiari, E. (2023). Management of type 2 diabetes in the new era. *Hormones, 22*(4), 677–684. https://doi.org/10.1007/S42000-023-00488-W.

Magliano, D., & Boyko, E. (2022). *IDF Diabetes Atlas*. https://europepmc.org/books/nbk581934 (accessed on 2nd February 2026).

Matoori, S. (2022). Diabetes and its complications. *ACS Pharmacology & Translational Science, 5*(8), 513–515. https://doi.org/10.1021/acsptsci.2c00122 (accessed on 2nd February 2026).

Mookiah, M. R. K., Acharya, U. R., Fujita, H., Tan, J. H., Chua, C. K., Bhandary, S. V., et al. (2015a). Application of different imaging modalities for diagnosis of diabetic macular edema: A review. *Computers in Biology and Medicine, 66*, 295–315. https://doi.org/10.1016/j.compbiomed.2015.09.012 (accessed on 2nd February 2026).

Noguerol, T. M., Alcalá, A. L., Beltrán, L. S., Cabrera, M. G., Cabrero, J. B., & Vilanova, J. C. (2017). Advanced MR imaging techniques for differentiation of neuropathic arthropathy and osteomyelitis in the diabetic foot. *Radiographics, 37*(4), 1161–1180. https://doi.org/10.1148/RG.2017160101.

Ogurtsova, K., Guariguata, L., Barengo, N. C., Lopez-Doriga Ruiz, P., Sacre, J. W., Karuranga, S., et al. (2022). IDF diabetes atlas: Global estimates of undiagnosed diabetes in adults for 2021. *Diabetes Research and Clinical Practice, 183*, 109118. https://www.sciencedirect.com/science/article/pii/S0168822721004770 (accessed on 2nd February 2026).

Ojo, O. A., Ibrahim, H. S., Rotimi, D. E., Ogunlakin, A. D., & Ojo, A. B. (2023). Diabetes mellitus: From molecular mechanism to pathophysiology and pharmacology. *Medicine in Novel Technology and Devices, 19*. https://doi.org/10.1016/j.medntd.2023.100247 (accessed on 2nd February 2026).

Ortiz-Martínez, M., González-González, M., Martagón, A. J., Hlavinka, V., Willson, R. C., & Rito-Palomares, M. (2022). Recent developments in biomarkers for diagnosis and screening of type 2 diabetes mellitus. *Current Diabetes Reports, 22*(3), 95–115. https://doi.org/10.1007/S11892-022-01453-4 (accessed on 2nd February 2026).

Owen, K., Turner, H., & Wass, J. (2022). *Oxford Handbook of Endocrinology & Diabetes*. OUP Oxford. https://books.google.com/books?hl=en&lr=&id=yPJbEAAAQBAJ&oi=fnd&pg=PP1&dq=diabetes&ots=2O_IzKcQ21&sig=5GX3pEfoRJlAB2hoPrfqZcUnZ24 (accessed on 2nd February 2026).

Patel, R., Sina, R. E., & Keyes, D. (2024). Lifestyle modification for diabetes and heart disease prevention. *StatPearls*. https://www.ncbi.nlm.nih.gov/books/NBK585052/ (accessed on 2nd February 2026).

Pectasides, M., & Kalva, S. P. (2011). Diabetes revealed: Multisystem danger. *American Journal of Roentgenology, 196*(2), 274–286. https://doi.org/10.2214/AJR.10.5922 (accessed on 2nd February 2026).

Petersen, B., Vesper, I., Pachwald, B., Dagenbach, N., Buck, S., Waldenmaier, D., et al. (2021). Diabetes management intervention studies: Lessons learned from two studies. *Trials, 22*(1). https://doi.org/10.1186/S13063-020-05017-3 (accessed on 2nd February 2026).

Pop-Busui, R., Januzzi, J. L., Bruemmer, D., Butalia, S., Green, J. B., Horton, W. B., et al. (2022). Heart failure: An underappreciated complication of diabetes. A consensus report of the American Diabetes Association. *Am Diabetes Assoc*. https://doi.org/10.2337/dci22-0014 (accessed on 2nd February 2026).

Sharma, K., Akre, S., Chakole, S., & Wanjari, M. B. (2022). Stress-induced diabetes: A review. *Cureus, 14*(9), e29142. https://www.ncbi.nlm.nih.gov/pmc/articles/PMC9561544/ (accessed on 2nd February 2026).

Skinner, T. C., Joensen, L., & Parkin, T. (2020). Twenty-five years of diabetes distress research. *Diabetic Medicine, 37*(3), 393–400. https://doi.org/10.1111/DME.14157 (accessed on 2nd February 2026).

Syed, F. Z. (2022). Type 1 diabetes mellitus. *Annals of Internal Medicine, 175*(3). https://www.acpjournals.org/doi/abs/10.7326/aitc202203150 (accessed on 2nd February 2026).

Tomic, D., Shaw, J. E., & Magliano, D. J. (2022). The burden and risks of emerging complications of diabetes mellitus. *Nature Reviews Endocrinology, 18*, 525–539. https://doi.org/10.1038/s41574-022-00690-7 (accessed on 2nd February 2026).

Vijan, S., & Hayward, R. A. (2004). Pharmacologic lipid-lowering therapy in type 2 diabetes mellitus: Background paper for the American College of Physicians. *Annals of Internal Medicine, 140*(8). https://doi.org/10.7326/0003-4819-140-8-200404200-00013 (accessed on 2nd February 2026).

Westman, E. C. (2021). Type 2 diabetes mellitus: A pathophysiologic perspective. *Frontiers in Nutrition, 8*. https://doi.org/10.3389/FNUT.2021.707371 (accessed on 2nd February 2026).

Widyahening, I. S., Khunti, K., Vos, R. C., & Chew, B. H. (2022). Editorial: Achieving effective management and treatment of diabetes mellitus in future primary care. *Frontiers in Endocrinology, 13*. https://doi.org/10.3389/FENDO.2022.854244/FULL (accessed on 2nd February 2026).

Zhang, J., Xu, J., Hu, X., Chen, Q., Tu, L., Huang, J., et al. (2017). Diagnostic method of diabetes based on support vector machine and tongue images. *BioMed Research International, 2017*. https://doi.org/10.1155/2017/7961494 (accessed on 2nd February 2026).

CHAPTER 4

Navigating Diabetes Complications and Comorbidities

MOHSIN VAHID KHAN,[1,*] MOHAMMAD RUMMAN,[1] GULAM RABBANI,[2] MOHD KAMIL HUSSAIN,[3] and NAFEES AHMAD[4]

[1]*Department of Biosciences, Integral University, Lucknow, Uttar Pradesh, India*

[2]*School of Chemical Engineering, Yeungnam University, Gyeongsan, Gyeongbuk, Republic of Korea*

[3]*Department of Chemistry, Government Raza Postgraduate College, Rampur, Uttar Pradesh, India*

[4]*Department of Chemistry, Integral University, Lucknow, Uttar Pradesh, India*

*Corresponding author

ABSTRACT

Diabetes mellitus (DM) is a chronic illness common worldwide. The World Health Organization (WHO) reports about 422 million people living with diabetes globally, causing around 1.5 million deaths annually. Lifestyle and environmental changes contribute to a steady increase in diabetes prevalence. DM can result from either inability to produce insulin (type 1 DM) or responding normally to insulin (type 2 DM), leading to sustained hyperglycemia. Hyperglycemia affects multiple organs including kidneys, heart, liver, eyes, and nervous system. One mechanism underlying secondary complications of hyperglycemia is enhanced lipid-peroxidation and increased production of reactive

Diabetes: Novel Insights and Therapies. Anas Islam and Badruddeen (Eds)

DOI: 10.1201/9781779644596-6

carbonyl species such as 4-hydroxy-2-nonenal (4-HNE), sufficient to damage multiple tissues. Other mechanisms include increased formation of advanced glycation end-products (AGEs), enhanced glycolytic flux, and increased activity of hexosamine pathway. Prolonged hyperglycemia in DM patients can lead to secondary complications and multiple comorbidities, including obesity, hypertension, dyslipidemia, heart disease, and neurological disorders. Proper management of DM is crucial to control hyperglycemia and prevent secondary complications. This chapter details comorbidities often reported in DM patients, presents known underlying molecular mechanisms, describes current management strategies, and provides novel perspectives on managing DM-associated secondary complications.

4.1 INTRODUCTION

The word *diabetes* originates from the Greek word *diabaino*, which means "to pass through" or "run through," while the Latin word *mellitus* is used in the sense of sweetness, meaning "honey." diabetes is a metabolic disorder that is expected to occupy the seventh position in the next five years, according to the WHO, as a major culprit of fatality (Mathers and Loncar, 2006). Since diabetes has been reported to induce impediments linked with several other ailments, including neuropathy, foot ulcers, and diabetic nephropathy, timely diagnosis of diabetes followed by treatment remains inexorable (Tan et al., 2018). The unremitted worldwide diabetes propagation shows its devastating face when comparing the increment of diabetic patient count in almost 35 years, spanning from 1980 to 2014. The diabetic patient number was less than 110 million in 1980 but reached 422 million in 2014, with approximately a four-times rise in reckoning, and is estimated to touch a record sum of 642 million in the next 15 years (Standl et al., 2019; WHO, 2017).

Diabetes has a rich and multifaceted history spanning centuries. The Ebers Papyrus, an ancient Egyptian medical document from about 1550 BC, contains the oldest known reference to diabetes and lists symptoms such as increased thirst and urination. The association between diabetes inception with young age and obesity correspondingly was first described by two great Indian physicians, Shushruta and Charaka, around 500–600 BC. During the Roman Empire, the physician Galen elaborated on Hippocrates' theories, further connecting diabetes to an imbalance in bodily fluids. In the Middle Ages, diabetes was often associated with a sweet taste in the urine, leading to the term 'mellitus' being added to its name (Ahmed, 2002; Sapra and Bhandari, 2023; *The Lancet*, 2017). The Greek physicians, Rufus of Ephesus and Galen, during the first and second century AD, respectively, in their treatises elucidated the features of a serious disease that might lead to death, known for causing debility, extreme thirstiness, and abnormal, excess urine production, polyuria. On observing the person with polyuria only for a couple of times, he named this health complication diarrhea of urine as diabetes diarrhea urinoma. Later on, renowned Greco-Roman physician Aretaeus, with the Cappadocian surname, coined the term "diabetes mellitus" in the second century AD. Aretaeus learned medicine in Alexandria while practicing in Rome, and his surname refers to the birthplace named Cappadocia (Karamanou et al., 2016; Laios et al., 2012).

In the 17th century, British physician Thomas Willis conducted pioneering experiments using a urinometer to measure the specific gravity of urine, which allowed for the diagnosis of diabetes. In the 18th century, the Scottish physician Matthew Dobson introduced the use of opium to alleviate the symptoms of diabetes. When German scientists Oskar Minkowski and Joseph von Mering identified the pancreas' involvement in diabetes in 1869, it was a significant advance. Their experiments on dogs demonstrated that removing the pancreas resulted in severe hyperglycemia and other diabetic symptoms. In a 19th-century doctoral thesis entitled "contribution to the microscopic anatomy of the pancreas" by German researcher Paul Langerhans, various types of cells constituting pancreatic islets were described. In 1893, Gustave Edouard Laguesse, a French histologist, conjectured the possibility of glycosuria treatment by an element produced by the islets of Langerhans, which could be correlated as insulin secretion occurs in the pancreas. He also termed the tissues of those regions involved in insulin secretion as the islets of Langerhans ("îlots de Langerhans") (Laguesse, 1893, 1895; Langerhans, 1869). Diabetes, especially referring to diabetes mellitus (DM), is one of the most prevalent metabolic disorders with incessantly raised blood glucose levels (BGLs) because of an anomalous glycogenolysis and gluconeogenesis pathway leading to hyperglycemia. The onset of hyperglycemic condition is directly associated with insulin secreted from beta cells of the pancreas and may lead to both acute as well as chronic impediments. The flawed metabolism of food components like carbohydrates, protein, and fats as a result of either unregulated insulin secretion leading to failure to meet the cellular demand, abnormal functioning due to abnormal structural alteration, or a combination of both states causes hyperglycemia (Roden and Shulman, 2019; Sacks et al., 2023). The cells control insulin expression as well as secretion in well-versed coordination since impairment at any step may cause diabetes-associated health complications. To maintain glucose homeostasis, proper secretion followed by functioning is obligatory. But homeostasis gets disturbed due to insulin resistance and/or erroneous insulin secretion and finally results in the onset of diabetes, which affects a huge number of populations across the globe. The hormone insulin, generated by the pancreas and controls blood sugar levels (BSLs), was successfully isolated in 1921 by Canadian scientists Frederick Banting and Charles Best (Ahmed, 2002; Sapra and Bhandari, 2023). This discovery revolutionized diabetes treatment, allowing for the injection of insulin to manage blood sugar and prevent complications. Since the discovery of insulin, significant advancements have been made in diabetes research and management. The invention of blood glucose meters in the 1970s enabled patients to monitor their BSLs at home. The development of insulin pumps and continuous glucose monitors further improved blood sugar control and reduced the risk of complications. Ongoing research continues to explore new treatments, technologies, and preventative measures to improve the lives of individuals living with diabetes.

4.2 CLASSIFICATION OF DIABETES

In 1979, for the first time, the National Diabetes Data Group (NDDG) published a classification of diabetes, although it was further modified within six years, that is, in 1985. However, for one year after the classification (up to 1980), the WHO validated this classification (Alberti and Zimmet, 1998; National Diabetes Data Group, 1979). Considering pharmacological methods opted to treat diabetic patients, NDDG categorized diabetes in two sets and devised the term insulin-dependent diabetes mellitus (IDDM) associated with patients with a slender physique requiring insulin for treatment with a chance of onset of ketosis. Meanwhile, patients with obesity being treated by other strategies like exercise and medications without the need for insulin and ketosis possibility were referred to as non-insulin-dependent diabetes mellitus (NIDDM).

After being in frequent use over the decade, both terms gradually tended to be obsolete and misclassified due to compounding evidence of other types of diabetes and the need for insulin even for NIDDM patients to achieve effective control over the diabetes (Leslie et al., 2021; N/A, 2018; Thunander et al., 2008).

The diabetes reported in childhood is popularly designated as type 1 diabetes mellitus, formerly entitled juvenile-onset diabetes, while diabetes onset in the adult population is termed type 2 diabetes mellitus (T2DM), previously known as adulthood-onset diabetes. But recent studies reveal that type 1 diabetes mellitus (T1DM) may not only commence in any stage, like adult-onset diabetes, but is rather most predominant and almost double that of juvenile-onset. The improper understanding concomitant with immune, metabolic, and genetic parameters of juvenile-onset as well as adulthood-onset diabetes may result in the ambiguity of diabetes classification. Therefore, in 1997, the International Expert Committee classified diabetes mellitus on the basis of etiology. Type 1 and type 2 are major categories of diabetes mellitus, and to avoid any confusion in reading the Roman numerals "I" or "II" as 1 or 2, the Arabic numeral system is used in the new classification system to designate diabetes classes as type 1 and type 2 (Mayfield, 1998). Type 2 diabetes is described as a condition of impairment in the secretion of insulin by pancreatic beta cells and insulin resistance as a result of heterogeneous genetic malady. This class of diabetes is most prevalent, and its occurrence is not only related to factors including obesity, lack of exercise, and aging, but rather allied with previous gestational background in females and diabetic family history. Furthermore, gestational diabetes mellitus (GDM) is not apparently observed before gestation as diabetes but is diagnosed either during the second or third trimester of pregnancy. Additionally, several "other specific types" of diabetes may be induced due to different factors, like after transplantation of organs, medication-induced diabetes while HIV treatment by using glucocorticoid, maturity-onset diabetes, as well as neonatal diabetes. Furthermore, maturity-onset diabetes in youth, abbreviated as MODY, has been reported with functionally impaired beta cells *via* chemical, infection, or chemically induced pancreatic dysfunction, genetic aberration, cystic fibrosis, pancreatitis, and in case of acromegaly. The classification of diabetes along with their characteristics is depicted in Table 4.1 (N/A, 1997, 2018; Lebovitz, 2001).

4.3 CHARACTERISTICS OF DIFFERENT TYPES OF DIABETES

4.3.1 TYPE 1 DIABETES

Mistaken targeting and killing of insulin-producing pancreatic beta cells by the body's immune system results in type 1 diabetes onset. Type 1 is related to the approximately complete damage of insulin-secreting pancreatic beta cells. The discerning damage of pancreatic beta cells may be caused by either T-cell interceded autoimmune disease or non-autoimmune factors, but in most cases, autoimmune disease is the culprit, which might be fatal in untreated conditions.

The onset of T1DM does not discriminate based on gender and ensues within two weeks, almost in a similar ratio in both males and females prior to the age of 25 years in 95% of the cases (Mayfield, 1998). Insulin, a hormone crucial for regulating BGLs, is no longer produced adequately, leading to hyperglycemia (high blood sugar). Although it can manifest at any age, this illness is often identified in childhood or adolescence. This chronic autoimmune illness, commonly referred to as juvenile diabetes or insulin-dependent diabetes, affects millions of people globally. Moreover, the precise etiology of type 1 diabetes is still unknown; meanwhile, scientists assume that it results from a complicated interaction between environmental factors and genetic susceptibility. A person's risk is increased if they have a first-degree relative who has the disease, which is one important factor in family history. There may be other contributing environmental variables, such as vitamin D insufficiency, exposure to certain chemicals, and viral infections.

The symptoms of type 1 diabetes, which frequently appear suddenly, include increased hunger, weariness, blurred vision, frequent urination (especially at night), excessive thirst, unexplained weight loss, and slow-healing wounds (Taplin and Barker, 2008). Diagnosis involves blood tests to measure BGLs, as well as HbA1c levels, which reflect average BSLs over the past 2–3 months. There is currently no cure for type 1 diabetes, requiring lifelong management to maintain healthy BGLs (Lahtela et al., 1997; Matsuyoshi et al., 2006). The current and promising treatment methods of T1DM revolve around several recently developed measures as shown in Table 4.2.

TABLE 4.1 Classification of Diabetes

Classification	Subordinate Type	Prevalence	Hallmarks	References
Type 1 diabetes mellitus (T1DM)	Type 1A	5–10%	Beta cell destruction due to cell-mediated autoimmune response, resulting in almost total insulin deficiency	Craig et al. (2009); Diagnosis and Classification of Diabetes Mellitus (2005)
	Type 1B		Idiopathic (not linked with autoimmune)	
	Others		Cystic fibrosis, pancreatitis, and pancreatectomy	
Type 2 diabetes mellitus (T2DM)	–	90–95%	Inadequate release of insulin by beta cells; absence of insulin function and insulin sensitivity	
Gestational diabetes mellitus (GDM)	–	1–14%	Glucose tolerance declines specifically in the third trimester of pregnancy; excessive thirst	
Genetic defects allied with beta cell functioning	Maturity-onset diabetes of the young (MODY) (HNF-4α (MODY1), Glucokinase (MODY2), HNF-1α (MODY3), insulin promoter factor-1 (IPF-1; MODY4), HNF-1β (MODY5), NeuroD1 (MODY6)), HNF-4α, HNF-1β, IPF-1, NeuroD1, others	–	Underexpression of various transcription factors of beta cells	
Genetic defect in insulin action	Type A insulin resistance, lipoatrophy, Rabson-Mendenhall syndrome, leprechaunism, others	–	Severe insulin resistance due to alterations in the insulin receptor	
Endocrine ailments linked to diabetes	Cushing's syndrome, somatostatinoma, acromegaly, hyperthyroidism, aldosteronoma, glucagonoma, phaeochromocytoma, others	–	Share features with type 2 diabetes mellitus (T2DM)	
Drugs- or compounds-induced diabetes	New-generation drugs and other compounds/ chemicals: diazoxide, glucocorticoids, nicotinic acid, pentamidine, α-interferon, β-adrenergic agonists	–	Generally presents as type 2 diabetes mellitus (T2DM)	

TABLE 4.2 Various Methods Employed for T1DM Treatment

Current Promising Methods	Description	References
Insulin therapy	Regular insulin injections or infusions are essential to regulate blood sugar. This includes various types of insulin with different durations and delivery methods, allowing for personalized management.	Aschner (2020)
Blood glucose monitoring	Frequent blood glucose checks are crucial for understanding individual responses to insulin and for making adjustments to treatment plans.	Gordon (2019)
Diet and exercise	Blood sugar control and overall health are greatly supported by a low-carbohydrate diet and regular physical activity.	Hamdy et al. (2001)
Complications monitoring	Regular screenings are essential for detecting potential complications such as kidney disease, nerve damage, eye disorders, and cardiovascular problems.	McGuffee et al. (2020)
Immunotherapy	Strategies aiming to suppress the immune response against the pancreas, potentially halting or reversing the destruction of beta cells.	Allen and Dayan (2021)
Islet transplantation	Replacing damaged beta cells with healthy ones from donors.	Shapiro et al. (2016)
Stem cell therapy	Utilizing stem cells to generate new insulin-producing cells.	Bani Hamad et al. (2021)
Artificial pancreas	Development of closed-loop systems that use real-time blood glucose monitoring to autonomously control insulin administration.	Boughton and Hovorka (2020)

4.3.2 *TYPE 2 DIABETES*

Hyperglycemia, or high blood sugar, is a hallmark of type 2 diabetes, a chronic metabolic illness. About 90% of cases of diabetes are of this kind, making it the most prevalent type. Insulin is a hormone that helps control BSLs; when the body grows resistant to it, type 2 diabetes occurs. This resistance leads to a buildup of glucose in the bloodstream. Type 2 diabetes is associated with a number of risk factors, such as a family history of the disease, obesity, physical inactivity, poor nutrition, age (more than 45), ethnicity (Native Americans, African Americans, and Hispanics), and so forth, (Galicia-Garcia et al., 2020; Roden and Shulman, 2019). Type 2 diabetes may not show any symptoms in its early stages. However, people may feel increased thirst, frequent urination, increased appetite, weariness, slow-healing wounds, tingling or numbness in their hands and feet, and impaired vision when their BSLs rise. Blood tests, such as the oral glucose tolerance test (OGTT), fasting blood glucose test, and HbA1c test, which calculates the average BSLs over the previous two to three months, are commonly used to identify type 2 diabetes (Blair, 2016).

Bringing BSLs down to a healthy range is the main objective of type 2 diabetes therapy. This can be accomplished by changing one's lifestyle to include less sugar and carbs in the diet, frequent exercise, and weight loss. To treat this illness, injections of insulin and oral drugs including metformin, sulfonylureas, and glitazones are frequently utilized (Fadini et al., 2017; Umpierrez and Korytkowski, 2016). Numerous consequences, such as heart disease, stroke, kidney failure, diabetic retinopathy, diabetic neuropathy, eye damage, and amputations, can result from uncontrolled type 2 diabetes (Hornquist et al., 1995). Many patients of type 2 diabetes can lead long, robust lives if they receive the right care and control their lifestyle. Effective management of the illness requires regular monitoring of BSLs, adherence to medication, and timely treatment of complications.

4.3.3 GESTATIONAL DIABETES

Globally, there is rising worry over gestational diabetes, a disease in which pregnant women have elevated BSLs. This transient kind of diabetes generally manifests in the second or third trimester of pregnancy and goes away after delivery. The exact cause remains uncertain, but hormonal changes and insulin resistance during pregnancy are believed to play a significant role (Genuth et al., 2018; Lebovitz, 2001). While gestational diabetes does not directly harm the baby, it can lead to complications like macrosomia (large baby), birth defects, and respiratory distress in newborns. For the mother, it increases the risk of preeclampsia, premature birth, and long-term health issues like type 2 diabetes after pregnancy. Early detection through routine blood glucose testing is crucial for managing gestational diabetes. Maintaining a nutritious diet, engaging in regular physical activity, and closely monitoring BSLs are crucial tactics for controlling the illness and lowering risks (Kim et al., 2002; Noctor et al., 2016). To keep blood sugar under control, insulin therapy could be required in some situations. Although gestational diabetes can be challenging, it is a manageable condition with appropriate care, promoting a healthy pregnancy and birth for both mother and baby.

4.4 INSULIN RESISTANCE AND DISPOSITION INDEX

Insulin resistance is considered a pioneer disorder in the progression of T2DM, and prior to hyperglycemia onset, the existence of insulin resistance has been reported in impending T2DM patients. The phenomenon of insulin resistance is employed as a prime indication for identifying individuals prone to T2DM development, since the occurrence of insulin resistance in a predisposed T2DM population may commence several years before, ranging from one to two decades, as evidenced by anatomical studies (Shulman, 2000). The anomalous and compromised response by distinct cells against internally secreted or exogenously introduced insulin is connoted as insulin resistance. It has been evidenced that individuals with insulin resistance are not only confined to the irregularities of glucose metabolism but also include impairment in other important metabolic pathways of biomolecules such as lipids and amino acids. However, insulin resistance remains majorly associated with irregularities in glucose metabolism *via* diminished insulin-mediated transport and further metabolism in skeletal muscle and adipocytes, besides lessened hepatic output and altered insulin suppression in adipocyte lipolysis.

Together with insulin resistance, a causal factor of pancreatic beta cell function failure is assumed to be raised insulin secretion requisition (Defronzo, 2009). For the prediction of T2DM progression, a term "disposition index" (DI) has been devised which qualitatively explains the equilibrium established to maintain glucose tolerance. The DI is used for indexing the functioning of pancreatic beta cells, which signifies insulin sensitivity. The establishment of equilibrium describing DI takes place at the time of regulating glucose tolerance, which gets disturbed during lowered insulin sensitivity but sustained by concurrent supplemented secretion of insulin (Pacini, 2006).

4.5 DIAGNOSTICS OF DIABETES

Diabetes is responsible for several health hitches, which further lead to other complications if they remain undiagnosed and untreated. Moreover, it is inevitable to be vigilant regarding patients' diabetic status, and diabetes screening can be performed by analyzing different parameters followed by hyperglycemic crises or by displaying hyperglycemic symptoms such as polydipsia, polyuria, or loss of weight due to unknown reasons. The feeling of elevated thirstiness, craving, and reiterated need of urination are diabetic symptoms, along with the most common symptom, that is, elevated plasma glucose level. It is worth mentioning that the diabetic status measuring values of various diagnostics tests varies from individual to individual. Diabetes is identified by the results of the A1C test, which measures the elevated glycosylated hemoglobin level, the OGTT, the random glucose test, or fasting plasma glucose (FPG) (Figure 4.1). The dissimilar metabolic state of glucose has revealed three groups, including normal, prediabetes, and diabetes, upon diagnosis under different conditions. These conditions include A1C, 2 hours plasma glucose (PG) while OGTT, and FPG. Prediabetes is referred to as two intermediate steps, namely impaired fasting glucose (IFG) along with impaired glucose tolerance (IGT), resulting in T2DM progression starting from normal glucose tolerance (NGT). The FPG level is determined post meal gap of eight hours to maintain no caloric intake prior to the test, while 2 hours plasma glucose measuring is done after two hours of 75 gm administered glucose. Similarly, random glucose level is diagnosed instantaneously without considering post meal lapse (ADA Professional Practice Committee, 2024; Siu, 2015; Vijan, 2010).

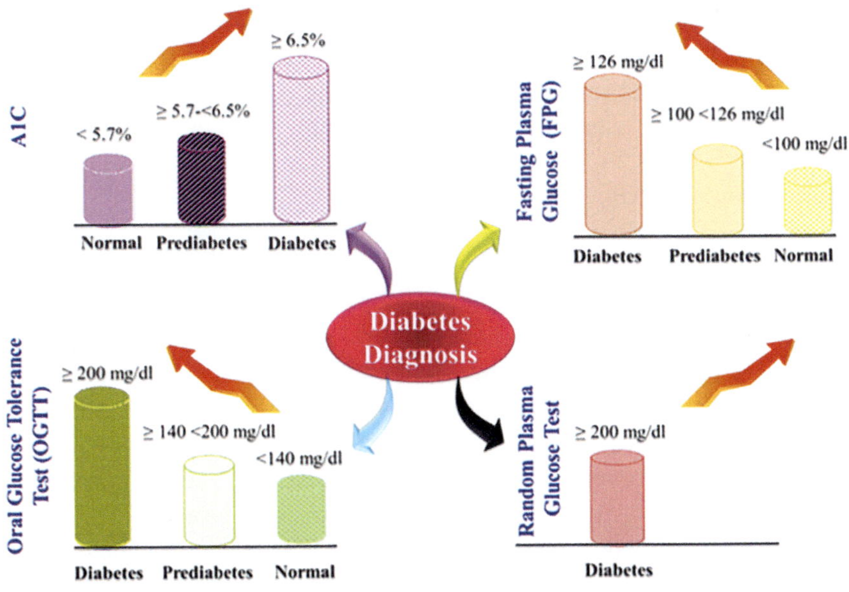

FIGURE 4.1 Diabetes diagnosis based on analysis of different parameters.

4.6 RISK FACTORS FOR TYPE 1 DIABETES MELLITUS (T1DM)

4.6.1 GENETIC FACTORS

Generally, the inception of T1DM in patients cannot directly be linked with heredity, and approximately 90% of T1DM patients do not show any first- or second-degree relation with disease onset (Anton et al., 2011). The chance of developing T1DM is high among diabetic patients' relatives, whereas for others, the lifetime possibility of diabetes remains approximately 0.4%. Furthermore, the risk of diabetes development is evident as it varies for children of male or female diabetic persons, ranging from 6–9% for male patients' children and 1.3–4% for children of females. Similarly, dizygotic twins exhibit a 6% T1DM permeance rate, which is very high in the case of identical twins (25–50%) and 6–7%, in almost the same range for siblings (Lee and Hwang, 2019). A substantial connection between genetic factors and T1DM has been established on the basis of 20,000 articles available on the National Center for Biotechnology Information (NCBI) database, focusing on investigating the link between genetic factors and T1DM. The analysis of genetic-associated studies reveals that genetic risk loci greater than 50 have been recognized as related to the immune system, especially human leukocyte antigen (HLA) encoding genes present in the region of the major histocompatibility complex (MHC) on the chromosome (Atkinson, 2012). The gene products linked with T1DM are known for performing functions such as the lowering of activation or signaling, the production or signaling of cytokines, an augmented response for antiviral as well as T1 interferon, and T cell formation along with antigen presentation (Li et al., 2015).

4.6.2 EPIGENETIC FACTORS

Notwithstanding the several factors contributing to T1DM onset, non-genetic factors, non-related with modification of DNA directly but potentially able to induce mitotically transmissible modification in expression of genes, are referred to as epigenetic factors. There are several mechanisms which not merely oversee the epigenetic effects but rather prompt each other via post-translational modification of histone protein, RNA-facilitated silencing of genes, and methylation of DNA molecule. The heritable epigenetic factors are not permanent but rather reversible as functions of alteration in environmental factors, and heritability of epigenetic factors in succeeding offspring occurs in somatic cells via conservation in some of the mitotic divisions. This explicit heritable alteration of chromatin governs the expression of gene and, against the environmental challenges, retorts pathologically as well as physiologically. The human leucocytes antigen (HLA) class I genes participate in progression of T1DM through following endogenous pathway for intracellular antigen processing and presentation to the T lymphocytes (Cerna, 2020; Nejentsev et al., 2007; Rose and Klose, 2014).

4.6.3 ENVIRONMENTAL FACTORS

The genetically susceptible population is prone to environmental factors-induced T1DM. Interestingly, environmental factors show a wide range of aspects with T1DM instigating potential and further augment the etiopathogenesis. Many physical properties of environmental factors are assumed to be developing or progressive causal elements of T1DM, such as the hotness of surrounding air, latitude of locality, and intensity and sunlight exposure. Bacterial, yeast-like fungal, and viral infections share a major segment of environmental factors associated with risk factors against T1DM. Following the corona pandemic, researchers have documented the significant contribution of the SARS-CoV-2 virus to the formation of type 1 diabetes by impairing insulin production that is dependent on glucose and by causing the infection-induced death and subsequent replication of pancreatic beta cells. Furthermore, viruses such as mumps virus, enterovirus, rubella virus, and Coxsackie virus have been found to be associated with T1DM (Abela and Fava, 2019; Zorena et al., 2022). The role of different food materials such as gluten in the initial months of the developmental phase has been substantiated experimentally and found to be very impactful in esteeming T1DM.

The genetically susceptible population is prone to environmental factor-induced T1DM. Interestingly, environmental factors encompass a wide range of aspects with the potential to instigate T1DM and further augment its etiopathogenesis. Many physical properties of environmental factors are assumed to be causative or progressive elements in the development of T1DM, such as ambient air temperature, latitude of the locality, and the intensity of sunlight exposure. Bacterial, yeast-like fungal, and viral infections constitute a major segment of the environmental risk factors associated with T1DM. Following the COVID-19 pandemic, researchers have documented the significant contribution of the SARS-CoV-2 virus to the development of type 1 diabetes by impairing glucose-dependent insulin production and causing infection-induced death and subsequent replication of pancreatic beta cells. Furthermore, viruses such as the mumps virus, enteroviruses, the rubella virus, and the Coxsackie virus have been found to be associated with T1DM (Abela and Fava, 2019; Zorena et al., 2022). The role of different food components, such as gluten, during the initial months of development has been substantiated experimentally and found to be highly influential in the development of T1DM.

4.7 RISK FACTORS FOR TYPE 2 DIABETES MELLITUS (T2DM)

4.7.1 GENETIC FACTOR

The various risk factors involved in the progression of T2DM have been categorized into non-modifiable and modifiable factors. Genetic character or family histories, along with ethnicity, are examples of non-modifiable risk factors, whereas lifestyle with less physical activity, a high caloric unhealthy diet, and obesity are known as modifiable factors. It has been observed that T2DM development differs in people of different geographical distributions and ethnicities. All races across the world develop T2DM, but prevalence is comparatively higher among Native Americans, Hispanics, African Americans, and other non-Caucasian populations (Galicia-Garcia et al., 2020; Hu, Manson et al., 2001). Moreover, along with thrifty genes, the Japanese population is assumed to possess several diabetic susceptible genes. This could be correlated by comparing the population of Western countries with Japanese people, since it has been evidenced that they exhibit lesser functionality of pancreatic cells, resulting in diminished insulin secretion potential (Kaku, 2010). The direct link between genetic factors and T2DM development has been strongly evidenced on the basis of a growing body of research.

The genetic factors cause impairment in the guiding system responsible for the metabolism of glucose molecules. As compared to dizygotic twins, monozygotic twins show a higher concordance rate for the onset of T2DM, which establishes a link between genetic factors and T2DM. The existence of over 50 diabetes–associated loci, mostly responsible for altering the function of pancreatic beta cells, has been recognized on the basis of genome-wide association studies (GWAS). It has been found that, regardless of the diabetes status of the parents, the relative risk for T2DM in a person is higher with a minimum of two siblings affected by T2DM. Similarly, on comparing children of diabetic and non-diabetic parents, it was revealed that, irrespective of whether the mother or father is diabetic, the offspring shows a risk of T2DM development more than thrice as high. Whereas, in the case of both diabetic parents, the chance of T2DM onset in children gets compounded six times more (Barnett et al., 1981; Meigs et al., 2000; Morris et al., 2012). The T2DM occurrence is reported at a lower body mass index (BMI) in Asian as well as Asian Americans as compared to the rest of the world, as it greatly varies among people with distinct body fat compositions or BMI levels (Araneta et al., 2015).

4.7.2 ENVIRONMENTAL FACTORS

Environmental factors play a critical and significant role in the progression of T2DM, which is again a modifiable factor and can be explained on the basis of the concept of the exposome. To differentiate the non-genetic environmental factors from non-modifiable ones, the term "exposome" was introduced in 2005 to represent the sum of environmental exposures that could trigger the onset of T2DM. The two categories of exposomes—internal and external—are further classifications for the exposome. Additionally, there exist two categories of external exposomes: the general external exposome and the specific external exposome. The general external exposome encompasses working as well as living spaces which have been physically created or developed around. Additionally, social interactions with groups of people with socioeconomic status, along with the availability and reasonability of food that directly connect with lifestyle, and the physical as well as chemical nature of the immediate surrounding are core examples of the general external exposome (Wild, 2005, 2012). The specific external exposome also includes several factors related to lifestyle. These lifestyle risk factors are involved in triggering T2DM, comprehending a wide range of aspects, and among all, obesity is considered the most imperative. Since obesity is also a heritable characteristic, it not only induces T2DM but rather facilitates the progression in approximately 90% of individuals. The potential lifestyle factors are smoking, consuming alcohol, a sedentary lifestyle, and a lack of physical work in the daily routine. Besides, some less discussed factors are the treatment of disease with certain medicines and experiencing momentous exposure of any kind of radiation, chemicals, or pollutants and nutrients related in improper amounts. Furthermore, other modifiable factors, including any specific disease, could also play a significant role in augmenting the prevalence of T2DM in patients. In obese adults, the major sleeping malady, obstructive sleep apnea (OSA), has been reported to be one of the most pertinent examples in affecting T2DM as well as prediabetes. The progression of diabetes and obesity are both correlated with more or less time of sleep (Pamidi and Tasali, 2012; Wild, 2012; Wu et al., 2014).

Since both the general exposome and specific exposome are linked and influence the internal exposome consecutively, that signifies assessment of a body's response against the challenges posed by the external exposome. The internal exposome is measured by analyzing the transcriptome, gut microbiome, metabolome, epigenetics, and transcriptome, and so forth. This analysis is accomplished by investigating the effects of modifiable lifestyles, such as the impact of smoking on the epigenome, or direct chemical screening via non-targeting. Smoking could trigger hyperglycemic conditions and insulin resistance since it is linked with elevated inflammation, oxidative stress, and obesity. It has been noticed that weight gain by new smoking quitters has shown an augmented risk in the advancement of T2DM (Guida et al., 2015; Niedzwiecki et al., 2019; Pan et al., 2015). The components of food material show an absolute influence on the T2DM progression, as it is evident that some fatty acids in the diet may expedite insulin resistance, whereas an augmented T2DM risk factor directly correlates with a higher glycemic index of a low-fiber diet. Obese people are highly prone to developing T2DM, and mild obesity in permutation with a high mass of visceral fat may show four to five times more chance of T2DM progression. The primary causal root of obesity is diet components such as reduced starch, high fat, low dietary fiber, the presence of high simple sugar, and lifestyle. Less muscle mass along with less physical workout with an unhealthy diet intensifies the obesity progression and leads to insulin resistance, which can be observed substantially as diabetic patients of high as well as middle-aged populations (Hu, van Dam et al., 2001; Liu et al., 2000). There are many consequences of deposited ectopic fat in organs like muscle and fat, such as inflammation in the islet of the pancreas, loss of beta cell functionality, and ultimately death of beta cells (van der Zijl et al., 2011). Furthermore, insulin resistance can be caused in insulin's target tissues, including organs like the liver, due to hepatitis C enterovirus infection (Feingold, 2000).

Air quality plays an imperative role in the progression of T2DM as a pollutant risk factor and may cause insulin resistance leading towards the disturbed proper glucose metabolic pathway followed by raised fasting glucose via augmentation in oxidative stress and systemic inflammation (Thiering and Heinrich, 2015).

4.7.3 EPIGENETICS

The heritable, cell-specific, and non-genetic modifications have proved the role of epigenetics in affecting the likelihood of T2DM onset, similar to the T1DM progression. The gene expression propensity by epigenetic factors is exhibited during embryonic development and during other stages of the life span. Furthermore, epigenetic changes may affect individuals in accordance with environmental interaction as dynamic expression alongside ancestral inheritance as static expression (Lacal and Ventura, 2018). It unravels the heterogeneous behavior of various cells and gene expression, even after possessing the same genetic content of humans. The growing body of evidence confirms that in distinct pathophysiological and physiological conditions, non-coding DNA regions are potentially regulated by epigenetics. Though the mechanism is still ambiguous, both excess and lack of a specific amount of nutrients in the intrauterine phase contribute to T2DM, cardiovascular disease (CVD), and obesity in the later phase of life by epigenetic modifications (Ainge et al., 2011; Capparelli and Iannelli, 2021; Zhou et al., 2018).

In recent years, several advanced and sensitive techniques have been developed to explore biomarkers for epigenetics linked with T2DM, like chromatin confirmation capture (3C)-derived assay chromatin immunoprecipitation (ChIP), especially to detect histone modification. The skeletal muscle cells and pancreatic islets from diabetic patients were selected to investigate the significance of epigenetics in T2DM development (Barres et al., 2009; Ling et al., 2008; Ma and Zhang, 2016). The studies confirmed the influence of modifications as a genuine culprit for T2DM and not a secondary disease. It is assumed that elevated glycated hemoglobin and glucose concentration endorse the methylation of DNA.

Investigation of three proteins—insulin, peroxisome proliferator-activated receptor-gamma coactivator alpha-1 (PGCα-1), and glucagon-like peptide-1 (GLP-1)—expressing genes, namely *INS*, *PDX1*, *PPARGC1A*, and the GLP-1 receptor, were performed against DNA methylation as compared to the pancreatic islets of non-diabetic, healthy persons. Ultimately, compromised insulin secretion takes place due to the under-expression of the above-mentioned set of three genes (Hall et al., 2013; Ling et al., 2008; Yang et al., 2011). Aging has been reported to be concomitant with T2DM onset, where DNA modification occurs in the form of methylation. Two spots on DNA—explicitly the NADH: ubiquinone oxidoreductase subunit B6 (NDUFB6) promoter for transcription factor binding and the CG nucleotide—are considered methylation-prone sites (Ling et al., 2007). Figure 4.2 portrays various risk factors responsible for the onset of both T1DM and T2DM.

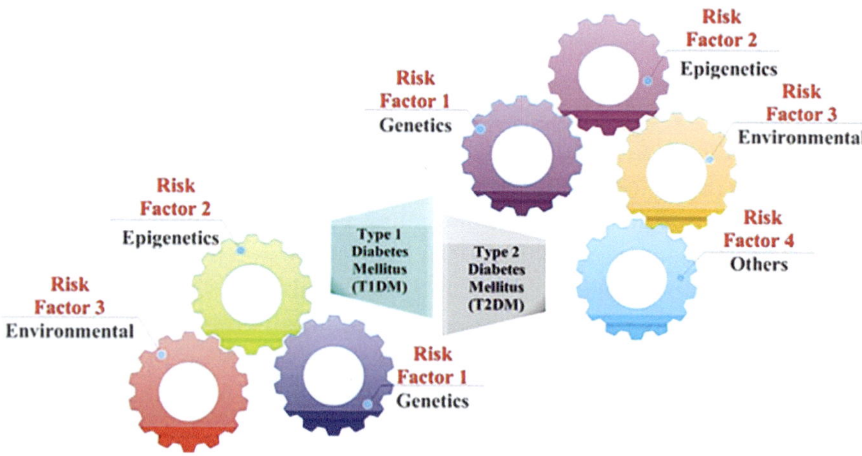

FIGURE 4.2 Representation of different factors associated with the progression of T1DM and T2DM.

4.7.4 OTHERS

Both the trivial and austere diabetes progression is connected with many disorders of the endocrine system. The adrenocorticotropic hormone (ACTH) overproduction in Cushing's disease and elevated plasma growth hormone causing overgrowth of face, feet, and bones in acromegaly are examples of endocrine disorders. According to the hypothesis of "fetal origin of disease" due to altered metabolism of glucose, in later phase of life, the chance of T2DM progression is very high for preterm babies with low weight during birth, which probably links with intrauterine growth restriction (Mericq et al., 2017).

4.8 PROTEIN AGGREGATION AND DIABETES

The improper folding of protein leads to a disordered conformation and causes the onset of several neurodegenerative and non-neurodegenerative diseases, collectively referred to as proteinopathies (Khan et al., 2018c). These protein aggregates are broadly categorized as amorphous and amyloid and detected by several aggregate-specific dyes microscopic investigation (Chandel et al., 2018; Khan et al., 2014, 2015, 2017, 2018a, b). Growing bodies of evidence have pieced together protein aggregation with diabetes progression. The process behind the development of T2DM is described by induced glucose alteration due to damaged islet cells of the pancreas. The damage of islet cells is caused by aggregation of amylin, also referred to as human islet amyloid polypeptide (hIAPP), due to misfolding followed by deposition mainly in the pancreas, besides many other organs such as the brain, kidney, liver, and even in circulating blood.

The unambiguous mechanism behind the amylin aggregation and deposition in organs is still debatable, but it connects the dots while distinguishing between T2DM progression from T1DM. The proteinaceous deposits from T2DM patient's pancreas were earlier reported as hyaline lesions. Chemical analysis of the amyloid revealed that the deposits are amylin neuropeptides from the calcitonin peptide family, made up of 37 amino acids and secreted from islets of the pancreas (Clark et al., 1996; Hassan et al., 2022; Westermark et al., 1987). The confirmation of amylin protein is highly sensitive against physical and chemical stress and undergoes aggregation in both *in vitro* and *in vivo*. The cytosolic as well as perinuclear dissemination of amylin aggregates has been observed in biopsy studies of diabetic patients' pancreatic islets. The accomplishment of alpha-helical and cytotoxic oligomers of amylin from the unfolded conformation of amylin takes place in response to the interaction of positively charged amylin with membranes or lipids containing negative charges. The alpha-helical conformation gains access to membrane permeation, while oligomers may induce apoptosis and alteration in islet functioning.

Amylin oligomers are also suggested to induce flaws in the secretion pathway, and after interaction with mitochondria, result in membrane disruption (Gurlo et al., 2010; Lin et al., 2007). Moreover, many case studies have revealed the formation of subcutaneous insulin aggregates, that is, amyloidosis, at the site of multiple injections when used as a therapeutic measure against T1DM and T2DM, and associated with impulsive hypoglycemia and chronic hyperglycemia. Such iatrogenic and localized insulin amyloids have been termed "AIns" by the Committee of Nomenclature of the International Society of Amyloidosis. The formation of insulin amyloid is not only related to poor diabetes management practices but rather puts an extra economic burden to employ more insulin than the prescribed dose, even to control the same glucose level.

Furthermore, surrounding tissues at the site of insulin administration may also be damaged due to the cytotoxic nature of aggregates and interactive behavior with blood components. This problem may get further compounded since several other modes of insulin administration, including injection and infusion, and even more advanced methods of insulin delivery via nebulization of powdered insulin protein, experience insulin amyloidosis. The formation of some non-inflammatory and painless protuberances underneath the skin may also be a result of insulin amyloidosis, along with discernible papules on the patient's body. In some patients, it has been observed that the insulin amyloidosis site remains preferable for administering insulin doses due to less painful insertion compared to other sites of injection (Lasagna-Reeves et al., 2010; Nilsson, 2016; Sipe et al., 2014).

There is a need for a clear distinction between insulin amyloids and lipohypertrophy, a subcutaneous extra fat accumulation causing insulin absorption impairment. The mandatory high dose of insulin due to amyloidosis in diabetic patients under treatment, as a consequence of a diminished rate of absorbance, results in unusual weight gain. The materialization of lipohypertrophy occurs in almost half of T1DM patients during treatment and may cause ambiguity in amyloidosis diagnosis. The determination of insulin amyloid at the site of frequent injection can be detected and distinguished from lipohypertrophy by a classical amyloid-specific dye, which potentially detects the presence of amyloid *in vivo* and also *in vitro* but does not interact with amorphous variants of protein aggregates (Khan et al., 2018a, b; Nilsson, 2016; Okamura et al., 2013).

4.9 DIABETIC COMORBIDITIES

Comorbidities can increase the complexity of managing diabetes. For instance, more medication may be required to regulate blood pressure and cholesterol in those with diabetes and CVD. Dialysis or a kidney transplant may be necessary for those with diabetes and chronic renal dysfunction. Comorbidities can also raise the chance of emergency department visits and hospital stays. Table 4.3 and Figure 4.3 summarize comorbidities directly linked with diabetic condition.

TABLE 4.3 List of Comorbidities Associated with Diabetes and Effects of Hyperglycemia

Comorbidity	Effects of Hyperglycemia	References
Cardiovascular diseases and heart failure	Damage to blood vessels, formation of atherosclerotic plaques, and thrombosis. Elevated levels of oxidative stress and the induction of several inflammatory pathways cause both extracellular and cellular damage, along with abnormal cardiac remodeling and both diastolic and systolic dysfunction.	Elendu et al. (2023); Mengstie et al. (2022); Tousoulis et al. (2014)
Stroke	Systemic inflammation, thickening of the capillary basement membrane, vascular endothelial dysfunction, and increased stiffness of early-age arteries.	Chen et al. (2016); Mosenzon et al. (2023); Zhu and Jiang (2023)
Renal diseases	Thickening of the glomerular basement membrane; mesangial expansion due to extracellular matrix accumulation; alterations in the number and/or density of glomerular epithelial cells (podocytes); broadening and effacement of the podocyte foot process; glomerulosclerosis; and tubulointerstitial fibrosis.	Bonner et al. (2020); Kumar et al. (2023); Reidy et al. (2014)
Neuropathy and retinopathy	Damage to nerves and microvasculature; neurodegeneration.	Coucha et al. (2015); Rasheed et al. (2021)
Dyslipidemia	Raised levels of hormone-sensitive lipase, which breaks down triglycerides and releases free fatty acids in adipose tissue.	Sztalryd and Kraemer (1995); Yanai et al. (2019)
Hypertension	Prolonged stress stimulates the sympathetic nervous system (SNS) and the hypothalamus-pituitary-adrenal (HPA-axis), increasing cortisol synthesis in the adrenal cortex and adrenaline and noradrenaline production in the adrenal medulla.	Ohishi (2018); Petrie et al. (2018)
Skin diseases	Immune system dysfunction and microvasculature damage.	Duff et al. (2015); Mendes et al. (2017)

4.9.1 CARDIOVASCULAR DISEASES (CVDS)

Cardiovascular disease (CVD) is one of the most typical complications of diabetes. Peripheral artery disease (PAD) and heart disease are conditions that diabetes makes more likely to occur. This is because diabetes has the potential to harm blood arteries and encourage the development of blood clots (Matheus et al., 2013). CVDs and diabetes have a complicated,

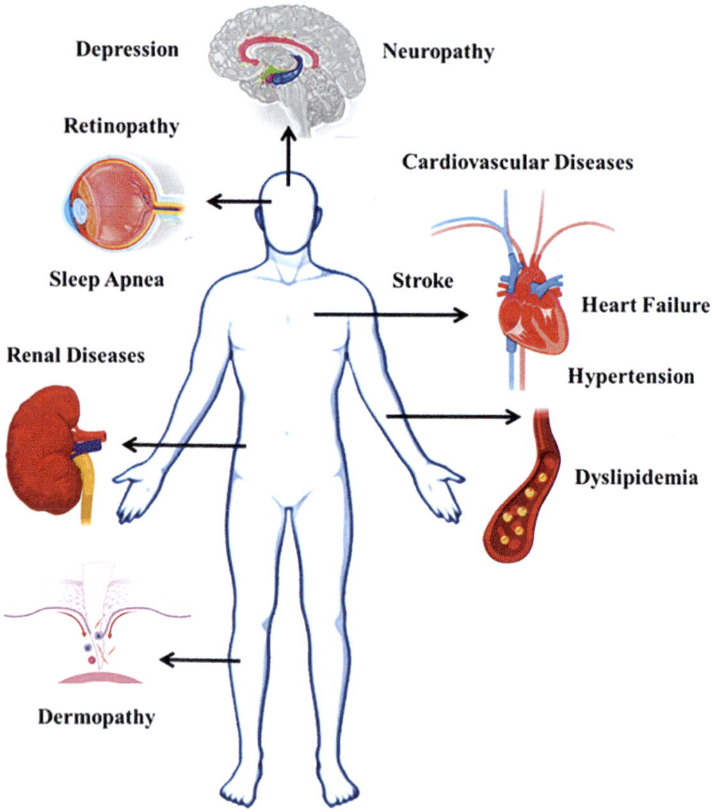

FIGURE 4.3 Schematic representation of diabetes-induced comorbidities and their consequences.

reciprocal interaction in which one condition both predisposes and exacerbates the other. Diabetes, which is defined by persistently high BSLs, accelerates atherosclerosis and raises the risk of CVDs, including peripheral arterial disease, coronary artery disease (CAD), and stroke, by causing endothelial dysfunction, inflammation, and oxidative stress. On the other hand, by decreasing insulin sensitivity, lowering glucose tolerance, and raising the risk of diabetic complications, CVDs can make diabetes treatment more difficult.

The underlying mechanisms involve shared risk factors, including obesity, physical inactivity, hypertension, dyslipidemia, and smoking. The elevated BGL in diabetes damages blood vessels, promotes the formation of atherosclerotic plaques, and increases the possibility of thrombosis, contributing to CAD and stroke (Shoelson et al., 2006). Additionally, diabetes impairs the body's ability to sense and respond to insulin, resulting in insulin resistance, which further exacerbates CVD risk (Czech, 2017). CVDs, in turn, can increase the severity and frequency of diabetic complications, including retinopathy, nephropathy, and neuropathy, due to the compromised blood flow and impaired oxygenation of tissues (Deshpande et al., 2008).

4.9.2 STROKE

For many reasons, people with diabetes have a higher risk of stroke. First, diabetes can damage blood vessels, making them more likely to become clogged or blocked (Rask-Madsen and King, 2013). Secondly, hypertension is an additional risk factor for stroke that can result from diabetes. Third, diabetes raises the chance of other illnesses, including heart disease and high cholesterol, which can also raise the risk of stroke (Pop-Busui et al., 2022). Individuals with diabetes who also have poor blood sugar management are at significantly greater risk of stroke. It is really two to four times more common for diabetics with poor blood sugar management to suffer a stroke than for those with adequate blood sugar control (Nanayakkara et al., 2021).

4.9.3 HEART FAILURE

Diabetes and heart failure, two seemingly separate conditions, are deeply intertwined, forming a dangerous cycle that significantly increases the risk of severe health complications and mortality. The presence of diabetes, regardless of type, significantly increases the risk of developing heart failure (Pop-Busui et al., 2022). This is due to the damaging effects of high blood sugar on the cardiovascular system. Chronic hyperglycemia leads to inflammation and thickening of the blood vessels, impairing blood flow and increasing strain on the heart.

This finally results in heart failure because it weakens the heart muscle and reduces its ability to pump blood throughout the body (Maack et al., 2018; Rubler et al., 1972). Conversely, heart failure can worsen diabetes control, creating a vicious cycle. The reduced blood flow from a weakened heart can lead to poor blood sugar regulation, further exacerbating hyperglycemia and accelerating the progression of both conditions (Murtaza et al., 2019). This complex relationship necessitates a multi-disciplinary approach to management, involving meticulous blood sugar control, strict adherence to cardiovascular health guidelines, and close monitoring of both conditions. In order to reduce the dangers and enhance the quality of life for those who bear this dual burden, early detection and management are essential.

4.9.4 RENAL DISEASES

Renal health is seriously threatened by diabetes, a chronic illness marked by increased BSLs. The persistently elevated blood sugar damages the small blood arteries in the kidneys, resulting in a series of issues called diabetic nephropathy (Cameron, 2006; Reutens, 2013). This insidious process begins with thickening of the glomerular basement membrane, the filtering unit of the kidney, restricting blood flow and impairing filtration. As the disease progresses, the glomeruli become scarred and damaged, resulting in proteinuria, the leakage of protein into the urine (Caramori et al., 2013; Fioretto and Mauer, 2007). This protein loss can cause edema and ultimately lead to kidney failure. Hypertension, a frequent companion of diabetes, further aggravates the damage by straining the delicate blood vessels (Han, 2012). The persistent damage to the kidneys can eventually lead to end-stage renal disease (ESRD), requiring dialysis or a kidney transplant to sustain life. Managing diabetes effectively through blood sugar control, blood pressure management, and healthy lifestyle choices is crucial in preventing and delaying the onset of diabetic nephropathy.

4.9.5 NEUROPATHY

Diabetic neuropathy, a debilitating complication of diabetes, arises from damaging of nerves due to elevated BSLs over time (Ashok et al., 2002). Damage to the nerves can result in a variety of symptoms, such as tingling, discomfort, weakness, and numbness, throughout the body. Peripheral neuropathy, the most prevalent kind, damages the nerves in the hands and feet and can result in burning, pins-and-needles sensation, or even loss of feeling (Bajaj and Banerji, 2004; Sadikot et al., 2004). Diabetic neuropathy may also impact the autonomic nervous system, regulating vital functions such as digestion, heart rate, and blood pressure, potentially leading to problems like gastroparesis, orthostatic hypotension, and erectile dysfunction. The severity and location of the nerve damage can vary greatly, with some individuals experiencing mild symptoms, while others suffer from severe pain and functional limitations. Effective management of diabetic neuropathy involves strict blood sugar control, management of pain and symptoms, and lifestyle modifications including regular exercise and a healthy diet (Cernea and Raz, 2021).

In order to stop more nerve damage and maintain quality of life, early identification and treatment are essential. While there is no cure for diabetic neuropathy, understanding and addressing the underlying cause of diabetes and its complications remains paramount in the prevention and management of this often-devastating condition. Diabetic neuropathy can be peripheral or autonomic (Levitt et al., 1996; Partanen et al., 1995). In peripheral neuropathy, diabetes damages nerves in the hands, feet, and legs, causing numbness, tingling, pain, and weakness (Bodman et al., 2024). Autonomic neuropathy affects nerves controlling involuntary functions, such as digestion, urinary function, and blood pressure regulation (Vinik et al., 2003).

4.9.6 RETINOPATHY

One of the main causes of adult blindness in affluent nations is diabetic retinopathy. It is a diabetic condition that impacts the blood vessels in the retina, the area at the back of the eye that is sensitive to light (Eisma et al., 2015; Sayin et al., 2015). Furthermore, diabetic retinopathy can lead to a variety of vision-associated difficulties, like blurred vision, double vision, and blind spots. In severe cases, it can lead to blindness (Wang et al., 2020). Nonproliferative diabetic retinopathy (NPDR) and proliferative diabetic retinopathy (PDR) are the two basic forms of diabetic retinopathy. The NPDR, or early stage of diabetic retinopathy, is defined by the formation of tiny aneurysms, or bulges, in the retina's blood vessels (Khan et al., 2017). PDR is a more severe form of diabetic retinopathy that is distinguished by the development of new blood vessels on the retina's surface. Vision issues may result from the fragility of these new blood vessels and their potential for blood leakage. A thorough eye examination that includes a fluorescein angiography and a dilated eye exam is used to identify diabetic retinopathy. The course of treatment for diabetic retinopathy is determined by the disease's stage (Mansour et al., 2020; Mounirou et al., 2022). Treatment for NPDR typically includes lifestyle changes, like controlling BSLs, blood pressure, and regular eye exams. Treatment for PDR may include laser therapy, eye injections, or surgery. To avoid visual loss, diabetic retinopathy must be identified and treated as soon as possible (Tomita et al., 2021). Regular eye exams are recommended for people with diabetes to screen for and monitor diabetic retinopathy.

4.9.7 HYPERTENSION (HIGH BLOOD PRESSURE)

Diabetes and hypertension, two seemingly distinct conditions, are often intertwined, creating a complex and potentially dangerous health scenario. Diabetes, a long-term metabolic disease marked by high blood sugar, frequently results in blood vessel damage, including kidney and heart damage. This damage intensifies the risk of developing hypertension, an ailment of consistently elevated blood pressure (Oparil et al., 2003; Petrie et al., 2018). In turn, hypertension further exacerbates the effects of diabetes, accelerating the damage to blood vessels and increasing the risk of heart attacks, strokes, and kidney failure (Meijer et al., 2012; Su et al., 2008). Each of these illnesses exacerbates the others, creating a vicious cycle that raises the likelihood of major health issues. This vicious cycle emphasizes how critical it is to treat both hypertension and diabetes with thorough care and early identification. Dietary and activity changes are essential for treating these disorders, and prescription drugs can help lower blood pressure and regulate blood sugar. The long-term health implications of diabetes and hypertension underscore the need for individuals to be proactive about their health, actively monitoring their blood sugar and blood pressure, and seeking professional medical advice to optimize their management and reduce the risks associated with these conditions (Cohen and Cohen, 2016).

4.9.8 DYSLIPIDEMIA (ABNORMAL CHOLESTEROL LEVELS)

Diabetes mellitus patients frequently develop diabetes-induced dyslipidemia, a complicated metabolic condition marked by anomalies in lipid metabolism (Chapman et al., 2011; Howard et al., 2000). Triglycerides (TGs) and lipoproteins containing apolipoprotein B (ApoB), such as very-low-density lipoprotein (VLDL) and intermediate-density lipoprotein (IDL), are primarily elevated in this dyslipidemic profile, whereas high-density lipoprotein (HDL) cholesterol levels are frequently decreased (Fox et al., 2015; Schofield et al., 2016). Insulin resistance and decreased insulin production are two of the several underlying processes of diabetes-induced dyslipidemia. Insulin resistance, a hallmark of type 2 diabetes, causes the liver to produce more VLDL-TGs and to have less lipoprotein lipase (LPL) activity, which lowers the amount of TG-rich lipoproteins that are cleared from the body (de Ferranti et al., 2014). Furthermore, increased lipolysis and the release of free fatty acids (FFAs) from adipose tissue can be caused by decreased insulin secretion, especially in type 1 diabetes, which exacerbates hypertriglyceridemia. The buildup of TG-rich lipoproteins and the creation of tiny, dense LDL particles—which are more vulnerable to oxidation and inflammation—as a result of these metabolic changes raise the risk of cardiovascular events.

4.9.9 SLEEP APNEA

Diabetes and sleep apnea are two common and often co-occurring health conditions. Low oxygen levels and interrupted sleep are the results of sleep apnea, a disease marked by frequent breathing pauses while sleeping. Several factors contribute to this link. Firstly, individuals with diabetes often have excess weight and obesity, known risk factors for sleep apnea. Individuals with diabetes are at an increased risk of developing sleep apnea, and the presence of sleep apnea can exacerbate diabetes management (Pamidi and Tasali, 2012; Wild, 2012; Young and Finn, 1998). Throughout sleep, the airway may get obstructed by the extra fat deposits in the throat and neck. Second, diabetes' high BGLs can cause tissue alterations and inflammation, which may worsen airway constriction (Tsalamandris et al., 2019).

The cyclical nature of these conditions is concerning: sleep apnea can worsen blood sugar control by disrupting sleep, leading to insulin resistance and increased risk of complications like hypoglycemia. Conversely, poor blood sugar control in diabetes can exacerbate sleep apnea by further contributing to inflammation and airway narrowing. This vicious cycle highlights the importance of early diagnosis and management of both conditions to prevent further complications and optimize overall health. Lifestyle changes such as quitting smoking and drinking, losing weight, and engaging in regular physical activity are all necessary for effective treatment. Continuous positive airway pressure (CPAP) therapy could be required in some situations to keep the airways open during sleep (Labarca et al., 2018). A balanced diet and strict blood sugar management with medication are essential for people with diabetes to properly manage their disease. Individuals can improve their general health, lower the chance of long-term issues, and increase their quality of life by treating sleep apnea and diabetes together.

4.9.10 DEPRESSION

Diabetes-induced depression is a major mental health issue that may profoundly impair the lives of those with diabetes (Chen et al., 2016; Roy and Lloyd, 2012). It has been estimated that up to 30% of people with diabetes experience depressive symptoms, which can range from mild feelings of sadness and hopelessness to severe episodes of major depression (Grigsby et al., 2002). Diabetes and depression have a complicated and reciprocal interaction in which the intensity and course of each illness is influenced by the other. People with diabetes may develop depression as a result of long-term stress, hormone abnormalities, and the psychological strain of managing a chronic illness (Herbert et al., 2006; Moulton et al., 2015).

Conversely, depression can worsen diabetes control by affecting medication adherence, diet, and exercise regimens, leading to further complications and a diminished quality of life. The presence of depression in diabetes not only compromises mental well-being but also increases the risk of cardiovascular events, diabetic retinopathy, nephropathy, and other diabetes-associated complications (Simon et al., 2007). Consequently, in order to improve general health outcomes and improve the quality of life for those with diabetes, early detection and appropriate therapy of depression are vital.

4.9.11 SKIN CONDITIONS

Diabetes can have a serious effect on the skin. Elevated BSLs have the potential to harm blood vessels and nerves, resulting in weakened skin integrity and heightened vulnerability to infections. Diabetes increases a person's risk of developing both common and uncommon skin disorders. One common manifestation is diabetic dermopathy, characterized by round or oval, reddish-brown spots, typically found on the lower legs

(Bustan et al., 2017; David et al., 2023). Another condition is necrobiosis lipoidica diabeticorum, which presents as raised, yellowish-brown patches or plaques, often on the shins and forearms (Boulton et al., 1988). Additionally, diabetes can intensify existing skin conditions such as eczema and psoriasis. Prolonged hyperglycemia can impair wound healing, making even minor cuts or abrasions more difficult to resolve, potentially leading to infections and complications (Dasari et al., 2021). Moreover, diabetic neuropathy can result in less sensation in the feet, which may aggravate infections or injuries over time. In order to maintain skin health, prevent infections, and swiftly address any skin issues, people with diabetes must practice proper skin care and regular skin monitoring.

4.10 MANAGEMENT STRATEGIES FOR DIABETES-ASSOCIATED COMORBIDITIES

A multifaceted strategy that tackles the underlying diabetes as well as the particular consequences is needed to manage diabetes-related comorbidities. This is careful blood glucose monitoring and following a customized diabetes care plan that calls for good food, frequent exercise, and weight control, among other lifestyle changes. For hypertension, blood pressure monitoring and medication adjustments are crucial (Possidente and Ongaro, 2001). Similarly, managing dyslipidemia includes monitoring cholesterol levels and employing statins or other lipid-lowering medications (Glasziou et al., 2008). Addressing diabetic retinopathy involves regular eye exams and potential laser treatment, while diabetic neuropathy necessitates pain management and lifestyle changes to reduce nerve damage (Cernea and Raz, 2021; Raman et al., 2021).

Furthermore, managing diabetic nephropathy requires strict blood pressure control, monitoring kidney function, and potentially medications to slow disease progression (Fineberg et al., 2013). Regular foot inspections, suitable footwear, and quick wound care are all part of managing foot issues. Comprehensive tests are essential for early detection, and prevention is still the key. Additionally, encouraging self-management abilities and enhancing therapy adherence depend heavily on patient education and support. Effective communication between patients and healthcare providers ensures personalized strategies are tailored to individual needs and ensures the best possible outcomes in managing diabetes-associated comorbidities.

4.11 CONCLUSION AND FUTURE PERSPECTIVES

The management of diabetes comorbidities is entering a transformative phase, marked by a growing comprehension of the intricate relationships that exist between diabetes and other concomitant diseases. Future perspectives in this area emphasize a holistic approach that integrates multifactorial strategies to address not only glycemic control but also the associated health complications. Technological innovations like telemedicine and continuous glucose monitoring (CGM) provide new possibilities for real-time data collection and individualized care, allowing medical professionals to customize patient regimens based on specific patient profiles. Beyond technology, there is an increasing emphasis on interdisciplinary collaboration among healthcare professionals. Future diabetes management paradigms will likely include coordinated efforts among endocrinologists, cardiologists, nephrologists, dietitians, and mental health professionals. This team-based care model aims to ensure that patients receive comprehensive treatment plans that recognize and target the unique challenges posed by comorbidities like CVD, obesity, and mental health disorders, which are prevalent in the diabetes population.

Furthermore, the emergence of precision medicine holds the potential to improve our comprehension of the genetic and environmental elements that contribute to diabetes and its associated conditions. Healthcare professionals can create specialized treatments and preventative measures that target the underlying causes of these disorders rather than just treating their symptoms by identifying certain biomarkers and risk factors. As research develops, we should expect novel pharmacological treatments that enhance renal function, cardiovascular health, and the general quality of life for diabetic patients in addition to controlling BSLs. The management of diabetes comorbidities will ultimately depend on a patient-centered strategy in which self-management and education are essential components. Patients will be more proactive in their healthcare journey and will have better results and improved management of their diabetes and related comorbidities if they are empowered by easily available tools and support networks. This shift towards a more integrated and personalized approach heralds a new era in diabetes care, emphasizing prevention, early intervention, and the importance of a multifaceted treatment strategy.

KEYWORDS

- **advanced glycation end-products**
- **continuous glucose monitoring**
- **continuous positive airway pressure**
- **diabetes mellitus**
- **free fatty acids**
- **healthcare**
- **hyperglycemia**
- **intermediate-density lipoprotein**
- **precision medicine**

REFERENCES

Abela, A. G., & Fava, S. (2019). Incidence of type 1 diabetes and distance from the sea: A descriptive epidemiological study. *J Diabetes, 11*(5), 345–347. https://doi.org/10.1111/1753-0407.12862 (accessed on 2nd February 2026).

Ahmed, A. M. (2002). History of diabetes mellitus. *Saudi Med J, 23*(4), 373–378.

Ainge, H. (2011). A systematic review on animal models of maternal high fat feeding and offspring glycemic control. *Int J Obes (Lond), 35*(3), 325–335. https://doi.org/ijo2010149 (accessed on 2nd February 2026).

Alberti, K. G., & Zimmet, P. Z. (1998). Definition, diagnosis and classification of diabetes mellitus and its complications. Part 1: Diagnosis and classification of diabetes mellitus. Provisional report of a WHO consultation. *Diabet Med, 15*(7), 539–553. https://doi.org/10.1002/(SICI)1096-9136(199807)15:7<539::AID-DIA668>3.0.CO;2-S (accessed on 2nd February 2026).

Allen, L. A., & Dayan, C. M. (2021). Immunotherapy for type 1 diabetes. *Br Med Bull, 140*(1), 76–90. https://doi.org/6459277 (accessed on 2nd February 2026).

American Diabetes Association Professional Practice Committee. (2024). Diagnosis and classification of diabetes: Standards of care in diabetes–2024. *Diabetes Care, 47*(Suppl 1), S20–S42. https://doi.org/10.2337/dc24-S002 (accessed on 2nd February 2026).

Anton, G. (2011). Type-specific human papillomavirus detection in cervical smears in Romania. *APMIS, 119*(1), 1–9. https://doi.org/10.1111/j.1600-0463.2010.02641.x (accessed on 2nd February 2026).

Araneta, M. R. (2015). Optimum BMI cut points to screen Asian Americans for type 2 diabetes. *Diabetes Care, 38*(5), 814–820. https://doi.org/dc14-2071 (accessed on 2nd February 2026).

Aschner, P. (2020). Insulin therapy in type 2 diabetes. *Am J Ther, 27*(1), e79–e90. https://doi.org/00045391-202001000-00009 (accessed on 2nd February 2026).

Ashok, S. (2002). Prevalence of neuropathy in type 2 diabetic patients attending a diabetes center in South India. *J Assoc Physicians India, 50*, 546–550.

Atkinson, M. A. (2012). The pathogenesis and natural history of type 1 diabetes. *Cold Spring Harb Perspect Med, 2*(11). https://doi.org/2/11/a007641 (accessed on 2nd February 2026).

Bajaj, M., & Banerji, M. A. (2004). Type 2 diabetes in South Asians: A pathophysiologic focus on the Asian-Indian epidemic. *Curr Diab Rep, 4*(3), 213–218. https://doi.org/10.1007/s11892-004-0026-4 (accessed on 2nd February 2026).

Bani Hamad, F. R. (2021). Efficacy of stem cell application in diabetes mellitus: Promising future therapy for diabetes and its complications. *Cureus, 13*(2), e13563. https://doi.org/10.7759/cureus.13563 (accessed on 2nd February 2026).

Barnett, A. H. (1981). Diabetes in identical twins: A study of 200 pairs. *Diabetology, 20*(2), 87–93. https://doi.org/10.1007/BF00262007 (accessed on 2nd February 2026).

Barres, R. (2009). Non-CpG methylation of the PGC-1alpha promoter through DNMT3B controls mitochondrial density. *Cell Metab, 10*(3), 189–198. https://doi.org/S1550-4131(09)00229-0 (accessed on 2nd February 2026).

Benson, V. S. (2010). Type 1 diabetes mellitus and components in drinking water and diet: A population-based, case-control study in Prince Edward Island, Canada. *J Am Coll Nutr, 29*(6), 612–624. https://doi.org/29/6/612 (accessed on 2nd February 2026).

Blair, M. (2016). Diabetes mellitus review. *Urol Nurs, 36*(1), 27–36.

Bodman, M. A. (2024). *Diabetic Peripheral Neuropathy*. https://doi.org/NBK442009 (accessed on 2nd February 2026).

Bonner, R. (2020). Diabetic kidney disease. *Prim Care, 47*(4), 645–659. https://doi.org/S0095-4543(20)30058-0 (accessed on 2nd February 2026).

Boughton, C. K., & Hovorka, R. (2020). The artificial pancreas. *Curr Opin Organ Transplant, 25*(4), 336–342. https://doi.org/00075200-202008000-00006 (accessed on 2nd February 2026).

Boulton, A. J. (1988). Necrobiosis lipidic diabeticorum: A clinicopathologic study. *J Am Acad Dermatol, 18*(3), 530–537. https://doi.org/S0190-9622(88)70076-6 (accessed on 2nd February 2026).

Bustan, R. S. (2017). Specific skin signs as a cutaneous marker of diabetes mellitus and the prediabetic state: A systematic review. *Dan Med J, 64*(1). https://doi.org/A5316 (accessed on 2nd February 2026).

Cameron, J. S. (2006). The discovery of diabetic nephropathy: From small print to center stage. *J Nephrol, 19*(Suppl 10), S75–S87.

Capparelli, R., & Iannelli, D. (2021). Role of epigenetics in type 2 diabetes and obesity. *Biomedicines, 9*(8). https://doi.org/biomedicines9080977 (accessed on 2nd February 2026).

Caramori, M. L. (2013). Renal lesions predict progression of diabetic nephropathy in type 1 diabetes. *J Am Soc Nephrol, 24*(7), 1175–1181. https://doi.org/ASN.2012070739 (accessed on 2nd February 2026).

Cerna, M. (2020). Epigenetic regulation in etiology of type 1 diabetes mellitus. *Int J Mol Sci, 21*(1). https://doi.org/ijms21010036 (accessed on 2nd February 2026).

Cernea, S., & Raz, I. (2021). Management of diabetic neuropathy. *Metabolism, 123*, 154867. https://doi.org/S0026-0495(21)00167-0 (accessed on 2nd February 2026).

Chandel, T. I. (2018). A mechanistic insight into protein–ligand interaction, folding, misfolding, aggregation and inhibition of protein aggregates: An overview. *Int J Biol Macromol, 106*, 1115–1129. https://doi.org/S0141-8130(17)33099-4 (accessed on 2nd February 2026).

Chapman, M. J. (2011). Triglyceride-rich lipoproteins and high-density lipoprotein cholesterol in patients at high risk of cardiovascular disease: Evidence and guidance for management. *Eur Heart J, 32*(11), 1345–1361. https://doi.org/ehr112 (accessed on 2nd February 2026).

Chen, R. (2016). Diabetes and stroke: Epidemiology, pathophysiology, pharmaceuticals and outcomes. *Am J Med Sci, 351*(4), 380–386. https://doi.org/S0002-9629(15)37933-7 (accessed on 2nd February 2026).

Chen, S. (2016). Association of depression with pre-diabetes, undiagnosed diabetes, and previously diagnosed diabetes: A meta-analysis. *Endocrine, 53*(1), 35–46. https://doi.org/10.1007/s12020-016-0869-x (accessed on 2nd February 2026).

Clark, A. (1996). Islet amyloid in type 2 (non-insulin-dependent) diabetes. *APMIS, 104*(1), 12–18. https://doi.org/10.1111/j.1699-0463.1996.tb00680.x (accessed on 2nd February 2026).

Cohen, J. B., & Cohen, D. L. (2016). Integrating out-of-office blood pressure in the diagnosis and management of hypertension. *Curr Cardiol Rep, 18*(11), 112. https://doi.org/10.1007/s11886-016-0780-3 (accessed on 2nd February 2026).

Coucha, M. (2015). Molecular mechanisms of diabetic retinopathy: Potential therapeutic targets. *Middle East Afr J Ophthalmol, 22*(2), 135–144. https://doi.org/MEAJO-22-135 (accessed on 2nd February 2026).

Craig, M. E. (2009). Definition, epidemiology and classification of diabetes in children and adolescents. *Pediatric Diabetes, 10*(Suppl 12), 3–12. https://doi.org/PDI568 (accessed on 2nd February 2026).

Czech, M. P. (2017). Insulin action and resistance in obesity and type 2 diabetes. *Nat Med, 23*(7), 804–814. https://doi.org/nm.4350 (accessed on 2nd February 2026).

Dahlquist, G. G. (1990). Dietary factors and the risk of developing insulin dependent diabetes in childhood. *BMJ, 300*(6735), 1302–1306. https://doi.org/10.1136/bmj.300.6735.1302 (accessed on 2nd February 2026).

Dasari, N. (2021). Updates in diabetic wound healing, inflammation, and scarring. *Semin Plast Surg, 35*(3), 153–158. https://doi.org/01305 (accessed on 2nd February 2026).

David, P. (2023). A comprehensive overview of skin complications in diabetes and their prevention. *Cureus, 15*(5), e38961. https://doi.org/10.7759/cureus.38961 (accessed on 2nd February 2026).

de Ferranti, S. D. (2014). Type 1 diabetes mellitus and cardiovascular disease: A scientific statement from the American Heart Association and American Diabetes Association. *Circulation, 130*(13), 1110–1130. https://doi.org/CIR.0000000000000034 (accessed on 2nd February 2026).

Defronzo, R. A. (2009). Banting Lecture. From the triumvirate to the ominous octet: A new paradigm for the treatment of type 2 diabetes mellitus. *Diabetes, 58*(4), 773–795. https://doi.org/58/4/773 (accessed on 2nd February 2026).

Deshpande, A. D. (2008). Epidemiology of diabetes and diabetes-related complications. *Phys Ther, 88*(11), 1254–1264. https://doi.org/ptj.20080020 (accessed on 2nd February 2026).

Duff, M. (2015). Cutaneous manifestations of diabetes mellitus. *Clin Diabetes, 33*(1), 40–48. https://doi.org/40 (accessed on 2nd February 2026).

Eisma, J. H. (2015). Current knowledge on diabetic retinopathy from human donor tissues. *World J Diabetes, 6*(2), 312–320. https://doi.org/10.4239/wjd.v6.i2.312 (accessed on 2nd February 2026).

Elendu, C. (2023). Heart failure and diabetes: Understanding the bidirectional relationship. *Medicine (Baltimore), 102*(37), e34906. https://doi.org/00005792-202309150-00025 (accessed on 2nd February 2026).

Fadini, G. P. (2017). SGLT2 inhibitors and diabetic ketoacidosis: Data from the FDA Adverse Event Reporting System. *Diabetology, 60*(8), 1385–1389. https://doi.org/10.1007/s00125-017-4301-8 (accessed on 2nd February 2026).

Feingold, K. R. (2000). *Atypical Forms of Diabetes*. https://doi.org/NBK279128 (accessed on 2nd February 2026).

Fineberg, D. (2013). Diabetic nephropathy: Diagnosis and treatment. *Nat Rev Endocrinol, 9*(12), 713–723. https://doi.org/nrendo.2013.184 (accessed on 2nd February 2026).

Fioretto, P., & Mauer, M. (2007). Histopathology of diabetic nephropathy. *Semin Nephrol, 27*(2), 195–207. https://doi.org/S0270-9295(07)00014-9 (accessed on 2nd February 2026).

Fox, C. S. (2015). Update on prevention of cardiovascular disease in adults with type 2 diabetes mellitus in light of recent evidence: A scientific statement from the American Heart Association and the American Diabetes Association. *Diabetes Care, 38*(9), 1777–1803. https://doi.org/dci15-0012 (accessed on 2nd February 2026).

Funda, D. P. (1999). Gluten-free diet prevents diabetes in NOD mice. *Diabetes Metab Res Rev, 15*(5), 323–327. https://doi.org/10.1002/(SICI)1520-7560(199909/10)15:5<323::AID-DMRR53>3.0.CO;2-P (accessed on 2nd February 2026).

Galicia-Garcia, U. (2020). Pathophysiology of type 2 diabetes mellitus. *Int J Mol Sci, 21*(17). https://doi.org/ijms21176275 (accessed on 2nd February 2026).

Genuth, S. M., Palmer, J. P., Nathan, D. M., Cowie, C. C., Casagrande, S. S., Menke, A., et al. (2018). Classification and diagnosis of diabetes. In *Diabetes in America* (3rd ed., Chapter 1). National Institute of Diabetes and Digestive and Kidney Diseases (US), Bethesda (MD).

Glasziou, P. P. (2008). Monitoring cholesterol levels: Measurement error or true change? *Ann Intern Med, 148*(9), 656–661. https://doi.org/148/9/656 (accessed on 2nd February 2026).

Gordon, C. (2019). Blood glucose monitoring in diabetes: Rationale and procedure. *Br J Nurs, 28*(7), 434–439. https://doi.org/10.12968/bjon.2019.28.7.434 (accessed on 2nd February 2026).

Grigsby, A. B. (2002). Prevalence of anxiety in adults with diabetes: A systematic review. *J Psychosom Res, 53*(6), 1053–1060. https://doi.org/S0022399902004178 (accessed on 2nd February 2026).

Guida, F. (2015). Dynamics of smoking-induced genome-wide methylation changes with time since smoking cessation. *Hum Mol Genet, 24*(8), 2349–2359. https://doi.org/ddu751 (accessed on 2nd February 2026).

Gurlo, T. (2010). Evidence for proteotoxicity in beta cells in type 2 diabetes: Toxic islet amyloid polypeptide oligomers form intracellularly in the secretory pathway. *Am J*

Patho, 176(2), 861–869. https://doi.org/S0002-9440(10)60398-7 (accessed on 2nd February 2026).

Hall, E. (2013). DNA methylation of the glucagon-like peptide 1 receptor (GLP1R) in human pancreatic islets. *BMC Med Genet, 14*, 76. https://doi.org/1471-2350-14-76 (accessed on 2nd February 2026).

Hamdy, O. (2001). Diet and exercise in type 2 diabetes mellitus. *Endocrinol Metab Clin North Am, 30*(4), 883–907. https://doi.org/S0889-8529(05)70220-6 (accessed on 2nd February 2026).

Han, H. C. (2012). Twisted blood vessels: Symptoms, etiology and biomechanical mechanisms. *J Vasc Res, 49*(3), 185–197. https://doi.org/000335123 (accessed on 2nd February 2026).

Hassan, S. (2022). Linking hIAPP misfolding and aggregation with type 2 diabetes mellitus: A structural perspective. *Biosci Rep, 42*(5). https://doi.org/231205 (accessed on 2nd February 2026).

Herbert, J. (2006). Do corticosteroids damage the brain? *J Neuroendocrinol, 18*(6), 393–411. https://doi.org/JNE1429 (accessed on 2nd February 2026).

Hornquist, J. O. (1995). Type II diabetes and quality of life: A review of the literature. *Pharmacoeconomics, 8*(Suppl 1), 12–16. https://doi.org/10.2165/00019053-199500081-00004 (accessed on 2nd February 2026).

Howard, B. V. (2000). LDL cholesterol as a strong predictor of coronary heart disease in diabetic individuals with insulin resistance and low LDL: The Strong Heart Study. *Arterioscler Thromb Vasc Biol, 20*(3), 830–835. https://doi.org/10.1161/01.atv.20.3.830 (accessed on 2nd February 2026).

Hu, F. B. (2001). Diet and risk of type II diabetes: The role of types of fat and carbohydrate. *Diabetology, 44*(7), 805–817. https://doi.org/10.1007/s001250100547 (accessed on 2nd February 2026).

Hu, F. B. (2001). Diet, lifestyle, and the risk of type 2 diabetes mellitus in women. *N Engl J Med, 345*(11), 790–797. https://doi.org/10.1056/NEJMoa010492 (accessed on 2nd February 2026).

Kaku, K. (2010). Pathophysiology of type 2 diabetes and its treatment policy. *JMAJ, 53*(1), 41–46.

Karamanou, M. (2016). Milestones in the history of diabetes mellitus: The main contributors. *World J Diabetes, 7*(1), 1–7. https://doi.org/10.4239/wjd.v7.i1.1 (accessed on 2nd February 2026).

Khan, A. (2017). Visual complications in diabetes mellitus: Beyond retinopathy. *Diabet Med, 34*(4), 478–484. https://doi.org/10.1111/dme.13296 (accessed on 2nd February 2026).

Khan, M. V. (2014). Fluoroalcohols-induced modulation and amyloid formation in conalbumin. *Int J Biol Macromol, 70*, 606–614. https://doi.org/S0141-8130(14)00502-9 (accessed on 2nd February 2026).

Khan, M. V. (2015). Non-fluorinated cosolvents: A potent amorphous aggregate inducer of metalloproteinase-conalbumin (ovotransferrin). *Int J Biol Macromol, 78*, 417–428. https://doi.org/S0141-8130(15)00259-7 (accessed on 2nd February 2026).

Khan, M. V. (2017). Polyols (glycerol and ethylene glycol) mediated amorphous aggregate inhibition and secondary structure restoration of metalloproteinase-conalbumin (ovotransferrin). *Int J Biol Macromol, 94*(Pt A), 290–300. https://doi.org/S0141-8130(16)31914-6 (accessed on 2nd February 2026).

Khan, M. V. (2018a). Biophysical insight reveals tannic acid as amyloid inducer and conformation transformer from amorphous to amyloid aggregates in Concanavalin A (ConA). *J Biomol Struct Dyn, 36*(5), 1261–1273. https://doi.org/10.1080/07391102.2017.1318718 (accessed on 2nd February 2026).

Khan, M. V. (2018b). Cationic surfactant mediated fibrillogenesis in bovine liver catalase: A biophysical approach. *J Biomol Struct Dyn, 36*(10), 2543–2557. https://doi.org/10.1080/07391102.2017.1363085 (accessed on 2nd February 2026).

Khan, M. V. (2018c). Protein folding, misfolding and aggregation: A tale of constructive to destructive assembly. *Int J Biol Macromol, 112*, 217–229. https://doi.org/S0141-8130(17)34415-X (accessed on 2nd February 2026).

Kim, C. (2002). Gestational diabetes and the incidence of type 2 diabetes: A systematic review. *Diabetes Care, 25*(10), 1862–1868. https://doi.org/10.2337/diacare.25.10.1862 (accessed on 2nd February 2026).

Kumar, M. (2023). The bidirectional link between diabetes and kidney disease: Mechanisms and management. *Cureus, 15*(9), e45615. https://doi.org/10.7759/cureus.45615 (accessed on 2nd February 2026).

Labarca, G. (2018). CPAP in patients with obstructive sleep apnea and type 2 diabetes mellitus: Systematic review and meta-analysis. *Clin Respir J, 12*(8), 2361–2368. https://doi.org/10.1111/crj.12915 (accessed on 2nd February 2026).

Lacal, I., & Ventura, R. (2018). Epigenetic inheritance: Concepts, mechanisms and perspectives. *Front Mol Neurosci, 11*, 292. https://doi.org/10.3389/fnmol.2018.00292 (accessed on 2nd February 2026).

Laguesse, D. E. (1895). Recherches sur l'histologie du pancréas chez le mouton. *J de l'anat et Physiol, 41*, 475–500.

Laguesse, G. E. (1893). Sur la formation des îlots de Langerhans dans le pancréas. *C. R. Soc. Biol., 45*, 819.

Lahtela, J. T. (1997). Severe antibody-mediated human insulin resistance: Successful treatment with the insulin analog lispro. A case report. *Diabetes Care, 20*(1), 71–73. https://doi.org/10.2337/diacare.20.1.71 (accessed on 2nd February 2026).

Laios, K. (2012). Aretaeus of Cappadocia and the first description of diabetes. *Hormones (Athens), 11*(1), 109–113. https://doi.org/10.1007/BF03401545 (accessed on 2nd February 2026).

Langerhans, P. (1869). *Beiträge zur mikroskopischen Anatomie der Bauchspeicheldrüse*. Inaugural-Dissertation, Medicine and Surgery. Berlin: Friedrich-Wilhelms.

Lasagna-Reeves, C. A. (2010). Inhaled insulin forms toxic pulmonary amyloid aggregates. *Endocrinology, 151*(10), 4717–4724. https://doi.org/en.2010-0457 (accessed on 2nd February 2026).

Lebovitz, H. E. (2001). Diagnosis, classification, and pathogenesis of diabetes mellitus. *J Clin Psychiatry, 62*(Suppl 27), 5–9; discussion 40–41.

Lee, H. S., & Hwang, J. S. (2019). Genetic aspects of type 1 diabetes. *Ann Pediatr Endocrinol Metab, 24*(3), 143–148. https://doi.org/10.6065/apem.2019.24.3.143 (accessed on 2nd February 2026).

Leslie, R. D. (2021). Adult-onset type 1 diabetes: Current understanding and challenges. *Diabetes Care, 44*(11), 2449–2456. https://doi.org/10.2337/dc21-0770 (accessed on 2nd February 2026).

Levitt, N. S. (1996). The natural progression of autonomic neuropathy and autonomic function tests in a cohort of people with IDDM. *Diabetes Care, 19*(7), 751–754. https://doi.org/10.2337/diacare.19.7.751 (accessed on 2nd February 2026).

Li, Y. R. (2015). Meta-analysis of shared genetic architecture across ten pediatric autoimmune diseases. *Nat Med, 21*(9), 1018–1027. https://doi.org/10.1038/nm.3933 (accessed on 2nd February 2026).

Lin, C. Y. (2007). Toxic human islet amyloid polypeptide (h-IAPP) oligomers are intracellular, and vaccination to induce anti-toxic oligomer antibodies does not prevent h-IAPP-induced beta-cell apoptosis in h-IAPP transgenic mice. *Diabetes, 56*(5), 1324–1332. https://doi.org/10.2337/db06-1579 (accessed on 2nd February 2026).

Ling, C. (2007). Genetic and epigenetic factors are associated with expression of respiratory chain component NDUFB6 in human skeletal muscle. *J Clin Invest, 117*(11), 3427–3435. https://doi.org/10.1172/JCI30938 (accessed on 2nd February 2026).

Ling, C. (2008). Epigenetic regulation of PPARGC1A in human type 2 diabetic islets and effect on insulin secretion. *Diabetology, 51*(4), 615–622. https://doi.org/10.1007/s00125-007-0916-5 (accessed on 2nd February 2026).

Liu, S. (2000). A prospective study of whole-grain intake and risk of type 2 diabetes mellitus in US women. *Am J Public Health, 90*(9), 1409–1415. https://doi.org/10.2105/ajph.90.9.1409 (accessed on 2nd February 2026).

Ma, F., & Zhang, C. Y. (2016). Histone modifying enzymes: Novel disease biomarkers and assay development. *Expert Rev Mol Diagn, 16*(3), 297–306. https://doi.org/10.1586/14737159.2016.1135057 (accessed on 2nd February 2026).

Maack, C. (2018). Heart failure and diabetes: Metabolic alterations and therapeutic interventions: A state-of-the-art review from the Translational Research Committee of the Heart Failure Association–European Society of Cardiology. *Eur Heart J, 39*(48), 4243–4254. https://doi.org/10.1093/eurheartj/ehy596 (accessed on 2nd February 2026).

Mansour, S. E. (2020). The evolving treatment of diabetic retinopathy. *Clin Ophthalmol, 14*, 653–678. https://doi.org/10.2147/OPTH.S236637 (accessed on 2nd February 2026).

Mathers, C. D., & Loncar, D. (2006). Projections of global mortality and burden of disease from 2002 to 2030. *PLoS Med, 3*(11), e442. https://doi.org/10.1371/journal.pmed.0030442 (accessed on 2nd February 2026).

Matheus, A. S. (2013). Impact of diabetes on cardiovascular disease: An update. *Int J Hypertense, 2013*, 653789. https://doi.org/10.1155/2013/653789 (accessed on 2nd February 2026).

Matsuyoshi, A. (2006). A case of slowly progressive type 1 diabetes with unstable glycemic control caused by unusual insulin antibody and successfully treated with steroid therapy. *Diabetes Res Clin Pract, 72*(3), 238–243. https://doi.org/10.1016/j.diabres.2005.10.018 (accessed on 2nd February 2026).

Mayfield, J. (1998). Diagnosis and classification of diabetes mellitus: New criteria. *Am Fam Physician, 58*(6), 1355–1362, 1369–1370.

McGuffee, A. E. (2020). Effects of routine checkups and chronic conditions on middle-aged patients with diabetes. *Adv Prev Med, 2020*, 4043959. https://doi.org/10.1155/2020/4043959 (accessed on 2nd February 2026).

Meigs, J. B. (2000). Parental transmission of type 2 diabetes: The Framingham Offspring Study. *Diabetes, 49*(12), 2201–2207. https://doi.org/10.2337/diabetes.49.12.2201 (accessed on 2nd February 2026).

Meijer, R. I. (2012). Insulin-induced microvascular recruitment in skin and muscle are related and both are associated with whole-body glucose uptake. *Microcirculation, 19*(6), 494–500. https://doi.org/10.1111/j.1549-8719.2012.00174.x (accessed on 2nd February 2026).

Mendes, A. L. (2017). Diabetes mellitus and the skin. *A Bras Dermatol, 92*(1), 8–20. https://doi.org/10.1590/abd1806-4841.20175514 (accessed on 2nd February 2026).

Mengstie, M. A. (2022). Molecular and cellular mechanisms in diabetic heart failure: Potential therapeutic targets. *Front Endocrinol (Lausanne), 13*, 947294. https://doi.org/10.3389/fendo.2022.947294 (accessed on 2nd February 2026).

Mericq, V. (2017). Long-term metabolic risk among children born premature or small for gestational age. *Nature Reviews Endocrinology, 13*(1), 50–62. https://doi.org/nrendo.2016.127 (accessed on 2nd February 2026).

Morris, A. P. (2012). Large-scale association analysis provides insights into the genetic architecture and pathophysiology of type 2 diabetes. *Nature Genetics, 44*(9), 981–990. https://doi.org/ng.2383 (accessed on 2nd February 2026).

Mosenzon, O. (2023). Diabetes and stroke: What are the connections? *Journal of Stroke, 25*(1), 26–38. https://doi.org/jos.2022.02306 (accessed on 2nd February 2026).

Moulton, C. D. (2015). Meta-analyses of structural regional cerebral effects in type 1 and type 2 diabetes. *Brain Imaging and Behavior, 9*(4), 651–662. https://doi.org/10.1007/s11682-014-9348-2 (accessed on 2nd February 2026).

Mounirou, B. A. M. (2022). Diabetic retinopathy: An overview of treatments. *Indian Journal of Endocrinology and Metabolism, 26*(2), 111–118. https://doi.org/IJEM-26-111 (accessed on 2nd February 2026).

Murtaza, G. (2019). Diabetic cardiomyopathy–A comprehensive updated review. *Progress in Cardiovascular Diseases, 62*(4), 315–326. https://doi.org/S0033-0620(19)30051-9 (accessed on 2nd February 2026).

N/A. (1997). Report of the Expert Committee on the Diagnosis and Classification of Diabetes Mellitus. *Diabetes Care, 20*(7), 1183–1197. https://doi.org/10.2337/diacare.20.7.1183 (accessed on 2nd February 2026).

N/A. (2005). Diagnosis and classification of diabetes mellitus. *Diabetes Care, 28*(Suppl 1), S37–S42. https://doi.org/28/suppl_1/s37 (accessed on 2nd February 2026).

N/A. (2018). Classification and diagnosis of diabetes: Standards of medical care in diabetes. *Diabetes Care, 41*(Suppl 1), S13–S27. https://doi.org/41/Supplement_1/S13 (accessed on 2nd February 2026).

Nanayakkara, N. (2021). Impact of age at type 2 diabetes mellitus diagnosis on mortality and vascular complications: Systematic review and meta-analyses. *Diabetology, 64*(2), 275–287. https://doi.org/10.1007/s00125-020-05319-w (accessed on 2nd February 2026).

National Diabetes Data Group. (1979). Classification and diagnosis of diabetes mellitus and other categories of glucose intolerance. *Diabetes, 28*(12), 1039–1057. https://doi.org/10.2337/diab.28.12.1039 (accessed on 2nd February 2026).

Nejentsev, S. (2007). Localization of type 1 diabetes susceptibility to the MHC class I genes HLA-B and HLA-A. *Nature, 450*(7171), 887–892. https://doi.org/nature06406 (accessed on 2nd February 2026).

Niedzwiecki, M. M. (2019). The exposome: Molecules to populations. *Annual Review of Pharmacology and Toxicology, 59*, 107–127. https://doi.org/10.1146/annurev-pharmtox-010818-021315 (accessed on 2nd February 2026).

Nilsson, M. R. (2016). Insulin amyloid at injection sites of patients with diabetes. *Amyloid, 23*(3), 139–147. https://doi.org/10.1080/13506129.2016.1179183 (accessed on 2nd February 2026).

Noctor, E. (2016). Abnormal glucose tolerance post-gestational diabetes mellitus as defined by the International Association of Diabetes and Pregnancy Study Groups criteria. *European Journal of Endocrinology, 175*(4), 287–297. https://doi.org/EJE-15-1260 (accessed on 2nd February 2026).

Ohishi, M. (2018). Hypertension with diabetes mellitus: Physiology and pathology. *Hypertension Research, 41*(6), 389–393. https://doi.org/10.1038/s41440-018-0034-4 (accessed on 2nd February 2026).

Okamura, S. (2013). Localized amyloidosis at the site of repeated insulin injection in a patient with type 2 diabetes. *Diabetes Care, 36*(12), e200. https://doi.org/36/12/e200 (accessed on 2nd February 2026).

Oparil, S. (2003). Pathogenesis of hypertension. *Annals of Internal Medicine, 139*(9), 761–776. https://doi.org/139/9/761 (accessed on 2nd February 2026).

Pacini, G. (2006). The hyperbolic equilibrium between insulin sensitivity and secretion. *Nutrition, Metabolism and Cardiovascular Diseases, 16*(Suppl 1), S22–S27. https://doi.org/S0939-4753(05)00244-9 (accessed on 2nd February 2026).

Pamidi, S., & Tasali, E. (2012). Obstructive sleep apnea and type 2 diabetes: Is there a link? *Frontiers in Neurology, 3*, 126. https://doi.org/10.3389/fneur.2012.00126 (accessed on 2nd February 2026).

Pan, A. (2015). Relation of active, passive, and quitting smoking with incident type 2 diabetes: A systematic review and meta-analysis. *The Lancet Diabetes & Endocrinology, 3*(12), 958–967. https://doi.org/S2213-8587(15)00316-2 (accessed on 2nd February 2026).

Partanen, J. (1995). Natural history of peripheral neuropathy in patients with non-insulin-dependent diabetes mellitus. *The New England Journal of Medicine, 333*(2), 89–94. https://doi.org/10.1056/NEJM199507133330203 (accessed on 2nd February 2026).

Petrie, J. R. (2018). Diabetes, hypertension, and cardiovascular disease: Clinical insights and vascular mechanisms. *Canadian Journal of Cardiology, 34*(5), 575–584. https://doi.org/S0828-282X(17)31214-X (accessed on 2nd February 2026).

Pop-Busui, R. (2022). Heart failure: An underappreciated complication of diabetes. A consensus report of the American Diabetes Association. *Diabetes Care, 45*(7), 1670–1690. https://doi.org/147048 (accessed on 2nd February 2026).

Possidente, K. J., & Ongaro, R. S. (2001). The role of home blood pressure monitoring in hypertension control. *Journal of Clinical Hypertension (Greenwich), 3*(3), 171–173. https://doi.org/JCH0450 (accessed on 2nd February 2026).

Raman, R. (2021). Diabetic retinopathy screening guidelines in India: All India Ophthalmological Society Diabetic Retinopathy Task Force and Vitreoretinal Society of

India Consensus Statement. *Indian Journal of Ophthalmology, 69*(3), 678–688. https://doi.org/301576 (accessed on 2nd February 2026).

Rasheed, R. (2021). Relationship between diabetic retinopathy and diabetic peripheral neuropathy–Neurodegenerative and microvascular changes. *Indian Journal of Ophthalmology, 69*(11), 3370–3375. https://doi.org/IndianJOphthalmol_2021_69_11_3370_329231 (accessed on 2nd February 2026).

Rask-Madsen, C., & King, G. L. (2013). Vascular complications of diabetes: Mechanisms of injury and protective factors. *Cell Metabolism, 17*(1), 20–33. https://doi.org/S1550-4131(12)00490-1 (accessed on 2nd February 2026).

Reidy, K. (2014). Molecular mechanisms of diabetic kidney disease. *Journal of Clinical Investigation, 124*(6), 2333–2340. https://doi.org/72271 (accessed on 2nd February 2026).

Reutens, A. T. (2013). Epidemiology of diabetic kidney disease. *Medical Clinics of North America, 97*(1), 1–18. https://doi.org/S0025-7125(12)00186-1 (accessed on 2nd February 2026).

Rewers, M., & Ludvigsson, J. (2016). Environmental risk factors for type 1 diabetes. *The Lancet, 387*(10035), 2340–2348. https://doi.org/S0140-6736(16)30507-4 (accessed on 2nd February 2026).

Roden, M., & Shulman, G. I. (2019). The integrative biology of type 2 diabetes. *Nature, 576*(7785), 51–60. https://doi.org/10.1038/s41586-019-1797-8 (accessed on 2nd February 2026).

Rose, N. R., & Klose, R. J. (2014). Understanding the relationship between DNA methylation and histone lysine methylation. *Biochemical et Biophysical Acta, 1839*(12), 1362–1372. https://doi.org/S1874-9399(14)00028-5 (accessed on 2nd February 2026).

Roy, T., & Lloyd, C. E. (2012). Epidemiology of depression and diabetes: A systematic review. *Journal of Affective Disorders, 142*(Suppl), S8–S21. https://doi.org/S0165-0327(12)70004-6 (accessed on 2nd February 2026).

Rubler, S. (1972). New type of cardiomyopathy associated with diabetic glomerulosclerosis. *American Journal of Cardiology, 30*(6), 595–602. https://doi.org/0002-9149(72)90595-4 (accessed on 2nd February 2026).

Sacks, D. B. (2023). Guidelines and recommendations for laboratory analysis in the diagnosis and management of diabetes mellitus. *Diabetes Care, 46*(10), e151–e199. https://doi.org/153425 (accessed on 2nd February 2026).

Sadikot, S. M. (2004). The burden of diabetes and impaired glucose tolerance in India using the WHO 1999 criteria: Prevalence of diabetes in India study (PODIS). *Diabetes Research and Clinical Practice, 66*(3), 301–307. https://doi.org/S0168-8227(04)00114-7 (accessed on 2nd February 2026).

Sapra, A., & Bhandari, P. (2023). *Diabetes*. https://doi.org/NBK551501 (accessed on 2nd February 2026).

Sayin, N. (2015). Ocular complications of diabetes mellitus. *World Journal of Diabetes, 6*(1), 92–108. https://doi.org/10.4239/wjd.v6.i1.92 (accessed on 2nd February 2026).

Schofield, J. D. (2016). Diabetes dyslipidemia. *Diabetes Therapy, 7*(2), 203–219. https://doi.org/10.1007/s13300-016-0167-x (accessed on 2nd February 2026).

Shapiro, A. M. (2016). Clinical pancreatic islet transplantation. *Nature Reviews Endocrinology, 13*(5), 268–277. https://doi.org/nrendo.2016.178 (accessed on 2nd February 2026).

Shoelson, S. E. (2006). Inflammation and insulin resistance. *Journal of Clinical Investigation, 116*(7), 1793–1801. https://doi.org/29069 (accessed on 2nd February 2026).

Shulman, G. I. (2000). Cellular mechanisms of insulin resistance. *Journal of Clinical Investigation, 106*(2), 171–176. https://doi.org/10583 (accessed on 2nd February 2026).

Simon, G. E. (2007). Cost-effectiveness of systematic depression treatment among people with diabetes mellitus. *Archives of General Psychiatry, 64*(1), 65–72. https://doi.org/64/1/65 (accessed on 2nd February 2026).

Sipe, J. D. (2014). Nomenclature 2014: Amyloid fibril proteins and clinical classification of the amyloidosis. *Amyloid, 21*(4), 221–224. https://doi.org/10.3109/13506129.2014.964858 (accessed on 2nd February 2026).

Siu, A. L. (2015). Screening for abnormal blood glucose and type 2 diabetes mellitus: U.S. Preventive Services Task Force Recommendation Statement. *Annals of Internal Medicine, 163*(11), 861–868. https://doi.org/2466368 (accessed on 2nd February 2026).

Standl, E. (2019). The global epidemics of diabetes in the 21st century: Current situation and perspectives. *European Journal of Preventive Cardiology, 26*(2_suppl), 7–14. https://doi.org/10.1177/2047487319881021 (accessed on 2nd February 2026).

Su, Y. (2008). Endothelial dysfunction in impaired fasting glycemia, impaired glucose tolerance, and type 2 diabetes mellitus. *American Journal of Cardiology, 102*(4), 497–498. https://doi.org/S0002-9149(08)00681-4 (accessed on 2nd February 2026).

Sztalryd, C., & Kraemer, F. B. (1995). Regulation of hormone-sensitive lipase in streptozotocin-induced diabetic rats. *Metabolism, 44*(11), 1391–1396. https://doi.org/0026-0495(95)90135-3 (accessed on 2nd February 2026).

Tan, S. Y. (2018). Type 1 and 2 diabetes mellitus: A review on current treatment approach and gene therapy as potential intervention. *Diabetes & Metabolic Syndrome: Clinical Research & Reviews, 13*(1), 364–372. https://doi.org/S1871-4021(18)30418-1 (accessed on 2nd February 2026).

Taplin, C. E., & Barker, J. M. (2008). Autoantibodies in type 1 diabetes. *Autoimmunity, 41*(1), 11–18. https://doi.org/789166784 (accessed on 2nd February 2026).

The Lancet (2017). Diabetes: A dynamic disease. *The Lancet, 389*(10085), 2163. https://doi.org/S0140-6736(17)31537-4 (accessed on 2nd February 2026).

Thiering, E., & Heinrich, J. (2015). Epidemiology of air pollution and diabetes. *Trends in Endocrinology & Metabolism, 26*(7), 384–394. https://doi.org/S1043-2760(15)00084-3 (accessed on 2nd February 2026).

Thunander, M. (2008). Incidence of type 1 and type 2 diabetes in adults and children in Kronoberg, Sweden. *Diabetes Research and Clinical Practice, 82*(2), 247–255. https://doi.org/S0168-8227(08)00334-3 (accessed on 2nd February 2026).

Tomita, Y. (2021). Updates on the current treatments for diabetic retinopathy and possibility of future oral therapy. *Journal of Clinical Medicine, 10*(20), Article 4666. https://doi.org/jcm10204666 (accessed on 2nd February 2026).

Tousoulis, D. (2014). Diabetes mellitus and heart failure. *European Cardiology, 9*(1), 37–42. https://doi.org/10.15420/ecr.2014.9.1.37 (accessed on 2nd February 2026).

Tsalamandris, S. (2019). The role of inflammation in diabetes: Current concepts and future perspectives. *European Cardiology, 14*(1), 50–59. https://doi.org/10.15420/ecr.2018.33.1 (accessed on 2nd February 2026).

Umpierrez, G., & Korytkowski, M. (2016). Diabetic emergencies–ketoacidosis, hyperglycemic hyperosmolar state and hypoglycemia. *Nature Reviews Endocrinology, 12*(4), 222–232. https://doi.org/nrendo.2016.15 (accessed on 2nd February 2026).

van der Zijl, N. J. (2011). Ectopic fat storage in the pancreas, liver, and abdominal fat depots: Impact on beta-cell function in individuals with impaired glucose metabolism. *Journal of Clinical Endocrinology & Metabolism, 96*(2), 459–467. https://doi.org/jc.2010-1722 (accessed on 2nd February 2026).

Vijan, S. (2010). In the clinic. Type 2 diabetes. *Annals of Internal Medicine, 152*(5), ITC3–1–15; quiz ITC3–16. https://doi.org/152/5/ITC3-1 (accessed on 2nd February 2026).

Vinik, A. I. (2003). Diabetic autonomic neuropathy. *Diabetes Care, 26*(5), 1553–1579. https://doi.org/10.2337/diacare.26.5.1553 (accessed on 2nd February 2026).

Wang, Y. (2020). Prevalence of and risk factors for diabetic retinopathy and diabetic macular edema in patients with early- and late-onset diabetes mellitus. *Ophthalmic Research, 65*(3), 293–299. https://doi.org/000508335 (accessed on 2nd February 2026).

Westermark, P. (1987). Amyloid fibrils in human insulinoma and islets of Langerhans of the diabetic cat are derived from a neuropeptide-like protein also present in normal islet cells. *Proceedings of the National Academy of Sciences of the United States of America, 84*(11), 3881–3885. https://doi.org/10.1073/pnas.84.11.3881 (accessed on 2nd February 2026).

Wild, C. P. (2005). Complementing the genome with an "exposome": The outstanding challenge of environmental exposure measurement in molecular epidemiology. *Cancer Epidemiology, Biomarkers & Prevention, 14*(8), 1847–1850. https://doi.org/14/8/1847 (accessed on 2nd February 2026).

Wild, C. P. (2012). The exposome: From concept to utility. *International Journal of Epidemiology, 41*(1), 24–32. https://doi.org/dyr236 (accessed on 2nd February 2026).

World Health Organization. (2017). *WHO Global Report on Diabetes*. World Health Organization.

Wu, Y. (2014). Risk factors contributing to type 2 diabetes and recent advances in the treatment and prevention. *International Journal of Medical Sciences, 11*(11), 1185–1200. https://doi.org/ijmsv11p1185 (accessed on 2nd February 2026).

Yanai, H. (2019). Diabetic dyslipidemia: Evaluation and mechanism. *Global Health & Medicine, 1*(1), 30–35. https://doi.org/10.35772/ghm.2019.01007 (accessed on 2nd February 2026).

Yang, B. T. (2011). Insulin promoter DNA methylation correlates negatively with insulin gene expression and positively with HbA(1c) levels in human pancreatic islets. *Diabetology, 54*(2), 360–367. https://doi.org/1967 (accessed on 2nd February 2026).

Young, T., & Finn, L. (1998). Epidemiological insights into the public health burden of sleep disordered breathing: Sex differences in survival among sleep clinic patients. *Thorax, 53*(Suppl 3), S16–S19. https://doi.org/10.1136/thx.53.2008.s16 (accessed on 2nd February 2026).

Zhou, Z. (2018). Epigenetic regulation of long non-coding RNAs in gastric cancer. *Oncotarget, 9*(27), 19443–19458. https://doi.org/23821 (accessed on 2nd February 2026).

Zhu, J., & Jiang, Y. (2023). Editorial: The role of diabetes in the pathophysiology and prognosis of ischemic stroke. *Frontiers in Endocrinology, 14*, 1207537. https://doi.org/10.3389/fendo.2023.1207537 (accessed on 2nd February 2026).

Zorena, K. (2022). Environmental factors and the risk of developing type 1 diabetes—Old disease and new data. *Biology (Basel), 11*(4), Article 608. https://doi.org/biology11040608 (accessed on 2nd February 2026).

PART III

Natural and Innovative Therapies

CHAPTER 5

Harnessing Nature: Exploring Natural Products in Diabetes Management

TAHREEN TAJ,[1] SWASTIK VERMA,[2] ASHWIN KOTNIS,[2] PRASHUL SETHI,[3] HIMANSHU SHARMA,[4] and SUMEL ASHIQUE[5,*]

[1]*Department of Pharmacology, Yenepoya Pharmacy College and Research Center, Yenepoya (Deemed to Be) University, Mangalore, Karnataka, India*

[2]*All India Institute of Medical Sciences, Bhopal, Madhya Pradesh, India*

[3]*Department of Pharmacology, College of Pharmacy, Shri Venkateswara University, Gajraula, Uttar Pradesh, India*

[4]*Department of Pharmacology, NIMS Institute of Pharmacy, NIMS University Rajasthan, Jaipur, Rajasthan, India*

[5]*Department of Pharmaceutical Technology, School of Health and Medical Sciences, Adamas University, Kolkata, West Bengal, India*

*Corresponding author

ABSTRACT

Diabetes mellitus (DM) is a leading cause of mortality, morbidity, and economic burden worldwide, with an increasing impact in low- and middle-income countries (LMICs). Despite the considerable advances in conventional treatment for diabetes for glycemic control and minimizing the complications of neuropathy, heart disease, and vascular disease, there is an increasing need for the discovery of natural products that can be harnessed for diabetes management, demonstrate good glycemic control with minimal adverse effects, and are easily available at an affordable cost.

Diabetes: Novel Insights and Therapies. Anas Islam and Badruddeen (Eds)

DOI: 10.1201/9781779644596-8

This chapter describes the complex gene-environment interactions in the multifactorial pathogenesis of diabetes mellitus, available conventional treatments, and their limitations, warranting the discovery of newer treatment regimens and the potential of natural products in the antidiabetic armamentarium. Further, the chapter delves into a comprehensive description of natural products, their sources, modes of action as antidiabetic medications, including their manufacturers, side effects, and ongoing clinical trials in humans and animals. This chapter concludes with the hope that integrating natural products with modern medicine can offer personalized and holistic strategies for diabetes management and improve health outcomes.

5.1 INTRODUCTION

The word diabetes mellitus (DM) was adopted from the Greek language, where "Diabetes" stands for siphon, meaning "to pass through," and "Mellitus" means "honeyed" or "sweet." The term signifies the presence of excess sugar in urine and blood, which is a cardinal symptom of the disease. In 250–300 BC, Apollonius of Memphis invented the word diabetes (Sapra et al., 2024). Diabetes mellitus is a group of metabolic disorders that share a common characteristic of chronic hyperglycemia (Petersmann et al., 2018). Diabetes mellitus is known for its traditional complications such as renal diabetic disease, stroke, coronary heart disease, heart failure, peripheral neuropathy, and peripheral vascular disease. Recently, a few obstacles have evolved in diabetes, such as infections, liver disease, functional and cognitive impairment, and cancer have been reported (Tomic et al., 2022). Since the expected 30 million cases in 1985 rose to 415 million in 2017, the global prevalence of diabetes mellitus has risen dangerously over the past decades (Fauci, 2018). According to the International Diabetes Federation (IDF), approximately 537 million adults aged 20–79 years are diagnosed with diabetes. This means that one in 10 persons has diabetes and is projected to increase to 643 million by 2030, and to 783 million by the year 2045. India and China are the countries with the largest diabetic burden in the world. Consequently, during this period, the global population is expected to grow by 20%, and the number of diabetics is predicted to increase by 46%. The prevalence of diabetes was 10.5% in 2021, and by 2045, it is expected to rise to 12.2%. Diabetes was anticipated to be marginally less common in women aged 20–79 years when compared to males (10.2% versus 10.8%). There were 17.7 million more men suffering from diabetes in the year 2021 than women. According to the IDF, nearly 1 in 2 adults are unaware that they are suffering from diabetes. The global prevalence estimates for 2021 indicate that impaired glucose tolerance (IGT) and impaired fasting glucose (IFG) are significant, and they are projected to increase by 2045 (IDF 2021). Some races are approximately 1.5–2 times more likely to develop diabetes in their lifetime, such as non-Hispanic Caucasians, African Americans, Native Americans, and Hispanics. Increased inactivity and poor intake practices have contributed to the simultaneous growth of diabetes and obesity, known as the diabetes epidemic (Gahete et al., 2018).

Diabetes mellitus is the most important cause of death worldwide; however, its influence fluctuates across different zones. In 2019, the death rate was found to be greater than before due to diabetes, which was 27.35 deaths per 100,000 as compared to 1990, which was 22.30 deaths per 100,000 (Jha et al., 2021). In 2021, nearly 6.7 million adults (20–79) were assessed to have died as a result of diabetes or complications. This is equivalent to 12.2% of the worldwide fatalities from all sources in this age range. Approximately 32.6% of all diabetes fatalities occur in individuals of employed age (under the age of 60), equivalent to 11.8% of total global responsibilities in adults under 60 (IDF, 2021). The largest contribution to deceases due to diabetes are from the Western Pacific, Middle East, and North Africa (IDF, 2021). 80% of demises occur due to diabetes in middle- and low-income countries, and the mortality rate is approximately double that of high-income countries. Diabetes is an important economic problem in countries, health systems, and families. The annual cost associated with diabetes in the United States is likely to be $327 billion, comprising $237 billion in direct medical expenditures and $90 billion in indirect costs stemming from the reduced productivity of individuals with diabetes (Gahete et al., 2018). Several different types of diabetes mellitus are thought to be affected by a multifaceted collaboration of genetics, in addition to ecological influences. It is initiated by poor insulin secretion, reduced insulin effectiveness, or both (Petersmann et al., 2018). According to the origin of diabetes mellitus, the variables associated with hyperglycemia include decreased insulin secretion, weakened glucose consumption, and elevated glucose generation (Longo et al., 2018). The enduring effects of diabetes mellitus include neuropathy, retinopathy, and nephropathy. People with diabetes are similarly at an increased risk of developing disorders including heart disease, peripheral vascular disease, cerebrovascular disease, obesity, nonalcoholic fatty liver disease (NAFLD) (WHO, 2019), and infectious diseases such as tuberculosis (WHO, 2019). Blood glucose levels (BGLs) are frequently maintained within a relatively small range of 70–120 mg/dl. According to the ADA and WHO, the diagnostic conditions for diabetes are as follows: a classic hyperglycemic patient symptom should have a plasma glucose level of at least 126 mg/dl at fasting, 200 mg/dl at random, 200 mg/dl after a 2-hour oral glucose tolerance test (OGTT) with a 75-gram loading dose, and a glycated hemoglobin (HbA1c) level of at least 6.5% (Gahete et al., 2018). The different forms of diabetes mellitus established for different etiologies are as follows (Figure 5.1):

1. **Type 1 Diabetes:** It is also referred to as insulin-dependent diabetes mellitus (IDDM). It is characterized by immune-mediated damage to the beta cells of the islets of Langerhans in the endocrine pancreas. This typically leads to absolute insulin deficiency. Onset is most common in children and young adults (Longo, 2018).
2. **Type 2 Diabetes:** Non-insulin-dependent diabetes mellitus (NIDDM) is the most common type of diabetes (WHO, 2019). It is considered by varying the grades of improper functions of beta cells and resistance to insulin. It may vary from insulin resistance with relative insulin deficit to predominantly insulin secretory weakness with insulin resistance (Fauci et al., 2018).
3. **Gestational Diabetes Mellitus (GDM):** This conventionally denotes uncharacteristic glucose tolerance with beginning or initial recognition throughout pregnancy. It is associated with obstetric and neonatal problems connected to greater child birth weight and is renowned as a risk factor for forthcoming cardiovascular diseases (CVDs) (Sweeting et al., 2022).
4. **Monogenic Diabetes**: This form of diabetes results from a mutation in a single gene. It is classified under the WHO classification of diabetes mellitus as a monogenic defect of beta-cell dysfunction and is characterized by a mutated gene followed by clinical syndrome. Clinical indicators of monogenic diabetes in beta cell dysfunction include maturity-onset diabetes of the young (MODY), permanent neonatal diabetes mellitus (PNDM), transient neonatal diabetes mellitus (TNDM), and hereditary syndromes where insulin-deficient diabetes is associated with particular clinical types (WHO, 2019).

5. **Maturity-Onset Diabetes of the Young (MODY):** MODY occurs due to genetic defects in the development or function of beta cells caused by mutations in (a) hepatocyte nuclear factor (HNF)-4α (MODY 1); (b) glucokinase (MODY 2); and (c) HNF-1α (MODY 3) (Longo et al., 2018). In addition, mutations in genes encoding insulin promoter factor-1, HNF-1β, and NeuroD1 may lead to other forms of MODY.

6. **Other Types:** Insulin mutations and mutations in ATP-sensitive potassium channel subunits can lead to persistent diabetes in neonates. Mitochondrial DNA mutations are also responsible for certain forms of diabetes. Additional pancreatic islet regulators or proteins, such as GATA4, KLF11, BLK, SLC2A2 (glucose transporter 2 [GLUT2]), GATA6, RFX6, GLIS3, and PAX4, and mutations in any of these genes may contribute to the development of different forms of diabetes. Exocrine pancreatic diseases may also lead to the progression of diabetes mellitus; these include pancreatitis, pancreatectomy, neoplasia, cystic fibrosis, hemochromatosis, and fibrocalcific pancreatopathy (Petersmann et al., 2018).

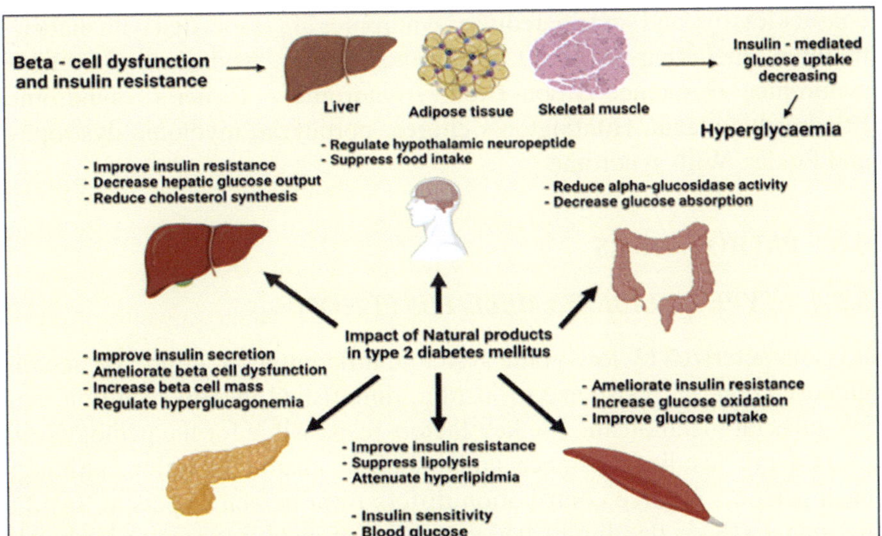

FIGURE 5.1 Role of natural products in type 2 diabetes mellitus.

Source: Reproduced from Rahman et al. (2022).

5.2 GENETIC DEFECTS IN INSULIN ACTION

It includes different mutations and syndromes characteristic of imperfections in the actions of insulin, such as Rabson-Mendenhall syndrome, type A insulin resistance, leprechaunism, and certain lipodystrophy syndromes (Longo et al., 2018).

5.2.1 ENDOCRINOPATHIES

Certain endocrine disorders, such as hyperthyroidism, Cushing's syndrome, glucagonoma, pheochromocytoma, acromegaly, somatostatinoma, and aldosteronoma, can also cause diabetes mellitus. It may also be induced by the use of glucocorticoids, Vacor (a rodenticide), nicotinic acid, diazoxide, β-adrenergic agonists, thiazides, calcineurin inhibitors, mTOR inhibitors, hydantoins, asparaginase, α-interferon, protease inhibitors, antipsychotics (atypical and others), and epinephrine, among others (Afify et al., 2023).

5.2.2 INFECTIOUS CAUSE

Certain microbes, such as congenital rubella, cytomegalovirus, and coxsackievirus, and some hereditary syndromes are associated with diabetes mellitus, including Wolfram syndrome, Down syndrome, Klinefelter syndrome, Laurence–Moon–Biedl syndrome, Turner's syndrome, Friedreich's ataxia, Huntington's chorea, porphyria, myotonic dystrophy, and Prader–Willi syndrome.

5.3 PATHOGENESIS

5.3.1 TYPE 2 DIABETES MELLITUS (T2DM)

It is characterized by low-grade systemic inflammation, improved hepatic glucose creation, resistance to insulin, diminished insulin secretion, and irregular fat metabolism. The key factors responsible for the pathogenesis of DM are insulin resistance and impaired insulin secretion, although each person's relative contribution differs from person to person. Insulin resistance (IR) is the diminished capability of insulin to act meritoriously on target tissues, specifically the liver, muscle, and fat. It is also affected by a combination of genetic vulnerability and obesity. Insulin resistance impairs glucose consumption by insulin-sensitive tissues and increases hepatic glucose output, leading to hyperglycemia. Improved hepatic glucose output mostly accounts for improved fasting plasma glucose (FPG) levels, whereas decreased peripheral glucose utilization results in postprandial hyperglycemia. A decrease in both the quantity and catalytic activity of insulin receptors is one of the most prevalent changes related to insulin resistance and an increased serine/threonine phosphorylation state in insulin receptor and insulin receptor substrate (IRS). Growth in tyrosine phosphatase activity, mainly PTP-1B, participates in receptor and IRS dephosphorylation, a reduction in PI3K and Akt kinase activity, and defects in GLUT-4 expression and function. These modifications cause a reduction in glucose uptake in the muscles and fat support modifications at the metabolic level. Hyperphosphorylation of IRS proteins on serine/threonine residues is an essential factor in the expansion of insulin resistance. IRS hyperphosphorylation transforms phosphorylation and activates Akt kinase by decreasing its interaction with PI3K and inhibiting its phosphorylation with tyrosine. Additionally, IRS phosphorylation at Ser/Thr residues accelerates its interruption. PKA, mTOR, JNK stress kinase, 70 kDa S6 ribosomal protein kinase, saturated fatty acids (SFA), amino acids, endothelin-1, pro-inflammatory cytokines, and angiotensin-II (Ang-II) are among the substances that increase kinase activity. MAPK phosphorylates IRS. (Gutiérrez-Rodelo et al., 2017).

5.3.2 OBESITY

Encourages the release of pro-inflammatory cytokines in response to an increase in macrophages invading adipose tissue, increasing SFA, and producing a condition of low-grade chronic inflammation. This causes IR due to IRS serine phosphorylation, PTP-1B expression, ceramide production, and GLUT-4 expression, leading to resistance to systemic insulin (Gutiérrez-Rodelo et al., 2017).

5.3.3 MITOCHONDRIAL DYSFUNCTION

It promotes lipid oxidation reduction due to a decrease in oxidative phosphorylation that leads to lipid accumulation that causes an increase in ceramide, which inhibits insulin signaling and promotes PKC activation that controls Akt dephosphorylation in addition to inactivation via PP2A, phosphorylating and preventing the insulin receptor and ceramides.

Moreover, the reduction of lipid oxidation produces reactive oxygen species (ROS), which in turn cause oxidative stress and injury to cells and mitochondria, eventually leading to apoptosis. ROS also leads to Ser/Thr kinase activation, leading to IR (Sangwung et al., 2020).

5.3.4 ENDOPLASMIC RETICULUM (ER)

Stress sensor kinases, including PERK, ATF-6, and IRE-1, are activated in the ER in response to misfolding. These proteins recognize protein misfolding and initiate the UPR pathway. Furthermore, these kinases stimulate inflammatory cytokine production. PERK promotes the release of NF-κB, generates inflammatory cytokines, such as TNF-α, IL-1β, and IL-6, and causes its translocation to the nucleus. As a concern, dissimilar serine kinases are activated, leading to IR. In addition, the IRE-1 kinases phosphorylate JNK, which in turn phosphorylates IRS-1 on Ser, which decreases the action of IRS-1 on other signaling proteins, primarily altering the MAP kinases and PI3K/Akt pathways, resulting in IR. The activation of NF-κB also takes place by the ATF-6 pathway, which causes the same response by pro-inflammatory cytokines, leading to IR (Gutiérrez-Rodelo et al., 2017).

5.3.5 BETA-CELL DYSFUNCTION

This leads to impaired insulin secretion, which is responsible for the pathogenesis of type 2 DM. Insulin secretion and sensitivity are linked. In type 2 DM, insulin secretion primarily increases in response to insulin resistance to preserve glucose tolerance. Glucose-accelerated secretion of insulin is the only part of the insulin secretory malfunction that is preferentially exaggerated at first, with a significantly reduced first secretory phase. At the beginning of type 2 diabetes, beta function is weakened by as much as 50%, even though the reactivity to further non-glucose secretagogues, comprising arginine, is integral. Improved pro-insulin secretion in type 2 diabetes is a replication of the abnormalities in pro-insulin processing. Furthermore, the deformity of insulin secretion progressed. It is unclear why the insulin secretory ability declines in patients with type 2 diabetes. It is assumed that problems in beta cell function, mass, and perhaps cellular individuality and differentiation status are triggered by insulin resistance. Individuals with type 2 diabetes over an extended period have a nearly 50%

reduction in beta cell mass and may also have deposits of islet amyloid fibrillar matter. Paradoxically, chronic hyperglycemia damages islet function ("glucose toxicity") and indicates the deterioration of hyperglycemia. Glycemic management is regularly associated with improved islet function. Moreover, increasing levels of free fatty acids (FFAs) ("lipotoxicity"), as well as local and systemic increases in pro-inflammatory cytokines due to an increase in islet-associated macrophages, may deteriorate islet function. Reduction in the level of glucagon-like peptide-1 (GLP-1) action may also contribute to decreased insulin secretion. Subsequently, insulin resistance can reduce glucose tolerance, and explicit diabetes requires beta cell malfunction. A substitute model has been proposed in which primary beta cell overstimulation results in insulin hypersecretion, which then indicates the progress of obesity and IR, and eventually to beta cell exhaustion (Esser et al., 2021). Epigenetics are emerging to play a role in the pathogenesis of diabetes. Investigations have scrutinized the methylation status of three genes, INS, PDX-1, and PPARGC1A, which are associated with insulin resistance. Pancreatic islets from type 2 DM patients displayed improved levels of DNA methylation and diminished expression of these genes. DNA Methylation and gene silencing of these genes result in alterations in insulin and glucagon secretion (Ling et al., 2008; Yang et al., 2011). In patients with type 2 diabetes mellitus (DM) and non-diabetic controls, pancreatic islets were examined for gene methylation and transcription levels. The investigators found 1649 CpG sites linked to 853 different genes. In islets of patients with type 2 diabetes, 102 differentially methylated genes, including CDKN1A, PDE7 B, SEPT9, and EXOC3L2-were also differently methylated. According to a functional study, these potential genes influence the production of insulin, glucagon secretion in α-cells, and exocytosis in pancreatic β-cells (Dayeh et al., 2014). Studies conducted on three genes (CAMK1D, TP53INP1, and ATP5G1) with conceivable regulatory mechanisms have been highlighted using epigenomic annotation data. These genes influence type 2 diabetes via epigenetic regulation of gene expression (Xue et al., 2018). According to recent research, changes in the expression of specific spliceosome constituents may have a causal relationship with IR, which precedes the development of type 2 DM in CVD patients. To stop the initial type 2 diabetes in clinical practice, the splicing machinery-associated molecular fingerprint may prove to be a useful non-invasive novel tool for early risk assessment (Gahete et al., 2018).

5.4 FACTORS RESPONSIBLE FOR DIABETES

Several risk factors, including genetic, environmental, dietary, and lifestyle factors, contribute to the improvement of type 2 DM (Dendup et al., 2018). These include overweight or obesity, physical inactivity, and certain races/ethnicities that are more prone to type 2 DM. Hypertension, dyslipidemia, and any history of CVD are risk factors for the emergence of type 2 diabetes.

5.4.1 OVERWEIGHT OR OBESE

BMI ≥ 25 kg/m^2 and ≥ 23 kg/m^2 in Asian Americans, or other ethnically appropriate descriptions for overweight, are certainly associated with an increased risk of developing type 2 DM. The potential mechanisms of obesity in type 2 DM include a high concentration of FFAs, altered adipokine expression (high expression of TNF-α and low levels of adiponectin), and low-grade inflammation, which lead to systemic insulin resistance (Klein et al., 2022). A BMI ≥ 25 kg/m^2 is associated with an 89% risk of developing diabetes-related complications (CDC, 2020).

5.4.2 PHYSICAL INACTIVITY

It is another habit of the younger generation that has led to an improved occurrence of type 2 DM. Modern lifestyles hurt people's health. It is usually supplemented by an intensification of stress levels, which interferes with the body's homeostasis. Studies have shown that physical inactivity leads to an increase in beta cell insufficiency, dyslipidemia, oxidative damage, mitochondrial dysfunction, and inflammation. This also led to an increase in the ceramide synthesis. All these features have led to the expansion of IR (Yaribeygi et al., 2021). An intake rich in saturated fats and trans fats is also a threat factor for type 2 DM. This leads to an increase in cholesterol levels, specifically an increase in low-density cholesterol (LDL) and very-low-density cholesterol (VLDL), and a decrease in high-density cholesterol (HDL). A significant risk factor is a triglyceride level >250 mg/dl (2.82 mmol/L) and/or an HDL cholesterol level <35 mg/dl (0.90 mmol/L). Genetics plays a key role in determining the susceptibility of an individual to develop type 2 DM. Certain race/ethnicities like African–American, Hispanic or Latino, Native American, Asian American, and Pacific Islander are more likely to progress to type

2 DM. According to the Centers for Disease Control and Prevention (CDC), the prevalence of type 2 DM among adults aged 18 years or older is 14.7% in American Indian/Alaska Native, 12.5% in Hispanics, and 11.7% in black and non-Hispanics respectively (CDC et al., 2020). The risk of emerging type 2 DM is significant if there is a family history for diabetes (parents or siblings with type 2 DM). If a mother, father, or both have type 2 diabetes, the assessed probability of being diagnosed with the disease doubles by approximately two to four times. According to previous studies, there is a higher chance of T2DM in the offspring of mothers with diabetes than in fathers with diabetes. The increased rate of disease transmission among mothers has been linked to both genetic (such as mutations in the mitochondria DNA) and environmental (such as the intrauterine environment) variables (Papazafiropoulou et al., 2017). In addition, newborns are at a risk of developing diabetes if they have a history of GDM. Formerly diagnosed with 5.7%–6.4% hemoglobin A1C, deprived glucose tolerance, or reduced fasting glucose are other factors that lead to type 2 DM. A history of CVD is also a major risk factor. Diabetes can be caused by long-term complications in two ways: small-vessel illness (microangiopathy), which mostly manifests as retinopathy, nephropathy, and neuropathy; and large-vessel sickness (macroangiopathy), which consists of atherosclerosis, ischemic heart disease, and lower extremity ischemia (Kumar et al., 2020). Hypertension (blood pressure ≥ 140/90 mm Hg) can also worsen the chronic manifestation of type 2 DM. There is a 68.4% risk of developing diabetes-related complications if the blood pressure is more than or equal to 140/90 mmHg or taking antihypertensive medication (CDC, 2020). Recent studies have shown that polycystic ovary syndrome and acanthosis nigricans may be rare risk factors for type 2 DM (Figure 5.2).

5.5 CONVENTIONAL TREATMENT APPROACHES: LIMITATIONS

Researchers have been working continuously in search of a proper cure for diabetes mellitus and obstacles to it and have been trying to find an effective way to minimize the side effects. Oral glucose-depressing treatments are the first-line management for type 2 diabetes when using pharmacologic treatments. Treatment improves glycemic control, diminishes "glucose toxicity" to beta cells, and may increase endogenous insulin secretion. Nevertheless, type 2 diabetes is an advanced illness that

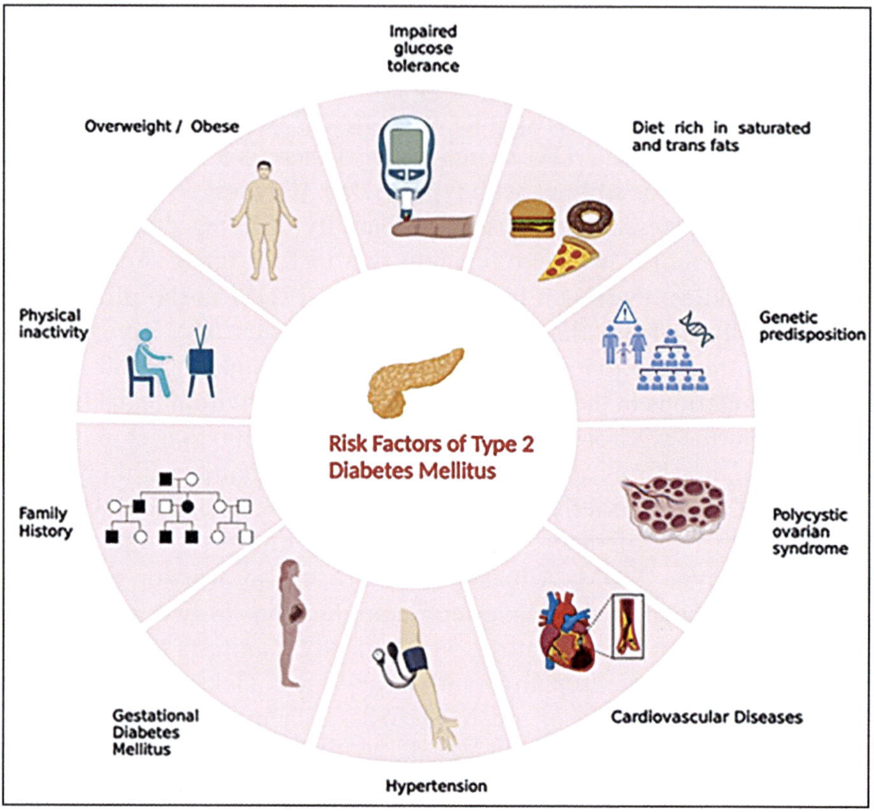

FIGURE 5.2 Risk factors of type 2 diabetes mellitus.

ultimately calls for a variety of treatment approaches, including insulin, for the mainstream population. In general, glucose-lowering agents have been used to target the pathophysiological process of type 2 DM. These comprised altered medication classes, rendering their modes of action. Glucagon-like peptide (GLP-1) agonists, alpha-glucosidase inhibitors, dipeptidyl peptides four (DPP-4) inhibitors, glinides or megalitinides, biguanides, sodium-glucose cotransporters-2 inhibitors, sulfonylurea, thiazolidinediones, glitazones, and insulin are among them (Undale et al., 2020). The oral medications available are biguanides, α-glucosidase inhibitors, dipeptidyl peptidase IV inhibitors, insulin secretagogues, sulfonylureas, non-sulfonylureas, sodium-glucose cotransporter 2 inhibitors, and thiazolidinediones.

5.5.1 BIGUANIDES

This class is represented by metformin, which slightly increases peripheral glucose consumption while reducing hepatic glucose synthesis. It passes into cells via carriers of organic cations and stimulates protein kinase, which is dependent on adenosine monophosphate (AMP). It improves insulin weakening in the liver, diminishes the action of glucagon, and reduces the process of formation and breakdown of glucose. It modifies the hepatocellular redox state, obstructs the glycerol-3-phosphate dehydrogenase mitochondrial redox transport catalyst, and decreases the amount of ATP produced by AMP, hepatic gluconeogenesis, lactate, the transformation of glycerol to glucose, and the activity of AMP-activated protein kinase (AMPK) (Mathu et al., 2021). Metformin progresses the lipid profile, reduces insulin and FPG levels, and causes slight weight loss. However, it has serious side effects. Metformin causes many adverse gastrointestinal effects including nausea, upset stomach, metallic taste, flatulence, and anorexia. Lactic acidosis has also been associated with treatment. The warning signs include fatigue, cold skin, muscle soreness, tiredness, disorientation, slow, irregular heartbeat, and stomach pain due to nausea and diarrhea (Jabade et al., 2022). A decrease in the pH of blood can cause non-specific signs and symptoms, including malaise, respiratory distress, elevated lactate levels, and anion gap acidosis (Mahmood et al., 2023). Risk factors include hepatic and renal weakened patients, the elderly, hypoxia, surgery, and alcoholism (Hsu et al., 2018). Patients with undiagnosed hypoxemia, unstable congestive heart failure (CHF), or mild renal insufficiency (glomerular filtration rate [GFR] $<$ 45 mL/min) should not use metformin. Patients who are unable to take anything orally should discontinue its use, as should those receiving radiographic contrast materials.

5.5.2 ALPHA-GLUCOSIDASE INHIBITORS

This group included acarbose, migitol, and vogilbose. By delaying glucose absorption, these inhibitors lower postprandial hyperglycemia and have no influence on insulin secretion or glucose utilization. By obstructing the enzyme in the lumen of the intestine that alters oligosaccharides into simple sugars, these medicines, when administered immediately before food, will lower the absorption of glucose. The foremost adverse effects (flatulence, diarrhea, and stomach distention) are associated with enlarged oligosaccharide transfer to the large bowel. These may increase the level of sulfonylurea and the incidence of hypoglycemia. It is necessary to avoid using antacids, in addition to bile acid resins, at the same time. Patients with gastroparesis, inflammatory bowel disease, or a blood creatinine level greater than 177 μmol/L (2 mg/dL) should not use these agents. While this class of mediators does not diminish HbA1c as effectively as other oral medicines, it is distinct in that it lowers the increase in blood sugar in later meals. The patient must take glucose if they experience hypoglycemia from additional diabetes management while taking these medications because it will slow down the breakdown and absorption of complex carbohydrates.

5.5.3 DIPEPTIDYL PEPTIDASE IV INHIBITORS

This group includes sitagliptin, vildagliptin, linagliptin, and alogliptin. These drugs prolong GLP-1 activity, leading to elevated insulin, and glucagon secretion will be decreased. There is also a side effect in that it is not effective in renal impairment and can lead to angioedema, urticaria, and immune-mediated dermatological effects.

5.5.4 INSULIN SECRETAGOGUES

These include mediators that disturb the ATP-sensitive potassium channel. It includes sulfonylureas, which reduce fasting and postprandial glucose levels. Sulfonylureas include glibornuride, gliclazide, glimepiride, and glipizide. It has a short onset of action and is inexpensive to use. Insulin secretagogues also enhance GLP-1 receptor signaling. Long-term consumption is associated with reduced microvascular and macrovascular complications. They are likely to cause hypoglycemia in the elderly. Weight gain and hypoglycemia are the two most common side effects of sulfonylureas. Weight gain is associated with the anabolic effects of higher and lower levels of insulin glycosuria. The safety of sulfonylureas in the cardiovascular system has been the subject of debate (Dahiru et al., 2022).

5.5.5 SODIUM-DEPENDENT GLUCOSE-LINKED CO-TRANSPORTER 2 (SGLT2) INHIBITORS

This cluster consisted of dapagliflozin, canagliflozin, empagliflozin, and ertugliflozin. In various tissues, the large protein cluster known as SGLTs facilitates the transfer of salt and glucose through cell plasma membranes. As this co-transporter is nearly completely conveyed in the kidney's proximal convoluted tubule, these medications reduce blood sugar levels (BSLs) by specifically blocking it. This results in a declined renal glucose threshold, inhibition of glucose reabsorption, and greater excretion of glucose in the urine. SGLT2 inhibitors also facilitated the re-absorption of sodium from the filtrate. Urine loses salt because of SGLT2 suppression. Since SGLT2 inhibitors diminish urine glucose levels, which specify diminished caloric intake, they cause weight reduction (between 2.8% and 3.9%) (Thomas et al., 2018). SGLT2 inhibitors, predominantly renin-angiotensin-aldosterone blockers, may cause acute kidney injury through effective volume depletion from increased diuresis and an excessive drop in transglomerular pressure. Additionally, the simultaneous use of medications that reduce medullary oxygenation, such as non-steroidal anti-inflammatory drugs along with radiocontrast agents, can induce renal medullary hypoxic damage, which is connected to enhanced distal tubular transport (Szalat et al., 2018).

5.5.6 THIAZOLIDINEDIONES

This treatment group included pioglitazone and rosiglitazone. Insulin resistance will decrease, and glucose utilization will increase. There was a 0.5–1.4% reduction in HbA1C. Adverse effects include peripheral edema, weight gain, CHF, fractures, and edema of the muscles. Treatment of type 2 DM is not limited to oral intake. Various medications can be administered via the parenteral route. These include amylin agonists, GLP-1 receptor agonists, and insulin administered via subcutaneous injection.

5.5.7 INSULIN

When considering type 2 diabetes, insulin should be taken into account as part of the first-line therapy, specifically for people who are hospitalized, unfavorably ill, lean, or severely underweight, or have essential renal or hepatic sicknesses that make oral glucose medications ineffective. After injection, it corresponds to the endogenous form, supporting the restoration of normal glucose levels and metabolism by triggering the glucose transporters of the cell membrane, which allows glucose to be absorbed into the cell. Insulin makes the synthesis of glucokinase which phosphorylates then drops the intracellular glucose in the liver besides enhances glycolysis by inducing hexokinase and 6-phosphofructokinase (Harvey et al., 2017). Based on the number of periods in which the highest action was noticed, exogenous insulin was classified as rapid-acting, short-acting, intermediate-acting, long-acting, or pre-mixed. When the attentiveness of insulin is highest in the blood, peak action occurs. Fast-acting products can be taken immediately before or immediately after food intake to provide an ideal insulin level. Their properties started to be noticeable within 5 to 15 min and remained for less than 5 h. The progression of short-acting insulin is between 0.5 and 1 h, and it takes 2 to 4 h for plasma concentrations to reach their maximum. For the persistence of meeting insulin requirements, these analogs ought to be directed 20 to 30 min before meals. The absorption rate of intermediate-acting insulin products is lower than that of predictable insulin because the insulin preparation encompasses protamine or zinc, which inhibit the hexamer from dissociating. They have an estimated duration of action of 20–24 hours. Long-term insulin analogs have an extensive interval of action for all insulin analogs, after engaging in activity for up to 36 h (Dahiru et al., 2022). The characteristic pre-mixed biphasic human insulin is mixed in a 30/70 or 50/50 ratio and comprises ordinary human insulin and neutral protamine Hagedorn (NPH). Certain insulin medications have adverse effects and contraindications. One of the most serious side effects is hypoglycemia, which can be fatal. Peripheral edema, weight gain, hypokalemia, and lipodystrophy, which can indicate skin shrinkage or hypertrophy, are additional problems associated with NPH insulin. Care should be taken to avoid hypokalemia and liver and kidney dysfunction (Aschner et al., 2021). Hypoglycemia is linked to insulin glargine, which manifests as diaphoresis, anxiety, nausea, shivering's, palpitations, tiredness, and poor concentration, among others. Convulsions, coma, unconsciousness, and even fatalities are possible consequences of extreme hypoglycemia. Insulin glargine may have various adverse effects at the site of injection and lipodystrophy at the injection site (Cunningham et al., 2022).

5.5.8 AMYLIN AGONISTS

These include injectable pramlintide, a soluble analog of human amylin. It slows gastric emptying and decreases glucagon secretion. Side effects include nausea, anorexia, and vomiting, which are dose-dependent and dissipate over time with the continuation of therapy (Qiao et al., 2017).

Observing BSLs supports the determination of differences in BSLs in diabetic patients. Tests conducted outside clinical facilities are denoted as capillary blood glucose (CBG) trials and others, such as BGL and BSL monitoring. CBG and plasma glucose venous blood tests can be performed in clinical facilities (Mathew et al., 2020) (Table 5.1).

TABLE 5.1 Overview of Natural Products to Overcome Diabetes

Name of Natural Products	Sources	Mechanism of Action	References
Tannins	Cereals, legumes, nuts, grapes, rice and oats, green tea, wine, beer, and coffee	Improve insulin sensitivity and inhibit alpha-glucosidase activity; adipocyte inhibition, glucose transport stimulation, and GLUT-4 translocation	Zhang et al. (2021)
Curcumin	*Curcuma longa* (turmeric), present in the rhizome	Lowers blood sugar levels after food intake and increases insulin sensitivity; obstructs alpha-glucosidase and alpha-amylase activities; inhibits lipid peroxidation and inflammatory cytokine levels along with NF-κB activation, supporting pancreatic cell viability	Alam et al. (2018); Oliveira et al. (2020); Xu et al. (2018)
Resveratrol	Grapes, peanuts, and berries	PPARγ receptor interaction, β-cell protection against oxidative stress, and increased insulin sensitivity through stimulation of deacetylase sirtuins 1–7	Blahova et al. (2021)
Lignans	Whole grains, legumes, coffee, wine, oilseeds, fruits, and vegetables	Decrease blood glucose levels and delay postprandial glucose absorption; diminish inflammation and oxidative stress; delay the onset of diabetes and improve glucose tolerance, insulin signaling, and insulin sensitivity	Blahova et al. (2021); Draganescu et al. (2021)
Anthocyanins	Berries such as blackberries, raspberries, cranberries, cherries, strawberries, and cabbages	Suppress free radical synthesis and lipid peroxidation, enhance insulin secretion, suppress alpha-glucosidase activity, and improve insulin resistance	Guo et al. (2018)
Quercetin	Apples, seeds, onions, berries, flowers, bark, and tea	Activates PI3K/Akt signaling pathways, promotes glucose absorption through an insulin-dependent MAPK mechanism, interacts with the PPARγ receptor, and inhibits alpha-glucosidase and alpha-amylase activities	Shi et al. (2019)

TABLE 5.1 *(Continued)*

Name of Natural Products	Sources	Mechanism of Action	References
Rutin	Oranges, grapefruits, lemons, limes, onions, apples, tea, and red wine	Modulates insulin secretion and positively affects the IRS-2/PI3K/Akt/GSK-3β signaling pathway	Liang et al. (2018)
Epigallocatechin gallate	Green tea from *Camellia sinensis*	Inhibits gluconeogenesis by upregulating insulin receptor tyrosine phosphorylation and downregulating phosphoenolpyruvate carboxykinase; enhances glucose-stimulated insulin secretion and exhibits antioxidant and anti-inflammatory properties	Orsolic et al. (2019); Wolfarm et al. (2006)
Kaempferol	Tea, vegetables, grapefruit, cruciferous *Ginkgo biloba*, and some edible berries	Prevents hyperglycemia progression and suppresses hepatic gluconeogenesis by decreasing pyruvate carboxylase activity	Alkhalidy et al. (2018)
Naringin	Citrus fruits such as oranges, grapefruit, and tomatoes	Increases glycogen concentration and hepatic glycolysis while decreasing hepatic gluconeogenesis; upregulates PPARγ, lowers blood glucose and cholesterol levels, and stimulates skeletal muscle expression of 5′ AMPK	Alam et al. (2014); Xu et al. (2018)
Garlic	Ripe bulb of *Allium sativum* Linn. (family Liliaceae)	Increases insulin secretion and sensitivity and reduces postprandial blood glucose levels	Emami et al. (2017)
Green tea	Leaves and buds of *Camellia sinensis*	Increases insulin binding and lowers glucose concentration; reduces blood glucose, improves insulin resistance, increases insulin secretion, and reduces diabetes-associated complications	Liu et al. (2013)
Strawberry	Fleshy receptacle of the strawberry plant	Decreases postprandial glucose concentrations and improves insulin sensitivity	Park et al. (2016)
Blackcurrant	Deciduous shrub in the family Grossulariaceae, producing edible berries	Lowers blood glucose levels and improves glucose tolerance; delays carbohydrate breakdown and prevents intestinal glucose absorption	Iizuka et al. (2018)
Rowanberry	Clusters of berries grown on the rowan tree	Inhibits alpha-glucosidase and alpha-amylase activities	Boath et al. (2012)

TABLE 5.1 *(Continued)*

Name of Natural Products	Sources	Mechanism of Action	References
Cornelian berry	Shrub from the dogwood family	Reduces blood glucose levels	Capcarova et al. (2019)
Bilberry	Fruit of the bilberry tree, consisting of small dark-blue berries	Decreases hyperglycemia, positively affects body weight gain, and inhibits alpha-amylase and alpha-glucosidase activities	Sidorova et al. (2018)
Carrot	–	Exhibits antidiabetic and anticholesterolemic effects	Kumar et al. (2020)
Sesame oil	Seeds of the sesame plant	Exhibits alpha-glucosidase inhibitory activity along with insulin-like effects	Alam et al. (2018)
Olive oil	Fruit of the olive tree (olives)	Improves β-cell function, insulin resistance, and adipocyte differentiation by combating oxidative stress and inflammation in pancreatic β-cells	Alkhatib et al. (2024)

5.6 NEED OF NATURAL PRODUCTS IN DIABETES MANAGEMENT

There have been both positive and negative implications of society's rapid development in the 21st century on people's lifestyles. For example, new risk factors have been associated with the development of chronic diseases such as T2DM, which has increased global mortality and morbidity (Vivó-Barrachina et al., 2022).

5.6.1 NATURAL PRODUCTS IN DIABETES MANAGEMENT

Hyperglycemia, cardiovascular events, renal and ophthalmic complaints, peripheral neuropathy, ulcers, and lower limb amputations are all symptoms of diabetes mellitus, a metabolic disorder caused by an imbalance of carbohydrates, lipids, and proteins (Maida et al., 2022). Its pathogenesis lies in insulin secretion and/or action. The most prevalent type of diabetes mellitus is type 2 DM. As insulin levels decrease, the insulin conflict in the body increases. Insulin synthesis from the pancreas is either inadequate or non-existent in patients with chronic type 1 diabetes (IDF, 2013). According to the IDF, an estimated 537 million individuals are diagnosed with diabetes worldwide (Rodríguez et al., 2022). To accomplish diabetes along with its complications, one must make lifestyle changes, take medications to reduce blood sugar, and seek specialized care. While traditional methods of diabetes care have made strides, there is a rising tide of concern in complementary and alternative medicine (CAM) treatments that promise to cure the condition while improving conventional methods (Serván et al., 2018). DM relies on natural substances and isolated chemicals (Pereira et al., 2023). The chemical and pharmacological effects of these compounds can vary; their main sources include different plants, fungi, marine organisms, and algae (Rey et al., 2015, 2019). For the management of blood glucose and the reduction of difficulties associated with diabetes, newer medications that consume natural products (Bernal et al., 2018). Both insulin-dependent diabetes mellitus (IDDM) and non-insulin-dependent diabetes mellitus (NIDDM) have traditionally been treated with herbal treatments. Hypoglycemic compounds derived from antidiabetic botanicals can augment the available current treatment options. Numerous modern health problems are rooted in traditional naturopathic medicines (Tiwari et al., 2015). According to the Ayurvedic *Sushruta Samhita*, which dates back to the fourth and fifth centuries BC, diabetes has been known since the Brahmic period (Thatte et al., 1989). Dietary indiscretion or a genetic predisposition can lead to diabetes (Thatte et al., 1989). Currently, herbal remedies are gaining popularity because they are inexpensive and have few side effects. Herbal remedies have long been a staple of traditional medicine, but little is known about how exactly these plants treat the illness (Tiwari et al., 2015). As alternatives to oral hypoglycemic drugs such as daonil, tolbutamide, and chlorpropamide, many plant-based bioactive medicines with hypoglycemic properties are equally effective. Full descriptions of other active chemicals produced from plants are still lacking (Bnouham et al., 2006). Because of their varied hypoglycemic and antihyperglycemic effects as well as their recognized therapeutic qualities, plants with antidiabetic characteristics are of interest to ethnobotanists (Grover et al., 2002). Pharmacological agents, lead compounds, and medicinal bioactive components originate from diverse plant species (Tiwari et al., 2015). Diabetes may have a natural cure in more conventional ways. According to Jung et al. (2006), certain plant species can reduce BGLs because of the abundance of bioactive compounds, such as terpenoids, flavonoids, phenolics, and coumarins. Plants of the family Liliaceae, genus *Allium*, species *Gymnema sylvestre*, species *Murraya koenigii*, species *Allium cepa, Withania somnifera* Dunal, *Ferula foetida* Linn., and the family Solanaceae have been found to possess antidiabetic characteristics in diabetes models. The significance of *G. sylvestre* in the treatment and management of diabetes has been extensively discussed in relation to its antidiabetic properties (Tiwari et al., 2014, 2015). One of the first antidiabetic therapeutic herbs recommended during the Middle Ages was *Galega officinalis* L. (Fabaceae). This plant, also termed goat rue, yielded a galega metabolite. It is a hazardous guanidine derivative. Nevertheless, this crucial fact helped create a precursor prototype for the biguanide-type hypoglycemic medication metformin. In addition to acarbose, miglitol, and voglibose, other natural compounds used to manage diabetes include pycnogenol, an aqueous extract of the Pinaceae family, and α-glucosidase inhibitors obtained from microbes. A useful technique for improving the field of systematic investigation of natural compounds as novel pharmaceuticals in commercial applications is ethnopharmacology. In addition to seaweed, fungi, and various mineral compounds, the primary substances evaluated were *Panax ginseng*, *Curcuma longa*, and *Trigonella foenum-graecum*. Many possible therapeutic targets have been identified, including α-amylase inhibition, effects on glucose transporters and uptake, increased insulin secretion, proliferation of pancreatic β-cells, and inhibition of proteins, such as tyrosine phosphatase (Pereira et al., 2023). Additionally, the metabolites that have been shown to be responsible for possible functions include polyphenols, organic acids, saponins, terpenes, and flavonoids. The main benefits of using these substances include improved insulin signaling, effects on lipid metabolism, fat reduction, α-glycosidase inhibition, glucose metabolism, antioxidant properties, and an impact on the intestinal microbiome. Concurrently, many pharmaceutical approaches have been developed, including solid (tablets, granules, etc.), liquid (syrups, solutions, etc.), heterodisperse (suspensions, etc.), and transmucosal adhesive (TLA) formulations. Finally, clinical efficacy studies and *in vitro* and *in vivo* safety and toxicity investigations were conducted (Rodríguez et al., 2022).

5.6.2 THE ADVANTAGES OF USING NATURAL SUBSTANCES AND THEIR DERIVATIVES IN THE MANAGEMENT OF DIABETES MELLITUS

Global healthcare systems are facing a significant problem in managing diabetes, a chronic metabolic illness that affects millions of people worldwide. Traditional treatment methods have drawbacks and side effects, as well as insufficient illness control, even if they can be beneficial to some degree. Consequently, individuals are increasingly interested in finding healthier and more efficient alternatives to traditional diabetes management methods (Andreozzi et al., 2020). Many researchers are now interested in the possibility of using natural chemicals or their derivatives to treat diabetes and its consequences. Many bioactive components with different pharmacological effects are housed in this chemical library. Plants, animals, fungi, and microbes are the natural sources from which they are derived. Investigating diabetic natural products can enable researchers to draw on both modern scientific and traditional medicinal knowledge, which can be a rich source of novel compounds (Pereira et al., 2023; Tsivileva et al., 2022). The various chemical compositions of natural products are one of their main advantages. Alkaloids, terpenoids, flavonoids, and phenolic compounds are only a few examples of a wide variety of physiologically active molecules found in the secondary metabolites produced by algae and plants. A multitude of molecular targets related to glucose homeostasis, insulin secretion, and insulin sensitivity can be modulated by drawing from this arsenal of diverse molecular designs (Sanches et al., 2023). Multiple pathways can be simultaneously affected by many natural chemicals, a phenomenon known as the pleiotropic effect. This is crucial in the complex pathophysiology of diabetes, which is characterized by dysregulation at multiple levels. Natural substances and their derivatives may provide synergistic effects in diabetes control because of their ability to simultaneously target numerous underlying pathways simultaneously (Pereira et al., 2023). By inducing inflammatory pathways and generating oxidative stress, uncontrolled hyperglycemia can cause microvascular and macrovascular complications. The anti-inflammatory and antioxidant activities of natural substances suggest that they could be useful in addressing these issues and maintaining human health (Akpoveso et al., 2023). Furthermore, natural pharmaceuticals often have a superior safety profile compared to manufactured pharmaceutical treatments. The extensive acceptance of these procedures over the years is evidence of the long history of usage and established safety in traditional medicine. This advantage in lowering the probability of adverse effects becomes even more crucial when dealing with diseases that require long-term management such as diabetes (Pereira et al., 2023). Several effective diabetes treatments originate from naturally occurring or derived chemicals. Their potential as materials for novel therapeutic techniques is enhanced by their diverse spectrum of effects, capacity to mitigate side effects, and distinctive chemical compositions. By utilizing the potential of natural components, we can expand the spectrum of therapeutic options and improve the results in patients with diabetes (Vivó-Barrachina et al., 2022). With an emphasis on their relevance and promise for future advancements, this review aims to provide a wide-ranging description of the function of natural substances in diabetes care (Pereira et al., 2023).

5.7 MARKETED NATURAL PRODUCT FORMULATIONS FOR DIABETES MANAGEMENT

A plethora of herbal antidiabetic remedies has emerged worldwide as a result of rigorous scientific investigations. Examples include Diabeta Plus, Diabecon®, and Glyoherb. Himalaya Herbal Healthcare's poly-herbal formulation Diabecon® is an effective product for managing diabetes. It aids in β-cell regeneration, provides protection against oxidative stress, and increases C-peptide levels. It reduces HbA1c, restores microalbuminuria to normal levels, and regulates lipid levels, similar to insulin. Owing to its antioxidant properties, Diabecon® may reduce the risks associated with diabetes (Kaur et al., 2014). Diabecon® decreased HbA1c more effectively than Hyponidd, Inolter, and Cogent DB, despite showing higher fasting insulin and C-peptide levels (Choudhury et al., 2018). Antioxidant and antihyperlipidemic qualities are also observed in the polyherbal antihyperglycemic drug glyo-herb. Medication reduces the risk of neuropathy, retinopathy, delays, or even cures it (Kaur et al., 2014). According to previous studies, streptozotocin (STZ)-induced type 1 diabetic mice show increased glucose tolerance and reduced blood glucose. Glyoherb treatment does not enhance STZ-induced liver and kidney function. Diabeta plus has many beneficial effects, including its ability to modulate the immune system, reduce hyperlipidemia, alleviate stress, and protect the liver (Kaur et al., 2014). Monotherapy for diabetes reduces or delays the onset of diabetes in persons who are at risk of developing the disease. When administered with oral hypoglycemics, it reduces resistance, pruritus, discomfort, and polyuria produced by diabetes (Choudhury et al., 2018) (Table 5.2).

TABLE 5.2 Herbal Products Being Sold in India for the Control of Diabetes

Sl. No.	Manufacturer	Medicine	Active Substances	Active Principles, Mechanism of Action, and Uses	References
1.	Admark Herbals Limited	Dia-care	Jambu Beej, Kadu, Sanjeevan Mool, Himej, Neem Chal, and Namejav	Dia-care offers 90-day and 18-month therapies for type 1 and type 2 diabetes. Treatment lasts for six cycles of 90 days and is consumed accordingly	Jonnalagadd et al. (2013); Manisha et al. (2007)
2.	Ayurvedic Cure and Ayurvedic Herbal Health Products	Dia-beta	*Acacia arabica* (black babul), *Tinospora cordifolia*, *Zingiber officinale* (ginger), *Momordica charantia* (bitter gourd), *Curcuma longa* (turmeric), *Azadirachta indica* (neem), *Gymnema sylvestre*, *Pterocarpus marsupium* (kino tree), *Vinca rosea* (periwinkle)	Plant-based antidiabetic formulation with immunomodulatory, antihyperlipidemic, antistress, and hepatoprotective properties; manages diabetes safely and effectively, helps overcome resistance to oral hypoglycemic medication, and improves weakness, unsteadiness, leg and body pain, polyuria, and pruritus	Jonnalagadd et al. (2013); Manisha et al. (2007)
3.	Ayurvedic Herbal Supplement	Pancreatic Tonic 180 cp	*Momordica charantia*, *Cinnamomum tamala*, *Pterocarpus marsupium*, *Syzygium cumini*, *Gymnema sylvestre*, *Trigonella foenum-graecum*, *Ficus racemosa*, *Aegle marmelos*, *Azadirachta indica*	Currently offered as a dietary supplement; pancreatic tonic is a botanical concoction of traditional Indian Ayurvedic herbs	Jonnalagadd et al. (2013); Manisha et al. (2007)
4.	Chakrapani Ayurveda	Ayurveda Alternative Herbal Formula to Diabetes	Jamun Gutli (*Syzygium cumini*), Karela (*Momordica charantia*), Pushkarmool (*Inula racemosa*), Gurmar (*Gymnema sylvestre*), Methika (*Trigonella foenum-graecum*), Guduchi (*Tinospora cordifolia*), Neem (*Azadirachta indica*)	Effective herbs that support insulin production, lower blood sugar, improve insulin sensitivity, strengthen pancreatic function, and aid in weight management, as recommended by Ayurveda	Jonnalagadd et al. (2013); Manisha et al. (2007)

TABLE 5.2 *(Continued)*

Sl. No.	Manufacturer	Medicine	Active Substances	Active Principles, Mechanism of Action, and Uses	References
5.	Garry and Sun Natural Remedies	Bitter Gourd Powder	Bitter gourd (*Momordica charantia*)	Treats diabetes, enhances immunity, purifies blood, and reduces blood sugar; acts as a laxative, hypoglycemic agent, tonic, stomachic, antibilious agent, and antidote; contains crystalline p-insulin, alkaloids, glycosides, saponins, phenolics, reducing sugars, oils, free acids, polypeptides, sterols, amino acids, and methionine	Jonnalagadd et al. (2013); Manisha et al. (2007)
6.		Gurmar Powder	Gurmar (*Gymnema sylvestre*)	Acts as an antidiabetic agent, cardiac stimulant, and diuretic; suppresses intestinal saccharide absorption, stimulates insulin secretion, lowers blood sugar, reduces glycosuria, and temporarily blocks sweet taste receptors	Jonnalagadd et al. (2013); Manisha et al. (2007)
7.	Himalaya	Diabecon	*Gymnema sylvestre*, *Pterocarpus marsupium*, *Casearia esculenta*, *Syzygium cumini*, *Asparagus racemosus*, *Glycyrrhiza glabra*, *Boerhavia diffusa*, *Ocimum sanctum*, *Sphaeranthus indicus*, *Tinospora cordifolia*, *Swertia chirata*, *Tribulus terrestris*, *Berberis aristata*, *Phyllanthus amarus*, *Gmelina arborea*, *Gossypium herbaceum*, *Aloe vera*, *Rumex maritimus*, Triphala, *Commiphora wightii*, *Momordica charantia*, shilajeet, *Abutilon indicum*, *Curcuma longa*, *Piper nigrum*	Improves hepatic and muscular glucagon levels, glucose utilization, C-peptide levels, and β-cell regeneration and repair; exhibits antioxidant properties, lowers HbA1c, normalizes microalbuminuria, modifies lipid profiles, and reduces long-term diabetic complications	Jonnalagadd et al. (2013); Manisha et al. (2007)

TABLE 5.2 *(Continued)*

Sl. No.	Manufacturer	Medicine	Active Substances	Active Principles, Mechanism of Action, and Uses	References
8.		Diasulin	*Tinospora cordifolia*, *Cassia auriculata*, *Momordica charantia*, *Curcuma longa*, *Emblica officinalis*, *Scoparia dulcis*, *Gymnema sylvestre*, *Syzygium cumini*, *Trigonella foenum-graecum*, *Coccinia indica*		Jonnalagadd et al. (2013); Manisha et al. (2007)
9.	Nature Beaute Sante	Diabecure	*Berberis vulgaris*, *Juglans regia*, *Erythraea centaurium*, *Taraxacum*, *Achillea millefolium*	Lowers blood sugar by enhancing pancreatic insulin secretion; complements diet and exercise to improve blood glucose control	Jonnalagadd et al. (2013); Manisha et al. (2007)
10.	Nature's Health Supply	Diabetes-Daily Care	Licorice root extract (20%), *Momordica* extract (7%), *Gymnema sylvestre* extract (25%), chromax, vanadium, fenugreek extract (50%), cinnamon extract (4%), alpha-lipoic acid	Effectively improves sugar metabolism	Jonnalagadd et al. (2013); Manisha et al. (2007)
11.	Plethico Laboratories	Syndrex	Extract from germinated fenugreek seeds	Germinated fenugreek seed extracts have been used in traditional formulations for approximately 1,000 years; the mechanism of action is under investigation in animal models and cultured islets	Jonnalagadd et al. (2013); Manisha et al. (2007)
12.	Swastik Formulations	Epinsulin	Vijaysar (*Pterocarpus marsupium*)	Epicatechin improves insulin release, glucose and lipid metabolism, erythrocyte osmotic fragility, neuropathy, and retinopathy; raises islet cAMP levels and helps prevent long-term diabetic complications when used with oral hypoglycemic drugs	Jonnalagadd et al. (2013); Manisha et al. (2007)

Source: Jonnalagadd et al. (2013); Manisha et al. (2007).

5.8 NATURAL SUBSTANCES UNDER CLINICAL TRIAL INVESTIGATION

This review restricts its scope to randomized clinical trials that have examined the use of natural remedies for the management of illnesses that have produced insufficient or preliminary outcomes, underscoring the need for additional studies and developments (Vivó-Barrachina et al., 2022) (Table 5.3).

5.9 NANOPARTICLE-LOADED NATURAL SUBSTANCES FOR DIABETES MANAGEMENT

The best nanoformulation of natural substances for MetS prevention or relief includes improved bioavailability, targeted drug delivery, prolonged along with controlled drug release, and a superior surface area toward volume ratio. These are some of the benefits of nanoformulations over traditional ones. Some of the side effects of nanoformulations compared to traditional formulations are related to their pharmacokinetic interaction, unpredictable stability, toxicity, short shelf life, and higher cost. Therefore, as an alternative to traditional medication delivery systems, nanoformulation and nanonization have been presented as potential solutions (Taghipour et al., 2019) (Table 5.4).

5.10 ANTI-DIABETIC ACTION OF NATURAL PRODUCTS AND ASSOCIATED EXPERIMENTAL STUDY (*IN-VIVO* MODEL)

In recent years, the exploration of potential antidiabetic agents from plant sources has surged, with over 1000 plants identified for their possible efficacy (Eddouks et al., 2005). However, the scientific evaluation of traditional medicinal plants to ascertain their safety, efficacy, and benefits as antidiabetic agents remains relatively limited, leaving a gap in understanding their true potential (Bnouham et al., 2006; Srinivasan et al., 2007). Comprehensive research encompassing animal methods, both *in vitro* and *in vivo*, is vital to unravel the mechanisms and analyze the effectiveness of these plants and their active ingredients (Vedtofte et al., 2010; Xiao et al., 2010). Given the heterogeneous properties of diabetes mellitus and its related conditions, a diverse array of animal models is essential for comprehensive investigation (Vedtofte et al., 2010; Xiao et al., 2010).

TABLE 5.3 Essential Characteristics of Selected Studies

Sl. No.	Clinical Trial Number	Main Compound	Research Type, Volunteers Involved, and Year	Status of Trial (Completed, Recruiting, Withdrawn)	Therapeutic Interventions	References
1.	IRCT2012101911168N	Dietary quercetin	Randomized clinical trial (2023)	Phase II completed; Phase III ongoing	Oral quercetin improved antioxidant status in patients with type 2 diabetes but did not improve glycemic control or lipid profile. Glycemic and hyperlipidemia management may benefit from dosage trials	Ostadmohammadi et al. (2019)
2.	US20040161247A1	DPP-4 inhibitor (70 mg sitagliptin) + 50 mg quercetin/kg	Randomized double-blind study with 110 participants (2022)	Phase II completed; Phase III ongoing	Improved metabolic profile and antioxidant status with enhanced glycemic management and anti-inflammatory effects	Eitah et al. (2019)
3.	06-VCN-VPP-2022	Sweet cherry and quercetin	Randomized double-blind study with 32 participants (2021)	Phase III ongoing	Administration of 200 mg sweet cherry quercetin/day in Wistar rats for 30 days lowered creatinine, blood glucose, and urinary microalbumin levels	Lachin et al. (2014)
4.	NCT02844803	Metformin and *Scutellaria baicalensis*	Randomized controlled trial with 17 participants (2020)	Completed	Glucose metabolism in patients with type 2 diabetes improved with *S. baicalensis* and metformin through modulation of gut microbiota	Vivó-Barrachina et al. (2022)
5.	NCT03211858	SAR-Asp	Randomized controlled trial with 580 participants (2020)	Completed	At 26 weeks, SAR-Asp demonstrated good glycemic control, safety, and immunogenicity comparable to commercial insulin aspart formulations and was well tolerated	Vivó-Barrachina et al. (2022)

TABLE 5.3 *(Continued)*

Sl. No.	Clinical Trial Number	Main Compound	Research Type, Volunteers Involved, and Year	Status of Trial (Completed, Recruiting, Withdrawn)	Therapeutic Interventions	References
6.	ACTRN12615000559516	Curcumin and LCn-3PUFA	Randomized controlled trial with 81 participants (2019)	Completed	Curcumin and LCn-3PUFA reduced triglycerides and insulin resistance, potentially lowering type 2 diabetes risk; no combined improvement in glycemic management was observed	Vivó-Barrachina et al. (2022)
7.	IRCT2016092730008N1	Iranian propolis	Randomized controlled trial with 94 participants (2019)	Completed	Iranian propolis influenced postprandial blood glucose, insulin levels, and insulin resistance; reductions in oxidative stress and inflammatory cytokines associated with chronic inflammation were observed	Zakerkish et al. (2019)
8.	UMIN000007361	Curcumin	Randomized controlled trial with 52 participants (2019)	Completed	Curcumin reduced oxidized LDL in non–insulin-dependent diabetics with impaired glucose tolerance; potential reduction in cardiovascular complications was observed, though long-term studies are needed	Vivó-Barrachina et al. (2022)
9.	138901203180N2	Hydroalcoholic extract of *Juglans regia* L. leaves	Randomized controlled trial with 39 participants (2018)	Completed	*J. regia* leaf extract did not affect glucose levels or HOMA-IR but reduced body weight and blood pressure; unexpectedly, the placebo (microcrystalline cellulose) reduced blood glucose	Vivó-Barrachina et al. (2022)
10.	NCT01471275	Metformin and a specially designed herbal formula (AMC)	Randomized controlled trial with 450 participants (2018)	Completed	Metformin and AMC improved glucose and lipid balance via modulation of gut microbiota, with increased *Blautia* and *Faecalibacterium*; magniferin and berberine trials were suggested	Vivó-Barrachina et al. (2022)

TABLE 5.3 *(Continued)*

Sl. No.	Clinical Trial Number	Main Compound	Research Type, Volunteers Involved, and Year	Status of Trial (Completed, Recruiting, Withdrawn)	Therapeutic Interventions	References
11.	CEN-20101016	Pinitol	Randomized controlled trial with 118 participants (2018)	Completed	Replacement of sucrose with a pinitol-fortified beverage may stimulate and regulate insulin secretion, potentially preventing diabetes and insulin resistance	Lambert et al. (2018)
12.	IRCT201502011157N9	Mixture of silymarin, nettle, and olibanum extracts	Randomized controlled trial with 60 participants (2017)	Completed	Supplementation reduced triglycerides and hyperglycemia; glycated hemoglobin, lipids, and fasting blood glucose decreased significantly, while cholesterol and blood pressure were unaffected	Vivó-Barrachina et al. (2022)

Source: Vivó-Barrachina et al. (2022).

TABLE 5.4 Brief Summary of the Results of Administering Natural-Based Nanodrugs in Various MetS Models

Sl. No.	Plant-Based Constituents	Herbal Nano Drugs	Description	References
1.	α-Eleostearic acid	Bitter gourd seed oil nanoemulsion	Suitable for diabetic management; exhibits antioxidant and ROS-scavenging properties. Alloxan-induced diabetic rats showed antidiabetic benefits. The nanoformulation had particle sizes <100 nm. Nanoemulsions with 0.25% and 1% α-eleostearic acid resulted in varying degrees of blood glucose reduction. By elevating PPAR-γ, α-eleostearic acid improved insulin sensitivity and glucose tolerance. GPx, SOD, and CAT levels increased significantly in plasma and liver samples	Paul et al. (2014)
2.	Baicalin	Nanostructured lipid carriers	Scavenges ROS and modulates antioxidant activity, reducing inflammation. Particle size was 92 ± 3.1 nm. In STZ-induced diabetic male Sprague–Dawley rats, baicalin and its nanoformulation reduced FBS, TC, HbA1c, and TG, improving glucose and lipid metabolism	Shi et al. (2016)
3.	Berberine tolerance	Solid lipid nanoparticles (SLNs)	Effectively treats diabetes. Diabetic mice were used. Particle size was 76.8 nm at a therapeutic dose of 100 mg/kg. Outcomes included reduced weight gain, improved insulin resistance, and lowered fasting blood glucose	Xue et al. (2013)
		O-Hexadecyl-dextran	Rat primary hepatocytes were tested for cytoprotection against glucose stress–induced apoptosis. Particle size ranged from 238 ± 18 nm, with doses of 0.125–2.0 mg. NP-treated cells showed reduced ROS, caspase activation, oxidative stress, and mitochondrial depolarization	Taghipour et al. (2019)
		Poly(lactic-co-glycolic acid)–polyvinyl alcohol block copolymers	Used to treat high LDL cholesterol. BBR chloride block copolymers altered PCSK-9 mRNA efficiently in Hep-G2 cells. Nanoformulations of 42–63 nm were used at 100 mg/kg	Taghipour et al. (2019)
4.	Capsicum oleoresin	Alginate double-layer nanoemulsion	Studied in 3T3-L1 cells and HF-diet–induced obese rats. Treatment with 1000 ng/mL reduced PPAR-γ and aP2 and lowered mRNA levels of HSL, CPT-1α, and fatty acid–binding proteins	Lee et al. (2017)

TABLE 5.4 *(Continued)*

Sl. No.	Plant-Based Constituents	Herbal Nano Drugs	Description	References
		Nanoemulsion	Used in HF-fed overweight rats. Administered at 0.1 mL/80 g body weight with particle sizes of 20–50 nm. Increased PPAR-α, UCP2, and CPT-1α gene expression and decreased adipogenic gene expression	Taghipour et al. (2019)
5.	Curcumin	Curcumin nanoemulsion	Used for hypertension and hypercholesterolemia. Studied *in vitro*. Nanoformulation particle size was 42.93 ± 29.85 nm. HMGR and ACE inhibition observed	Taghipour et al. (2019)
		Curcumin nanoparticles@ gelatin microspheres/ hydrogel	Diabetic wound model using STZ-induced diabetic rats. Particle size ranged from 4 to 8 μm. Increased GSH and decreased ROS	Liu et al. (2018)
		PBLG–PEG–PBLG	Used in diabetic rats and H9C2 cells for diabetes and cardiomyopathy. Nanoformulation (30 nm) administered at 20 mg/kg increased H_2S, CaSR, CSE, and CaM levels	Taghipour et al. (2019)
		PEGMA–DMAEMA–MAO	Used in STZ-induced diabetic rats for peripheral neuropathy. Nanoformulation (4 mg/kg) reduced IL-1β, p-Akt, and P2Y12 receptor levels in DRG SGCs	Taghipour et al. (2019)
		PLGA-based NPs with Q10	STZ-induced diabetic rats treated with 100 mg/kg nanoformulation (237 ± 6 nm). Reduced CRP, IL-6, triglycerides, total cholesterol, and increased HDL	Taghipour et al. (2019)
		PLGA–PVA polymers	STZ-induced diabetic cataract model. Nanoformulation (2 mg/day; 282 ± 5.72 nm) reduced VEGF and increased bioavailability	Taghipour et al. (2019)
		Pluronic nanomicelles	STZ-induced diabetic rats treated with 100 mg/kg nanoformulation (333 ± 6 nm). Increased NKx6 and Pdx-1 expression	Taghipour et al. (2019)

TABLE 5.4 *(Continued)*

Sl. No.	Plant-Based Constituents	Herbal Nano Drugs	Description	References
		Self-emulsifying drug delivery system	STZ-induced diabetic rats treated at 66.7 mg/kg with 170 nm particles. Reduced TNF-α and IL-6 levels	Taghipour et al. (2019)
6.	Emodin	Nanoemodin transferosome	HF-diet–induced obese rats treated with nanoformulation (292.2 nm). Increased ATGL expression, decreased G0S2, and reduced body weight and adipocyte size	Taghipour et al. (2019)
		PEGMA–DMAEMA–MAMMAM	Used in diet-induced T2DM rats with low-dose STZ. Nanoformulation (1 mg/mL) reduced TNF-α, P2X3 receptor, and ERK1/2 phosphorylation in DRG	Taghipour et al. (2019)
7.	Gymnemic acid	Nanosuspension	Diabetes-induced rat model. Lowered blood glucose levels	Ravichandran et al. (2014)
8.	Myricitrin	SLNs	Hyperglycemic myotube cells and STZ–nicotinamide-induced T2DM animals treated with 76.1 nm nanoformulation. Increased SOD, muscle glycogen, GLUT4, and Bcl-2/Bax ratio	Taghipour et al. (2019)
9.	Naringenin	Alginate-coated chitosan core–shell	STZ-induced diabetic rats treated with 150–300 nm particles. Toxicity-free and effective	Taghipour et al. (2019)
10.	Quercetin	Quercetin nanorods	Alloxan-induced diabetic rats treated with 15.4 nm particles at 20 mg/kg. Reduced FBG, G6Pase, FBPase, CAT, SOD, ALP, ALT, and AST; increased GSH and –SH	Taghipour et al. (2019)
		(QUE/P) NP	Diabetic nephropathy rat model. Nanoformulation (32 nm; 10 mg/kg) caused ICAM-1 downregulation [113]	Taghipour et al. (2019)
		Nanoemulsion	BALB/c mice with oxaliplatin-induced neuro- and hepatotoxicity treated with 20 mg/kg nanoformulation; reduced inflammation and apoptosis	Taghipour et al. (2019)
		PLGA NPs	STZ-induced diabetic rats treated with 150 mg/kg nanoformulation (179.9 ± 11.2 nm). Increased CAT and SOD levels and reduced drug dosage	Taghipour et al. (2019)

TABLE 5.4 *(Continued)*

Sl. No.	Plant-Based Constituents	Herbal Nano Drugs	Description	References
		pH-sensitive chitosan–alginate core–shell	STZ-induced diabetic rats and HT29 cells treated with 20 mg/kg nanoformulation. Reduced AST, ALT, and ALP levels	Taghipour et al. (2019)
11.	Resveratrol	Nanocapsule	HF-diet–induced diabetic mice treated with 207 nm particles. Controlled systolic and diastolic blood pressure	Taghipour et al. (2019)
12.	–	Nanoliposomes	STZ-induced diabetic cells treated with resveratrol (30 μg/mL; 215 nm). Increased GSH-Px and SOD	Yücel et al. (2018)
13.	Scutellarin	Amphiphilic chitosan derivatives (Chit-DC-VB12)	STZ-induced diabetic rats and Caco-2 cells treated with 150–250 nm nanoformulation. Downregulated VEGF, vWF, and VEGFR2	Taghipour et al. (2019)
14.	Silybin	PLGA polymers	STZ-induced hyperglycemic rats treated. Regenerative and antioxidant effects on β-cell membrane permeability observed	Das et al. (2014)
15.	Stevioside	Pluronic F-68 copolymer-based PLA nanoparticles	*In vitro* release model. Nanoformulation (10 mg; 110–130 nm) improved controlled release, bioavailability, and intestinal absorption	Taghipour et al. (2019)

Rodents, in particular, have been extensively utilized in diabetes research because of their short induction time, cost-effectiveness, and availability of genetic mutation models, making them a preferred choice for conducting research (Stranahan et al., 2010; Sugii et al., 2009; Sugrue et al., 2010). Nevertheless, challenges persist regarding the effective evaluation of active ingredients owing to differences in hepatic metabolism systems and variations in species sensitivity (Bnouham et al., 2006; Ro et al., 2010; Seo et al., 2009; Serreze et al., 2010; Sordi et al., 2010; Wei et al., 2010; Wu et al., 2009). These complexities underscore the necessity for rigorous evaluation methodologies to harness the full potential of therapeutic plants for combating diabetes.

5.10.1 *IN VIVO* ANIMAL MODELS FOR DIABETIC MELLITUS

Various chemical, genetic, or surgical alterations are some of the interferences that may lead to the improvement of diabetes mellitus. Experiments on diabetes normally employ mice; however, there have been occasions in which larger animals have been used to induce diabetes (Fernández-Millán et al., 2009; Matsui-Inohara et al., 2009; Matsumoto et al., 2009). Using a large animal surgical model, pancreatectomy has been successfully performed on a particular canine (Kretschmer et al., 1977). Previous studies have utilized animals that are sensitive to the disease to induce diabetes (Hutchinson, 1998; Stewart et al., 1993).

Based on the type of diabetes induction, it is feasible to further refine the categorization of diabetic models according to their characteristics. The following is a list of animal models that has been further refined.

- A spontaneously generated diabetic model (for example, a CBA/Ca mouse, *ob/ob* mouse, or another comparable model).
- A diabetic model that has been developed through experimentation, such as through the use of drugs such as alloxan or streptozotocin (STZ), or through surgical operations such as pancreatectomy.

5.10.1.1 *SPONTANEOUS MODELS*

Spontaneous models of diabetes, which are characterized by the spontaneous development of hyperglycemia without any external intervention, mimic certain aspects of human diabetes. Two such methods are the biobreeding (BB) rat model and the non-obese diabetic (NOD) mouse model.

NOD mice progress to autoimmune-mediated type 1 diabetes, pancreatic islets exhibiting lymphocytic infiltration, and progressive destruction of beta cells (Anderson et al., 2005). BB rats, on the other hand, spontaneously progress to type 1-like diabetes due to the autoimmune devastation of pancreatic beta cells (Makino et al., 1980). These models are responsible for understanding the immunological mechanisms underlying the pathogenesis of diabetes but may not fully recapitulate the heterogeneity of human diabetes.

5.10.1.2 CHEMICALLY INDUCED MODELS

Chemically induced models involve the administration of toxic agents to disrupt pancreatic beta cell function and induce hyperglycemia. STZ and alloxan are commonly used for this purpose. STZ selectively destroys pancreatic beta cells by inducing DNA alkylation, which results in insulin deficiency and hyperglycemia (Szkudelski et al., 2001). Alloxan induces beta-cell necrosis through the generation of ROS, leading to impaired insulin secretion impairment (Lenzen et al., 2008). These models allow for the study of insulin-deficiency-driven diabetes and are widely used to evaluate antidiabetic agents.

5.10.1.3 SURGICALLY INDUCED MODELS

Surgically induced models involve pancreatic manipulation to induce diabetes. Partial pancreatectomy, commonly performed in rodents, reduces beta-cell mass and impairs insulin secretion, leading to hyperglycemia. While surgical models allow for the controlled induction of diabetes and investigation of beta-cell regeneration mechanisms, they are associated with surgical complications and variability in outcomes (Bonner-Weir, 2000). Additionally, pancreatectomy models may not fully replicate the multifactorial etiology of human diabetes.

5.10.1.4 DIET-INDUCED MODELS

Diet-induced models involve the induction of diabetes through fat- or sugar-rich diets, causing obesity, insulin resistance, and glucose intolerance. These models closely resemble the pathophysiology of type 2 diabetes, mimicking the human condition considered by insulin resistance and relative insulin insufficiency. Rodent models fed high-fat diets develop obesity, dyslipidemia, and insulin resistance, followed by beta-cell dysfunction and hyperglycemia (Surwit et al., 1988). Although diet-induced models capture key aspects of type 2 diabetes, they may not fully replicate the chronic progressive nature of the disease.

5.10.1.5 GENETICALLY ENGINEERED MODELS

Genetically engineered models involve manipulation of specific genes associated with the pathogenesis of diabetes to induce the disease phenotype. Transgenic and knockout mouse models targeting genes are under insulin signaling; beta-cell function and glucose metabolism have been developed. For example, leptin-deficient (*ob/ob*) and leptin receptor–deficient (*db/db*) mice exhibit obesity, insulin resistance, and hyperglycemia owing to defects in leptin signaling (Coleman, 1978). Similarly, knockout models targeting genes, such as IRS and glucokinase, provide insights into the molecular mechanisms underlying diabetes development (Stoffel and Duncan, 1997). Genetically engineered models allow the investigation of specific molecular pathways implicated in diabetes and offer opportunities for targeted therapeutic interventions.

5.10.1.6 HYBRID MODELS

Hybrid models encompass a grouping of various approaches to induce diabetes, allowing researchers to mimic specific aspects of the disease. For example, combining a fat-rich diet with low-dose STZ administration in rodents results in a model that closely resembles type 2 diabetes, with obesity, insulin resistance, and damaged beta cells (Wang et al., 2012). Similarly, combining genetic modifications with chemical induction or dietary manipulation allows the generation of models that better mimic the complexity of human diabetes phenotypes.

5.10.1.7 VIRUS-INDUCED DIABETES MODEL

Some data suggest that viruses and autoimmune illnesses that damage particular beta cells may contribute to the enlargement of type 1 diabetes in children and adolescents (Craighead et al., 1978). Research indicates that a virus known as encephalomyocarditis, a D-variant virus, has the potential to damage pancreatic beta cells in the pancreas (Giron et al., 1983; Yoon et al., 1980). Adult mice of two different types, male ICR Swiss and male C3H/HeJ, are susceptible to viral infection. Compared to the latter, the former is more likely to result in the development of diabetes. Further validation of the study was achieved through the use of cyclosporine, a potent immunosuppressant, as a pretreatment protocol. It has been demonstrated that the induction of immunosuppressants has more severe consequences in diabetes in both cases (Gould et al., 1985).

5.10.1.8 ADVANTAGES AND LIMITATIONS

Every *in vivo* animal model of diabetes has unique advantages and limitations. Spontaneous models capture the autoimmune etiology of type 1 diabetes but lack genetic control and exhibit variable disease onset. Chemically induced models allow for controlled induction of diabetes but may not fully replicate the chronic progressive nature of the disease. Surgically induced models provide insights into beta cell regeneration but are associated with surgical complications and variability. Diet-induced models closely resemble type 2 diabetes but may not fully replicate the multifactorial etiology of the disease. Genetically engineered models offer targeted manipulation of specific genes but may exhibit phenotypic differences from human diabetes. Hybrid models combine different approaches to better mimic human disease phenotypes but may be more complex to develop and characterize.

5.10.1.9 RELEVANCE IN DIABETES RESEARCH

In vivo animal models play an important role in elucidating the pathophysiology of diabetes, exploring potential therapeutic interventions, and estimating the well-being and effectiveness of novel treatments. Spontaneous models provide insights into autoimmune mechanisms, whereas chemically induced models allow for the evaluation of antidiabetic agents. Surgically induced models offer opportunities for studying beta-cell regeneration, whereas diet-induced models mimic the metabolic disturbances of type 2 diabetes. Genetically engineered models facilitate the investigation of the specific molecular pathways involved in the pathogenesis of diabetes. Hybrid models combine different approaches to better replicate human disease phenotypes and offer opportunities for translational research.

5.10.2 ANTIDIABETIC ACTIVITY OF NATURAL SUBSTANCES

Diabetes mellitus (DM) presents a significant global health challenge, driving the search for effective therapeutic strategies. Amidst this pursuit, natural products have emerged as promising candidates owing to their varied chemical constituents and pharmacological properties. From alkaloids to polysaccharides, marine-derived compounds, and microbial metabolites, a plethora of natural sources offer compounds with potential antidiabetic activity.

5.10.2.1 PLANT-DERIVED COMPOUNDS

5.10.2.1.1 Alkaloids

Nitrogen-containing alkaloids are abundant in plants and exhibit diverse pharmacological activities. Several alkaloids have shown promising antidiabetic effects. Berberine, derived from various *Berberis* species, has garnered significant attention owing to its ability to improve insulin sensitivity, enhance glucose uptake, and inhibit hepatic gluconeogenesis (Dong et al., 2012). Metformin, originally obtained from the plant *Galega officinalis*, shares structural similarities with berberine and is a widely prescribed antidiabetic medication (Bailey and Day, 2004).

5.10.2.1.2 Flavonoids

Polyphenolic compounds are present in fruits, vegetables, and medicinal plants. These compounds exhibit potent antioxidant and anti-inflammatory activities, making them attractive candidates for diabetes management. Quercetin, apigenin, and epigallocatechin gallate (EGCG) are among the flavonoids with established antidiabetic effects. They improve insulin secretion, enhance insulin sensitivity, and protect pancreatic beta cells from oxidative stress-induced damage (Eid et al., 2017; Pu et al., 2013).

5.10.2.1.3 Polyphenols

Polyphenols, including those found in fruits, vegetables, tea, and wine, represent a variety of compounds found in plant-based diets and beverages.

Resveratrol, a polyphenol abundant in grapes and red wine, has been extensively studied for its potential antidiabetic properties. It activates various signaling pathways involved in glucose metabolism, enhances insulin sensitivity, and reduces oxidative stress and inflammation under diabetic conditions (Timmers et al., 2011). Similarly, curcumin, the active component of turmeric, exhibits antidiabetic effects through multiple mechanisms, including the inhibition of gluconeogenesis and modulation of insulin signaling pathways (Aggarwal et al., 2007).

5.10.2.1.4 Polysaccharides

Polysaccharides are complex carbohydrates found in various plant sources, including mushrooms, seaweeds, and medicinal herbs. These compounds have gained attention owing to their immunomodulatory and antidiabetic properties. Polysaccharides derived from medicinal mushrooms such as *Ganoderma lucidum* and *Cordyceps sinensis* have shown promising antidiabetic effects. They stimulate insulin secretion, enhance glucose uptake, and protect pancreatic beta cells from oxidative stress (Patel, 2012).

5.10.2.1.5 Terpenoids

Terpenoids are a class of substances present in essential oils and resinous exudates of plants. They display a variety of biological functions, such as antidiabetic effects. Terpenoids from plants such as *Gymnema sylvestre* and *Momordica charantia* have been studied for their potential to reduce BSLs and improve insulin sensitivity (Kang et al., 2016). Additionally, essential oils containing terpenoids have shown promising results in animal studies for controlling diabetes (Aprotosoaie et al., 2014).

5.10.2.2 MARINE-DERIVED COMPOUNDS

5.10.2.2.1 Marine algae

Marine algae, including brown, red, and green varieties, are excellent sources of bioactive compounds including polysaccharides, polyphenols, and pigments. Among these, polysaccharides such as alginate and fucoidan have shown significant antidiabetic activity. Alginate, derived from brown algae, exhibits hypoglycemic effects by inhibiting carbohydrate digestion and absorption, thereby decreasing postprandial BSLs (Fitton et al., 2011). Fucoidan, a sulfated polysaccharide found in brown seaweeds, demonstrates insulin-sensitizing properties and improves glucose uptake in the skeletal muscle and adipose tissue (Kim et al., 2010).

5.10.2.2.2 Marine sponges

Marine sponges, characterized by their remarkable biodiversity, produce a wide range of secondary metabolites with diverse pharmacological activities. Compounds isolated from marine sponges, such as manzamine A and halitoxin, have shown promising antidiabetic effects. Manzamine A increases insulin sensitivity and glucose absorption by exerting a strong inhibitory action on protein tyrosine phosphatase 1 B (PTP1B), a crucial enzyme in insulin signaling (Kobayashi et al., 1991). Similarly, halitoxin exhibits glucose-lowering properties by activating the AMPK pathway, which regulates glucose and lipid metabolism in cells (Du et al., 2015).

5.10.2.2.3 Marine microorganisms

Marine microorganisms, including bacteria, fungi, and microalgae, are a vast and relatively unexplored source of bioactive compounds. These microorganisms produce an array of secondary metabolites with diverse pharmacological activities, including anti-diabetic effects. Compounds isolated from marine bacteria and fungi, such as diketopiperazines and polyketides, have shown promising hypoglycemic and insulin-sensitizing properties in preclinical studies (Singh et al., 2011). Additionally, microalgal extracts containing bioactive peptides and polysaccharides have shown the potential to improve glucose metabolism and insulin sensitivity (El-Fawal et al., 2015).

5.10.2.2.4 Marine fish and invertebrates

Marine fishes and invertebrates, including mollusks, crustaceans, and fish species, produce bioactive peptides and proteins with potential therapeutic applications. These peptides exhibit diverse biological activities, including antidiabetic effects. Bioactive peptides isolated from marine sources have shown inhibitory activity against dipeptidyl peptidase-4 (DPP-4), an enzyme deprived of incretin hormones, thereby enhancing insulin secretion and improving glycemic control (Jayawardena et al., 2012).

5.10.2.3 FUNGAL COMPOUNDS

5.10.2.3.1 Polysaccharides

Fungi, particularly mushrooms, are renowned for their polysaccharide content, which exhibits various biological activities, including antidiabetic effects. Polysaccharides, such as β-glucans, isolated from medicinal mushrooms, such as *Ganoderma lucidum* and *Cordyceps sinensis*, have shown promising hypoglycemic properties (Patel et al., 2012). These polysaccharides stimulate insulin secretion, enhance glucose uptake, and improve insulin sensitivity, thereby contributing to improved glycemic control.

5.10.2.3.2 Terpenoids

A diverse class of compounds, terpenoids, which are abundant in fungal species, exhibit a wide range of biological activities, including antidiabetic effects. *Ganoderma* species, commonly known as reishi mushrooms, produce terpenoids with hypoglycemic and antihyperlipidemic properties (Sanodiya et al., 2009). These terpenoids regulate glucose metabolism, enhance insulin sensitivity, and reduce lipid accumulation, thereby offering potential therapeutic benefits for diabetes management.

5.10.2.3.3 Sterols

Sterols are lipid-like molecules found in fungi that possess various pharmacological activities, including antidiabetic effects. Ergosterol, a sterol compound found in fungi, has demonstrated insulin-sensitizing properties in preclinical studies (Hossain et al., 2017). Additionally, ergosterol derivatives have shown promising hypoglycemic effects by enhancing glucose uptake and inhibiting gluconeogenesis in diabetic animal models.

5.10.2.3.4 Peptides and proteins

Fungi produce bioactive peptides and proteins with potential therapeutic applications and antidiabetic effects. Peptide derivatives from fungal sources have shown inhibitory activity against key enzymes involved in carbohydrate metabolism, such as α-glucosidase and α-amylase, resulting in a decrease in postprandial glucose levels (Bischoff et al., 1995). Additionally, certain fungal proteins exhibit insulin-mimetic properties that enhance cellular glucose uptake and metabolism.

5.10.2.3.5 Microbial compounds

1. **Probiotics:** Certain strains of probiotics, notably *Lactobacillus* and *Bifidobacterium* species, modulate gut microbiota composition, reduce inflammation, and progress gut barrier tasks, thereby affecting glucose metabolism and insulin (Cani and Delzenne et al., 2011).
2. **Short-Chain Fatty Acids (SCFAs):** SCFAs, created by fermentation of nutritive fiber by gut microbiota, play a crucial role in glucose homeostasis by stimulating incretin secretion, enhancing insulin sensitivity, and promoting energy expenditure (den Besten et al., 2013). Exploration of these natural products as potential antidiabetic agents offers a promising possibility for innovative and beneficial interventions. These compounds, sourced from plants, marine organisms, fungi, and microbes, exhibit diverse mechanisms of action that target numerous aspects of the pathophysiology of diabetes. However, additional investigations are warranted to explain their mechanisms of action, optimize dosage regimens, and evaluate safety profiles for clinical translation. Additionally, exploring the synergistic interactions between natural substances and conventional antidiabetic drugs holds promise for enhancing therapeutic outcomes (Table 5.5).

TABLE 5.5 Anti-Diabetic Effects of Natural Products in *In Vivo* Models

Sl. No.	Natural Product	*In Vivo* Model	References
1.	Metformin	Chemically induced diabetic rats	Zhang et al. (2018)
2.	Berberine	High-fat diet–induced diabetic mice	Yin et al. (2015)
3.	Curcumin	Streptozotocin-induced diabetic rats	Ejaz et al. (2009)
4.	Resveratrol	Zucker diabetic fatty rats	Brasnyó et al. (2011)
5.	Cinnamon extract	Alloxan-induced diabetic rats	Qin et al. (2010)
6.	*Gymnema sylvestre* extract	Alloxan-induced diabetic rats	Baskaran et al. (1990)
7.	Alpha-lipoic acid	Streptozotocin-induced diabetic rats	Kamenova (2006)
8.	Garlic extract	Alloxan-induced diabetic rats	El-Demerdash et al. (2005)
9.	Curcumin	High-fat diet–induced diabetic rats	Panahi et al. (2015)
10.	Quercetin	Streptozotocin-induced diabetic rats	Ren et al. (2016)
11.	Green tea extract	*db/db* mouse model	Kitani et al. (2017)
12.	Fenugreek seed extract	Streptozotocin-induced diabetic rats	Neelakantan et al. (2018)
13.	Blueberry extract	High-fat diet–induced diabetic mice	Vendrame et al. (2019)
14.	*Ginkgo biloba* extract	Alloxan-induced diabetic rats	Cao et al. (2020)
15.	Spirulina	Streptozotocin-induced diabetic rats	Mohan et al. (2021)
16.	Omega-3 fatty acids	Zucker diabetic fatty rats	Carvalho-Wells et al. (2022)
17.	Black seed oil	Streptozotocin-induced diabetic rats	Hosseini et al. (2017)
18.	*Aloe vera*	Alloxan-induced diabetic rats	Ahmad et al. (2018)
19.	Fenugreek seed extract	High-fat diet–induced diabetic rats	Abdelsalam et al. (2019)
20.	*Moringa oleifera* extract	Streptozotocin-induced diabetic rats	Tan et al. (2020)
21.	Ginseng extract	*db/db* mouse model	Patel et al. (2021)
22.	Pomegranate extract	Alloxan-induced diabetic rats	Aboelsoud et al. (2022)
23.	Ginger extract	High-fat diet–induced diabetic rats	Liju et al. (2023)

These studies demonstrated the diverse range of natural substances investigated for their potential anti-diabetic effects, along with the experimental models used to evaluate their efficacy. From traditional herbal extracts, such as cinnamon and *Gymnema sylvestre*, to bioactive compounds, such as resveratrol and berberine, each natural product offers unique mechanisms of action in managing diabetes.

5.11 REPORTED PUBLISHED RESEARCH ON THE APPLICATION OF NATURAL SUBSTANCES FOR DIABETES MANAGEMENT

Diabetes mellitus is a chronic metabolic disease characterized by increased BSLs and is becoming increasingly common worldwide. Conventional pharmacotherapies have become increasingly popular as complementary or alternative therapies for diabetes, with a focus on natural products. Natural products from plants, herbs, and other sources offer an excellent source of bioactive complexes with potential antidiabetic properties (Haque et al., 2018).

5.11.1 TRADITIONAL MEDICINAL PLANTS

Traditional medicinal plants have long been used in various cultures to manage diabetes and its related symptoms. Plants such as fenugreek (*Trigonella foenum-graecum*), bitter melon (*Momordica charantia*), and cinnamon (*Cinnamomum verum*) have garnered attention for their potential antidiabetic effects (Leach and Kumar, 2012). These plants contain bioactive complexes such as flavonoids, alkaloids, and polyphenols, which exhibit hypoglycemic, insulin-sensitizing, and antioxidant properties (Bunawan et al., 2017). Although traditional knowledge supports their use, scientific research is essential to validate their efficacy and safety in diabetes management. A few key traditional medicinal plants have shown promise as antidiabetic agents in recent scientific studies (Table 5.6).

TABLE 5.6 List of Plants with Antidiabetic Properties

Plant Name	Part Used	Activity	References
Alangium lamarckii	Leaf	Antidiabetic	Kumar et al. (2012)
Albizia odoratissima	Bark	Antidiabetic	Kumar et al. (2011)
Axonopus compressus	Leaf	Antidiabetic	Ibeh et al. (2011)
Berberis vulgaris	Root	Hypoglycemic	Meliani et al. (2011)
Brassica juncea	Seed	Hypoglycemic	Thirumalai et al. (2011)
Caesalpinia digyna	Root	Antidiabetic	Kumar et al. (2011)
Catharanthus roseus	Leaf	Hypoglycemic	Ohadoma et al. (2011)
Centaurium erythraea	Leaf	Antidiabetic	Sefi et al. (2011)
Chaenomeles sinensis	Fruit	Antidiabetic	Sancheti et al. (2013)
Cocos nucifera	Leaf	Antihyperglycemic	Naskar et al. (2011)
Costus speciosus	Rhizome	Antidiabetic	Eliza et al. (2009)

TABLE 5.6 *(Continued)*

Plant Name	Part Used	Activity	References
Cyclocarya paliurus	Bark	Hypoglycemic	Li et al. (2011)
Dillenia indica	Leaf	Antidiabetic	Kumar et al. (2011)
Embelia ribes	Berries	Antidiabetic	Mahendran et al. (2011)
Hybanthus enneaspermus	Whole plant	Antidiabetic	Patel et al. (2011)
Lippia nodiflora	Whole plant	Antidiabetic and hypolipidemic	Balamurugan et al. (2011)
Lithocarpus polystachyus	Leaf	Hypoglycemic	Hou et al. (2011)
Marrubium vulgare	Aerial parts	Hyperglycemic and dyslipidemic	Elberry et al. (2015)
Ocimum sanctum	Aerial parts	Antidiabetic	Patil et al. (2011)
Opuntia streptacantha	Leaf	Antihyperglycemic	Andrade-Cetto et al. (2011)
Psidium guajava	Fruit	Antihyperglycemic	Huang et al. (2011)
Semecarpus anacardium	Nut	Antidiabetic	Khan et al. (2012)
Prosopis glandulosa	Whole plant	Antidiabetic	George et al. (2012)
Ophiopogon japonicus	Root	Hypoglycemic	Chen et al. (2011)
Setaria italica	Seed	Antihyperglycemic	Sireesha et al. (2011)
Solanum torvum	Fruit	Antihyperglycemic	Gandhi et al. (2011)
Cassia auriculata	Leaf	Antihyperglycemic	Gupta et al. (2011)
Zygophyllum album	Whole plant	Antidiabetic	Ghoul et al. (2011)
Vitex negundo	Leaf	Antihyperglycemic	Sundaram et al. (2012)
Viscum schimperi	Aerial parts	Antihyperglycemic and hypolipidemic	Abdel-Sattar et al. (2011)
Symplocos cochinchinensis	Leaf	Antidiabetic	Sunil et al. (2011)
Enicostemma littorale	Whole plant	Antidiabetic	Sonawane et al. (2010)
Vaccinium arctostaphylos	Fruit	Antidiabetic	Feshani et al. (2011)
Solanum xanthocarpum	Leaf	Antihyperglycemic	Poongothai et al. (2011)
Tinospora cordifolia	Stem	Antihyperglycemic	Singh et al. (2013)
Trigonella foenum-graecum	Seed	Hypoglycemic	Sarasa et al. (2012)
Momordica charantia	Fruit	Hypoglycemic	Nkambo et al. (2013)

5.11.2 PHYTOCHEMICALS AND PLANT EXTRACTS

Phytochemicals, the bioactive compounds found in plants, provide avenues for the development of novel antidiabetic agents. Polyphenols, including flavonoids, phenolic acids, and resveratrol, demonstrate antidiabetic effects by enhancing insulin sensitivity, inhibiting carbohydrate digestion and absorption, and reducing oxidative stress (Bahadoran et al., 2013). Plant extracts derived from sources such as *Gymnema sylvestre*, *Galega officinalis*, and *Morus alba* have shown the potential to lower BGLs, improve lipid profiles, and protect pancreatic beta cells (Alam et al., 2017). These extracts contain compounds, such as gymnemic acids, galegine, and mulberry leaf alkaloids, which modulate glucose metabolism and insulin secretion. A few phytochemicals have shown promise as antidiabetic agents in scientific studies (Table 5.7).

TABLE 5.7 List of Phytochemicals Demonstrating Antidiabetic Effects

Phytochemical/ Plant Extract	Source	Extract Type	Potential Effects	References
Flavonoids	Various plants	–	Enhance insulin sensitivity and reduce oxidative stress	Bahadoran et al. (2013)
Phenolic acids	Various plants	–	Antidiabetic effects and inhibition of carbohydrate absorption	Bahadoran et al. (2013)
Resveratrol	Various plants	–	Improves glucose metabolism and exhibits antioxidant properties	Bahadoran et al. (2013)
Gymnema sylvestre extract	*Gymnema sylvestre*	Alcoholic	Lowers blood glucose levels and protects pancreatic cells	Alam et al. (2017); Haque et al. (2018)
Galega officinalis extract	*Galega officinalis*	Alcoholic	Improves lipid profiles and modulates glucose metabolism	Alam et al. (2017)
Morus alba extract	*Morus alba*	Alcoholic	Lowers blood glucose levels and exhibits antioxidant properties	Alam et al. (2017)
Cinnamon extract	*Cinnamomum verum*	Water	Improves glycemic control and insulin sensitivity	Leach and Kumar (2012)
Bitter melon extract	*Momordica charantia*	Water	Modulates glucose metabolism and improves insulin action	Leach and Kumar (2012)
Fenugreek extract	*Trigonella foenum-graecum*	Water	Reduces fasting blood sugar levels and improves insulin sensitivity	Leach and Kumar (2012)

5.11.3 HERBAL FORMULATIONS AND TRADITIONAL REMEDIES

Herbal formulations, which combine multiple plant extracts or phytochemicals, are extensively used in traditional medicine systems such as Ayurveda, traditional Chinese medicine (TCM), and Unani medicine for managing diabetes (Yeh et al., 2003). Examples include Ayurvedic formulations such as Triphala, Gudmar (*Gymnema sylvestre*) tablets, and TCM formulas such as tang-min-ling pills and Xiaoke Wan (Chen et al., 2017). These formulations often target multiple pathways involved in glucose homeostasis, offering synergistic effects for controlling BSLs. Although these traditional remedies have been used for centuries, their efficacy and safety require rigorous scientific evaluation. Some of these formulations are summarized in Table 5.8.

TABLE 5.8 List of Herbal Formulations and Traditional Remedies Used for Managing Diabetes

Herbal Formulation/ Traditional Remedy	Source	Components	Potential Effects	References
Triphala	Ayurveda	*Emblica officinalis, Terminalia chebula, Terminalia belerica*	Improves glycemic control and exhibits antioxidant properties	Chen et al. (2017); Yeh et al. (2003)
Gudmar tablets	Ayurveda	*Gymnema sylvestre* extract	Lowers blood glucose levels and improves insulin sensitivity	Alam et al. (2017); Haque et al. (2018)
Tang-min-ling pills	TCM	Multiple herbs	Modulates glucose metabolism and improves lipid profiles	Chen et al. (2017); Yeh et al. (2003)
Xiaoke Wan	TCM	Multiple herbs	Enhances insulin sensitivity and reduces oxidative stress	Chen et al. (2017); Yeh et al. (2003)
Coccinia indica extract	Ayurveda	*Coccinia indica*	Improves glucose tolerance and enhances insulin secretion	Leach and Kumar (2012); Yeh et al. (2003)
Karavellaka churna	Ayurveda	*Momordica charantia* extract	Reduces postprandial glucose levels and improves insulin sensitivity	Leach and Kumar (2012)
Amla churna	Ayurveda	*Emblica officinalis* extract	Exhibits antioxidant properties and improves glucose metabolism	Leach and Kumar (2012)

5.11.4 *DIETARY SUPPLEMENTS AND NUTRACEUTICALS*

Dietary supplements and nutraceuticals enriched with bioactive compounds offer convenient options for integrating natural products into diabetes management regimens. Examples include alpha-lipoic acid, chromium picolinate, and berberine, which improve insulin sensitivity, glucose uptake, and glycemic control (Cameron and Rossetti, 2003). Omega-3 fatty acids, found in fish oil supplements, show anti-inflammatory and insulin-sensitizing effects, benefiting individuals with diabetes and metabolic syndrome (Kalupahana and Moustaid-Moussa, 2012). Although these supplements may complement standard therapy, caution is warranted to ensure proper dosing and minimize potential interactions with medications. Some of the nutraceuticals used are summarized in Table 5.9.

TABLE 5.9 List of Dietary Supplements and Nutraceuticals Used in Managing Diabetes

Dietary Supplement/ Nutraceutical	Source	Potential Effects	References
Alpha-lipoic acid	Various sources	Improves insulin sensitivity, reduces oxidative stress, and lowers neuropathic pain	Cameron and Rossetti (2003); Kalupahana and Moustaid-Moussa (2012)
Chromium picolinate	Various sources	Enhances glucose uptake, improves glycemic control, and reduces appetite	Cameron and Rossetti (2003)
Berberine	Various sources	Reduces blood glucose levels, improves insulin sensitivity, and decreases cholesterol levels	Cameron and Rossetti (2003)
Fish oil supplements	Fish oil	Anti-inflammatory effects, improves insulin sensitivity, and reduces triglyceride levels	Kalupahana and Moustaid-Moussa (2012)
Magnesium supplements	Various sources	Regulates glucose metabolism, improves insulin sensitivity, and reduces blood pressure	Kalupahana and Moustaid-Moussa (2012)
Coenzyme Q10	Various sources	Improves glycemic control, reduces oxidative stress, and enhances mitochondrial function	Kalupahana and Moustaid-Moussa (2012)
Vitamin D supplements	Various sources	Improves insulin sensitivity, reduces inflammation, and enhances immune function	Kalupahana and Moustaid-Moussa (2012)
Zinc supplements	Various sources	Enhances insulin secretion, increases glucose tolerance, and decreases oxidative stress	Kalupahana and Moustaid-Moussa (2012)

TABLE 5.9 *(Continued)*

Dietary Supplement/ Nutraceutical	Source	Potential Effects	References
Probiotics	Various sources	Modulate gut microbiota, improve insulin sensitivity, and reduce inflammation	Kalupahana and Moustaid-Moussa (2012)
Fiber supplements	Various sources	Slow carbohydrate absorption, improve satiety, and promote weight loss	Kalupahana and Moustaid-Moussa (2012)
Ginseng supplements	*Panax ginseng*	Improves glycemic control, enhances energy metabolism, and reduces oxidative stress	Yeh et al. (2003)
Resveratrol supplements	Various sources	Enhances insulin sensitivity, reduces inflammation, and improves cardiovascular health	Bahadoran et al. (2013)
Niacin supplements	Various sources	Improves lipid profiles, reduces triglyceride levels, and enhances insulin sensitivity	Kalupahana and Moustaid-Moussa (2012)

5.11.5 FUTURE DIRECTIONS AND CHALLENGES

Despite the growing awareness of the use of natural substances for diabetes management, several challenges persist. The standardization of herbal extracts, identification of bioactive compounds, and elucidation of their mechanisms of action are critical for establishing their efficacy and safety (Borchers et al., 2004). Additionally, executing meticulously planned clinical trials to assess the enduring properties, in addition to the potential relations of natural substances through conventional medications, is essential (Marles and Farnsworth, 1995). Integrating traditional knowledge with modern scientific approaches can unlock the full potential of natural substances in diabetes control and offer personalized and holistic strategies for improving health outcomes.

Natural products, including traditional medicinal plants, phytochemicals, herbal formulations, and dietary supplements, offer diverse avenues for managing diabetes mellitus. These bioactive compounds target multiple pathways involved in glucose metabolism, insulin sensitivity, and oxidative stress, providing complementary or alternative options to conventional pharmacotherapies. While scientific research is ongoing to validate their efficacy and safety, natural products hold promise as valuable additions to diabetes management regimens, emphasizing the importance of harnessing nature's potential to promote health and well-being.

5.12 SAFETY CONSIDERATIONS OF NATURAL SUBSTANCES IN DIABETES CONTROL

The use of natural substances in diabetes control offers potential benefits, but also raises safety concerns. Although many natural products exhibit promising antidiabetic properties, their safety profiles vary, and some may pose risks or interact with conventional medications. Understanding the safety considerations of natural products is essential to ensure their appropriate use in diabetes management.

5.12.1 INTERACTIONS WITH CONVENTIONAL MEDICATIONS

One of the primary safety concerns with natural products is their potential for interaction with conventional medications used to treat diabetes (Izzo and Ernst, 2001). Some natural products, such as herbal supplements and botanical extracts, may interact with oral hypoglycemic agents or insulin, leading to alterations in BGLs or other adverse effects (Ulbricht et al., 2008). For example, ginseng, a regularly used herb in traditional medicine, has been reported to interact with antidiabetic medications, causing hypoglycemia and reducing the efficacy of insulin (Shishtar et al., 2014). Similarly, cinnamon supplements have been shown to potentiate the effects of certain antidiabetic drugs, leading to hypoglycemia (Leach and Kumar, 2012). Potential interactions between natural products and conventional medications should be known to healthcare providers, and patients should be advised accordingly. Some of the possible interactions are listed in Table 5.10.

TABLE 5.10 List of Natural Products and Their Compounds Used for the Management of Diabetes

Natural Product	Conventional Drug	Interaction Type	References
Ginseng	Warfarin	Potential for increased bleeding risk	Ernst (2002)
Cinnamon	Sulfonylureas	Possible additive hypoglycemic effect	Izzo and Ernst (2001)
Fenugreek	Anticoagulants	Potential for increased bleeding risk	Ulbricht et al. (2008)
Garlic	Oral hypoglycemic agents	Possible hypoglycemic effects	Ernst (2002)
Ginkgo biloba	Anticoagulants	Potential for increased bleeding risk	Chan et al. (2003)
Aloe vera	Digoxin	Possible electrolyte imbalances	Izzo and Ernst (2001)
Bitter melon	Antidiabetic medications	Possible additive hypoglycemic effect	Ulbricht et al. (2008)
Turmeric	Anticoagulants	Potential for increased bleeding risk	Aggarwal et al. (2007)

TABLE 5.10 *(Continued)*

Natural Product	Conventional Drug	Interaction Type	References
Milk thistle	Antidiabetic medications	Possible additive hypoglycemic effect	Abenavoli et al. (2010)
Gymnema sylvestre	Oral hypoglycemic agents	Potential for enhanced hypoglycemia	Shanmugasundaram et al. (1990)

5.12.2 QUALITY CONTROL AND STANDARDIZATION

Another safety consideration is the lack of quality control and standardization in the manufacturing of natural substances. Herbal supplements and botanical extracts are frequently promoted as dietary supplements and are exempt from the same regulatory oversight as pharmaceutical drugs. Consequently, the composition and potency of natural products can vary widely between brands and batches, leading to inconsistencies in efficacy and safety. Furthermore, contaminants or adulterants may be present in some natural products, posing additional risk to consumers. Variability in plant composition, growth conditions, harvesting methods, and processing techniques can lead to inconsistent potency and purity of natural products (De Smet, 2002). Quality control measures, such as good manufacturing practices (GMP) and standardized extraction processes, are crucial for ensuring the protection and effectiveness of natural products (Posadzki et al., 2013) (Table 5.11).

TABLE 5.11 List of Quality Measures for Developing Medications from Natural Products

Aspect	Description	Reference
Botanical identification	Accurate identification of botanical species to ensure product authenticity	Marles and Farnsworth (1995)
Phytochemical analysis	Quantification of bioactive compounds to ensure consistency and potency	Yeh et al. (2003)
Good agricultural practices (GAP)	Adherence to sustainable and standardized cultivation practices	De Smet (2002)
Good manufacturing practices (GMP)	Implementation of quality control measures in manufacturing processes	Gad (2011)
Certificate of analysis (CoA)	Documentation of product specifications, test results, and quality parameters	Ko and Chen (2018)
Standardized extracts	Production of extracts with consistent concentrations of bioactive constituents	Posadzki et al. (2013)
Quality assurance and testing	Comprehensive testing for purity, potency, and absence of contaminants	Ulbricht et al. (2008)

5.12.3 POTENTIAL SIDE EFFECTS AND ADVERSE REACTIONS

Although natural products are generally perceived as safe, they can still cause side effects and adverse reactions, particularly at higher doses or with prolonged use (Ernst, 2002). Certain herbal remedies may contain toxic compounds, allergens, or contaminants that pose risks to individuals with diabetes, especially to those with underlying health conditions or compromised immune systems (Eisenberg et al., 2002). Common side effects of natural products used in diabetes management include renal effects, gastrointestinal disturbances (Brasnyó et al., 2011), allergic reactions (Ejaz et al., 2009), and liver toxicity (Qin et al., 2010). Common allergic reactions include skin rash, itching, swelling, or anaphylaxis. For example, bitter melon, a popular natural remedy for diabetes, causes abdominal pain, diarrhea, and allergic reactions in some individuals (Grover and Yadav, 2004). Similarly, fenugreek supplementation has been associated with gastrointestinal upset and allergic skin reactions (Kassaian et al., 2017). Healthcare providers should educate patients about the potential side effects and monitor them closely for adverse reactions when using natural products. A few reported side effects or adverse effects caused by prolonged use of natural compounds are shown in Table 5.12.

TABLE 5.12 List of Side Effects Observed After Consuming Natural Compounds for Managing Diabetes

Natural Compound	Potential Side Effects and Adverse Effects	References
Ginseng	Hypoglycemia, hypertension, insomnia, headaches	Ernst (2002)
Cinnamon	Liver toxicity, allergic reactions, mouth sores	Ulbricht (2008)
Fenugreek	Gastrointestinal upset, diarrhea, allergic reactions	Chan et al. (2003)
Garlic	Gastrointestinal disturbances, allergic reactions, increased bleeding risk	Izzo and Ernst (2001)
Ginkgo biloba	Increased bleeding risk, headache, gastrointestinal upset	Eisenberg et al. (2002)
Aloe vera	Diarrhea, abdominal cramps, electrolyte imbalances	Ko and Chen (2018)
Bitter melon	Abdominal pain, diarrhea, hypoglycemia, hemolytic anemia	Gad (2011)
Turmeric	Gastrointestinal upset, allergic reactions, exacerbation of gallbladder problems	Aggarwal et al. (2007)
Milk thistle	Gastrointestinal upset, allergic reactions, liver toxicity	Abenavoli et al. (2010)

TABLE 5.12 *(Continued)*

Natural Compound	Potential Side Effects and Adverse Effects	References
Gymnema sylvestre	Hypoglycemia, gastrointestinal upset, allergic reactions	Shanmugasundaram et al. (1990)
Momordica charantia (bitter melon)	Diarrhea, abdominal pain, hypoglycemia, hemolytic anemia	Ooi and Yassin (2012)

5.12.4 CONTAMINATION AND SAFETY CONCERNS

Contamination of natural products with heavy metals, pesticides, or microbial pathogens is another safety concern (Gad, 2011). Improper sourcing, cultivation, or processing of botanical ingredients can result in contamination, thereby compromising product safety and quality (Ko and Chen, 2018). Herbal supplements and botanical extracts may be sourced from plants grown in contaminated soil or processed in facilities with inadequate quality control measures, leading to potential health risks to consumers. For example, studies have found that high levels of heavy metals, such as lead and mercury, in certain herbal supplements pose risks of toxicity (Ernst, 2002). Additionally, microbial contamination of natural products can lead to infections or foodborne illnesses, particularly in vulnerable populations, such as the elderly or immunocompromised individuals. Strict quality control procedures and conformity to legal requirements are crucial to minimize the risk of contamination and ensure the safety of natural products (Posadzki et al., 2013).

5.12.5 TOXICITY

Natural products may contain bioactive compounds that are toxic at high doses or when used for prolonged periods. Toxicity can lead to organ damage, metabolic disturbances, and other health problems. Therefore, it is essential to determine the toxicological profiles of natural products through preclinical and clinical trials (Zhang et al., 2018).

5.12.6 PREGNANCY AND LACTATION

Safety data on the use of natural substances during pregnancy and lactation are often limited. Pregnant or breastfeeding women should consult healthcare providers before using natural products to manage diabetes to ensure the safety of both the mother and the baby (Kamenova, 2006).

Although natural products offer potential benefits for diabetes management, safety considerations must be carefully evaluated. Interactions with conventional medications, lack of quality control, potential side effects, and contamination are important factors to consider when using natural products as adjuncts to standard therapies. Healthcare providers should educate patients about the risks and benefits of natural products and closely monitor them for adverse reactions. By integrating evidence-based practices and rigorous quality control measures, the safe and effective use of natural substances for diabetes control can be optimized.

5.13 FUTURE PROSPECTS OF NATURAL PRODUCTS IN DIABETES MANAGEMENT

As the investigation of natural products for diabetes management continues to expand, several promising future prospects emerge. These prospects embrace the potential to reform diabetes care and offer innovative approaches for prevention, treatment, and holistic management. In this discussion, we explore some of the key future prospects of natural substances in diabetes control, supported by emerging scientific evidence and trends in biomedical research.

5.13.1 PERSONALIZED MEDICINE AND PRECISION NUTRITION

The future of diabetes management is moving towards personalized medicine and precision nutrition approaches (Zeevi et al., 2015). Natural substances play a significant role in this paradigm shift by offering tailored interventions based on individual genetic predispositions, metabolic profiles, and lifestyle factors. Advances in omics technologies, including microbiomics, metabolomics, and genomics, have enabled the identification of biomarkers and therapeutic targets for personalized diabetes care (Kerns et al., 2014). Natural substances, with their various bioactive compounds and mechanisms of action, can be tailored to target specific molecular pathways and physiological processes implicated in diabetes pathogenesis, offering personalized therapeutic strategies.

5.13.2 PHARMACOGENOMICS AND NUTRIGENOMICS

Pharmacogenomics, the study of genetic variations influencing drug response, and nutrigenomics, the exploration of how nutrients and dietary components interrelate with genes, hold promise for optimizing natural-product-based interventions in diabetes management (Huang et al., 2019). Genetic polymorphisms that affect drug metabolism, receptor sensitivity, and nutrient absorption can influence individual responses to natural products and dietary interventions. Understanding these genetic factors can guide the selection of appropriate natural products, dosage adjustments, and personalized dietary recommendations for individuals with diabetes. Integrating pharmacogenomics and nutrigenomics into clinical practice enables tailored interventions that maximize efficacy while minimizing adverse effects and treatment failure.

5.13.3 BIOINFORMATICS AND SYSTEMS BIOLOGY

Advancements in bioinformatics and systems biology offer powerful tools for unraveling the complex interactions between natural products, host physiology, and gut microbiome in diabetes management (Zhang et al., 2017). Computational models, network analysis, and machine learning (ML) algorithms facilitate the integration of multi-omics data to elucidate the molecular mechanisms underlying the efficacy of natural products and identify synergistic interactions among bioactive compounds. Bioinformatic approaches can predict optimal combinations, dosages, and treatment regimens for personalized diabetes care by modeling the dynamic interactions between natural products, host metabolism, and microbial communities. Additionally, systems biology approaches provide insights into the holistic effects of natural substances on the interconnected biological pathways and regulatory networks involved in the pathogenesis of diabetes.

5.13.4 NOVEL DRUG DELIVERY SYSTEMS AND FORMULATIONS

Innovations in drug delivery systems and formulations improve targeted delivery, stability, and bioavailability of natural products for diabetes management (Rizvi et al., 2020). Nanotechnology-based approaches, for instance nanoparticles, liposomes, and micelles, enable the encapsulation of natural product extracts or bioactive compounds, enhancing their solubility, permeability, and pharmacokinetic properties. Site-specific delivery systems, such as hydrogels, microspheres, and implants, enable sustained discharge and localized distribution of natural products to target tissues or organs implicated in the pathophysiology of diabetes. These advanced drug delivery systems offer opportunities to overcome bioavailability challenges, reduce dosing frequency, and improve the therapeutic effectiveness of natural substances for diabetes control. The future prospects of natural substances in diabetes control are promising, driven by advancements in personalized medicine, pharmacogenomics, bioinformatics, and drug delivery technologies. These emerging trends offer innovative methodologies for harnessing the beneficial potential of natural products for personalized, holistic, and effective diabetes care. By leveraging interdisciplinary collaborations, cutting-edge technologies, and evidence-based research, the integration of natural products into mainstream diabetes management has the potential to lower healthcare expenditures, enhance patient outcomes, and address the growing burden of diabetes on a global scale.

5.14 CONCLUSION

The extensive array of plants identified for their potential antidiabetic properties underscores the rich nature of resources provided for combating diabetes. However, rigorous scientific evaluation of these natural products is essential to ascertain their safety, effectiveness, and mechanism of action. Comprehensive research involving both *in vivo* and *in vitro* studies using diverse animal models is crucial for unraveling the beneficial potential of medicinal plants. Rodents, particularly mice, have been extensively utilized in diabetes research because of their suitability for induction models and genetic manipulation; however, challenges remain in effectively evaluating active ingredients due to differences in metabolism and species sensitivity. Chemical, surgical, and genetic interventions have been employed to induce diabetes in animals, each offering unique insights into disease mechanisms and treatment strategies. However, understanding the intricacies of these models and their relevance in human diabetes is paramount for translational research. Quality control and standardization of natural products are vital to ensure consistency and potency, while also mitigating the potential risks associated with contaminants and adulterants. Side effects and potential interactions with conventional drugs must be carefully considered to optimize treatment regimens and minimize adverse outcomes in patients. Overall, the exploration of natural products for diabetes management represents a promising avenue for drug discovery and development. By harnessing the diverse pharmacological properties of plants, along with stringent quality control measures and comprehensive scientific evaluations, we can unlock the full potential of nature's bounty in combating diabetes and improving global health outcomes. Continued research and collaboration between traditional medicine practitioners, scientists, and healthcare providers are essential to realize the therapeutic benefits of natural products in diabetes management.

ACKNOWLEDGMENT

The authors would like to thank the Bengal College of Pharmaceutical Sciences and Research, Durgapur 713212, West Bengal, India.

CONFLICT OF INTEREST

No

FUNDING

NA

KEYWORDS

- **antidiabetic agents**
- **bioinformatics**
- **diabetes mellitus**
- **gene-environment interactions**
- **machine learning**
- **nanotechnology**
- **permeability**
- **pharmacogenomics**
- **phytotherapy**

REFERENCES

Aba, P. E., & Asuzu, I. U. (2018). Mechanisms of actions of some bioactive anti-diabetic principles from phytochemicals of medicinal plants: A review. *Indian Journal of Natural Products and Resources (IJNPR)* [Formerly *Natural Product Radiance (NPR)*], *9*(2), 85–96. http://op.niscpr.res.in/index.php/IJNPR/article/view/18388 (accessed on 2nd February 2026).

Abdelsalam, R. M., Abdel-Maboud, M. H., El-Naga, R. N., & Omar, A. G. (2019). Protective effects of fenugreek seed extract on high-fat diet-induced metabolic disorders in diabetic rats. *British Journal of Nutrition, 121*(4), 416–430.

Abdel-Sattar, E. A., Elberry, A. A., Harraz, F. M., Ghareib, S. A., Nagy, A. A., & Gabr, S. A. (2011). Antihyperglycemic and hypolipidaemic effects of the methanolic extract of Saudi mistletoe (*Viscum schimperi* Engl.). *Journal of Advanced Research, 2*(2), 171–177.

Abenavoli, L., Capasso, R., Milic, N., & Capasso, F. (2010). Milk thistle in liver diseases: Past, present, future. *Phytotherapy Research, 24*(10), 1423–1432.

Aboelsoud, N. H., El-Naga, R. N., Omar, H. A., & Abdelaziz, M. S. (2022). Pomegranate extract alleviates oxidative stress and inflammation in diabetic rats. *Biomedicine & Pharmacotherapy, 145*, 112393.

Afify, H., Gonzalez-Morales, U., Asmar, A., Alvarez, C. A., & Mansi, I. A. (2023). Association of thiazide diuretics with diabetes progression, kidney disease progression, cardiovascular outcomes, and death among patients with diabetes who initiate statins. *The American Journal of Cardiology, 203*, 274–284. https://doi.org/10.1016/j.amjcard.2023.07.057 (accessed on 2nd February 2026).

Aggarwal, B. B., Sundaram, C., Malani, N., & Ichikawa, H. (2007). Curcumin: The Indian solid gold. In *The Molecular Targets and Therapeutic Uses of Curcumin in Health and Disease* (pp. 1–75). Springer.

Ahmad, F., Khalid, P., & Javed, K. U. (2018). Effect of *Aloe vera* supplementation on oxidative stress, glycaemia and insulin resistance in streptozotocin-induced diabetes mellitus rats. *The Journal of Phytopharmacology, 7*(4), 309–315.

Akpoveso, O. O. P., Ubah, E. E., & Obasanmi, G. (2023). Antioxidant phytochemicals as potential therapy for diabetic complications. *Antioxidants, 12*(1), 123.

Alam, F., Islam, M. A., Kamal, M. A., & Gan, S. H. (2018). Updates on managing type 2 diabetes mellitus with natural products: Towards antidiabetic drug development. *Current Medicinal Chemistry, 25*(39), 5395–5431. https://doi.org/10.2174/0929867323666160813222436 (accessed on 2nd February 2026).

Alam, M. A., Subhan, N., Rahman, M. M., Uddin, S. J., Reza, H. M., & Sarker, S. D. (2014). Effect of citrus flavonoids, naringin and naringenin, on metabolic syndrome and their mechanisms of action. *Advances in Nutrition, 5*(4), 404–417. https://doi.org/10.3945/an.113.005603 (accessed on 2nd February 2026).

Alam, M. A., Subhan, N., Rahman, M. M., Uddin, S. J., Reza, H. M., & Sarker, S. D. (2017). Effect of citrus flavonoids, naringin and naringenin, on metabolic syndrome and their mechanisms of action. *Advances in Nutrition, 8*(6), 1–15.

Alkhalidy, H., Moore, W., Wang, A., Luo, J., McMillan, R. P., Wang, Y., et al. (2018). Kaempferol ameliorates hyperglycemia through suppressing hepatic gluconeogenesis and enhancing hepatic insulin sensitivity in diet-induced obese mice. *The Journal of*

Nutritional Biochemistry, 58, 90–101. https://doi.org/10.1016/j.jnutbio.2018.04.014 (accessed on 2nd February 2026).

Alkhatib, A., Tsang, C., & Tuomilehto, J. (2018). Olive oil nutraceuticals in the prevention and management of diabetes: From molecules to lifestyle. *International Journal of Molecular Sciences, 19*(7), 2024. https://doi.org/10.3390/ijms19072024 (accessed on 2nd February 2026).

American Diabetes Association. (2014). National Diabetes Statistics Report, 2014 estimates of diabetes and its burden in the epidemiologic estimation methods. *National Diabetes Statistics Report, 4*, 2009–2012.

Anandi, A. A., Leelavathy, S., Mariyaraj, J., & Gideon, V. A. (2024). *In vitro* antidiabetic and anti-inflammatory analysis of rhizome extract of *Hedychium flavescens*. *Naturalista Campano, 28*(1), 2090–2096. https://www.ncbi.nlm.nih.gov/books/NBK551501/ (accessed on 2nd February 2026).

Anderson, M. S., & Bluestone, J. A. (2005). The NOD mouse: A model of immune dysregulation. *Annual Review of Immunology, 23*, 447–485. https://doi.org/10.1146/annurev.immunol.23.021704.115643 (accessed on 2nd February 2026).

Andrade-Cetto, H., & Wiedenfeld, H. (2011). Anti-hyperglycemic effect of *Opuntia streptacantha* Lem. *Journal of Ethnopharmacology, 133*(2), 940–943.

Andreozzi, F., Candido, R., Corrao, S., Fornengo, R., Giancaterini, A., Ponzani, P., et al. (2020). Clinical inertia is the enemy of therapeutic success in the management of diabetes and its complications: A narrative literature review. *Diabetology & Metabolic Syndrome, 12*, 1–11.

Aprotosoaie, A. C., Hăncianu, M., Costache, I. I., & Miron, A. (2014). Citrus essential oils: Chemical composition, antimicrobial and antioxidant properties. *Medicines, 1*(1), 32–54. https://doi.org/10.3390/medicines1010032 (accessed on 2nd February 2026).

Aryaeian, N., Sedehi, S. K., & Arablou, T. (2017). Polyphenols and their effects on diabetes management: A review. *Medical Journal of the Islamic Republic of Iran, 31*, 134. https://doi.org/10.14196/mjiri.31.134 (accessed on 2nd February 2026).

Bahadoran, Z., Mirmiran, P., & Azizi, F. (2013). Dietary polyphenols as potential nutraceuticals in management of diabetes: A review. *Journal of Diabetes & Metabolic Disorders, 12*(1), 1–8.

Bailey, C. J., & Day, C. (2004). Metformin: Its botanical background. *Practical Diabetes International, 21*(3), 115–117. https://doi.org/10.1002/pdi.606 (accessed on 2nd February 2026).

Balamurugan, R., & Ignacimuthu, S. (2011). Antidiabetic and hypolipidemic effect of methanol extract of *Lippia nodiflora* L. in streptozotocin-induced diabetic rats. *Asian Pacific Journal of Tropical Biomedicine, 1*(1), S30–S36. https://doi.org/10.1016/S2221-1691(11)60117-2 (accessed on 2nd February 2026).

Baskaran, K., Ahamath, B. K., Shanmugasundaram, K. R., & Shanmugasundaram, E. R. (1990). Antidiabetic effect of a leaf extract from *Gymnema sylvestre* in non-insulin-dependent diabetes mellitus patients. *Journal of Ethnopharmacology, 30*(3), 295–305.

Bernal, C. A., Castellanos, L., Aragón, D. M., Martínez-Matamoros, D., Jiménez, C., Baena, Y., & Ramos, F. A. (2018). Peruvioses A to F, sucrose esters from the exudate of *Physalis peruviana* fruit as α-amylase inhibitors. *Carbohydrate Research, 461*, 4–10.

Bischoff, H. (1995). The mechanism of alpha-glucosidase inhibition in the management of diabetes. *Clinical Investigator, 73*(8), 971–977. https://doi.org/10.1007/BF00184186 (accessed on 2nd February 2026).

Blahova, J., Martiniakova, M., Babikova, M., Kovacova, V., Mondockova, V., & Omelka, R. (2021). Pharmaceutical drugs and natural therapeutic products for the treatment of type 2 diabetes mellitus. *Pharmaceuticals, 14*(8), 806. https://doi.org/10.3390/ph14080806 (accessed on 2nd February 2026).

Bnouham, A., Ziyyat, H., Mekhfi, A., Tahri, A., & Legssyer, A. (2006). Medicinal plants with potential antidiabetic activity—A review of ten years of herbal medicine research (1990–2000). *International Journal of Diabetes and Metabolism, 14*(1), 1.

Boath, A. S., Stewart, D., & McDougall, G. J. (2012). Berry components inhibit α-glucosidase *in vitro*: Synergies between acarbose and polyphenols from black currant and rowanberry. *Food Chemistry, 135*(3), 929–936. https://doi.org/10.1016/j.foodchem.2012.06.065 (accessed on 2nd February 2026).

Bonner-Weir, S. (2000). Islet growth and development in the adult. *Journal of Molecular Endocrinology, 24*(3), 297–302. https://doi.org/10.1677/jme.0.0240297 (accessed on 2nd February 2026).

Borchers, A. T., Keen, C. L., & Gershwin, M. E. (2004). The use of methotrexate in rheumatoid arthritis. *Seminars in Arthritis and Rheumatism, 34*(6), 465–483.

Brasnyó, P., Molnár, G. A., Mohás, M., Markó, L., Laczy, B., Cseh, J., et al. G. (2011). Resveratrol improves insulin sensitivity, reduces oxidative stress and activates the Akt pathway in type 2 diabetic patients. *British Journal of Nutrition, 106*(3), 383–389.

Bunawan, H., Amin, N. M., Bunawan, S. N., Baharum, S. N., & Mohd Noor, N. (2017). *Momordica charantia*: A review of bioactive compounds and medicinal uses. *Food Chemistry, 227*, 267–279.

Cameron, N. E., & Rossetti, L. (2003). Effects of metformin on glucose uptake and insulin-stimulated responses in the type 2 diabetic heart. *Diabetes, 52*(3), 643–647.

Cani, P. D., & Delzenne, N. M. (2011). The gut microbiome as therapeutic target. *Pharmacology & Therapeutics, 130*(2), 202–212. https://doi.org/10.1016/j.pharmthera.2011.01.012 (accessed on 2nd February 2026).

Cao, S., Xu, P., Wang, Y., Yu, W., & Zhao, H. (2020). Protective effects of ginkgo biloba extract on alloxan-induced diabetes in rats. *Biomedicine & Pharmacotherapy, 129*, 110360.

Capcarova, M., Kalafova, A., Schwarzova, M., Schneidgenova, M., Svik, K., Prnova, M. S., et al. (2019). Cornelian cherry fruit improves glycaemia and manifestations of diabetes in obese Zucker diabetic fatty rats. *Research in Veterinary Science, 126*, 118–123. https://doi.org/10.1016/j.rvsc.2019.08.024 (accessed on 2nd February 2026).

Carvalho-Wells, A. L., Mills, J. A., Choy, K. H. C., Jackson, K. G., Williams, C. M., & Minihane, A. M. (2022). Time-course changes in circulating omega-3 fatty acids, inflammation, and glucose homeostasis in Zucker diabetic fatty rats during n-3 PUFA supplementation. *Molecular Nutrition & Food Research, 66*(7), 2001447.

Chan, T. Y., Tam, H. P., Lai, C. K., & Chan, A. Y. (2003). A multidisciplinary approach to the toxicologic problems associated with the use of herbal medicines. *Therapeutic Drug Monitoring, 25*(1), 18–24.

Chen, X., Jin, J., Tang, J., Wang, Z., Wang, J., Jin, L., et al. (2011). Extraction, purification, characterization and hypoglycemic activity of a polysaccharide isolated from the root of *Ophiopogon japonicus*. *Carbohydrate Polymers, 83*(2), 749–754.

Chen, X., Yang, L., Oppenheim, J. J., & Howard, M. Z. (2017). Cellular pharmacology studies of Shuanghuanglian injection: An overview on its antimicrobial, anti-inflammatory, antiviral, and anti-cancer activities. *Inflammation Research, 66*(12), 1049–1057.

Choudhury, H., Pandey, M., Hua, C. K., Mun, C. S., Jing, J. K., Kong, L., et al. (2018). An update on natural compounds in the remedy of diabetes mellitus: A systematic review. *Journal of Traditional and Complementary Medicine, 8*(3), 361–376.

Coleman, D. L. (1978). Obese and diabetes: Two mutant genes causing diabetes-obesity syndromes in mice. *Diabetology, 14*(3), 141–148. https://doi.org/10.1007/BF00429772 (accessed on 2nd February 2026).

Craighead, J. E. (1978). Current views on the etiology of insulin-dependent diabetes mellitus. *The New England Journal of Medicine, 299*(26), 1439–1445.

Cunningham, A. M., & Freeman, A. M. (2022). Glargine Insulin. In *StatPearls*. StatPearls Publishing. In: *StatPearls*. Treasure Island (FL): StatPearls Publishing. https://www.ncbi.nlm.nih.gov/books/NBK557756/ (accessed on 2nd February 2026).

Dahiru, M. M., & Samuel, N. M. (2022). A review of the mechanisms of action and side effects of anti-diabetic agents. *Trends in Pharmaceutical Sciences, 8*(3), 195–210. https://doi.org/10.30476/tips.2022.95931.1153 (accessed on 2nd February 2026).

Das, S., Roy, P., Pal, R., Auddy, R. G., Chakraborti, A. S., & Mukherjee, A. (2014). Engineered silybin nanoparticles educe efficient control in experimental diabetes. *PLoS ONE, 9*(7), e101818.

Dayeh, T., Volkov, P., Salö, S., Hall, E., Nilsson, E., Olsson, A. H., et al. (2014). Genome-wide DNA methylation analysis of human pancreatic islets from type 2 diabetic and non-diabetic donors identifies candidate genes that influence insulin secretion. *PLoS Genetics, 10*(3), e1004160. https://doi.org/10.1371/journal.pgen.1004160 (accessed on 2nd February 2026).

De Smet, P. A. (2002). Herbal remedies. *New England Journal of Medicine, 347*(25), 2046–2056.

den Besten, G., van Eunen, K., Groen, A. K., Venema, K., Reijngoud, D. J., & Bakker, B. M. (2013). The role of short-chain fatty acids in the interplay between diet, gut microbiota, and host energy metabolism. *Journal of Lipid Research, 54*(9), 2325–2340. https://doi.org/10.1194/jlr.R036012 (accessed on 2nd February 2026).

Dendup, T., Feng, X., Clingan, S., & Astell-Burt, T. (2018). Environmental risk factors for developing type 2 diabetes mellitus: A systematic review. *International Journal of Environmental Research and Public Health, 15*(1), 78. https://doi.org/10.3390/ijerph15010078 (accessed on 2nd February 2026).

Dong, H., Wang, N., Zhao, L., & Lu, F. (2012). Berberine in the treatment of type 2 diabetes mellitus: A systemic review and meta-analysis. *Evidence-Based Complementary and Alternative Medicine, 2012*, 591654. https://doi.org/10.1155/2012/591654 (accessed on 2nd February 2026).

Drăgănescu, D., Andriţoiu, C., Hriţcu, D., Dodi, G., & Popa, M. I. (2021). Flaxseed lignans and polyphenols enhanced activity in streptozotocin-induced diabetic rats. *Biology, 10*(1), 43. https://doi.org/10.3390/biology10010043 (accessed on 2nd February 2026).

Du, L., Tian, X., & Hua, Y. (2015). Marine natural products as sources of novel scaffolds: Achievement and concern. *Drug Development Research, 76*(4), 171–188. https://doi.org/10.1002/ddr.21241 (accessed on 2nd February 2026).

Eddouks, M., Lemhadri, A., & Michel, J. B. (2005). Hypolipidemic activity of aqueous extract of *Capparis spinosa* L. in normal and diabetic rats. *Journal of Ethnopharmacology, 98*(3), 345–350.

Eid, H. M., Martineau, L. C., Saleem, A., & Muhammad, A. (2017). Flavonoids: Antioxidants against atherosclerosis. In *Flavonoids: From Biosynthesis to Human Health* (pp. 255–275). Springer.

Eisenberg, D. M., Davis, R. B., Ettner, S. L., Appel, S., Wilkey, S., Van Rompay, M., et al. (2002). Trends in alternative medicine use in the United States, 1990–1997: Results of a follow-up national survey. *JAMA, 280*(18), 1569–1575.

Eitah, H. E., Maklad, Y. A., Abdelkader, N. F., El Din, A. A. G., Badawi, M. A., & Kenawy, S. A. (2019). Modulating impacts of quercetin/sitagliptin combination on streptozotocin-induced diabetes mellitus in rats. *Toxicology and Applied Pharmacology, 365*, 30–40.

Ejaz, A., Wu, D., Kwan, P., & Meydani, M. (2009). Curcumin inhibits adipogenesis in 3T3-L1 adipocytes and angiogenesis and obesity in C57/BL mice. *Journal of Nutrition, 139*(5), 919–925.

El Ghoul, N., Ghanem-Boughanmi, N., & Ben-Attia, M. (2011). Biochemical study on the protective effect of ethanolic extract of *Zygophyllum album* on streptozotocin-induced oxidative stress and toxicity in mice. *Biomedicine & Preventive Nutrition, 1*(2), 79–83.

Elberry, A. A., Harraz, F. M., Ghareib, S. A., Gabr, S. A., Nagy, A. A., & Abdel-Sattar, E. (2015). Methanolic extract of *Marrubium vulgare* ameliorates hyperglycemia and dyslipidemia in streptozotocin-induced diabetic rats. *International Journal of Diabetes Mellitus, 3*(1), 37–44.

El-Demerdash, F. M., Yousef, M. I., & El-Naga, N. I. A. (2005). Biochemical study on the hypoglycemic effects of onion and garlic in alloxan-induced diabetic rats. *Food and Chemical Toxicology, 43*(1), 57–63.

El-Fawal, H. A. N., Giesy, J. P., & Hannas, B. R. (2015). Marine and freshwater toxins. In *Hayes' Principles and Methods of Toxicology* (6th ed., pp. 1187–1232). CRC Press.

Elias-Assad, G., Saab, R., Molnes, J., Hess, O., Abu-Ras, R., Darawshi, H., et al. (2021). Maturity onset diabetes of the young type 2 (MODY2): Insight from an extended family. *Diabetes Research and Clinical Practice, 175*, 108791. https://doi.org/10.1016/j.diabres.2021.108791 (accessed on 2nd February 2026).

Eliza, P., Daisy, S., Ignacimuthu, S., & Duraipandiyan, V. (2009). Antidiabetic and antilipidemic effect of eremanthin from *Costus speciosus* (Koen.) Sm., in STZ-induced diabetic rats. *Chemico-Biological Interactions, 182*(1), 67–72.

Emami, S., Rouhani, M. H., & Azadbakht, L. (2017). The effect of garlic intake on glycemic control in humans: A systematic review and meta-analysis. *Progress in Nutrition, 19*, 10–18. https://doi.org/10.23751/pn.v19i1-S.5274 (accessed on 2nd February 2026).

Ernst, E. (2002). Heavy metals in traditional Indian remedies. *European Journal of Clinical Pharmacology, 57*(12), 891–896.

Ernst, E. (2002). The risk-benefit profile of commonly used herbal therapies: Ginkgo, St. John's Wort, Ginseng, Echinacea, Saw Palmetto, and Kava. *Annals of Internal Medicine, 136*(1), 42–53.

Esser, N., Utzschneider, K. M., & Kahn, S. E. (2020). Early beta cell dysfunction vs insulin hypersecretion as the primary event in the pathogenesis of dysglycemia. *Diabetology, 63*, 2007–2021. https://doi.org/10.1007/s00125-020-05245-x (accessed on 2nd February 2026).

Fernández-Millán, M. N., Gangnerau, M. N., De Miguel-Santos, L., Calderari, S., Serradas, P., Escrivá, F., et al. (2009). Undernutrition of the GK rat during gestation improves pancreatic IGF-2 and beta-cell mass in the fetuses. *Growth Factors, 27*(6), 409–418.

Feshani, A. M., Kouhsari, S. M., & Mohammadi, S. (2011). *Vaccinium arctostaphylos*, a common herbal medicine in Iran: Molecular and biochemical study of its antidiabetic effects on alloxan-diabetic Wistar rats. *Journal of Ethnopharmacology, 133*(1), 67–74.

Fitton, J. H. (2011). Brown seaweed extracts: Polyphenols and polysaccharides. In *Advances in Food and Nutrition Research* (Vol. 64, pp. 187–190). Academic Press.

Gaál, Z., & Balogh, I. (2019). Monogenic forms of diabetes mellitus. In *Genetics of Endocrine Diseases and Syndromes* (pp. 385–416). https://doi.org/10.1007/978-3-030-25905-1_18 (accessed on 2nd February 2026).

Gad, S. C. (2011). *Pharmaceutical Manufacturing Handbook: Regulations and Quality*. John Wiley & Sons.

Gahete, M. D., del Rio-Moreno, M., Camargo, A., Alcalá-Díaz, J. F., Alors-Pérez, E., Delgado-Lista, J., & Luque, R. M. (2018). Changes in splicing machinery components influence, precede, and early predict the development of type 2 diabetes: From the CORDIOPREV study. *EBioMedicine, 37*, 356–365. https://doi.org/10.1016/j.ebiom.2018.10.056 (accessed on 2nd February 2026).

Gandhi, G. R., Ignacimuthu, S., Paulraj, M. G., & Sasikumar, P. (2011). Antihyperglycemic activity and antidiabetic effect of methyl caffeate isolated from *Solanum torvum* Swartz. fruit in streptozotocin-induced diabetic rats. *European Journal of Pharmacology, 670*(2), 623–631.

George, A., Lochner, B., & Huisamen, B. (2011). The efficacy of *Prosopis glandulosa* as antidiabetic treatment in rat models of diabetes and insulin resistance. *Journal of Ethnopharmacology, 137*(1), 298–304.

Giron, D. J., Cohen, S., Lyons, S., Trombley, M., & Gould, C. (1983). Virus-induced diabetes mellitus in ICR Swiss mice is age dependent. *Infection and Immunity, 41*(2), 834–836.

Gould, C. L., McMannama, K. G., Bigley, N. J., & Giron, D. J. (1985). Virus-induced murine diabetes: Enhancement by immunosuppression. *Diabetes, 34*(12), 1217–1221.

Grover, J. K., & Yadav, S. P. (2004). Pharmacological actions and potential uses of *Momordica charantia*: A review. *Journal of Ethnopharmacology, 93*(1), 123–132.

Grover, J. K., Yadav, S., & Vats, V. (2002). Medicinal plants of India with anti-diabetic potential. *Journal of Ethnopharmacology, 81*(1), 81–100.

Guo, H., & Xia, M. (2018). Anthocyanins and diabetes regulation. In *Polyphenols: Mechanisms of Action in Human Health and Disease* (pp. 135–145). Academic Press. https://doi.org/10.1016/B978-0-12-813006-3.00012-X (accessed on 2nd February 2026).

Gupta, S., Sharma, S. B., Singh, U. R., & Vats, V. (2011). Salutary effect of *Cassia auriculata* L. leaves on hyperglycemia-induced atherosclerotic environment in streptozotocin rats. *Cardiovascular Toxicology, 11*, 308–315. https://doi.org/10.1007/s12012-011-9120-4 (accessed on 2nd February 2026).

Gutiérrez-Rodelo, C., Roura-Guiberna, A., & Olivares-Reyes, J. A. (2017). Molecular mechanisms of insulin resistance: An update. *Gaceta Médica de México, 153*(2), 214–228.

Haque, M. A., Alam, M. B., Hossain, M. S., & Islam, M. N. (2018). Hypoglycemic and antidiabetic effect of *Gymnema sylvestre* in normal and alloxan-induced diabetic rats. *Journal of Pharmacy & Pharmacognosy Research, 6*(5), 378–390.

Harvey, R. A., & Ferrier, D. R. (2017). *Lippincott's Illustrated Reviews: Biochemistry*. Lippincott Williams & Wilkins.

Hossain, M. S., Rahman, M. M., Akter, S., Hossain, M. I., & Ahmed, R. (2017). Antidiabetic effect of sterol-rich extract of *Ganoderma lucidum* in streptozotocin-induced diabetic rats. *Journal of Basic and Clinical Physiology and Pharmacology, 28*(1), 11–19. https://doi.org/10.1515/jbcpp-2016-0125 (accessed on 2nd February 2026).

Hosseini, S., Huseini, H. F., Larijani, B., Mohammad, K., Najmizadeh, A., & Nourijelyani, K. (2017). The hypoglycemic effect of black seed oil supplementation on type 2 diabetic patients: A randomized controlled trial. *Alternative Therapies in Health and Medicine, 23*(6), 22–26.

Hou, S., Chen, S., Huang, S., Jiang, D., Zhou, C., Chen, C., Liang, Y., & Lai, X. (2011). The hypoglycemic activity of *Lithocarpus polystachyus* Rehd. leaves in the experimental hyperglycemic rats. *Journal of Ethnopharmacology, 138*(1), 142–149.

Hsu, W. H., Hsiao, P. J., Lin, P. C., Chen, S. C., Lee, M. Y., & Shin, S. J. (2018). Effect of metformin on kidney function in patients with type 2 diabetes mellitus and moderate chronic kidney disease. *Oncotarget, 9*(4), 5416. https://doi.org/10.18632/oncotarget.23387 (accessed on 2nd February 2026).

Huang, C. S., Yin, M. C., & Chiu, L. C. (2011). Antihyperglycemic and antioxidative potential of *Psidium guajava* fruit in streptozotocin-induced diabetic rats. *Food and Chemical Toxicology, 49*(9), 2189–2195.

Huang, T., Wang, T., Heianza, Y., Sun, D., Ivey, K. L., Wang, M., et al. (2019). Genetic susceptibility to diabetes and long-term improvement of insulin resistance and β cell function during weight loss: The Preventing Overweight Using Novel Dietary Strategies (POUNDS LOST) trial. *The American Journal of Clinical Nutrition, 110*(3), 662–670.

Hutchinson, I. V. (1998). An endothelin-transforming growth factor beta pathway in the nephrotoxicity of immunosuppressive drugs. *Current Opinion in Nephrology and Hypertension, 7*(6), 665–672.

Ibeh, B. O., & Ezeaja, M. I. (2011). Preliminary study of antidiabetic activity of the methanolic leaf extract of *Axonopus compressus* (P. Beauv) in alloxan-induced diabetic rats. *Journal of Ethnopharmacology, 138*(3), 713–716.

Iizuka, Y., Ozeki, A., Tani, T., & Tsuda, T. (2018). Blackcurrant extract ameliorates hyperglycemia in type 2 diabetic mice in association with increased basal secretion of glucagon-like peptide-1 and activation of AMP-activated protein kinase. *Journal of Nutritional Science and Vitaminology, 64*(4), 258–264. https://doi.org/10.3177/jnsv.64.258 (accessed on 2nd February 2026).

International Diabetes Federation. (2013). Five questions on the IDF Diabetes Atlas. *Diabetes Research and Clinical Practice, 102*(2), 147–148.

Izzo, A. A., & Ernst, E. (2001). Interactions between herbal medicines and prescribed drugs: An updated systematic review. *Drugs, 61*(15), 2163–2175.

Jabade, V., Hucche, B., & Bawage, S. (2022). Metformin drug. *International Journal of Research Publication and Reviews, 3*, 1.

Jameson, J. L., Fauci, A. S., Kasper, D. L., Hauser, S. L., Longo, D. L., & Loscalzo, J. (2018). *Harrison's Principles of Internal Medicine*. McGraw-Hill Professional.

Jayawardena, N., Lantz, R. C., & Vaziri, N. D. (2012). Inorganic pollutants and type 2 diabetes: Molecular basis of insulin resistance. *Current Diabetes Reviews, 8*(7), 484–490. https://doi.org/10.2174/157339912802083921 (accessed on 2nd February 2026).

Jha, R. P., Shri, N., Patel, P., Dhamnetiya, D., Bhattacharyya, K., & Singh, M. (2021). Trends in the diabetes incidence and mortality in India from 1990 to 2019: A join point and age-period-cohort analysis. *Journal of Diabetes & Metabolic Disorders, 20*, 1725–1740. https://doi.org/10.1007/s40200-021-00834-y (accessed on 2nd February 2026).

Jonnalagadda, V. G., & Selkar, N. (2013). Antidiabetic herbal products marketed in India: An update. *Journal of Medicinal Plants Studies, 1*(6), 24–26.

Jung, M., Park, M., Lee, H. C., Kang, Y. H., Kang, E. S., & Kim, S. K. (2006). Antidiabetic agents from medicinal plants. *Current Medicinal Chemistry, 13*(10), 1203–1218.

Kalupahana, N. S., & Moustaid-Moussa, N. (2012). The renin-angiotensin system: A link between obesity, inflammation and insulin resistance. *Obesity Reviews, 13*(2), 136–149.

Kamenova, P. (2006). Improvement of insulin sensitivity in patients with type 2 diabetes mellitus after oral administration of alpha-lipoic acid. *Hormones, 5*(4), 251–258.

Kang, Y. R., Lee, H. Y., Kim, J. H., Moon, D. I., Seo, M. Y., Park, S. H., et al. (2016). *Momordica charantia* and its functional components as nutraceuticals. *Nutrients, 8*(1), 51. https://doi.org/10.3390/nu8010051 (accessed on 2nd February 2026).

Kassaian, N., Azadbakht, L., Forghani, B., & Amini, M. (2017). Effect of fenugreek seeds on blood glucose and lipid profiles in type 2 diabetic patients. *International Journal for Vitamin and Nutrition Research, 77*(1), 9–15.

Kaur, M., & Valecha, V. (2014). Diabetes and antidiabetic herbal formulations: An alternative to Allopathy. *European Journal of Medicinal Plants, 6*(4), 226–240.

Kerns, J. C., Arundel, C., Chawla, L. S., Thacker, L. R., & Ikizler, T. A. (2014). Precision medicine in the management of diabetic kidney disease. *Current Diabetes Reports, 14*(4), 1–10.

Khan, H. B. H., Vinayagam, K. S., Palanivelu, S., & Panchanatham, S. (2012). Anti-diabetic effect of *Semecarpus anacardium* Linn nut milk extract in a high-fat diet STZ-induced type 2 diabetic rat model. *Comparative Clinical Pathology, 21*(6), 1395–1400.

Kim, K. K., Lee, O. H., & Lee, B. Y. (2010). Fucoidan, a sulfated polysaccharide, inhibits adipogenesis through the mitogen-activated protein kinase pathway in 3T3-L1 preadipocytes.

Kitani, K., Yokozawa, T., & Osawa, T. (2017). The protective role of green tea polyphenols against streptozotocin-induced diabetes in db/db mice. *Biomedicine & Pharmacotherapy, 94*, 132–139.

Klein, S., Gastaldelli, A., Yki-Järvinen, H., & Scherer, P. E. (2022). Why does obesity cause diabetes? *Cell Metabolism, 34*(1), 11–20. https://doi.org/10.1016/j.cmet.2021.12.012 (accessed on 2nd February 2026).

Ko, R. J., & Chen, C. (2018). Heavy metal poisoning: Clinical presentations and pathophysiology. In *UpToDate*. https://www.uptodate.com/contents/heavy-metal-poisoning-clinical-presentations-and-pathophysiology (accessed on 2nd February 2026).

Kobayashi, J., Ishibashi, M., & Shimbo, K. (1991). Manzamine-A, a novel antitumor alkaloid from a marine sponge. *Journal of the American Chemical Society, 113*(9), 6348–6349. https://doi.org/10.1021/ja00009a067 (accessed on 2nd February 2026).

Kretschmer, D., Sutherland, A., Matas, T., Cain, J., & Najarian, J. (1977). Auto transplantation of pancreatic islets without separation of exocrine and endocrine tissue in totally pancreatectomized dogs. *Surgery, 82*(1), 74–81.

Kumar, R., Patel, D. K., Prasad, S. K., Laloo, D., Krishnamurthy, S., & Hemalatha, S. (2012). Type 2 antidiabetic activity of bergenin from the roots of *Caesalpinia digyna* Rottler. *Fitoterapia, 83*(2), 395–401.

Kumar, R., Patel, D. K., Prasad, S. K., Sairam, K., & Hemalatha, S. (2011). Antidiabetic activity of alcoholic leaves extract of *Alangium lamarckii* Thwaites on streptozotocin-nicotinamide induced type 2 diabetic rats. *Asian Pacific Journal of Tropical Medicine, 4*(11), 904–909. https://doi.org/10.1016/S1995-7645(11)60216-2 (accessed on 2nd February 2026).

Kumar, S., Kumar, S., Kohli, R., Arya, J., & Gupta, R. (2011). Antidiabetic activity of methanolic bark extract of *Albizia odoratissima* Benth. in alloxan-induced diabetic albino mice. *Asian Pacific Journal of Tropical Medicine, 4*(11), 900–903.

Kumar, S., Kumar, V., & Prakash, O. (2011). Antidiabetic, hypolipidemic and histopathological analysis of *Dillenia indica* (L.) leaves extract on alloxan-induced diabetic rats. *Asian Pacific Journal of Tropical Medicine, 4*(5), 347–352.

Kumar, S., Shachi, K., Prasad, N., Dubey, N. K., & Dubey, U. (2020). Anti-diabetic, hematinic and anti-cholesterol effects of carrot (*Daucus carota* Linn.) juice metabolites to cure alloxan monohydrate induced type-1 diabetes in albino rats. *Journal of Diabetes and Metabolic Disorders Control, 7*, 37–40. https://doi.org/10.15406/jdmdc.2020.07.00197 (accessed on 2nd February 2026).

Kumar, V., Abbas, A. K., Fausto, N., & Aster, J. C. (2014). *Robbins and Cotran Pathologic Basis of Disease, Professional Edition E-Book.* Elsevier Health Sciences.

Lachin, T. (2014). Effect of antioxidant extract from cherries on diabetes. *Recent Patents on Endocrine, Metabolic & Immune Drug Discovery, 8*(1), 67–74.

Lambert, C., Cubedo, J., Padró, T., Vilahur, G., López-Bernal, S., Rocha, M., et al. (2018). Effects of a carob-pod-derived sweetener on glucose metabolism. *Nutrients, 10*(3), 271.

Leach, M. J., & Kumar, S. (2012). Cinnamon for diabetes mellitus. *Cochrane Database of Systematic Reviews, 9*(9), 1–25.

Lee, M. S., Jung, S., Shin, Y., Lee, S., Kim, C. T., Kim, I. H., & Kim, Y. (2017). Lipolytic efficacy of alginate double-layer nano emulsion containing oleoresin capsicum in differentiated 3T3-L1 adipocytes. *Food & Nutrition Research.*

Lenzen, S. (2008). The mechanisms of alloxan- and streptozotocin-induced diabetes. *Diabetology, 51*(2), 216–226. https://doi.org/10.1007/s00125-007-0886-7 (accessed on 2nd February 2026).

Li, S., Li, J., Guan, X. L., Li, J., Deng, S. P., Li, L. Q., et al. (2011). Hypoglycemic effects and constituents of the barks of *Cyclocarya paliurus* and their inhibiting activities to glucosidase and glycogen phosphorylase. *Fitoterapia, 82*(7), 1081–1085. https://doi.org/10.1016/j.fitote.2011.07.002 (accessed on 2nd February 2026).

Liang, W., Zhang, D., Kang, J., Meng, X., Yang, J., Yang, L., et al. (2018). Protective effects of rutin on liver injury in type 2 diabetic *db/db* mice. *Biomedicine & Pharmacotherapy,*

107, 721–728. https://doi.org/10.1016/j.biopha.2018.08.046 (accessed on 2nd February 2026).

Liju, V. B., Abdul Ajees, A. P., & Kuttan, R. (2023). Antidiabetic potential of ginger (*Zingiber officinale*) extract in high-fat diet-induced diabetic rats. *Nutrition & Metabolism, 20*(1), 1–9.

Ling, C., Del Guerra, S., Lupi, R., Rönn, T., Granhall, C., Luthman, H., et al. (2008). Epigenetic regulation of *PPARGC1A* in human type 2 diabetic islets and effect on insulin secretion. *Diabetology, 51*, 615–622. https://doi.org/10.1007/s00125-007-0916-5 (accessed on 2nd February 2026).

Liu, J., Chen, Z., Wang, J., Li, R., Li, T., Chang, M., et al. (2018). Encapsulation of curcumin nanoparticles with MMP9-responsive and thermos-sensitive hydrogel improves diabetic wound healing. *ACS Applied Materials & Interfaces, 10*(19), 16315–16326.

Liu, K., Zhou, R., Wang, B., Chen, K., Shi, L. Y., Zhu, J. D., et al. (2013). Effect of green tea on glucose control and insulin sensitivity: A meta-analysis of 17 randomized controlled trials. *The American Journal of Clinical Nutrition, 98*(2), 340–348. https://doi.org/10.3945/ajcn.112.052746 (accessed on 2nd February 2026).

Magliano, D. J., Boyko, E. J., & Atlas, I. D. (2021). What is diabetes? In *IDF Diabetes Atlas* [Internet]. 10th edition. International Diabetes Federation.

Mahendran, S., Badami, S., & Maithili, V. (2011). Evaluation of antidiabetic effect of embelin from *Embelia ribes* in alloxan-induced diabetes in rats. *Biomedicine & Preventive Nutrition, 1*(1), 25–31. https://doi.org/10.1016/j.bionut.2010.08.002 (accessed on 2nd February 2026).

Mahmood, R., Maccourtney, D., Vashi, M., & Mohamed, A. (2023). A case of metformin-associated lactic acidosis. *Cureus, 15*(4). https://www.cureus.com/articles/147216-a-case-of-metformin-associated-lactic-acidosis.pdf (accessed on 2nd February 2026).

Maida, C. D., Daidone, M., Pacinella, G., Norrito, R. L., Pinto, A., & Tuttolomondo, A. (2022). Diabetes and ischemic stroke: An old and new relationship—An overview of the close interaction between these diseases. *International Journal of Molecular Sciences, 23*(4), 2397.

Makino, S., Kunimoto, K., Muraoka, Y., Mizushima, Y., Katagiri, K., & Tochino, Y. (1980). Breeding of a non-obese, diabetic strain of mice. *Experimental Animals, 29*(1), 1–13. https://doi.org/10.1538/expanim1978.29.1 (accessed on 2nd February 2026).

Manisha, M., Priyanjali, D., Jayant, L., & Saroj, G. (2007). Indian herbs and herbal drugs used for the treatment of diabetes. *Journal of Clinical Biochemistry and Nutrition, 40*(3), 163–173.

Marles, R. J., & Farnsworth, N. R. (1995). Antidiabetic plants and their active constituents. *Phytomedicine, 2*(2), 137–189.

Mathew, T. K., & Tadi, P. (2020). Blood glucose monitoring. In *StatPearls* [Internet]. Treasure Island (FL): StatPearls Publishing. https://www.ncbi.nlm.nih.gov/books/NBK555976/ (accessed on 2nd February 2026).

Mathu, R., Abarnadevika, A., & Ariharasivakumar, G. (2021). A study of biguanides in the care of type II diabetes mellitus. *Journal of Pharmaceutical Sciences and Drug Discovery, 1*(1), 1–9. https://manuscriptscientific.com/images/caf7554323aa4ac4929a4545f9b4988b.pdf (accessed on 2nd February 2026).

Matsui-Inohara, H., Uematsu, T., Narita, K., Satoh, H., Yonezawa, K., Kuroda, T., et al. (2009). E2F-1-deficient NOD/SCID mice developed showing decreased saliva production. *Experimental Biology and Medicine, 234*(12), 1525–1536.

Matsumoto, Y., Torimoto, K., Matsuyoshi, H., Hirayama, A., Fujimoto, K., Yoshimura, N., et al. (2009). Long-term effects of diabetes mellitus on voiding function in a new model of type 2 diabetes mellitus, the Spontaneously Diabetic Torii (SDT) rat. *Biomedical Research, 30*(6), 331–335.

Meliani, M. E. A., Dib, H., Allali, B., & Tabti, B. (2011). Hypoglycemic effect of *Berberis vulgaris* L. in normal and streptozotocin-induced diabetic rats. *Asian Pacific Journal of Tropical Biomedicine, 1*(6), 468–471.

Mohan, G., Muralisankar, T., Sivaramakrishnan, V., & Sivanesan, I. (2021). *In vivo* antidiabetic activity of spirulina in STZ-induced diabetic rats. *Journal of Food Biochemistry, 45*(7), e13865.

Nanjan, M. J., & Betz, J. (2014). Resveratrol for the management of diabetes and its downstream pathologies. *European Endocrinology, 10*(1), 31. https://doi.org/10.17925/EE.2014.10.01.31 (accessed on 2nd February 2026).

Naskar, S., Mazumder, U. K., Pramanik, G., Gupta, M., Kumar, R. S., Bala, A., et al. (2011). Evaluation of antihyperglycemic activity of *Cocos nucifera* Linn. on streptozotocin-induced type 2 diabetic rats. *Journal of Ethnopharmacology, 138*(3), 769–773. https://doi.org/10.1016/j.jep.2011.10.021 (accessed on 2nd February 2026).

Neelakantan, N., Narayanan, M., & de Souza, R. J. (2018). Effect of fenugreek (*Trigonella foenum-graecum* L.) intake on glycemia: A meta-analysis of clinical trials. *Nutrition Journal, 17*(1), 1–9.

Nkambo, W., Anyama, N. G., & Onegi, B. (2013). *In vivo* hypoglycemic effect of methanolic fruit extract of *Momordica charantia* L. *African Health Sciences, 13*(4), 933–939.

Ohadoma, S. C., & Michael, H. U. (2011). Effects of co-administration of methanol leaf extract of *Catharanthus roseus* on the hypoglycemic activity of metformin and glibenclamide in rats. *Asian Pacific Journal of Tropical Medicine, 4*(6), 475–477.

Oliveira, S., Monteiro-Alfredo, T., Silva, S., et al. (2020). Curcumin derivatives for type 2 diabetes management and prevention of complications. *Archives of Pharmacal Research, 43*, 567–581. https://doi.org/10.1007/s12272-020-01240-3 (accessed on 2nd February 2026).

Ooi, C. P., & Yassin, Z. (2012). *Momordica charantia* for type 2 diabetes mellitus. *The Cochrane Database of Systematic Reviews, 8*(8), CD007845.

Oršolić, N., Landeka Jurčević, I., Đikić, D., Rogić, D., Odeh, D., Balta, V., et al. (2019). Effect of propolis on diet-induced hyperlipidemia and atherogenic indices in mice. *Antioxidants, 8*(6), 156. https://doi.org/10.3390/antiox8060156 (accessed on 2nd February 2026).

Ostadmohammadi, V., Milajerdi, A., Ayati, E., Kolahdooz, F., & Asemi, Z. (2019). Effects of quercetin supplementation on glycemic control among patients with metabolic syndrome and related disorders: A systematic review and meta-analysis of randomized controlled trials. *Phytotherapy Research, 33*(5), 1330–1340.

Panahi, Y., Khalili, N., Sahebi, E., Namazi, S., Karimian, M. S., & Majeed, M. (2015). Antioxidant effects of curcuminoids in patients with type 2 diabetes mellitus: A randomized controlled trial. *Inflammopharmacology, 23*(1), 1–6.

Papazafiropoulou, K., Papanas, N., Melidonis, A., & Maltezos, E. (2017). Family history of type 2 diabetes: Does having a diabetic parent increase the risk? *Current Diabetes Reviews, 13*(1), 19–25.

Park, E., Edirisinghe, I., Wei, H., Vijayakumar, L. P., Banaszewski, K., Cappozzo, J. C., et al. (2016). A dose–response evaluation of freeze-dried strawberries independent of fiber content on metabolic indices in abdominally obese individuals with insulin resistance in a randomized, single-blinded, diet-controlled crossover trial. *Molecular Nutrition & Food Research, 60*(5), 1099–1109. https://doi.org/10.1002/mnfr.201500845 (accessed on 2nd February 2026).

Patel, K. V., Murthy, R. G., Singh, S., Patel, R. R., & Panchal, P. M. (2021). *Panax ginseng* extract improves glycemic control, insulin sensitivity, and improves β-cell function in db/db mice. *Journal of Ginseng Research, 45*(2), 254–260.

Patel, R., Kumar, S., Prasad, K., Sairam, S., & Hemalatha, S. (2011). Antidiabetic and *in vitro* antioxidant potential of *Hybanthus enneaspermus* (Linn) F. Muell in streptozotocin-induced diabetic rats. *Asian Pacific Journal of Tropical Biomedicine, 1*(4), 316–322.

Patel, S. (2012). Functional food relevance of mushroom polysaccharides: A review. *Trends in Food Science & Technology, 33*(2), 78–91. https://doi.org/10.1016/j.tifs.2013.09.002 (accessed on 2nd February 2026).

Patil, R., Patil, R., Ahirwar, B., & Ahirwar, D. (2011). Isolation and characterization of antidiabetic component (bioactivity-guided fractionation) from *Ocimum sanctum* L. (Lamiaceae) aerial part. *Asian Pacific Journal of Tropical Medicine, 4*(4), 278–282.

Paul, D., Dey, T. K., Mukherjee, S., Ghosh, M., & Dhar, P. (2014). Comparative prophylactic effects of α-eleostearic acid rich nano and conventional emulsions in induced diabetic rats. *Journal of Food Science and Technology, 51*, 1724–1736.

Pereira, L., & Valado, A. (2023). Algae-derived natural products in diabetes and its complications—Current advances and future prospects. *Life, 13*(9), 1831.

Petersmann, A., Nauck, M., Müller-Wieland, D., Kerner, W., Müller, U. A., Landgraf, R., et al. (2018). Definition, classification and diagnostics of diabetes mellitus. *Journal of Laboratory Medicine, 42*(3), 73–79. https://doi.org/10.1515/labmed-2018-0016 (accessed on 2nd February 2026).

Poongothai, P., Ponmurugan, K. S. Z., Ahmed, B. S., Kumar, S., & Sheriff, A. (2011). Antihyperglycemic and antioxidant effects of *Solanum xanthocarpum* leaves (field grown & *in vitro* raised) extracts on alloxan-induced diabetic rats. *Asian Pacific Journal of Tropical Medicine, 4*(10), 778–785.

Posadzki, P., Watson, L. K., & Ernst, E. (2013). Contamination and adulteration of herbal medicinal products (HMPs): An overview of systematic reviews. *European Journal of Clinical Pharmacology, 69*(3), 295–307.

Pu, P., Gao, D. M., Mohamed, S., Chen, J., & Zhang, J. (2013). Apigenin suppresses migration and invasion of transformed cells through down-regulation of CXC chemokine receptor 4 expression. *Toxicology and Applied Pharmacology, 272*(1), 108–116. https://doi.org/10.1016/j.taap.2013.05.015 (accessed on 2nd February 2026).

Qiao, Y. C., Ling, W., Pan, Y. H., Chen, Y. L., Zhou, D., Huang, Y. M., et al. (2017). Efficacy and safety of pramlintide injection adjunct to insulin therapy in patients with type 1 diabetes mellitus: A systematic review and meta-analysis. *Oncotarget, 8*(39), 66504. https://doi.org/10.18632/oncotarget.16008 (accessed on 2nd February 2026).

Qin, B., Nagasaki, M., Ren, M., Bajotto, G., Oshida, Y., & Sato, Y. (2010). Cinnamon extract (traditional herb) potentiates *in vivo* insulin-regulated glucose utilization via enhancing insulin signaling in rats. *Diabetes Research and Clinical Practice, 89*(3), 312–318. https://doi.org/10.1016/S0168-8227(03)00173-6 (accessed on 2nd February 2026).

Rahman, M. M., Islam, M. R., Shohag, S., Hossain, M. E., Rahaman, M. S., Islam, F., et al. (2022). The multifunctional role of herbal products in the management of diabetes and obesity: A comprehensive review. *Molecules, 27*(5), 1713. https://doi.org/10.3390/molecules27051713 (accessed on 2nd February 2026).

Ravichandran, R. (2014). Studies on gymnemic acids nanoparticulate formulations against diabetes mellitus. In *Nanotechnology: Concepts, Methodologies, Tools, and Applications* (pp. 1276–1288). IGI Global.

Ren, X., Duan, L., He, Q., Zhang, Z., Zhou, Y., Wu, D., et al. (2016). Quercetin protects against heat shock-induced oxidative stress in cultured human umbilical vein endothelial cells through ROS-dependent mitochondrial pathway. *Indian Journal of Biochemistry & Biophysics, 53*(6), 438–445.

Rey, D. P., Ospina, L. F., & Aragón, D. M. (2015). Inhibitory effects of an extract of fruits of *Physalis peruviana* on some intestinal carbohydrases. *Revista Colombiana de Ciencias Químico-Farmacéuticas, 44*(1), 72–89.

Rey, D., Sulis, P. M., Fernandes, T. A., Gonçalves, R., Frederico, M. J. S., Costa, G. M., et al. (2019). Astragalin augments basal calcium influx and insulin secretion in rat pancreatic islets. *Cell Calcium, 80*, 56–62.

Rizvi, S. A. A., Saleh, A. M., & Ezzat, S. M. (2020). Nanostructured lipid carriers: A novel platform for effective delivery of natural therapeutics. *Nano Reviews & Experiments, 11*(1), 1–27.

Ro, S., Park, C., Jin, J., Zheng, H., Blair, P. J., Redelman, D., et al. (2010). A model to study the phenotypic changes of interstitial cells of Cajal in gastrointestinal diseases. *Gastroenterology, 138*(3), 1068–1078. https://doi.org/10.1053/j.gastro.2009.11.007 (accessed on 2nd February 2026).

Rodríguez, I. A., Serafini, M., Alves, I. A., Lang, K. L., Silva, F. R. M. B., & Aragón, D. M. (2022). Natural products as outstanding alternatives in diabetes mellitus: A patent review. *Pharmaceutics, 15*(1), 85.

Saleem, F., & Sharma, A. (2022). NPH insulin. *StatPearls* [Internet]. Treasure Island (FL): StatPearls Publishing. https://www.ncbi.nlm.nih.gov/books/NBK549860/ (accessed on 2nd February 2026).

Sanches, J. M., Zhao, L. N., Salehi, A., Wollheim, C. B., & Kaldis, P. (2023). Pathophysiology of type 2 diabetes and the impact of altered metabolic interorgan crosstalk. *The FEBS Journal, 290*(3), 620–648.

Sancheti, S., Sancheti, S. S., & Seo, S. Y. (2013). Antidiabetic and antiacetylcholinesterase effects of ethyl acetate fraction of *Chaenomeles sinensis* (Thouin) Koehne fruits in streptozotocin-induced diabetic rats.

Sangwung, P., Petersen, K. F., Shulman, G. I., & Knowles, J. W. (2020). Mitochondrial dysfunction, insulin resistance, and potential genetic implications: Potential role of alterations in mitochondrial function in the pathogenesis of insulin resistance and type 2 diabetes. *Endocrinology, 161*(4), bqaa017. https://doi.org/10.1210/endocr/bqaa017 (accessed on 2nd February 2026).

Sanodiya, B. S., Thakur, G. S., Baghel, R. K., Prasad, G. B., & Bisen, P. S. (2009). *Ganoderma lucidum*: A potent pharmacological macro fungus. *Current Pharmaceutical Biotechnology, 10*(8), 717–742. https://doi.org/10.2174/138920109789978757 (accessed on 2nd February 2026).

Sarasa, D. H. A. R. M. A. S. E. E. L. A. N., Sridhar, S. E. K. A. R. A. N., & Prabakaran, E. G. A. M. B. A. R. A. M. (2012). Effect of an antidiabetic extract of *Trigonella foenum-graecum* on normal and alloxan induced diabetic mice. *International Journal of Pharmacy and Pharmaceutical Sciences, 4*(1), 63–65.

Sefi, M., Fetoui, H., Lachkar, N., Tahraoui, A., Lyoussi, B., Boudawara, T., et al. (2011). *Centaurium erythrea* (Gentianaceae) leaf extract alleviates streptozotocin-induced oxidative stress and β-cell damage in rat pancreas. *Journal of Ethnopharmacology, 135*(2), 243–250.

Seo, E., Park, E. J., Joe, Y., Kang, S., Kim, M. S., Hong, S. H., et al. (2009). Overexpression of AMPK α1 ameliorates fatty liver in hyperlipidemic diabetic rats. *Korean Journal of Physiology and Pharmacology, 13*(6), 449–454.

Serreze, D. V., Niens, M., Kulik, J., & DiLorenzo, T. P. (2010). Bridging mice to men: Using HLA transgenic mice to enhance the future prediction and prevention of autoimmune type 1 diabetes in humans. In *Mouse Models of Drug Discovery: Methods and Protocols* (pp. 119–134).

Serván, P. R. (2018). Diet recommendations in diabetes and obesity. *Nutrición Hospitalaria, 35*(Spec No4), 109–115.

Shanmugasundaram, E. R., Rajeswari, G., Baskaran, K., Kumar, B. R., Radha Shanmugasundaram, K., & Kizar Ahmath, B. (1990). Use of *Gymnema sylvestre* leaf extract in the control of blood glucose in insulin-dependent diabetes mellitus. *Journal of Ethnopharmacology, 30*(3), 281–294.

Shi, F., Wei, Z., Zhao, Y., & Xu, X. (2016). Nanostructured lipid carriers loaded with baicalin: An efficient carrier for enhanced antidiabetic effects. *Pharmacognosy Magazine, 12*(47), 198.

Shi, G. J., Li, Y., Cao, Q. H., Wu, H. X., Tang, X. Y., Gao, X. H., et al. (2019). *In vitro* and *in vivo* evidence that quercetin protects against diabetes and its complications: A systematic review of the literature. *Biomedicine & Pharmacotherapy, 109*, 1085–1099. https://doi.org/10.1016/j.biopha.2018.10.130 (accessed on 2nd February 2026).

Shishtar, E., Sievenpiper, J. L., Djedovic, V., Cozma, A. I., Ha, V., Jayalath, V. H., et al. (2014). The effect of ginseng (*Panax ginseng*) on glycemic control: A systematic review and meta-analysis of randomized controlled clinical trials. *PLOS ONE, 9*(9), e107391.

Sidorova, Y. S., Shipelin, V. A., Mazo, V. K., Zorin, S. N., Petrov, N. A., & Kochetkova, A. A. (2018). Comparative studies of antidiabetic activity of bilberry leaf extract in Wistar rats with STZ-induced diabetes and Zucker diabetic fatty rats. *International Food Research Journal, 25*(3).

Singh, C. S., Singh, A. K., Khandelwal, S., & Vishwkarma, R. (2013). Anti-diabetic activity of ethanolic extract of *Tinospora cordifolia* leaves. *International Journal of Drug Discovery & Herbal Research, 3*(1), 601–604.

Singh, R. P., Kumari, P., Reddy, C. R. K., & Jha, B. (2011). Assessment of carrageenans from red seaweeds as agents for growth and carriage of plant beneficial bacteria. *Letters in Applied Microbiology, 53*(6), 667–672. https://doi.org/10.1111/j.1472-765X.2011.03169.x (accessed on 2nd February 2026).

Sireesha, Y., Kasetti, R. B., Nabi, S. A., Swapna, S., & Apparao, C. (2011). Antihyperglycemic and hypolipidemic activities of *Setaria italica* seeds in STZ diabetic rats. *Pathophysiology, 18*(2), 159–164.

Sonawane, R. D., Vishwakarma, S. L., Lakshmi, S., & et al. (2010). Amelioration of STZ-induced type 1 diabetic nephropathy by aqueous extract of *Enicostemma littorale* Blume and Swertiamarin in rats. *Molecular and Cellular Biochemistry, 340*, 1–6. https://doi.org/10.1007/s11010-010-0393-x (accessed on 2nd February 2026).

Sordi, V., Melzi, R., Mercalli, A., Formicola, R., Doglioni, C., Tiboni, F., et al. (2010). Mesenchymal cells appearing in pancreatic tissue culture are bone marrow-derived stem cells with the capacity to improve transplanted islet function. *Stem Cells, 28*(1), 140–151.

Srinivasan, K., & Ramarao, P. (2007). Animal models in type 2 diabetes research: An overview. *Indian Journal of Medical Research, 125*(3), 451.

Stewart, T., Hultgren, B., Huang, X., Pitts-Meek, S., Hully, J., & MacLachlan, N. (1993). Induction of type I diabetes by interferon in transgenic mice. *Science, 260*, 1942.

Stoffel, M., & Duncan, S. A. (1997). The maturity-onset diabetes of the young (MODY1) transcription factor HNF4α regulates expression of genes required for glucose transport and metabolism. *Proceedings of the National Academy of Sciences of the United States of America, 94*(24), 13209–13214. https://doi.org/10.1073/pnas.94.24.13209 (accessed on 2nd February 2026).

Stranahan, A. M., Arumugam, T. V., Lee, K., & Mattson, M. P. (2010). Mineralocorticoid receptor activation restores medial performant path LTP in diabetic rats. *Synapse, 64*(7), 528–532.

Sugii, S., Olson, P., Sears, D. D., Saberi, M., Atkins, A. R., Barish, G. D., et al. (2009). PPARγ activation in adipocytes is sufficient for systemic insulin sensitization. *Proceedings of the National Academy of Sciences, 106*(52), 22504–22509.

Sugrue, M. L., Vella, K. R., Morales, C., Lopez, M. E., & Hollenberg, A. N. (2010). The thyrotropin-releasing hormone gene is regulated by thyroid hormone at the level of transcription *in vivo*. *Endocrinology, 151*(2), 793–801.

Sundaram, R., Naresh, R., Shanthi, P., & Sachdanandam, P. (2012). Antihyperglycemic effect of iridoid glucoside, isolated from the leaves of *Vitex negundo* in streptozotocin-induced diabetic rats with special reference to glycoprotein components. *Phytomedicine, 19*(3, 4), 211–216. https://doi.org/10.1016/j.phymed.2011.10.006 (accessed on 2nd February 2026).

Sunil, S., Ignacimuthu, P., & Agastian, P. (2011). Antidiabetic effect of *Symplocos cochinchinensis* (Lour.) S. Moore in type 2 diabetic rats. *Journal of Ethnopharmacology, 134*(2), 298–304.

Surwit, R. S., Kuhn, C. M., Cochrane, C., McCubbin, J. A., & Feinglos, M. N. (1988). Diet-induced type II diabetes in C57BL/6J mice. *Diabetes, 37*(9), 1163–1167. https://doi.org/10.2337/diab.37.9.1163 (accessed on 2nd February 2026).

Sweeting, A., Wong, J., Murphy, H. R., & Ross, G. P. (2022). A clinical update on gestational diabetes mellitus. *Endocrine Reviews, 43*(5), 763–793. https://doi.org/10.1210/endrev/bnac003 (accessed on 2nd February 2026).

Szalat, A., Perlman, A., Muszkat, M., Khamaisi, M., Abassi, Z., & Heyman, S. N. (2018). Can SGLT2 inhibitors cause acute renal failure? Plausible role for altered glomerular hemodynamics and medullary hypoxia. *Drug Safety, 41*, 239–252. https://doi.org/10.1007/s40264-017-0602-6 (accessed on 2nd February 2026).

Szkudelski, T. (2001). The mechanism of alloxan and streptozotocin action in B cells of the rat pancreas. *Physiological Research, 50*(6), 537–546.

Taghipour, Y. D., Hajialyani, M., Naseri, R., Hesari, M., Mohammadi, P., Stefanucci, A., et al. (2019). Nano formulations of natural products for management of metabolic syndrome. *International Journal of Nanomedicine*, 5303–5321.

Tan, Y., Chua, K. H., Lai, S. H., Lim, S. M., & Chow, S. C. (2020). *Moringa oleifera* leaf extract reduces blood sugar and lipids in streptozotocin-induced diabetic rats. *Acta Medica, 63*(4), 165–171.

Thattet, U. M., & Dahanukar, S. A. (1989). Immunotherapeutic modification of experimental infections by Indian medicinal plants. *Phytotherapy Research, 3*(2), 43–49.

Thirumalai, T., Therasa, S. V., Elumalai, E., & David, E. (2011). Hypoglycemic effect of *Brassica juncea* (seeds) on streptozotocin-induced diabetic male albino rat. *Asian Pacific Journal of Tropical Biomedicine, 1*(4), 323–325.

Thomas, M. C., & Cherney, D. Z. (2018). The actions of SGLT2 inhibitors on metabolism, renal function and blood pressure. *Diabetologia, 61*, 2098–2107. https://doi.org/10.1007/s00125-018-4669-0 (accessed on 2nd February 2026).

Timmers, S., Konings, E., Bilet, L., Houtkooper, R. H., van de Weijer, T., Goossens, G. H., et al. (2011). Calorie restriction-like effects of 30 days of resveratrol supplementation on energy metabolism and metabolic profile in obese humans. *Cell Metabolism, 14*(5), 612–622. https://doi.org/10.1016/j.cmet.2011.10.002 (accessed on 2nd February 2026).

Tiwari, P. (2015). Recent trends in therapeutic approaches for diabetes management: A comprehensive update. *Journal of Diabetes Research, 2015*. https://doi.org/10.1155/2015/340838 (accessed on 2nd February 2026).

Tiwari, P., Mishra, B. N., & Sangwan, N. S. (2014). Phytochemical and pharmacological properties of *Gymnema sylvestre*: An important medicinal plant. *BioMed Research International, 2014*. https://doi.org/10.1155/2014/830285 (accessed on 2nd February 2026).

Tomic, D., Shaw, J. E., & Magliano, D. J. (2022). The burden and risks of emerging complications of diabetes mellitus. *Nature Reviews Endocrinology, 18*(9), 525–539. https://doi.org/10.1038/s41574-022-00690-7 (accessed on 2nd February 2026).

Tsivileva, O. M., Koftin, O. V., & Evseeva, N. V. (2022). Coumarins as fungal metabolites with potential medicinal properties. *Antibiotics, 11*(9), 1156. https://doi.org/10.3390/antibiotics11091156 (accessed on 2nd February 2026).

Ulbricht, C., Basch, E., Burke, D., Cheung, L., Ernst, E., Giese, N., et al. (2008). An evidence-based systematic review of herb and supplement interactions by the Natural Standard Research Collaboration. *Expert Opinion on Drug Safety, 7*(1), 13–32.

Undale, V. R., Kurkute, S. S., & Jadhav, S. S. (2020). Curcumin potentiates therapeutic efficacy of metformin: A preclinical study in STZ-NA induced hyperglycemia in Wistar rats. *Research Journal of Pharmacy and Technology, 13*(6), 2591–2596. http://dx.doi.org/10.5958/0974-360X.2020.00461.8 (accessed on 2nd February 2026).

Vargas-Uricoechea, H., & Aschner, P. (2021). Comparative efficacy and safety of basal insulins: A review. *Diabetes & Metabolic Syndrome: Clinical Research & Reviews, 15*(6), 102318. https://doi.org/10.1016/j.dsx.2021.102318 (accessed on 2nd February 2026).

Vedtofte, T. B., Bodvarsdottir, T. S., Gotfredsen, C. F., Karlsen, A. E., Knudsen, L. B., & Heller, R. S. (2010). Liraglutide, but not vildagliptin, restores normoglycemia and insulin content in the animal model of type 2 diabetes, *Psammomys obesus*. *Regulatory Peptides, 160*(1), 106–114.

Vendrame, S., Daugherty, A., Kristo, A. S., Riso, P., & Klimis-Zacas, D. (2019). Wild blueberry (*Vaccinium angustifolium*)-enriched diet improves dyslipidemia and modulates the expression of genes related to lipid metabolism in obese Zucker rats. *British Journal of Nutrition, 121*(11), 1231–1241.

Vivó-Barrachina, L., Rojas-Chacón, M. J., Navarro-Salazar, R., Belda-Sanchis, V., Pérez-Murillo, J., Peiró-Puig, A., et al. (2022). The role of natural products on diabetes mellitus treatment: A systematic review of randomized controlled trials. *Pharmaceutics, 14*(1), 101.

Wang, X., Ge, A., Cheng, M., Guo, F., Zhao, M., & Zhou, X. (2012). A model of type 2 diabetes in rats using high-fat diet with low doses of streptozotocin. *Chinese Journal of Pharmacology and Toxicology, 26*(5), 458–463. https://doi.org/10.3867/j.issn.1000-3002.2012.05.007 (accessed on 2nd February 2026).

Wei, D., Li, J., Shen, M., Jia, W., Chen, N., Chen, T., et al. (2010). Cellular production of n-3 PUFAs and reduction of n-6-to-n-3 ratios in the pancreatic β-cells and islets enhance insulin secretion and confer protection against cytokine-induced cell death. *Diabetes, 59*(2), 471–478.

Wolfram, S., Raederstorff, D., Preller, M., Wang, Y., Teixeira, S. R., Riegger, C., et al. (2006). Epigallocatechin gallate supplementation alleviates diabetes in rodents. *The Journal of Nutrition, 136*(10), 2512–2518. https://doi.org/10.1093/jn/136.10.2512 (accessed on 2nd February 2026).

World Health Organization. (2019). *Classification of Diabetes Mellitus*. World Health Organization.

Wu, G. Z., Hong, G., Zhang, W. P., & Zhang, H. B. (2009). Effect of 1-[4-[2-(4-bromobenzenesulfonamino) ethyl] phenylsulfonyl]-3-(trans-4-methylcyclohexyl) urea (i4), a new synthetic sulfonylurea compound, on glucose metabolism *in vivo* and *in vitro*. *Arzneimittelforschung, 59*(11), 550–556.

Xiao, Y., Lv, S., Lin, S., Jin, L., Zhang, Y., Wang, X., et al. (2010). Cardiac protection by basic fibroblast growth factor from ischemia/reperfusion-induced injury in diabetic rats. *Biological & Pharmaceutical Bulletin, 33*(3), 444–449.

Xu, L., Li, Y., Dai, Y., & Peng, J. (2018). Natural products for the treatment of type 2 diabetes mellitus: Pharmacology and mechanisms. *Pharmacological Research, 130*, 451–465. https://doi.org/10.1016/j.phrs.2018.01.015 (accessed on 2nd February 2026).

Xue, A., Wu, Y., Zhu, Z., Zhang, F., Kemper, K. E., Zheng, Z., et al. (2018). Genome-wide association analyses identify 143 risk variants and putative regulatory mechanisms for type 2 diabetes. *Nature Communications, 9*(1), 2941. https://doi.org/10.1038/s41467-018-04951-w (accessed on 2nd February 2026).

Xue, M., Yang, M. X., Zhang, W., Li, X. M., Gao, D. H., Ou, Z. M., et al. (2013). Characterization, pharmacokinetics, and hypoglycemic effect of berberine-loaded solid lipid nanoparticles. *International Journal of Nanomedicine*, 4677–4687.

Yang, B. T., Dayeh, T. A., Kirkpatrick, C. L., Taneera, J., Kumar, R., Groop, L., et al (2011). Insulin promoter DNA methylation correlates negatively with insulin gene expression and positively with HbA1c levels in human pancreatic islets. *Diabetologia, 54*, 360–367. https://doi.org/10.1007/s00125-010-1967-6 (accessed on 2nd February 2026).

Yaribeygi, H., Maleki, M., Sathyapalan, T., Jamialahmadi, T., & Sahebkar, A. (2021). Pathophysiology of physical inactivity-dependent insulin resistance: A theoretical mechanistic review emphasizing clinical evidence. *Journal of Diabetes Research, 2021*. https://doi.org/10.1155/2021/7796727 (accessed on 2nd February 2026).

Yeh, G. Y., Eisenberg, D. M., Kaptchuk, T. J., & Phillips, R. S. (2003). Systematic review of herbs and dietary supplements for glycemic control in diabetes. *Diabetes Care, 26*(4), 1277–1294.

Yin, J., Xing, H., & Ye, J. (2015). Efficacy of berberine in patients with type 2 diabetes mellitus. *Metabolism, 57*(5), 712–717.

Yoon, J., McClintock, P., Onodera, T., & Notkins, A. (1980). Virus-induced diabetes mellitus. XVIII. Inhibition by a nondiabetogenic variant of encephalomyocarditis virus. *Journal of Experimental Medicine, 152*(4), 878–892.

Yücel, Ç., Karatoprak, G. Ş., & Aktaş, Y. (2018). Nano liposomal resveratrol as a novel approach to treatment of diabetes mellitus. *Journal of Nanoscience and Nanotechnology, 18*(6), 3856–3864.

Zakerkish, M., Jenabi, M., Zaeemzadeh, N., Hemmati, A. A., & Neisi, N. (2019). The effect of Iranian propolis on glucose metabolism, lipid profile, insulin resistance, renal function and inflammatory biomarkers in patients with type 2 diabetes mellitus: A randomized double-blind clinical trial. *Scientific Reports, 9*(1), 7289.

Zeevi, D., Korem, T., Zmora, N., Israeli, D., Rothschild, D., Weinberger, A., et al. (2015). Personalized nutrition by prediction of glycemic responses. *Cell, 163*(5), 1079–1094.

Zhang, H., Colclough, K., Gloyn, A. L., & Pollin, T. I. (2021). Monogenic diabetes: A gateway to precision medicine in diabetes. *The Journal of Clinical Investigation, 131*(3). https://doi.org/10.1172/JCI142244 (accessed on 2nd February 2026).

Zhang, Q., Xiao, X., Feng, K., Wang, T., Li, W., Yuan, T., et al. (2018). Metformin improves lipid metabolism disorders through reducing the expression of microsomal triglyceride transfer protein in OLETF rats. *Biological & Pharmaceutical Bulletin, 41*(3), 355–362.

Zhang, Y. S., Khademhosseini, A., & Arneri, A. (2017). Emerging technologies in engineering approaches to diabetes management. *Advanced Healthcare Materials, 6*(13), 1700695.

CHAPTER 6

Revolutionizing Diabetes Care with Nanotechnology Innovations

PURBA MANDAL,[1] ADITYA SINGH,[1] JUBER AKHTAR,[1,*] and PERWEZ ALAM[2]

[1]*Faculty of Pharmacy, Integral University, Dasauli, Lucknow, Uttar Pradesh, India*

[2]*Department of Pharmacognosy, College of Pharmacy, King Saud University, Riyadh, Kingdom of Saudi Arabia*

*Corresponding author

ABSTRACT

Diabetes mellitus (DM) is a chronic metabolic disorder characterized by elevated blood glucose levels (BGLs) due to defects in insulin production, insulin action, or both. Nanotechnology has emerged as a revolutionary tool for diabetes care, offering potential solutions in areas such as glucose monitoring, insulin delivery, and tissue regeneration. This chapter explores the latest nanotechnology-based advancements in diabetes management, highlighting their efficacy, safety, and potential clinical applications. The integration of nanotechnology with emerging fields such as gene editing and artificial intelligence (AI) holds promise for personalized and precision medicine in diabetes treatment. However, the challenges related to safety, scalability, and regulatory concerns remain critical.

6.1 INTRODUCTION

Diabetes mellitus (DM) is a chronic condition characterized by high blood sugar/glucose levels owing to insufficient insulin production or failure to

Diabetes: Novel Insights and Therapies. Anas Islam and Badruddeen (Eds)

DOI: 10.1201/9781779644596-9

utilize insulin when it is produced (*The Lancet*, 2023). There are three main classifications of this condition: type 1, type 2, and gestational diabetes (Figure 6.1, Table 6.1). Insulin production is inhibited by autoimmune diseases that cause type 1 diabetes (Di Miglio et al., 2018; Katsarou et al., 2017). Diabetes affects people of all ages, sexes, and geographic locations and is one of the most common causes of death and morbidity worldwide. More than 90% of diabetes cases are type 2, which is affected by both environmental and inherited factors (*The Lancet*, 2023). Both type 1 and type 2, the most prevalent forms of DM, have diagnostic standards. Type 1 diabetes is primarily caused by autoimmune destruction of pancreatic beta cells (Ahmad et al., 2022). Sedentary lifestyle and obesity are associated with type 2 diabetes (*The Lancet*, 2023). Both the mother and fetus are at an increased risk of difficulties during pregnancy and delivery if they have gestational diabetes. By 2025, just over 1% of women, as well as fewer men, will have achieved worldwide targets for halting the growth of diabetes (Ahmad et al., 2022; Sun et al., 2022).

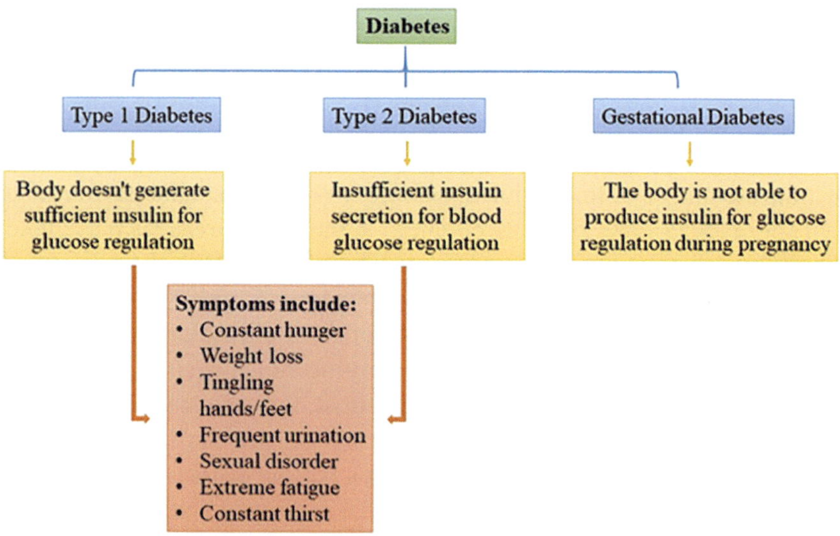

FIGURE 6.1 Classification of diabetes.

Diabetes affects 240 million people globally, with 105% of the population managing the disease. The IDF estimates that 537 million people are currently managing the disease, resulting in a healthcare expense of $966 billion in 2021. The cost is predicted to rise to over $1054 billion by 2045,

TABLE 6.1 Diabetes Can Be Categorized Using the Main Categories

Diabetes Type	Alternate Name	Key Characteristics	References
Type 1 diabetes (T1D)	Insulin-dependent diabetes (IDDM)	Caused by the destruction of β-cells, resulting in absolute insulin deficiency. The process is primarily linked to immune-mediated or unknown mechanisms	ADA (2011); Sharma et al. (2024)
Type 2 diabetes (T2D)	Non–insulin-dependent diabetes (NIDDM)	Characterized by insulin resistance combined with a progressive reduction in insulin secretion	ADA (2011); Sharma et al. (2024)
Gestational diabetes mellitus	–	Identified during the second or third trimester of pregnancy, typically without clear indications of preexisting diabetes	ADA (2011); Sharma et al. (2024)
Other specific types of diabetes	–	Includes diabetes related to genetic anomalies in β-cell function, insulin action, pancreatic diseases, endocrine disorders, infections, or rare immune conditions	ADA (2011); Mobasseri et al. (2020); Sharma et al. (2024)

with the prevalence of diabetes expected to increase to 643 million by 2030 and 783 million by 2045 (Hossain et al., 2024; Laraeni et al., 2021; Ong et al., 2021).

India, China, the United States, Italy, Indonesia, Japan, Pakistan, Brazil, Russia, and Bangladesh are the 10 nations with the highest rates of diabetes. The prevalence is expected to increase to 643 million people worldwide by 2030, mostly as a result of a 150% increase in developing nations, with Qatar being the most affected (Hossain et al., 2024; Laraeni et al., 2021).

Africa, with a diabetes prevalence of 4.5%, is expected to experience an increase of 129% in diabetes cases by 2045, resulting in approximately 55 million cases. The region also had the highest proportion of undiagnosed cases (53.6%). Despite only dedicating 1.3% of global expenditure on diabetes, Africa hosts approximately 4.5% of the global population affected by the disease (Hossain et al., 2024).

Approximately 387 million individuals worldwide suffer from DM, a complicated and non-transmissible endocrine illness that is expected to increase significantly, impacting over 640 million people by 2040. The illness is characterized by high blood levels of fat and glucose, as well as oxidative stress, which can cause persistent problems with the kidneys, eyes, nerves, and blood vessels, among other organs (Giovannini et al., 2016).

Type 2 diabetes mellitus (T2DM) is an illness with several causes connected to both polygenic and environmental variables, making a solution difficult due to genetic polymorphisms and other risk factors (WHO, 2016; Wu et al., 2014). Type 1 diabetes mellitus (T1DM) is becoming more common each year despite the fact that obesity-linked T2DM accounts for the majority of cases. Although both types of diabetes are associated with a lower BGL and prolonged risk of circulatory system problems, approximately 10% of patients with diabetes have T1DM (Aloke et al., 2022; Rask-Madsen et al., 2013).

Normoglycemia can reduce diabetes-related complications, but hypoglycemia in T1DM patients limits the attainment of near-normoglycemia. Unaware diabetics are vulnerable to T1DM, hindering their ability to achieve the necessary glycemic control (Aloke et al., 2022; Callejas et al., 2013).

Currently, the primary therapeutic regimens for type 2 diabetes include insulin injections and oral administration of hypoglycemic agents; however, these methods are often accompanied by side effects (DeFronzo et al., 2016; Palmer et al., 2016). Insulin is crucial for managing insulin-deficient DM, but maintaining tight glycemic control without negative side effects, such as low blood glucose and weight gain, remains a challenge, emphasizing the need for alternative techniques or adjuncts (Aloke et al., 2022; The DCCT Research Group, 1988, 1997).

6.2 UNDERSTANDING GENETIC PERSPECTIVES OF DIABETES MELLITUS

The organized structure of the human genome, which is made up of 30 billion nucleotide base pairs with substantial inter-individual variation, is better understood owing to the human genome project. The genetic analysis of common illnesses and their characteristics has advanced significantly over the last 10 years thanks to genome-wide association studies (GWAS). Previously, the pathogenic relevance of a gene and its related products was used to determine the hereditary basis of illnesses using the candidate gene approach. Hundreds of genes and genetic loci linked to type 1 and type 2 diabetes have been identified and investigated via the use of candidate gene along with GWAS techniques (Grant, 2019).

1. **Type 1 Diabetes Mellitus (T1DM):** This is a disorder in which pancreatic cells are damaged by the immune system, necessitating the use of an external source of insulin-secreting pancreatic cells. Autoantigens such as insulin, zinc transporter protein, protein tyrosine phosphatase, and glutamic acid decarboxylase (GAD) isoforms are indicative of type 1 diabetes mellitus. Hereditary susceptibility to T1D may be influenced by more than 20 different genetic regions. T1DM is caused by mutations in the human leukocyte complex (HLA) genes, DR and DQ, on chromosome 6 (Grant et al., 2019; Morran et al., 2015). The disorder is most strongly associated with differences in these genes, which are located on many chromosomes. Insulin-dependent diabetes (IDDM1) has also been associated with stress and environmental variables, such as viral infections. A significant portion of the heritable risk of type 1 diabetes (T1D) is ascribed to HLA class II genes, including IDDM1. The risk of type 1 diabetes is independently increased by more genes in the central, class I, and extended class I regions (Noble and Valdes, 2011; Steck and Rewers, 2011).

2. **Type 2 Diabetes Mellitus (T2DM):** A polygenic condition called T2DM is characterized by a decrease in insulin production with pancreatic cell failure, which prevents glucose from entering fat, muscle, or liver cells. It is mostly inherited and can last years without treatment, which might have long-term consequences. T2DM is influenced by a number of unknown variables such as age, physical inactivity, sedentary lifestyle, tobacco use, and binge drinking. T2DM risk is also influenced by genetic factors. Individuals with T1DM and T2DM are genetically predisposed to the disease, and T1DM is more likely to be inherited. The main risk factor for type 2 diabetes is the interplay between many genes spread throughout the genome (Galicia-Garcia et al., 2020). It is essential to understand how mutations in insulin receptor genes affect the body (Ali, 2013; Prasad and Groop, 2015).

3. **Genetic Variance in Other Specific Types of Diabetes:** Neurocognitive impairment is associated with obesity, metabolic syndrome, insulin resistance, and systemic metabolic dysfunction, such as diabetes. Patients with Alzheimer's disease (AD) have reduced insulin levels and neuronal insulin receptors, which

interfere with the insulin-signaling cascade and cause insulin resistance (Nguyen et al., 2020; Stoeckel et al., 2016). Cognitive impairment has been linked to brain dysfunction and abnormalities in lipids, proteins, carbohydrates, and fat. As T2DM advances to AD, neuroendocrine dysfunction known as T3D develops. It is linked to a number of conditions, including inflammation, acetylcholine esterase activity, the effect of the ApoE4A genotype on synaptic flexibility, and vascular alterations in the brain capillaries (Ortiz et al., 2022).

6.3 NANOTECHNOLOGY: A PARADIGM SHIFT IN DIABETES CARE

Nanotechnology has the potential to develop accurate and medically useful implantable and wearable sensing technologies, particularly for diabetes diagnosis. Diabetic blood sugar level (BSL) tests require regular checks to prevent dangerous BGLs. The development of wearable and implanted sensing devices that provide accurate and continuous medical data is possible using nanotechnology (Dias and Cunha, 2018).

Nanotechnology is commonly utilized in diabetes diagnosis using microphysiometers or implantable sensors (Rauf et al., 2016). Microphysiometers made from multi-walled carbon nanotubes can detect insulin levels through the electrical transfer of electrons produced during insulin oxidation (Bruen et al., 2017). Nanostructured implanted sensors employ fluorescent-molecule-coated polyethylene glycol beads to monitor BSLs (Chen et al., 2017).

Sensor microchips are being created to continually monitor important bodily functions, including temperature, pulse, and blood sugar. The creation of a microchip-based test to distinguish between the two primary types of diabetes is made possible by microchips implanted under the skin, which provides a constant signal (Mannino et al., 2019). Traditional techniques for diagnosing type-1 diabetes are costly, sluggish, and only available in well-equipped medical facilities; the microchip-based test represents a portable, affordable alternative (Kahanovitz et al., 2017).

Nanotechnology has the potential to revolutionize medicine by enabling access to clinically relevant cells and by analyzing small volumes of analytes, with properties such as nanoscale carbon being stronger than steel, highly malleable, fluorescent, and electrically conductive (Pickup et al., 2008). Nanotechnology has significantly improved diabetes treatment by improving the glucose sensor technology, enabling accurate insulin dosing, and improving diabetes management. Advances in nanomedicine have enabled more frequent blood glucose measurements and robust insulin delivery systems that can detect fluctuations and automatically modulate insulin release to maintain normoglycemia, thereby improving patient health and quality of life (DiSanto et al., 2015).

6.3.1 *ADVANTAGES OF NANOTECHNOLOGY IN HEALTHCARE*

Nanotechnology has revolutionized diabetes management by providing real-time, sensitive, and minimally invasive glucose monitoring, which is crucial for precise insulin administration and treatment optimization. Biosensors based on nanotechnology have the potential to improve patient care and insulin detection (Mandal et al., 2023). Examples include wearable devices that employ nanosensors for continuous glucose monitoring (CGM), which eliminates the need for periodic fingerstick testing (Huang et al., 2020). For the detection of blood glucose, quantum dot nanoparticles provide increased sensitivity and specificity (Chen et al., 2014). Simple and quick colorimetric assays based on nanoparticles are appropriate for point-of-care monitoring in environments with limited resources (Brasiunas et al., 2021). Graphene and carbon nanotubes are two nanomaterials that are used in electrochemical biosensors to increase the sensitivity and responsiveness of glucose detection (Zhu et al., 2012). By offering sensitive and accurate monitoring, these cutting-edge techniques enable people to make knowledgeable decisions regarding their treatment course and way of life. The use of nanotechnology in blood sugar monitoring and insulin delivery has transformed the treatment of diabetes, empowering people to make informed decisions about their course of action and way of life.

Nanocarrier-based drug delivery in healthcare offers several benefits, including:

1. **Improved Bioavailability:** Nanocarriers can enhance drug absorption and bioavailability by protecting them from degradation in the gastrointestinal tract (Dixit et al., 2023).
2. **Enhanced Targeting:** To improve medication distribution to the targeted areas, nanocarriers can be developed to target certain tissues or cells, such as insulin-resistant tissues or pancreatic beta cells (El-Dakroury et al., 2023).

3. **Reduced Side Effects:** Nanocarriers that deliver drugs to specific tissues can reduce side effects, reduce off-target effects, and enhance patient tolerability (Patel et al., 2017).

4. **Sustained Release:** The frequency of drug administration can be decreased using nanocarriers, which provide regulated, sustained drug release that produces more consistent and lasting therapeutic effects (Natarajan et al., 2014).

6.4 NANOTECHNOLOGY INNOVATIONS TRANSFORMING DIABETES MANAGEMENT

Bioelectronics has become a crucial medical tool for evaluating physiological indicators, particularly in conditions such as diabetes, renal failure, heart disease, diabetic foot, and stroke. Early-stage diabetes can be difficult to identify, necessitating continuous urine and blood glucose monitoring for its prevention and early treatment (Zhang et al., 2018).

6.4.1 MONITORING OF URINE GLUCOSE

Elevated urinary glucose levels are problematic because they may be a sign of diabetes. The first urine glucose meter manufactured in Japan was used in 1996 to measure urine glucose levels between 0 and 500 mg/dL in a systematic manner (Miyashita et al., 2009; Su et al., 2012). Carbon nanotubes (CNTs) have also been investigated for the detection of urine glucose. Because CNTs dissolve in biopolymer chitosan (CS) aqueous solutions, urine glucose can be detected without any issues. With a broad measuring range of 0–2000 mg/dL, a fast response time of 6 s, and resistance to interference, Kimura Group's UG-201 urine glucose meter is remarkably sensitive and performs very well (Zhang et al., 2004).

Wang et al. (2020) developed a colorimetric assay for ALS urine glucose detection using quantitative H_2O_2 and a smartphone ambient light sensor (Wang et al., 2020). Using an enzyme biofuel cell (EBFC), Zhang et al. (2021) developed a flexible, self-powered biosensor that could identify the makeup of urine when fastened to a nappy. The biosensor system, which included an EBFC, a power management system, and a light-emitting diode, was able to detect the quantity of glucose in the urine of diabetic patients without the need for external power (Zhang et al., 2021). Lee et al. (2021) developed a paper sensor for red blood cell membranes (RBCMs) using polyaniline nanoparticles (PAni-NPs), which are highly selective, noninvasive, and user-friendly (Thakur et al., 2014). The glucose transporter-1 protein in RBCM functions as an advanced filter that transfers glucose while rejecting other molecules. The paper sensor was approximately 85% more selective than the uncoated paper sensors and could detect urine glucose concentrations between 0 and 10 mg/mL (0–56 mM) (Ji et al., 2011; Lee et al., 2021).

6.4.2 MONITORING BLOOD GLUCOSE

Given its simplicity of collection and the abundance of indicators, blood is the preferred sample for disease-related markers. However, successful post-meal glucose control requires more than monitoring fasting plasma glucose (FPG) levels. According to recent studies, reducing postprandial plasma glucose is essential for lowering hemoglobin A1c (HbA1c), a measure of the advancement of diabetes. Self-monitoring is an effective method for managing BGLs in patients with diabetes (Cui et al., 2000; Niu et al., 2018; Zhang et al., 2021) (Table 6.2).

TABLE 6.2 Comparison of Glucose Monitoring Technologies

Technology	Description	Key Features	Accuracy and Standards	References
Glucometer	Portable devices using finger pricks to measure blood glucose	Uses glucose oxidase (GOx) or glucose dehydrogenase (GDH) with mediators such as ferrocene or hexacyanoferrate	95% of readings must be within 15 mg/dL (0.83 mM) or 15% of the reference value at 100 mg/dL (5.6 mM)	Heller and Feldman (2008); Tonyushkina and Nichols (2009); Vashist et al. (2011); Yoo et al. (2010)
Colorimetric strip	Flexible, self-powered device that monitors glucose levels in real-time using piezoelectricity and enzyme reactions	Incorporates GOx@ ZnO nanowires; converts mechanical energy into electrical signals for biosensing	Provides real-time monitoring; quantitative precision is not always guaranteed	Zhu et al. (2017)
Ames reflectance meter	Early glucose meter using reflected light from a reagent strip for semiquantitative glucose measurement	Uses color comparison against a chart after applying blood to a reagent pad; includes initial and refined models	Reflocheck demonstrated cost savings and good correlation in diabetes screening trials	Forrest et al. (1987)

6.5 NANOSENSORS FOR PRECISE GLUCOSE MONITORING

Diabetes, a major worldwide health issue, affects 24 million Americans and might impact 44.1 million by 2034 (Huang et al., 2009). Serious side effects of the illness include blindness, cardiovascular problems, and lower-limb amputations. Patients must use a sensor test strip and a finger-prick sample to track their BGLs to control them. These sensors report glucose concentrations via electrochemical enzymatic measurements using screen-printed electrodes (Wang, 2008). They allow for quick and precise measurements without laboratory analysis, but they have drawbacks, such as uncomfortable sampling, missed sampling time points, and analyses that are not performed while the patient is in bed (Burge et al., 2008).

New commercial solutions concentrate on continuous glucose measurements to overcome these restrictions. Continuous monitoring is also a goal of early-stage nanotechnology research that utilizes nanosensors and nanomaterials. Owing to their small size, high surface area/volume ratios, and improved optical characteristics, nanomaterials and nanosensors provide a number of advantages. These characteristics have been used by researchers to enhance the precision, dimensions, durability, and usefulness of diabetic treatment sensors (Cash and Clark, 2010).

Recent developments in nanosensors and nanomaterials for diabetes treatment include electrochemical glucose biosensors (including nanomaterials), electrochemical biosensors applied to clinical samples, and glucose detection. While other diabetes targets have been targeted using nanotechnology, the focus remains on glucose detection (Lee et al., 2007; Vaddiraju et al., 2009).

Nanotechnology has been utilized to incorporate glucose sensors into devices, offering advantages such as a higher surface area and improved catalytic activity. These sensors can be implanted like the current technology for continuous monitoring but face drawbacks such as fouling and decreased sensor life due to immune foreign body response. Nanofabrication methods have the potential to produce injectable, long-lasting nanoscale glucose sensors. However, because these sensors lack clinical data and represent a significant departure from the continuous monitoring sensors already in use, further studies are required before they can be widely used.

With benefits including increased surface area, effective electron transfer, and extra catalytic processes, nanotechnology is being used in diabetes sensors to improve glucose detection. The ability of carbon nanotubes (CNTs) to transmit electrons and their large surface areas make them a preferred modification. More enzyme immobilization and signal production are possible when a highly porous nanofiber is immobilized on glucose oxidase because it has a larger electronic surface area than bulk metal electrodes (Zhu et al., 2010).

To create nanocomposites for glucose detection, CNTs can be combined with other nanomaterials or polymers to enhance their catalytic activity. Recently, CNTs and gold nanoparticles have been assembled layer-by-layer to create nanocomposite membranes, while metal nanoparticles of platinum, silver, gold/platinum, and non-metals such as silica and composites of iron and silica oxide have been used. CNT membranes can be placed on nanostructured electrodes, such as titanium dioxide (TiO_2) nanotube arrays or electrodes modified by alumina coatings (Baby and Ramaprabhu, 2010; Gopalan et al., 2009; Pang et al., 2009; Zhang et al., 2010).

Different types of nanostructured electrodes, such as ZnO arranged in nanowire and nanotube arrays, can enhance traditional macrostructured electrodes (Usman et al., 2010). Compared with traditional electrodes, nanowire arrays made of ruthenium and gold have a larger surface area and better electrochemical interrogation. Nanoparticles, such as those of gold, platinum, and palladium, can be used to create nanostructures in addition to producing nanoscale characteristics on the electrode surface (Santhosh et al., 2009).

Magnetic nanoparticles, generally manufactured from iron oxide, have also been employed for glucose sensors, easing the assembly of GOx-labeled nanoparticles with the electrode and permitting the development of conductive nanoparticles on the surface of the electrode (Li et al., 2009). The application of polymers has a range of electrochemical characteristics, such as the ability to operate at different potentials, which reduces electrochemical interference from typical electroactive substances found in blood, resulting in nonspecific results when using conventional electrochemical detection techniques.

6.6 NANOPARTICLE-BASED DRUG DELIVERY SYSTEMS IN DIABETES CARE

Nanoparticles are small, biodegradable, biocompatible, and contain drugs such as peptides and oligonucleotides. They can be administered orally or parenterally, act as drug carriers, protect drugs from environmental conditions, and transport them to target body compartments. By delivering oligonucleotides to regulate gene expression, non-viral cell transfection can be performed both *in vivo* and *in vitro* (Figure 6.2) (Mitchell et al., 2021).

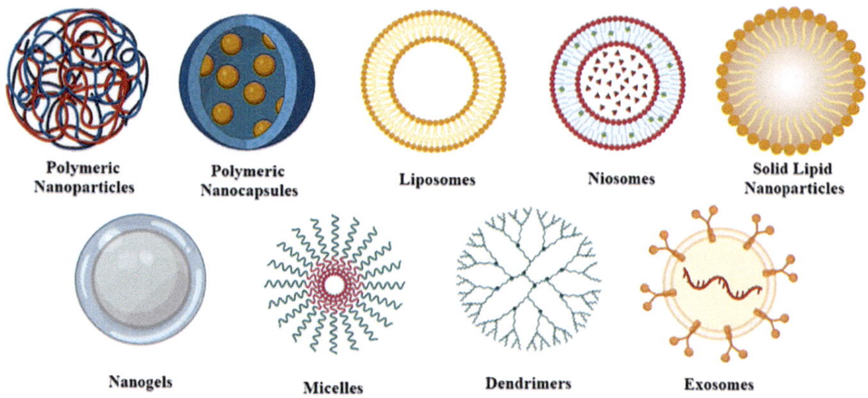

FIGURE 6.2 Nanoparticles used in the management of diabetes.

6.6.1 POLYMERIC NANOPARTICLES

Colloidal drug delivery methods, known as nanoparticles (NPs), have particles ranging in size from 10 to 1000 nm. They may assume the shape of a matrix system, in which the drug is distributed throughout the particles, or a reservoir system, in which the drug is contained in a cavity encircled by a polymeric membrane (Mudshinge et al., 2011). The main advantage of NPs is their enhanced bioavailability, bypassing first-pass metabolism, resulting in a reduced dose and minimal toxicity to non-target cells. Targeted drug delivery using NPs also reduces side effects, increases locoregional concentration, and facilitates quick action. However, NPs have several toxicity concerns, including accidental inhalation, oxidative stress-related inflammatory reactions, access to the central nervous system through olfactory receptors, or direct uptake through the blood-brain barrier. NPs also have limitations such as unpredictable stability, low shelf life, and high manufacturing costs (Davatgaran et al., 2017).

Polymeric nanoparticles are solid polymer matrices that contain either natural or synthetic drugs. They are released through the destabilization of body fluids. Hydrophilic matrices based on polysaccharides and proteins are suitable for releasing hydrophilic molecules, such as insulin. Hydrophobic matrices based on PLA or PLGA are destabilized by biodegradation following slow water penetration. These matrices are used for both hydrophilic and lipophilic drugs, ensuring prolonged drug delivery over time (Afsharzadeh et al., 2018).

6.6.2 POLYMERIC NANOCAPSULES

Polymeric nanocapsules are solid shells containing liquid phases such as serum albumin. These must be crosslinked to prevent solubilization in aqueous bodily fluids. Albumin nanocapsules contain hydrophobic liquids, such as vegetable oils, which are suitable for encapsulating lipophilic drugs. PLA or PLGA shells have an aqueous internal liquid phase, making them suitable for encapsulating hydrophilic drugs, such as insulin and biologics (Purohit et al., 2023).

6.6.3 LIPOSOMES

Liposomes are vesicles made of phospholipid bilayers containing an aqueous phase that is ideal for hydrophilic and hydrophobic drugs. The choice of phospholipid type and its mixing with other lipid molecules can alter the physicochemical characteristics of the liposome surface, affecting the release characteristics across different administration sites and body compartments (Sercombe et al., 2015).

Because of their internal structure, liposomes—spherical vesicles with lipid bilayers that include an aqueous phase—are efficient delivery systems for hydrophilic medications like insulin. Their composition and production techniques affect their biocompatibility and biodegradability. Recent research has shown that liposomes with certain properties, such as a negative surface charge and a size range of 150–210 nm, may raise insulin concentrations and lower BGLs *in vivo* (Yazdi et al., 2020; Zhao et al., 2020). Changes like functionalization with cell-penetrating peptides (CPPs) have the potential to increase stability and endocytosis-mediated absorption. Through folate receptor-mediated endocytosis, folate-targeted PEGylated liposomes intended for insulin administration have shown improved bioavailability and cell uptake (Von Zuben et al., 2021). Liposomal chitosan gel, developed for wound healing with encapsulated insulin, exhibits stability and sustained release, showing potential clinical benefits (Dawoud et al., 2019). Elastic liposomes containing sodium-glycodeoxycholate (SGDC) markedly improved insulin penetration via buccal tissues. For self-regulated insulin delivery, novel strategies like glucose-sensitive multivesicular liposomes using the double emulsion method have promise (Bashyal et al., 2021). The possibility of using liposomes made from camel milk's fat globule membrane (MFGM) as insulin carriers was investigated by Shafiq et al. (2023). The research team of Wu et al. (2023) explored liposomes containing arginine–insulin complexes (AINS) inside cysteine-modified alginate (Cys-Alg) hydrogels, which resulted in liposome-in-alginate hydrogels (AINS-Lip-Gel). The study showed that intestinal permeation with AINS reached approximately 2.0-fold more compared to free insulin, while AINS-Lip achieved a 6.0-fold increase (Wu et al., 2023).

6.6.4 NIOSOMES

Niosomes, synthetic microscopic vesicles composed of cholesterol and non-ionic surfactants, are a promising class of drug delivery vehicles. They offer sustained and prolonged release profiles, accommodating substances with varying solubility. Niosomes can be categorized as large, small, and multilamellar vesicles, offering enhanced drug entrapment efficiency and controlled release kinetics (Yang et al., 2011). They have shown promising results in vaginal delivery systems for insulin, reducing BGLs and providing sustained hypoglycemic effects. In a previous study, niosomes made from polyoxyethylene alkyl ethers (Brij™) were developed for insulin encapsulation to protect insulin against enzymatic degradation. These niosomes have the potential to be sustained-release oral dosage forms for insulin delivery (Pardakhty et al., 2007).

6.6.5 SOLID LIPID NANOPARTICLES

Solid lipid nanoparticles (SLNs) exist as submicron carriers consisting of solid lipids, including purified triacylglycerols and waxes, as well as acylglycerols and surfactant mixtures. The submicron carriers demonstrate both biodegradable properties, and they provide advantages for commercial production operations. A drug release profile can be predictably controlled through the composition-based character of degradation processes. Multiple insulin-loaded SLN formulations exist that use lecithin and polyoxyethylene esters of 12-hydroxystearic acid as their surfactant components. Research shows that diabetic rats received hypoglycemic benefits from VB12-coated gel-core SLNs, which protected insulin from rapid dissolution under low pH conditions (Suhail et al., 2019). Insulin-protecting cationic SLNs retain stability and continue releasing drug substances while maintaining stability in media environments (Elshaarani et al., 2020). Muntoni et al. (2021) delivered insulin glargine into SLNs, which were transformed into stable solid oral formulations for improved shelf durability. The hypoglycemic effects of the products were examined in healthy rat models and diabetic rat models, where the capsule formulation demonstrated the most promising outcomes (Muntoni et al., 2021).

6.6.6 NANOGELS

A network of polymer chains with basic or acidic groups that absorb and hold onto many aqueous solutions make up nanogels, which are hydrogels at the nanoscale. They are of various types, including synthetic, natural, hybrid, neutral, anionic, or cationic, depending on their surface charge. Nanogels can internally load biological cargo and externally conjugate to different molecules via functional group bonds (Zhao et al., 2016).

The research team of Baloch et al. (2022) developed a new method to deliver insulin through the mouth by developing insulin-intercalated graphene oxide (In@GO NgC) nanogel composites. Releases of the drug under simulated intestinal conditions reached enhanced levels, followed by resistance against enzymatic breakdown exceeding 6 h (Baloch et al., 2022).

The group of Muddassir et al. (2019) synthesized hydroxyethyl methacrylate (HEMA) nanogels through emulsion polymerization before assessing them as delivery devices for oral insulin treatment. The characterization research showed HEMA nanogels maintain a stable structure and prolonged circulation period, display low levels of uptake by macrophages, and exhibit excellent stability properties. The *in vivo* findings showed that insulin inside HEMA nanogels gained better intestinal absorption and maintained BGLs for 12 hours after administration following ingestion (Mudassir et al., 2019).

The team of Chou et al. (2016) created an insulin delivery system through injected self-assembled CHC nanoparticles blended with lysozyme for extended basal insulin delivery. Experiments within petri dishes showed both precise degradation abilities and insulin release patterns of CHC-lysozyme gel, which verified its potential safe interaction with degradation byproducts. The injectable system shows potential value as a new long-acting insulin delivery technique which could enhance treatment compliance while lowering the issues related to standard insulin therapy (Chou et al., 2016).

6.6.7 MICELLES

Nanocarriers based on polymeric micelles find widespread application because they maintain hydrophobic cores surrounded by hydrophilic outer areas. Different techniques exist to boost insulin-loading efficiency and maintain stability of hydrophilic insulin while addressing the technical challenges involved with encapsulation. The hypoglycemic effect of glucose and H_2O_2 dual-responsive polymeric micelles *in vivo* is now possible because of innovative insulin delivery approaches that maintain high levels of biocompatibility (Caturano et al., 2024; Liu et al., 2020).

The research team of Bahman created an SMA poly-(styrene-co-maleic acid) micellar system for oral insulin delivery to overcome degradation challenges and improve intestinal insulin absorption. The research team used pH-dependent encapsulation to place insulin within SMA micelles while measuring their characteristics through dynamic light scattering and HPLC. *In vitro* analysis of Caco-2 cells and *ex vivo* rat intestinal section examinations alongside *in vivo* tests using diabetic mice validated the glucose uptake promotion by SMA-insulin (Bahman et al., 2020).

Han et al. (2020) developed a zwitterionic micelle platform that enables drug penetration through intestinal mucus and enhances epithelial absorption via transporters. An oral insulin prototype encapsulated in enteric-coated capsules exhibited high oral bioavailability (>40%), customizable insulin action profiles, promising long-term safety, and significant advances in oral protein drug delivery (Han et al., 2020).

Italiya et al. (2019) developed an orally active nanoformulation for lisofylline (LSF), encapsulated as an ester prodrug into biodegradable polymeric micelles (LSF-LA PLMs), enhancing its pharmacokinetic profile and improving oral bioavailability (Italiya et al., 2019). Hu et al. (2019) explored amphiphilic pH-sensitive block copolymers as carriers for oral insulin delivery, synthesizing them via ARGET ATRP and self-assembling into pH-responsive cationic polymeric micelles (PCPMs) (Hu et al., 2019).

6.6.8 *DENDRIMERS*

Dendrimers are synthetic polymers produced by the reaction of methyl acrylate with diamine. Owing to their regular construction, molecules designed to attain certain qualities can be effectively functionalized on their surfaces (Wang et al., 2022). For example, the modification of PEG can improve stabilization and prevent macrophage attack (Zeng et al., 2019). The caproyl-modified G2 PAMAM dendrimer enhances pulmonary insulin absorption via both transcellular and paracellular pathways (Kamalden et al., 2017). PEG-based amphiphilic dendrimers exhibit stability at acidic pH and reduce BGLs (Rodríguez-Morales et al., 2021). To improve diabetes control, Xian et al. (2024) created a nanoscale complex with autonomous insulin therapy that is sensitive to glucose levels. To create an injectable insulin depot, they used a synthetic dendrimer carrier and altered it to a high-affinity glucose-binding motif. When BGLs in diabetic pigs were increased, serum insulin concentrations increased in response to the nanocomplex, which kept blood glucose under control for at least a week (Xian et al., 2024).

6.6.9 *EXOSOMES*

Exosomes are vesicles with membranes that can be anywhere in size between 30 and 150 nm, and are composed of lipids and proteins. Their function as cargo agents for delivery and their interactions with target cells are physiological. Exosomes generated from the pancreas of patients with type 2 diabetes have been shown to affect the survival and death of pancreatic β-cells through the miRNAs they carry (Castaño et al., 2020). Exosomes improve cellular glucose transport and metabolism, making them promising candidates for use in insulin-delivery systems. Wu et al. (2022) examined the possibility of using milk-derived exosomes as oral drug delivery systems and discovered that EXO@INS had a stronger and longer-lasting hypoglycemic impact than insulin administered subcutaneously. Active multi-targeting absorption mechanisms, pH adaptation during gastrointestinal transit, activation of ERK1/2 and p38 MAPK signaling pathways, and efficient intestinal mucus penetration are characteristics of milk-derived exosomes (Wu et al., 2022).

6.7 NANOMATERIAL-BASED ADMINISTRATIONS IN DIABETES CARE

6.7.1 *ORAL ADMINISTRATION*

Although the intestinal epithelium significantly hinders insulin absorption, oral insulin delivery is the most practical method to control diabetes (Shah et al., 2016). Although gastric enzymes help break down the stomach and transport insulin, the active ingredient must be embedded in a protective matrix (Patra et al., 2018). The optimal choice is a combination of calcium phosphate, polyethylene glycol, insulin, and casein. Polymer-based nanoparticle strategies are considered to be more efficient than conventional oral and intravenous methods for insulin delivery. Insulin delivery systems are composed of pH-sensitive biodegradable polymers encircled by nanoporous membranes that permit the regulated release of insulin. Insulin polymeric nanoparticles are orally administered to animals using insulin-loaded nanopellets (Mansoor et al., 2019).

Insulin carriers are being researched, including co-polymers, such as N-dimethylaminoethyl methacrylate, polyurethanes, polyanhydrides, polyacrylic acids, and polyacrylamide. To efficiently transport insulin, hydrogels and microspheres can function as protease inhibitors and permeability enhancers (Wu et al., 2019). Insulin intestinal absorption has been demonstrated to be improved by chitosan nanoparticles more than by aqueous solutions. Insulin-encapsulated chitosan nanoparticles, enhanced with a mucoadhesive chitosan coating, extend their stay in the small intestine and facilitate the absorption of insulin through the paracellular route into the bloodstream (Marques et al., 2020).

6.7.2 *INHALATION*

The innovative insulin system utilizing nanotechnology emphasizes inhalation rather than injection, facilitating the regulated release of insulin into the bloodstream. Inhaler systems provide a gentle environment characterized by low enzyme levels and neutral pH, in contrast to the gastrointestinal route (Bajracharya et al., 2019). Common inhaler systems include dry powder formulations and solutions (Xia et al., 2019). The incorporation of insulin into nanoparticles enables the inhalation of a dry powder formulation directly into the lungs, preventing the degradation of insulin. Regular lung function tests are necessary before treatment, which increases the overall cost. According to Di et al. (2014), a focused ultrasound system (FUS)-triggered injectable polymeric nanoparticle-crosslinked network-based controlled insulin delivery system was able to manage BGLs in type 1 diabetic mice. Chitosan nanoparticles are regarded as an effective option for creating an inhalation delivery system aimed at treating type 2 diabetes because they have the potential to improve insulin absorption. Innovative composite nanomaterials made from poly(methylmethacrylate)-grafted carboxylated chitosan appeared to improve the effectiveness of regulated insulin release (Jaafar and Hamid, 2019).

6.7.3 NANOPUMP

The nanopump is a powerful medical device that comprises a volumetric pump and check valves integrated onto micro-electromechanical systems (MEMS) or nanoelectromechanical systems (NEMS) chips. The chip consists of three layers: a silicon-on-insulator (SOI) layer containing micromachined pump components and Pyrex cover plates. The major function of the pump is to administer insulin, which may continuously maintain stable BGLs and provide low doses of medicine over a long period of time (Shirin et al., 2019).

6.7.4 ARTIFICIAL PANCREAS

The development of an artificial pancreas system that includes a continuous glucose meter, glucose monitor, and insulin infusion pump could potentially provide a permanent solution for patients with diabetes. The initial idea, first demonstrated in 1974, involved a sensor electrode measuring BGLs, which was then fed into a small computer (Allen and Gupta, 2019). The infusion pump was activated, allowing insulin to enter the bloodstream from a small reservoir. To shield transplanted cells from the immune system and promote the flow of glucose, insulin, and oxygen, a silicon box filled with animal pancreatic beta cells was utilized (Cito et al., 2018). Patients with diabetes can have a box made of material the size of nanopores implanted beneath their skin. This allows insulin and glucose to block larger immune system molecules. A smart insulin patch with more than 100 microneedles loaded with insulin and glucose-sensing enzymes has the potential to develop insulin delivery technology (Veiseh and Langer, 2015). A nanorobot with internal chambers for selective insulin release and surface glucose sensors is a current research project (Yu et al., 2015).

6.8 COMPLICATIONS OF DIABETES

Diabetes can lead to significant problems and is usually split into microvascular and macrovascular forms. Damage to the renal, nervous, and eye systems is an example of microvascular problems, while stroke, heart disease, and peripheral vascular disease are examples of macrovascular complications. Peripheral vascular diseases can result in non-healable bruises, gangrene, and amputation. Pregnancy-related problems include teeth issues, pneumonia, inadequate immunity against influenza, and macrosomia. Patients with type 1 and type 2 diabetes may have comparable consequences, but the number and timing of these events may differ (Figure 6.3) (Zheng et al., 2018).

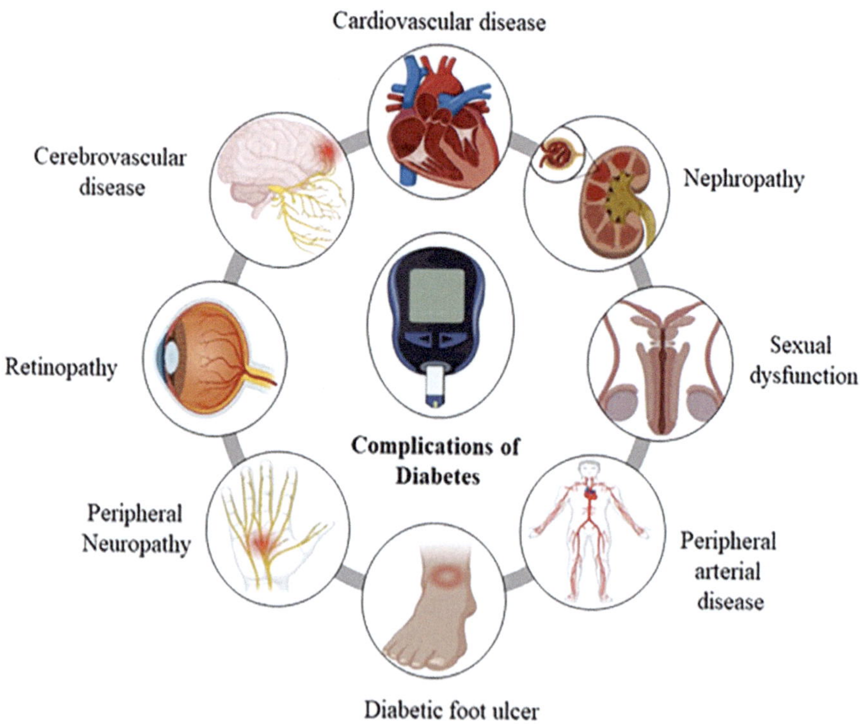

FIGURE 6.3 Complications of diabetes.

6.8.1 DIABETIC NEPHROPATHY (DN)

Chronic kidney disease (CKD), commonly referred to as nephropathy, is a slow-developing illness that lowers the glomerular filtration rate (GFR) and causes proteinuria. Given the critical role that the kidneys play in regulating blood pressure and preserving cardiovascular health, it is a serious health concern (Lim, 2014). The kidneys play a crucial role in diabetes by regulating fluid and salt levels, which are vital for blood pressure control and the maintenance of cardiovascular health. Nephropathy is influenced by various physiological changes, including changes in toxin filtration into the blood, kidney regulation of fluid balance and blood pressure, and activation of vitamin D cells in the kidneys. Glomerular hyperfiltration, caused by blood pressure changes, can lead to severe kidney damage; however, diabetics with normal or higher filtration rates are better protected against end-stage kidney disease.

Proteinuria, the accumulation of albumin in the urine, is linked to renal hemodynamic changes and glomerular filtration difficulties. Early diabetic conditions often cause hyperplasia and hypertrophy of the kidney, with the proximal tubule constituting > 90% of the cortical mass. Tubular interstitial fibrosis, the development of the extracellular matrix in the tubular kidney, significantly contributes to renal disease progression in patients (Faselis et al., 2020).

6.8.2 DIABETIC RETINOPATHY (DR)

Diabetic macular edema (DME) and proliferative diabetic retinopathy (PDR) are the main causes of diabetic retinopathy, which is a leading cause of blindness or visual loss. Oxidative stress, growth factor stimulation, inflammation, and PKC and hexosamine pathways are among the mechanisms through which DR advances. It is thought to be caused by diabetic retinal neurodegeneration (DRN) and is the most common vascular disease. According to a meta-analysis of 35 studies published between 1980 and 2008, the prevalence of DR and PDR among people with diabetes was 2.2%–12.7% globally and 3.4%–12.3%, respectively (Himasa et al., 2022). Blood hypertension, blood sugar, and dyslipidemia are risk factors for the development of DR. PDR and non-proliferative diabetic retinopathy (NPDR) are two types of DR. There are three types of NPDR: mild, moderate, and severe. Microaneurysms and hemorrhages are the causes of mild NPDR, but retinal hypoxia and severe lesions result from severe NPDR. Later stages of DR are characterized by extensive hemorrhage, and the proliferative stage of DR increases the risk of vision loss by forming new blood vessels on the retina that may burst unexpectedly or after exercise. Remission occurs after neovascularization for fibrous tissue development (Raghav et al., 2022).

6.8.3 DIABETIC PERIPHERAL NEUROPATHY (DPN)

DPN causes malfunction of the peripheral nervous system, leading to symptoms including burning, tingling, and numbness. It is a common subtype with serious side effects. Elevated BGLs harm small blood arteries that provide oxygen and nutrients to nerves, damaging the autonomic and distal sensory nerve fibers. Impaired motor, sensory, and autonomic nervous systems (ANS) are frequently associated with DPN. Sorbitol buildup, oxidative stress, PKC, glycosylation end products, disruption of hexosamine and polymerase pathways, and neurovascular destruction are some of the factors that contribute to nerve damage. This is associated with insufficient endothelial cell function and repair processes (Raghav et al., 2022).

6.8.4 SEXUAL DYSFUNCTION

Patients with T2DM frequently experience sexual dysfunction, which has a major negative effect on their quality of life. Erectile dysfunction (ED), which affects at least three months of sexual activity, is a diagnostic tool and an early indicator of the consequences of diabetes. Half of the diabetic people develop erectile dysfunction within 10 years of receiving a diabetes diagnosis, making them more likely to experience it than non-diabetics. In T2DM, ED may manifest early. Women with diabetes are more likely to experience sadness, and BMI is the sole factor associated with female sexual dysfunction (FSD) is BMI. Reduced sexual desire, decreased arousal, dyspareunia, and trouble experiencing orgasmic consequences are hallmarks of FSD. FSD is more common in women with type 2 diabetes; however, its etiology and risk factors are unknown (Raghav et al., 2022).

6.8.5 HEART STROKE AND HEART DISEASES

Ischemic heart disease and stroke are the primary causes of fatalities in diabetes, accounting for 65% of the fatalities. The mortality rate under these conditions is two to four times greater in those with diabetes. Cardiovascular disease (CVD) risk factors include hypertension and hyperlipidemia. Glycemic control, renin-angiotensin-receptor enforcement, and antiplatelet medication are among the management and treatment approaches recommended for patients with diabetes. Diabetes-related diastolic dysfunction can harm the heart in the absence of hypertension or coronary artery disease (CAD). In both type 1 and type 2 diabetes, the strongest indicator of the risk of CVD is long-term blood glucose control, as assessed by HbA1C measurements (Raghav et al., 2022).

6.8.6 DIABETIC FOOT ULCER (DFU)

Diabetic foot ulcers (DFU) are a serious health issue for people with diabetes because they can have detrimental effects on their physical and mental health and increase the risk of recurrence, amputation, and death. DFUs occur below the ankle, and 68% die after limb amputation. 80% of these cases were caused by impaired arterial blood flow. Peripheral neuropathies, vascular insufficiency, and decreased infection resistance are the main conditions associated with DFU. Oxidative stress contributes to the complexity of this problem. Diabetic foot problems are often caused by physical or mechanical damage, which results in skin ulcers. In patients with diabetes, inflammatory cells migrate and exert less force at the ulcer site, and leukocytes, fibroblasts, and neutrophils perform worse. Diabetes, high blood pressure, hyperlipidemia, and smoking are additional risk factors for foot ulcers. Males who have had diabetes or ulcers for more than 10 years, vascular and neurological conditions, smoking, sedentary lifestyles, and inadequate glycemic management are among the risk factors (Raghav et al., 2022).

6.9 NANOENGINEERED BIOMATERIALS FOR TISSUE REGENERATION IN DIABETES CARE

The largest organ in the human body, the skin, controls body temperature and essential processes. Although injured skin heals on its own, diabetic people and those with larger damaged regions require treatment to speed up wound closure and lower morbidity rates. This section discusses the pathology, medical needs, and current therapies for patients with diabetic foot and burn, highlighting the high demand for regenerative skin scaffolds (Mclaughlin et al., 2016).

6.9.1 WOUND HEALING

Prolonged bleeding is a significant issue in patients with diabetes, with 15% reporting this condition and 20% undergoing limb amputation. Traditional therapeutic methods are ineffective owing to continuous molecular changes in wound healing. Diabetic wound healing involves four phases: hemostasis, inflammation, proliferation, and remodeling. Nanotechnology is being explored as a potential solution to resolve the complications associated with diabetic wound closure (Sharma et al., 2023).

Diabetic wounds pose a serious risk to the health of diabetic patients, as they might result in amputation and persistent, uncontrollable ulcers. Blood glucose management, surgical debridement, skin transplantation, wound dressing, and hyperbaric oxygen therapy are some examples of traditional therapies. The limited therapeutic benefits of current diabetic wound treatments call for the creation of more potent, painless, and scar-free therapies. Owing to their capacity to transport medications, absorb cells, and regulate drug distribution over time, nanoparticles have been used as physiologically active delivery systems (Haque et al., 2021).

EGF and its receptors are lacking in diabetic wounds, which results in poor tissue regeneration and complicated wound healing. Vascular endothelial growth factor (VEGF) and epidermal growth factor (EGF) are essential for wound healing. EGF-containing nanoparticles are more effective (Chu et al., 2010).

In diabetic wounds, VEGFR2 mRNA expression is elevated. Curcumin, a naturally occurring hydrophobic polyphenol with antibacterial, antioxidant, anti-inflammatory, and anticancer properties, increases VEGF production, collagen deposition, wound healing rate, and granulation tissue development (Chereddy et al., 2015). Sesamol is a phenolic compound with anti-inflammatory, antioxidant, and anti-hyperglycemic properties. It promotes wound healing by enhancing extracellular matrix (ECM) deposition and reducing inflammation. Additionally, melatonin, an indoleamine that effectively scavenges reactive oxygen species (ROS), was tested for its healing properties through topical application in diabetic rats (Gourishetti et al., 2020).

6.9.2 DIABETIC FOOT AND THE ROLE OF TISSUE ENGINEERING

Diabetic foot infections (DFI) significantly contribute to DFU, leading to hospitalization and lower limb amputation. The current treatment guidelines for DFI involve antimicrobial therapy, surgical procedures, or revascularization, along with non-surgical wound care therapies, such as custom shoes and orthotics (Uçkay et al., 2015). Wound healing is a multifaceted biological process that involves angiogenesis, inflammation, chemotaxis, and tissue remodeling. Chronic wounds cause inflammation owing to bacterial colonization, which is exacerbated in diabetic patients, leading to early tissue degradation and a never-ending cycle of wound healing, resulting in impaired healing (Tam et al., 2013).

A wound care specialist evaluated the severity of DFU, followed by debridement and ongoing assessment of the wound area for potential surgical reconstruction. Soft-tissue repair can range from allowing the wound to heal naturally by utilizing microsurgical flaps to aid the healing process. Advancements in skin substitutes, including cadaver skin, xenografts, and synthetic options, have significantly enhanced their quality and regenerative abilities, providing temporary remedies, particularly for extensive wounds with irregular shapes (Baum et al., 2006).

Mechanical harvesting of donor skin, discoloration, infection risk, discomfort, and scarring are some of the disadvantages of autologous grafting and flap transplantation. Most autologous grafts merely apply epidermal covering, which results in a scarred donor site and a wound barrier that is not completely functional (Tam et al., 2013).

Recently, there has been an increase in biocompatible healing products designed for skin regeneration, including skin grafts and wound dressings (Tam et al., 2013). Amniotic membranes show potential as treatment options, yet their susceptibility to infection and scarcity hinders their viability as a conclusive solution for DFU. Currently, lab-created living tissue-engineered products such as Apligraf® and Dermagraft® are used to address DFU, as these engineered materials stimulate an angiogenic response in the wound, thereby enhancing the healing process. Additionally, therapies such as hyperbaric oxygen and negative pressure have surfaced as possible nonsurgical alternatives for DFU treatment; however, clinical evidence does not entirely support their effectiveness (Gurtner et al., 2008).

6.10 CHALLENGES AND CONSIDERATIONS

Precision treatment for diabetes uses medicine, diagnostics, and best practices to meet individual needs. However, there are barriers to its broad application, including skepticism regarding diabetes treatment strategies, medicines, genetic medicine, and precision medicine. The restricted capacity to discern relationships is contingent upon the frequency of genetic variations, magnitude of intended effects, and size of the sample (Shaffer et al., 2012).

Pharmacogenomics is effective in detecting unusual diabetic side effects in small studies, but larger sample sizes are needed as research advances towards whole-exome and whole-genome sequencing (Lee et al., 2014). Pharmacogenomic alterations can have significant clinical effects when grouped within a gene or pathway. However, genomics faces challenges in the management of dosage regimens in diabetes and cardiovascular medicine. Practical considerations include organizing and integrating genomic data to form an EHR and developing clinical decision-support tools for informed treatment decisions. Although several groups have contributed to model systems, more data are needed for future handling (Auwerx et al., 2022; Hicks et al., 2016). Nanotechnology-based medication systems offer numerous advantages, but they also have certain limitations and issues (Table 6.3).

TABLE 6.3 Key Challenges and Considerations That will Enhance Nanotechnology Integration in Diabetes Care

Challenges	Description
Concerns about toxicity and biocompatibility	Ensuring the safety of nanoparticles is essential, as their prolonged presence may lead to toxicity and undesirable side effects.
Regulatory requirements	Developing standardized evaluation protocols and clear regulations is vital for the safe progression of nanotechnology solutions.
Ethical considerations	Addressing ethical aspects, including patient autonomy, confidentiality, and equitable distribution of innovative therapies, is critical.
Patient acceptance and cost	Educating patients and promoting accessibility are key to fostering trust and ensuring the affordability of advanced treatments.
Sustained stability	The practical application of nanocarriers requires the maintenance of their integrity over time.
Interactions between drugs and combination therapies	The effective management of diabetes requires a thorough understanding of potential drug interactions and the optimization of combination therapies.
Outcome	The effective incorporation of nanotechnology into diabetes management can be improved by tackling these challenges.

6.11 FUTURE DIRECTIONS AND OPPORTUNITIES

It is anticipated that rising incidence, more serious consequences, and higher expenditures will impact diabetes care in the future. Globally, the prevalence of diabetes is predicted to increase from 285 million to 435 million by 2030, and from 6.6% in 2010. Preventing diabetes is crucial, as one in three US babies will develop the disease. The current healthcare cost is more than $174 billion. To enhance diabetes care, improved care models, especially financial models, are required. The current healthcare system often lacks resources for patient self-management, which results in limited education and support. One of the biggest obstacles to reaching evidence-based patient objectives is clinical inertia, which occurs when doctors do not accelerate treatment, and patients do not reach the desired outcomes.

The increasing use of CGM, personal health records, and shared patient portals poses risks to diabetes care providers. To address this issue, better management systems with filters and alerts are required. Primary care physicians are crucial to the healthcare delivery system, and any reorganization should focus on the primary care settings. Nanotechnology and nanoparticles are revolutionizing diabetes management by enabling the early detection and diagnosis of diabetes-associated biomarkers through imaging techniques. Advanced insulin delivery systems that incorporate nanoparticles, such as liposomes or polymer-based carriers, provide a responsive mechanism for insulin release, minimizing the risk of hypoglycemia, and enhancing glycemic control. Nano-sized drug formulations incorporating lipids or polymers have the potential to improve drug bioavailability, stability, and effectiveness, thereby enabling personalized treatment regimens with reduced side effects.

To address the underlying causes of diabetes, nanoparticles are being utilized in the development of artificial pancreas systems that combine automated insulin administration with CGM to restore and repair pancreatic beta cells. By offering tailored therapies based on a person's genetic and molecular profile, nanotechnology is transforming into personalized medicine. Patients with diabetes and medical professionals can receive real-time feedback from wearable devices that use nanoparticles for CGM. Nanotechnology has the potential to optimize drug delivery and minimize side effects in diabetes medications; however, addressing safety concerns, regulatory considerations, and ethical implications is crucial for successful clinical application. Researchers are developing nanomedicines for precise insulin delivery, addressing challenges such as oral bioavailability, immunogenicity, and production consistency. To guarantee consistent nanoparticle production, protective coatings, surface alterations, and sophisticated manufacturing processes have been investigated. The main goal is to create next-generation nanocarriers with improved targeting capabilities.

Real-time monitoring of insulin distribution and therapeutic efficacy is possible by the incorporation of biosensors and enhanced imaging into nanomedicine platforms. This enables individualized treatment plans and intersects with new areas such as gene editing and regenerative medicine. Research on glucose-responsive insulin (GRI) release nanosystems has gained considerable attention, utilizing glucose-sensitive components to trigger insulin release during hyperglycemic episodes. Ongoing collaboration among multidisciplinary research teams, along with continued funding for preclinical and clinical trials, is essential for advancing these innovations toward practical clinical applications. Diabetes treatment might greatly benefit from nanotechnology; however, issues including accessibility, cost-effectiveness, scalability, and safety must be resolved. Interdisciplinary cooperation between researchers, engineers, physicians, and regulatory bodies is essential for innovation and patient-centered care. Nanotechnology-driven diabetic treatment solutions can be developed and adopted more quickly thanks to emerging technologies like AI and digital health platforms.

6.12 CONCLUSION

Nanotechnology offers a groundbreaking approach to diabetes management and provides innovative solutions for insulin delivery, glucose monitoring, and tissue regeneration. While these advancements hold significant potential, challenges, such as safety concerns, cost-effectiveness, and accessibility, must be addressed. Collaborative efforts among multidisciplinary research teams, clinicians, and regulatory bodies are essential for successful clinical translation of nanotechnology-driven diabetes treatments. Additionally, emerging technologies such as AI can further enhance the development and application of personalized diabetes care solutions, ensuring better patient outcomes and quality of life.

KEYWORDS

- **artificial intelligence**
- **diabetes mellitus**
- **digital health platforms**
- **glucose monitoring**
- **insulin delivery**
- **nanotechnology**
- **personalized medicine**
- **tissue regeneration**

REFERENCES

Afsharzadeh, M., Hashemi, M., Mokhtarzadeh, A., Abnous, K., & Ramezani, M. (2018). Recent advances in co-delivery systems based on polymeric nanoparticle for cancer treatment. *Artificial Cells, Nanomedicine, and Biotechnology, 46*, 1095–1110. https://doi.org/10.1080/21691401.2017.1376675 (accessed on 2nd February 2026).

Ahmad, E., Lim, S., Lamptey, R., Webb, D. R., & Davies, M. J. (2022). Type 2 diabetes. *Lancet, 400*, 1803–1820. https://doi.org/10.1016/S0140-6736(22)01655-5 (accessed on 2nd February 2026).

Ali, O. (2013). Genetics of type 2 diabetes. *World Journal of Diabetes, 4*, 114–123. https://doi.org/10.4239/wjd.v4.i4.114 (accessed on 2nd February 2026).

Allen, N., & Gupta, A. (2019). Current diabetes technology: Striving for the artificial pancreas. *Diagnostics, 9*, 31. https://doi.org/10.3390/diagnostics9010031 (accessed on 2nd February 2026).

Aloke, C., Egwu, C. O., Aja, P. M., Obasi, N. A., Chukwu, J., Akumadu, B. O., et al. (2022). Current advances in the management of diabetes mellitus. *Biomedicines, 10*, 2436. https://doi.org/10.3390/biomedicines10102436 (accessed on 2nd February 2026).

American Diabetes Association. (2011). Diagnosis and classification of diabetes mellitus. *Diabetes Care, 34*(Supplement 1), S62–S69. https://doi.org/10.2337/dc11-S062 (accessed on 2nd February 2026).

Auwerx, C., Sadler, M. C., Reymond, A., & Kutalik, Z. (2022). From pharmacogenetics to pharmaco-omics: Milestones and future directions. *HGG Advances, 3*, 100100. https://doi.org/10.1016/j.xhgg.2022.100100 (accessed on 2nd February 2026).

Baby, T. T., & Ramaprabhu, S. (2010). SiO_2 coated Fe_3O_4 magnetic nanoparticle dispersed multiwalled carbon nanotubes based amperometric glucose biosensor. *Talanta, 80*, 2016–2022. https://doi.org/10.1016/j.talanta.2009.11.010 (accessed on 2nd February 2026).

Bahman, F., Taurin, S., Altayeb, D., Taha, S., Bakhiet, M., & Greish, K. (2020). Oral insulin delivery using poly(styrene co-maleic acid) micelles in a diabetic mouse model.

Pharmaceutics, 12, 1026. https://doi.org/10.3390/pharmaceutics12111026 (accessed on 2nd February 2026).

Bajracharya, R., Song, J. G., Back, S. Y., & Han, H. K. (2019). Recent advancements in non-invasive formulations for protein drug delivery. *Computational and Structural Biotechnology Journal, 17*, 1290–1308. https://doi.org/10.1016/j.csbj.2019.09.004 (accessed on 2nd February 2026).

Baloch, S. G., Shaikh, H., Shah, S., Memon, S., & Memon, A. A. (2022). Synthesis of an insulin intercalated graphene oxide nanogel composite: Evaluation of its release profile and stability for oral delivery of insulin. *Nanoscale Advances, 4*, 2303–2312. https://doi.org/10.1039/D1NA00887K (accessed on 2nd February 2026).

Bashyal, S., Seo, J. E., Keum, T., Noh, G., Lamichhane, S., & Lee, S. (2021). Development, characterization, and *ex vivo* assessment of elastic liposomes for enhancing the buccal delivery of insulin. *Pharmaceutics, 13*, 565. https://doi.org/10.3390/pharmaceutics13040565 (accessed on 2nd February 2026).

Baum, C. L., & Arpey, C. J. (2005). Normal cutaneous wound healing: Clinical correlation with cellular and molecular events. *Dermatologic Surgery, 31*, 674–686; discussion 686. https://doi.org/10.1111/j.1524-4725.2005.31612 (accessed on 2nd February 2026).

Brasiunas, B., Popov, A., Ramanavicius, A., & Ramanaviciene, A. (2021). Gold nanoparticle based colorimetric sensing strategy for the determination of reducing sugars. *Food Chemistry, 351*, 129238. https://doi.org/10.1016/j.foodchem.2021.129238 (accessed on 2nd February 2026).

Bruen, D., Delaney, C., Florea, L., & Diamond, D. (2017). Glucose sensing for diabetes monitoring: Recent developments. *Sensors, 17*, 1866. https://doi.org/10.3390/s17081866 (accessed on 2nd February 2026).

Burge, M. R., Mitchell, S., Sawyer, A., & Schade, D. S. (2008). Continuous glucose monitoring: The future of diabetes management. *Diabetes Spectrum, 21*, 112–119. https://doi.org/10.2337/diaspect.21.2.112 (accessed on 2nd February 2026).

Callejas, D., Mann, C. J., Ayuso, E., Lage, R., Grifoll, I., Roca, C., et al. (2013). Treatment of diabetes and long-term survival after insulin and glucokinase gene therapy. *Diabetes, 62*, 1718–1729. https://doi.org/10.2337/db12-1113 (accessed on 2nd February 2026).

Cash, K. J., & Clark, H. A. (2010). Nano sensors and nanomaterials for monitoring glucose in diabetes. *Trends in Molecular Medicine, 16*, 584–593. https://doi.org/10.1016/j.molmed.2010.08.002 (accessed on 2nd February 2026).

Castaño, C., Mirasierra, M., Vallejo, M., Novials, A., & Párrizas, M. (2020). Delivery of muscle-derived exosomal miRNAs induced by HIIT improves insulin sensitivity through down-regulation of hepatic FoxO1 in mice. *Proceedings of the National Academy of Sciences of the United States of America, 117*, 30335–30343. https://doi.org/10.1073/pnas.2016112117 (accessed on 2nd February 2026).

Caturano, A., Nilo, R., Nilo, D., Russo, V., Santonastaso, E., Galiero, R., et al. (2024). Advances in nanomedicine for precision insulin delivery. *Pharmaceuticals, 17*, 945. https://doi.org/10.3390/ph17070945 (accessed on 2nd February 2026).

Chen, C., Zhao, X. L., Li, Z. H., Zhu, Z. G., Qian, S. H., & Flewitt, A. J. (2017). Current and emerging technology for continuous glucose monitoring. *Sensors, 17*, 182. https://doi.org/10.3390/s17010182 (accessed on 2nd February 2026).

Chen, S., Hai, X., Chen, X. W., & Wang, J. H. (2014). *In situ* growth of silver nanoparticles on graphene quantum dots for ultrasensitive colorimetric detection of H_2O_2 and glucose.

Analytical Chemistry, 86, 6689–6694. https://doi.org/10.1021/ac501497d (accessed on 2nd February 2026).

Chereddy, K. K., Lopes, A., Koussoroplis, S., Payen, V., Moia, C., Zhu, H., et al. (2015). Combined effects of PLGA and vascular endothelial growth factor promote the healing of non-diabetic and diabetic wounds. *Nanomedicine: Nanotechnology, Biology, and Medicine, 11*, 1975–1984. https://doi.org/10.1016/j.nano.2015.07.006 (accessed on 2nd February 2026).

Chou, H. S., Larsson, M., Hsiao, M. H., Chen, Y. C., Röding, M., Nydén, M., et al. (2016). Injectable insulin-lysozyme-loaded nanogels with enzymatically-controlled degradation and release for basal insulin treatment: *In vitro* characterization and *in vivo* observation. *Journal of Controlled Release, 224*, 33–42. https://doi.org/10.1016/j.jconrel.2015.12.036 (accessed on 2nd February 2026).

Chu, Y., Yu, D., Wang, P., Xu, J., Li, D., & Ding, M. (2010). Nanotechnology promotes the full-thickness diabetic wound healing effect of recombinant human epidermal growth factor in diabetic rats. *Wound Repair and Regeneration, 18*, 499–505. https://doi.org/10.1111/j.1524-475X.2010.00612.x (accessed on 2nd February 2026).

Cito, M., Pellegrini, S., Piemonti, L., & Sordi, V. (2018). The potential and challenges of alternative sources of β cells for the cure of type 1 diabetes. *Endocrine Connections, 7*, R114–R125. https://doi.org/10.1530/EC-18-0012 (accessed on 2nd February 2026).

Cui, G., Kim, S. J., Choi, S. H., Nam, H., Cha, G. S., & Paeng, K. J. (2000). A disposable amperometric sensor screen printed on a nitrocellulose strip: A glucose biosensor employing lead oxide as an interference-removing agent. *Analytical Chemistry, 72*, 1925–1929. https://doi.org/10.1021/ac991213d (accessed on 2nd February 2026).

Davatgaran-Taghipour, Y., Masoomzadeh, S., Farzaei, M. H., Bahramsoltani, R., Karimi-Soureh, Z., et al. (2017). Polyphenol nano formulations for cancer therapy: Experimental evidence and clinical perspective. *International Journal of Nanomedicine, 12*, 2689–2702. https://doi.org/10.2147/IJN.S131973 (accessed on 2nd February 2026).

Dawoud, M. H. S., Yassin, G. E., Ghorab, D. M., & Morsi, N. M. (2019). Insulin mucoadhesive liposomal gel for wound healing: A formulation with sustained release and extended stability using quality by design approach. *AAPS PharmSciTech, 20*, 158. https://doi.org/10.1208/s12249-019-1363-6 (accessed on 2nd February 2026).

De Souza Von Zuben, E., Eloy, J. O., Araujo, V. H. S., Gremião, M. P. D., & Chorilli, M. (2021). Insulin-loaded liposomes functionalized with cell-penetrating peptides: Influence on drug release and permeation through porcine nasal mucosa. *Colloids and Surfaces A, 622*, 126624. https://doi.org/10.1016/j.colsurfa.2021.126624 (accessed on 2nd February 2026).

DeFronzo, R., Fleming, G. A., Chen, K., & Bicsak, T. A. (2016). Metformin-associated lactic acidosis: Current perspectives on causes and risk. *Metabolism: Clinical and Experimental, 65*, 20–29. https://doi.org/10.1016/j.metabol.2015.10.014 (accessed on 2nd February 2026).

Di, J., Price, J., Gu, X., Jiang, X., Jing, Y., & Gu, Z. (2014). Ultrasound-triggered regulation of blood glucose levels using injectable nano-network. *Advanced Healthcare Materials, 3*, 811–816. https://doi.org/10.1002/adhm.201300490 (accessed on 2nd February 2026).

Dias, D., & Paulo Silva Cunha, J. P. (2018). Wearable health devices—Vital sign monitoring, systems and technologies. *Sensors, 18*, 2414. https://doi.org/10.3390/s18082414 (accessed on 2nd February 2026).

DiMeglio, L. A., Evans-Molina, C., & Oram, R. A. (2018). Type 1 diabetes. *Lancet, 391*, 2449–2462. https://doi.org/10.1016/S0140-6736(18)31320-5 (accessed on 2nd February 2026).

DiSanto, R. M., Subramanian, V., & Gu, Z. (2015). Recent advances in nanotechnology for diabetes treatment. *Wiley Interdisciplinary Reviews: Nanomedicine and Nanobiotechnology, 7*, 548–564. https://doi.org/10.1002/wnan.1329 (accessed on 2nd February 2026).

Dixit, P. V., Mishra, D. K., Sharma, S., & Gautam, R. K. (2023). Nanocarriers and diabetes: New vistas and the way ahead. *Current Pharmaceutical Biotechnology, 24*, 1420–1429. https://doi.org/10.2174/1389201024666221227140728 (accessed on 2nd February 2026).

El-Dakroury, W. A., Zewail, M. B., & Amin, M. M. (2023). Design, optimization, and *in-vivo* performance of glipizide-loaded O-carboxymethyl chitosan nanoparticles in insulin resistant/type 2 diabetic rat model. *Journal of Drug Delivery Science and Technology, 79*, 104040. https://doi.org/10.1016/j.jddst.2022.104040 (accessed on 2nd February 2026).

Elshaarani, T., Yu, H., Wang, L., Lin, L., Wang, N., ur Rahman Naveed, K., et al. (2020). Dextran-crosslinked glucose responsive nanogels with a self-regulated insulin release at physiological conditions. *European Polymer Journal, 125*, 109505. https://doi.org/10.1016/j.eurpolymj.2020.109505 (accessed on 2nd February 2026).

Faselis, C., Katsimardou, A., Imprialos, K., Deligkaris, P., Kallistratos, M., & Dimitriadis, K. (2020). Microvascular complications of type 2 diabetes mellitus. *Current Vascular Pharmacology, 18*, 117–124. https://doi.org/10.2174/1570161117666190502103733 (accessed on 2nd February 2026).

Forrest, R. D., Jackson, C. A., & Yudkin, J. S. (1987). Screening for diabetes mellitus in general practice using a reflectance meter system. The Islington diabetes survey. *Diabetes Research, 6*, 119–122.

Galicia-Garcia, U., Benito-Vicente, A., Jebari, S., Larrea-Sebal, A., Siddiqi, H., Uribe, K. B., et al. (2020). Pathophysiology of type 2 diabetes mellitus. *International Journal of Molecular Sciences, 21*, 6275. https://doi.org/10.3390/ijms21176275 (accessed on 2nd February 2026).

GBD 2021 Diabetes Collaborators. (2023). Global, regional, and national burden of diabetes from 1990 to 2021, with projections of prevalence to 2050: A systematic analysis for the Global Burden of Disease Study 2021. *Lancet, 402*, 203–234. https://doi.org/10.1016/S0140-6736(23)01301-6 (accessed on 2nd February 2026).

Giovannini, P., Howes, M. J. R., & Edwards, S. E. (2016). Medicinal plants used in the traditional management of diabetes and its sequelae in Central America: A review. *Journal of Ethnopharmacology, 184*, 58–71. https://doi.org/10.1016/j.jep.2016.02.034 (accessed on 2nd February 2026).

Gopalan, A. I., Lee, K. P., Ragupathy, D., Lee, S. H., & Lee, J. W. (2009). An electrochemical glucose biosensor exploiting a polyaniline grafted multiwalled carbon nanotube/perfluoro sulfonate ionomer–silica nanocomposite. *Biomaterials, 30*, 5999–6005. https://doi.org/10.1016/j.biomaterials.2009.07.047 (accessed on 2nd February 2026).

Gourishetti, K., Keni, R., Nayak, P. G., Jitta, S. R., Bhaskaran, N. A., Kumar, L., et al. (2020). Sesamol-loaded PLGA nanosuspension for accelerating wound healing in diabetic foot ulcer in rats. *International Journal of Nanomedicine, 15*, 9265–9282. https://doi.org/10.2147/IJN.S268941 (accessed on 2nd February 2026).

Grant, S. F. A. (2019). The TCF7L2 locus: A genetic window into the pathogenesis of Type 1 and type 2 diabetes. *Diabetes Care, 42*, 1624–1629. https://doi.org/10.2337/dci19-0001 (accessed on 2nd February 2026).

Gurtner, G. C., Werner, S., Barrandon, Y., & Longaker, M. T. (2008). Wound repair and regeneration. *Nature, 453*, 314–321. https://doi.org/10.1038/nature07039 (accessed on 2nd February 2026).

Han, X., Lu, Y., Xie, J., Zhang, E., Zhu, H., Du, H., et al. (2020). Zwitterionic micelles efficiently deliver oral insulin without opening tight junctions. *Nature Nanotechnology, 15*, 605–614. https://doi.org/10.1038/s41565-020-0693-6 (accessed on 2nd February 2026).

Haque, S. T., Saha, S. K., Haque, E., & Biswas, N. (2021). Nanotechnology-based therapeutic applications: *In vitro* and *in vivo* clinical studies for diabetic wound healing. *Biomaterials Science, 9*, 7705–7747. https://doi.org/10.1039/D1BM01211H (accessed on 2nd February 2026).

Heller, A., & Feldman, B. (2008). Electrochemical glucose sensors and their applications in diabetes management. *Chemical Reviews, 108*, 2482–2505. https://doi.org/10.1021/cr068069y (accessed on 2nd February 2026).

Hicks, J. K., Dunnenberger, H. M., Gumpper, K. F., Haidar, C. E., & Hoffman, J. M. (2016). Integrating pharmacogenomics into electronic health records with clinical decision support. *American Journal of Health-System Pharmacy, 73*, 1967–1976. https://doi.org/10.2146/ajhp160030 (accessed on 2nd February 2026).

Himasa, F. I., Singhal, M., Ojha, A., & Kumar, B. (2022). Prospective for diagnosis and treatment of diabetic retinopathy. *Current Pharmaceutical Design, 28*, 560–569. https://doi.org/10.2174/1381612827666211115154907 (accessed on 2nd February 2026).

Hossain, J., Al-Mamun, M., & Islam, M. R. (2024). Diabetes mellitus, the fastest growing global public health concern: Early detection should be focused. *Health Science Reports, 7*, e2004. https://doi.org/10.1002/hsr2.2004 (accessed on 2nd February 2026).

Hu, W. Y., Wu, Z. M., Yang, Q. Q., Liu, Y. J., Li, J., & Zhang, C. Y. (2019). Smart pH-responsive polymeric micelles for programmed oral delivery of insulin. *Colloids and Surfaces B: Bio Interfaces, 183*, 110443. https://doi.org/10.1016/j.colsurfb.2019.110443 (accessed on 2nd February 2026).

Huang, C., Hao, Z., Qi, T., Pan, Y., & Zhao, X. (2020). An integrated flexible and reusable graphene field effect transistor nano sensor for monitoring glucose. *Journal of Materiomics, 6*, 308–314. https://doi.org/10.1016/j.jmat.2020.02.002 (accessed on 2nd February 2026).

Huang, E. S., Basu, A., O'Grady, M., & Capretta, J. C. (2009). Projecting the future diabetes population size and related costs for the U.S. *Diabetes Care, 32*, 2225–2229. https://doi.org/10.2337/dc09-0459 (accessed on 2nd February 2026).

Italiya, K. S., Basak, M., Mazumdar, S., Sahel, D. K., Shrivastava, R., Chitkara, D., et al. (2019). Scalable self-assembling micellar system for enhanced oral bioavailability and efficacy of lisofylline for treatment of Type-I diabetes. *Molecular Pharmaceutics, 16*, 4954–4967. https://doi.org/10.1021/acs.molpharmaceut.9b00833 (accessed on 2nd February 2026).

Jaafar, M. H. M., & Hamid, K. A. (2019). Chitosan-coated alginate nanoparticles enhanced absorption profile of insulin via oral administration. *Current Drug Delivery, 16*, 672–686. https://doi.org/10.2174/1567201816666190620110748 (accessed on 2nd February 2026).

Ji, P., Murata-Hori, M., & Lodish, H. F. (2011). Formation of mammalian erythrocytes: Chromatin condensation and enucleation. *Trends in Cell Biology, 21*, 409–415. https://doi.org/10.1016/j.tcb.2011.04.003 (accessed on 2nd February 2026).

Kahanovitz, L., Sluss, P. M., & Russell, S. J. (2017). Type 1 diabetes—A clinical perspective. *Point of Care: The Journal of Near-Patient Testing & Technology, 16*, 37–40. https://doi.org/10.1097/POC.0000000000000125 (accessed on 2nd February 2026).

Kamalden, T. A., Macgregor-Das, A. M., Kannan, S. M., Dunkerly-Eyring, B., Khaliddin, N., Xu, Z., et al. (2017). Exosomal MicroRNA-15a transfer from the pancreas augments diabetic complications by inducing oxidative stress. *Antioxidants and Redox Signaling, 27*, 913–930. https://doi.org/10.1089/ars.2016.6844 (accessed on 2nd February 2026).

Katsarou, A., Gudbjörnsdottir, S., Rawshani, A., Dabelea, D., Bonifacio, E., Anderson, B. J., et al. (2017). Type 1 diabetes mellitus. *Nature Reviews Disease Primers, 3*, 17016. https://doi.org/10.1038/nrdp.2017.16 (accessed on 2nd February 2026).

Laraeni, Y., Danuyanti, I. G. A. N., Resnhaleksmana, E., Pauzi, I., Mataram, I. K. A., & Agustini, N. P. (2021). High antioxidant level in *Cajanus sajan* reduces blood glucose level and improves blood lipid profile of rats as diabetes mellitus models. *International Journal of Health Sciences, 5*. https://doi.org/10.29332/ijhs.v5n1.725 (accessed on 2nd February 2026).

Lee, S. H., Lee, H., Park, J. S., Choi, H., Han, K. Y., Seo, H. S., et al. (2007). A novel approach to ultrasensitive diagnosis using supramolecular protein nanoparticles. *FASEB Journal, 21*, 1324–1334. https://doi.org/10.1096/fj.06-7303com (accessed on 2nd February 2026).

Lee, S., Abecasis, G. R., Boehnke, M., & Lin, X. (2014). Rare-variant association analysis: Study designs and statistical tests. *American Journal of Human Genetics, 95*, 5–23. https://doi.org/10.1016/j.ajhg.2014.06.009 (accessed on 2nd February 2026).

Lee, T., Kim, I., Cheong, D. Y., Roh, S., Jung, H. G., Lee, S. W., et al. (2021). Selective colorimetric urine glucose detection by paper sensor functionalized with polyaniline nanoparticles and cell membrane. *Analytica Chimica Acta, 1158*, 338387. https://doi.org/10.1016/j.aca.2021.338387 (accessed on 2nd February 2026).

Li, J., Wei, X., & Yuan, Y. (2009). Synthesis of magnetic nanoparticles composed by Prussian Blue and glucose oxidase for preparing highly sensitive and selective glucose biosensor. *Sensors and Actuators B: Chemical, 139*, 400–406. https://doi.org/10.1016/j.snb.2009.03.004 (accessed on 2nd February 2026).

Lim, A. K. (2014). Diabetic nephropathy–complications and treatment. *International Journal of Nephrology and Renovascular Disease, 7*, 361–381. https://doi.org/10.2147/IJNRD.S40172 (accessed on 2nd February 2026).

Liu, X., Li, C., Lv, J., Huang, F., An, Y., Shi, L., & Ma, R. (2020). Glucose and H_2O_2 dual-responsive polymeric micelles for the self-regulated release of insulin. *ACS Applied Bio Materials, 3*, 1598–1606. https://doi.org/10.1021/acsabm.9b01185 (accessed on 2nd February 2026).

Mandal, D., Sarmah, J. K., & Gupta, J. (2023). NanoRevolution: Pioneering applications of nanotechnology in Type II diabetes care. *Engineering Proceedings, 56*(1), 56. https://doi.org/10.3390/ASEC2023-15312 (accessed on 2nd February 2026).

Mannino, G. C., Andreozzi, F., & Sesti, G. (2019). Pharmacogenetics of type 2 diabetes mellitus, the route toward tailored medicine. *Diabetes/Metabolism Research and Reviews, 35*, e3109. https://doi.org/10.1002/dmrr.3109 (accessed on 2nd February 2026).

Mansoor, S., Kondiah, P. P. D., Choonara, Y. E., & Pillay, V. (2019). Polymer-based nanoparticle strategies for insulin delivery. *Polymers, 11*, 1380. https://doi.org/10.3390/polym11091380 (accessed on 2nd February 2026).

Marques, C., Som, C., Schmutz, M., Borges, O., & Borchard, G. (2020). How the lack of chitosan characterization precludes implementation of the safe-by-design concept. *Frontiers in Bioengineering and Biotechnology, 8*, 165. https://doi.org/10.3389/fbioe.2020.00165 (accessed on 2nd February 2026).

McLaughlin, S., Podrebarac, J., Ruel, M., Suuronen, E. J., McNeill, B., & Alarcon, E. I. (2016). Nano-engineered biomaterials for tissue regeneration: What has been achieved so far? *Frontiers in Materials, 3*. https://doi.org/10.3389/fmats.2016.00027 (accessed on 2nd February 2026).

Mitchell, M. J., Billingsley, M. M., Haley, R. M., Wechsler, M. E., Peppas, N. A., & Langer, R. (2021). Engineering precision nanoparticles for drug delivery. *Nature Reviews Drug Discovery, 20*, 101–124. https://doi.org/10.1038/s41573-020-0090-8 (accessed on 2nd February 2026).

Miyashita, M., Ito, N., Ikeda, S., Murayama, T., Oguma, K., & Kimura, J. (2009). Development of urine glucose meter based on micro-planar amperometric biosensor and its clinical application for self-monitoring of urine glucose. *Biosensors and Bioelectronics, 24*, 1336–1340. https://doi.org/10.1016/j.bios.2008.07.072 (accessed on 2nd February 2026).

Mobasseri, M., Shirmohammadi, M., Amiri, T., Vahed, N., Hosseini Fard, H., & Ghojazadeh, M. (2020). Prevalence and incidence of type 1 diabetes in the world: A systematic review and meta-analysis. *Health Promotion Perspectives, 10*, 98–115. https://doi.org/10.34172/hpp.2020.18 (accessed on 2nd February 2026).

Morran, M. P., Vonberg, A., Khadra, A., & Pietropaolo, M. (2015). Immunogenetics of type 1 diabetes mellitus. *Molecular Aspects of Medicine, 42*, 42–60. https://doi.org/10.1016/j.mam.2014.12.004 (accessed on 2nd February 2026).

Mudassir, J., Darwis, Y., Muhamad, S., & Khan, A. A. (2019). Self-assembled insulin and nanogels polyelectrolyte complex (Ins/NGs-PEC) for oral insulin delivery: Characterization, lyophilization and *in-vivo* evaluation. *International Journal of Nanomedicine, 14*, 4895–4909. https://doi.org/10.2147/IJN.S199507 (accessed on 2nd February 2026).

Mudshinge, S. R., Deore, A. B., Patil, S., & Bhalgat, C. M. (2011). Nanoparticles: Emerging carriers for drug delivery. *Saudi Pharmaceutical Journal, 19*, 129–141. https://doi.org/10.1016/j.jsps.2011.04.001 (accessed on 2nd February 2026).

Muntoni, E., Anfossi, L., Milla, P., Marini, E., Ferraris, C., Capucchio, M. T., et al. (2021). Glargine insulin loaded lipid nanoparticles: Oral delivery of liquid and solid oral dosage forms. *Nutrition, Metabolism, and Cardiovascular Diseases, 31*, 691–698. https://doi.org/10.1016/j.numecd.2020.09.020 (accessed on 2nd February 2026).

Natarajan, J. V., Nugraha, C., Ng, X. W., & Venkatraman, S. (2014). Sustained-release from nanocarriers: A review. *Journal of Controlled Release, 193*, 122–138. https://doi.org/10.1016/j.jconrel.2014.05.029 (accessed on 2nd February 2026).

Niu, Z., Zhang, W., Yu, C., Zhang, J., & Wen, Y. (2018). Recent advances in biological sample preparation methods coupled with chromatography, spectrometry and electrochemistry analysis techniques. *TrAC Trends in Analytical Chemistry, 102*, 123–146. https://doi.org/10.1016/j.trac.2018.02.005 (accessed on 2nd February 2026).

Noble, J. A., & Valdes, A. M. (2011). Genetics of the HLA region in the prediction of type 1 diabetes. *Current Diabetes Reports, 11*, 533–542. https://doi.org/10.1007/s11892-011-0223-x (accessed on 2nd February 2026).

Ortiz, G. G., Huerta, M., González-Usigli, H. A., Torres-Sánchez, E. D., Delgado-Lara, D. L., Pacheco-Moisés, F. P., et al. (2022). Cognitive disorder and dementia in type 2 diabetes mellitus. *World Journal of Diabetes, 13*, 319–337. https://doi.org/10.4239/wjd.v13.i4.319 (accessed on 2nd February 2026).

Palmer, S. C., Mavridis, D., Nicolucci, A., Johnson, D. W., Tonelli, M., Craig, J. C., et al. (2016). Comparison of clinical outcomes and adverse events associated with glucose-lowering drugs in patients with type 2 diabetes: A meta-analysis. *JAMA, 316*, 313–324. https://doi.org/10.1001/jama.2016.9400 (accessed on 2nd February 2026).

Pang, X., He, D., Luo, S., & Cai, Q. (2009). An amperometric glucose biosensor fabricated with Pt nanoparticle-decorated carbon nanotubes/TiO_2 nanotube arrays composite. *Sensors and Actuators B: Chemical, 137*, 134–138. https://doi.org/10.1016/j.snb.2008.09.051 (accessed on 2nd February 2026).

Pardakhty, A., Varshosaz, J., & Rouholamini, A. (2007). *In vitro* study of polyoxyethylene alkyl ether niosomes for delivery of insulin. *International Journal of Pharmaceutics, 328*, 130–141. https://doi.org/10.1016/j.ijpharm.2006.08.002 (accessed on 2nd February 2026).

Patel, K., Atkinson, C., Tran, D., & Nadig, S. N. (2017). Nanotechnological approaches to immunosuppression and tolerance induction. *Current Transplantation Reports, 4*, 159–168. https://doi.org/10.1007/s40472-017-0146-9 (accessed on 2nd February 2026).

Patra, J. K., Das, G., Fraceto, L. F., Campos, E. V. R., Rodriguez-Torres, M. D. P., Acosta-Torres, L. S., et al. (2018). Nano based drug delivery systems: Recent developments and future prospects. *Journal of Nanobiotechnology, 16*, 71. https://doi.org/10.1186/s12951-018-0392-8 (accessed on 2nd February 2026).

Pickup, J. C., Zhi, Z. L., Khan, F., Saxl, T., & Birch, D. J. S. (2008). Nanomedicine and its potential in diabetes research and practice. *Diabetes/Metabolism Research and Reviews, 24*, 604–610. https://doi.org/10.1002/dmrr.893 (accessed on 2nd February 2026).

Prasad, R. B., & Groop, L. (2015). Genetics of type 2 diabetes—Pitfalls and possibilities. *Genes, 6*, 87–123. https://doi.org/10.3390/genes6010087 (accessed on 2nd February 2026).

Purohit, D., Jalwal, P., Manchanda, D., Saini, S., Verma, R., Kaushik, D., et al. (2023). Nanocapsules: An emerging drug delivery system. *Recent Patents on Nanotechnology, 17*, 190–207. https://doi.org/10.2174/1872210516666220210113256 (accessed on 2nd February 2026).

Raghav, S. S., Kumar, B., Sethiya, N. K., & Kaul, A. (2022). A mechanistic insight on phytoconstituents delivering hypoglycemic activity: A comprehensive overview. *Future*

Pharmacology, 2, 511–546. https://doi.org/10.3390/futurepharmacol2040032 (accessed on 2nd February 2026).

Rask-Madsen, C., & King, G. L. (2013). Vascular complications of diabetes: Mechanisms of injury and protective factors. *Cell Metabolism, 17*, 20–33. https://doi.org/10.1016/j.cmet.2012.11.012 (accessed on 2nd February 2026).

Rauf, S., Hayat Nawaz, M. A., Badea, M., Marty, J. L., & Hayat, A. (2016). Nano-engineered biomimetic optical sensors for glucose monitoring in diabetes. *Sensors, 16*, 1931. https://doi.org/10.3390/s16111931 (accessed on 2nd February 2026).

Rodríguez-Morales, B., Antunes-Ricardo, M., & González-Valdez, J. (2021). Exosome-mediated insulin delivery for the potential treatment of diabetes mellitus. *Pharmaceutics, 13*, 1870. https://doi.org/10.3390/pharmaceutics13111870 (accessed on 2nd February 2026).

Santhosh, P., Manesh, K. M., Uthayakumar, S., Komathi, S., Gopalan, A. I., & Lee, K. P. (2009). Fabrication of enzymatic glucose biosensor based on palladium nanoparticles dispersed onto poly(3,4-ethylenedioxythiophene) nanofibers. *Bioelectrochemistry, 75*, 61–66. https://doi.org/10.1016/j.bioelechem.2008.12.001 (accessed on 2nd February 2026).

Sercombe, L., Veerati, T., Moheimani, F., Wu, S. Y., Sood, A. K., & Hua, S. (2015). Advances and challenges of liposome assisted drug delivery. *Frontiers in Pharmacology, 6*, 286. https://doi.org/10.3389/fphar.2015.00286 (accessed on 2nd February 2026).

Shaffer, J. R., Feingold, E., & Marazita, M. L. (2012). Genome-wide association studies: Prospects and challenges for oral health. *Journal of Dental Research, 91*, 637–641. https://doi.org/10.1177/0022034512446968 (accessed on 2nd February 2026).

Shafiq, S., Siddiq Abduh, M., Iqbal, F., Kousar, K., Anjum, S., & Ahmad, T. (2024). A novel approach to insulin delivery via oral route: Milk fat globule membrane derived liposomes as a delivery vehicle. *Saudi Journal of Biological Sciences, 31*, 103945. https://doi.org/10.1016/j.sjbs.2024.103945 (accessed on 2nd February 2026).

Shah, R. B., Patel, M., Maahs, D. M., & Shah, V. N. (2016). Insulin delivery methods: Past, present and future. *International Journal of Pharmaceutical Investigation, 6*, 1–9. https://doi.org/10.4103/2230-973X.176456 (accessed on 2nd February 2026).

Sharma, R., Borah, S. J., Bhawna, Kumar, S., Gupta, A., Kumari, V., Kumar, R., et al. (2023). Emerging trends in nano-based antidiabetic therapeutics: A path to effective diabetes management. *Materials Advances, 4*, 3091–3113. https://doi.org/10.1039/D3MA00159H (accessed on 2nd February 2026).

Sharma, R., Musyuni, P., Majeed, J., & Aggarwal, G. (2024). Challenges and opportunities in precision therapy for diabetic patients. *Health Sciences Review, 12*, 100190. https://doi.org/10.1016/j.hsr.2024.100190 (accessed on 2nd February 2026).

Shirin, A., Della Rossa, F., Klickstein, I., Russell, J., & Sorrentino, F. (2019). Optimal regulation of blood glucose level in Type I diabetes using insulin and glucagon. *PLOS ONE, 14*, e0213665. https://doi.org/10.1371/journal.pone.0213665 (accessed on 2nd February 2026).

Steck, A. K., & Rewers, M. J. (2011). Genetics of type 1 diabetes. *Clinical Chemistry, 57*, 176–185. https://doi.org/10.1373/clinchem.2010.148221 (accessed on 2nd February 2026).

Stoeckel, L. E., Arvanitakis, Z., Gandy, S., Small, D., Kahn, C. R., Pascual-Leone, A., et al. (2016). Complex mechanisms linking neurocognitive dysfunction to insulin resistance and other metabolic dysfunction. *F1000Research, 5*, 353. https://doi.org/10.12688/f1000research.8300.2 (accessed on 2nd February 2026).

Su, L., Feng, J., Zhou, X., Ren, C., Li, H., & Chen, X. (2012). Colorimetric detection of urine glucose based $ZnFe_2O_4$ magnetic nanoparticles. *Analytical Chemistry, 84*, 5753–5758. https://doi.org/10.1021/ac300939z (accessed on 2nd February 2026).

Suhail, M., Rosenholm, J. M., Minhas, M. U., Badshah, S. F., Naeem, A., Khan, K. U., et al. (2019). Nanogels as drug-delivery systems: A comprehensive overview. *Therapeutic Delivery, 10*, 697–717. https://doi.org/10.4155/tde-2019-0010 (accessed on 2nd February 2026).

Sun, H., Saeedi, P., Karuranga, S., Pinkepank, M., Ogurtsova, K., Duncan, B. B., et al. (2022). IDF Diabetes Atlas: Global, regional and country-level diabetes prevalence estimates for 2021 and projections for 2045. *Diabetes Research and Clinical Practice, 183*, 109119. https://doi.org/10.1016/j.diabres.2021.109119 (accessed on 2nd February 2026).

Ta, Q. T. H., & Nguyen, T. K. O. (2020). Type 3 diabetes and its role implications in Alzheimer's disease. *International Journal of Molecular Sciences, 21*, 3165. https://doi.org/10.3390/ijms21093165 (accessed on 2nd February 2026).

Tam, J., Wang, Y., Farinelli, W. A., Jiménez-Lozano, J., Franco, W., Sakamoto, F. H., et al. (2013). Fractional skin harvesting: Autologous skin grafting without donor-site morbidity. *Plastic and Reconstructive Surgery Global Open, 1*, e47. https://doi.org/10.1097/GOX.0b013e3182a85a36 (accessed on 2nd February 2026).

Thakur, B., Amarnath, C. A., & Sawant, S. N. (2014). Pectin coated polyaniline nanoparticles for an amperometric glucose biosensor. *RSC Advances, 4*, 40917–40923. https://doi.org/10.1039/C4RA05264A (accessed on 2nd February 2026).

The DCCT Research Group. (1988). Weight gain associated with intensive therapy in the Diabetes Control and Complications Trial. *Diabetes Care, 11*, 567–573. https://doi.org/10.2337/diacare.11.7.567 (accessed on 2nd February 2026).

The Diabetes Control and Complications Trial Research Group. (1997). Hypoglycemia in the Diabetes Control and Complications Trial. *Diabetes, 46*, 271–286. https://doi.org/10.2337/diab.46.2.271 (accessed on 2nd February 2026).

The Lancet. (2023). Diabetes: A defining disease of the 21st century. *Lancet, 401*, 2087. https://doi.org/10.1016/S0140-6736(23)01296-5 (accessed on 2nd February 2026).

Tonyushkina, K., & Nichols, J. H. (2009). Glucose meters: A review of technical challenges to obtaining accurate results. *Journal of Diabetes Science and Technology, 3*, 971–980. https://doi.org/10.1177/193229680900300446 (accessed on 2nd February 2026).

Trofimov, A. D., Ivanova, A. A., Zyuzin, M. V., & Timin, A. S. (2018). Porous inorganic carriers based on silica, calcium carbonate and calcium phosphate for controlled/modulated drug delivery: Fresh outlook and future perspectives. *Pharmaceutics, 10*, 167. https://doi.org/10.3390/pharmaceutics10040167 (accessed on 2nd February 2026).

Uçkay, I., Aragón-Sánchez, J., Lew, D., & Lipsky, B. A. (2015). Diabetic foot infections: What have we learned in the last 30 years? *International Journal of Infectious Diseases, 40*, 81–91. https://doi.org/10.1016/j.ijid.2015.09.023 (accessed on 2nd February 2026).

Usman Ali, S. M. U., Nur, O., Willander, M., & Danielsson, B. (2010). A fast and sensitive potentiometric glucose microsensor based on glucose oxidase coated ZnO nanowires grown on a thin silver wire. *Sensors and Actuators B: Chemical, 145*, 869–874. https://doi.org/10.1016/j.snb.2009.12.072 (accessed on 2nd February 2026).

Vaddiraju, S., Tomazos, I., Burgess, D. J., Jain, F. C., & Papadimitrakopoulos, F. (2010). Emerging synergy between nanotechnology and implantable biosensors: A review. *Biosensors and Bioelectronics, 25*, 1553–1565. https://doi.org/10.1016/j.bios.2009.12.001 (accessed on 2nd February 2026).

Vashist, S. K., Zheng, D., Al-Rubeaan, K., Luong, J. H. T., & Sheu, F. S. (2011). Technology behind commercial devices for blood glucose monitoring in diabetes management: A review. *Analytica Chimica Acta, 703*, 124–136. https://doi.org/10.1016/j.aca.2011.07.024 (accessed on 2nd February 2026).

Veiseh, O., & Langer, R. (2015). Diabetes: A smart insulin patch. *Nature, 524*, 39–40. https://doi.org/10.1038/524039a (accessed on 2nd February 2026).

Wang, J. (2008). Electrochemical glucose biosensors. *Chemical Reviews, 108*, 814–825. https://doi.org/10.1021/cr068123a (accessed on 2nd February 2026).

Wang, J., Li, B., Qiu, L., Qiao, X., & Yang, H. (2022). Dendrimer-based drug delivery systems: History, challenges, and latest developments. *Journal of Biological Engineering, 16*, 18. https://doi.org/10.1186/s13036-022-00298-5 (accessed on 2nd February 2026).

Wang, T. T., Zhang, Y., Li, Q., Zhou, Y., & Liu, Z. (2020). Label-free colorimetric detection of urine glucose based on color fading using smartphone ambient-light sensor. *Chemosensors, 8*, 10. https://doi.org/10.3390/chemosensors8010010 (accessed on 2nd February 2026).

World Health Organization. (2016). *Global Report on Diabetes*. World Health Organization. https://iris.who.int/handle/10665/204871 (accessed on 2nd February 2026).

Wu, H., Nan, J., Yang, L., Park, H. J., & Li, J. (2023). Insulin-loaded liposomes packaged in alginate hydrogels promote the oral bioavailability of insulin. *Journal of Controlled Release, 353*, 51–62. https://doi.org/10.1016/j.jconrel.2022.11.032 (accessed on 2nd February 2026).

Wu, J. Z., Yang, Y., Li, S., Shi, A., Song, B., Niu, S., et al. (2019). Glucose-sensitive nanoparticles based on poly(3-acrylamidophenylboronic acid-block-N-vinylcaprolactam) for insulin delivery. *International Journal of Nanomedicine, 14*, 8059–8072. https://doi.org/10.2147/IJN.S220936 (accessed on 2nd February 2026).

Wu, L., Wang, L., Liu, X., Bai, Y., Wu, R., Li, X., et al. (2022). Milk-derived exosomes exhibit versatile effects for improved oral drug delivery. *Acta Pharmaceutica Sinica B, 12*, 2029–2042. https://doi.org/10.1016/j.apsb.2021.12.015 (accessed on 2nd February 2026).

Wu, Y., Ding, Y., Tanaka, Y., & Zhang, W. (2014). Risk factors contributing to type 2 diabetes and recent advances in the treatment and prevention. *International Journal of Medical Sciences, 11*, 1185–1200. https://doi.org/10.7150/ijms.10001 (accessed on 2nd February 2026).

Xia, Y., Su, Y., Wang, Q., Yang, C., Tang, B., Zhang, Y., et al. (2019). Preparation, characterization, and pharmacodynamics of insulin-loaded fumaryl diketopiperazine microparticle dry powder inhalation. *Drug Delivery, 26*, 650–660. https://doi.org/10.1080/10717544.2019.1631408 (accessed on 2nd February 2026).

Xian, S., Xiang, Y., Liu, D., Fan, B., Mitrová, K., Ollier, R. C., et al. (2024). Insulin–dendrimer nanocomplex for multi-day glucose-responsive therapy in mice and swine. *Advanced Materials, 36*, e2308965. https://doi.org/10.1002/adma.202308965 (accessed on 2nd February 2026).

Yang, R., Gao, R., Li, F., He, H., & Tang, X. (2011). The influence of lipid characteristics on the formation, *in vitro* release, and *in vivo* absorption of protein-loaded SLN prepared by the double emulsion process. *Drug Development and Industrial Pharmacy, 37*, 139–148. https://doi.org/10.3109/03639045.2010.497151 (accessed on 2nd February 2026).

Yazdi, J. R., Tafaghodi, M., Sadri, K., Mashreghi, M., Nikpoor, A. R., Nikoofal-Sahlabadi, S., et al. (2020). Folate targeted pegylated liposomes for the oral delivery of insulin: *In vitro* and *in vivo* studies. *Colloids and Surfaces. B, Bio Interfaces, 194*, 111203. https://doi.org/10.1016/j.colsurfb.2020.111203 (accessed on 2nd February 2026).

Yoo, E. H., & Lee, S. Y. (2010). Glucose biosensors: An overview of use in clinical practice. *Sensors, 10*, 4558–4576. https://doi.org/10.3390/s100504558 (accessed on 2nd February 2026).

Yu, J., Zhang, Y., Ye, Y., DiSanto, R., Sun, W., Ranson, D., et al. (2015). Microneedle-array patches loaded with hypoxia-sensitive vesicles provide fast glucose-responsive insulin delivery. *Proceedings of the National Academy of Sciences of the United States of America, 112*, 8260–8265. https://doi.org/10.1073/pnas.1505405112 (accessed on 2nd February 2026).

Zeng, Z., Qi, D., Yang, L., Liu, J., Tang, Y., Chen, H., et al. (2019). Stimuli-responsive self-assembled dendrimers for oral protein delivery. *Journal of Controlled Release, 315*, 206–213. https://doi.org/10.1016/j.jconrel.2019.10.049 (accessed on 2nd February 2026).

Zhang, J., Liu, J., Su, H., Sun, F., Lu, Z., & Su, A. (2021). A wearable self-powered biosensor system integrated with diaper for detecting the urine glucose of diabetic patients. *Sensors and Actuators. Part B, 341*, 130046. https://doi.org/10.1016/j.snb.2021.130046 (accessed on 2nd February 2026).

Zhang, M., Smith, A., & Gorski, W. (2004). Carbon nanotube−chitosan system for electrochemical sensing based on dehydrogenase enzymes. *Analytical Chemistry, 76*, 5045–5050. https://doi.org/10.1021/ac049519u (accessed on 2nd February 2026).

Zhang, W., Zhang, L., Gao, H., Yang, W., Wang, S., Xing, L., et al. (2018). Self-powered implantable skin-like glucometer for real-time detection of blood glucose level *in vivo*. *Nano-Micro Letters, 10*, 32. https://doi.org/10.1007/s40820-017-0185-x (accessed on 2nd February 2026).

Zhang, Y., Guo, G., Zhao, F., Mo, Z., Xiao, F., & Zeng, B. (2010). A novel glucose biosensor based on glucose oxidase immobilized on AuPt nanoparticle–carbon nanotube–ionic liquid hybrid coated electrode. *Electroanalysis, 22*, 223–228. https://doi.org/10.1002/elan.200900306 (accessed on 2nd February 2026).

Zhang, Y., Sun, J., Liu, L., & Qiao, H. (2021). A review of biosensor technology and algorithms for glucose monitoring. *Journal of Diabetes and its Complications, 35*, 107929. https://doi.org/10.1016/j.jdiacomp.2021.107929 (accessed on 2nd February 2026).

Zhao, D., Shi, X., Liu, T., Lu, X., Qiu, G., & Shea, K. J. (2016). Synthesis of surfactant-free hydroxypropyl methylcellulose nanogels for controlled release of insulin. *Carbohydrate Polymers, 151*, 1006–1011. https://doi.org/10.1016/j.carbpol.2016.06.055 (accessed on 2nd February 2026).

Zhao, R., Lu, Z., Yang, J., Zhang, L., Li, Y., & Zhang, X. (2020). Drug delivery system in the treatment of diabetes mellitus. *Frontiers in Bioengineering and Biotechnology, 8*, 880. https://doi.org/10.3389/fbioe.2020.00880 (accessed on 2nd February 2026).

Zheng, Y., Ley, S. H., & Hu, F. B. (2018). Global aetiology and epidemiology of type 2 diabetes mellitus and its complications. *Nature Reviews. Endocrinology, 14*, 88–98. https://doi.org/10.1038/nrendo.2017.151 (accessed on 2nd February 2026).

Zhu, X., Sarwar, M., Yue, Q., Chen, C., & Li, C. Z. (2017). Biosensing of DNA oxidative damage: A model of using glucose meter for non-glucose biomarker detection. *International Journal of Nanomedicine, 12*, 979–987. https://doi.org/10.2147/IJN.S125437 (accessed on 2nd February 2026).

Zhu, Z., Garcia-Gancedo, L., Flewitt, A. J., Xie, H., Moussy, F., & Milne, W. I. (2012). A critical review of glucose biosensors based on carbon nanomaterials: Carbon nanotubes and graphene. *Sensors, 12*, 5996–6022. https://doi.org/10.3390/s120505996 (accessed on 2nd February 2026).

Zhu, Z., Song, W., Burugapalli, K., Moussy, F., Li, Y. L., & Zhong, X. H. (2010). Nano-yarn carbon nanotube fiber based enzymatic glucose biosensor. *Nanotechnology, 21*, 165501. https://doi.org/10.1088/0957-4484/21/16/165501 (accessed on 2nd February 2026).

CHAPTER 7

Decoding the Genomic Foundations of Diabetes

RAJA CHAKRAVERTY,[1,*] IRYNA VLASENKO,[2] and SHAMBO SAMRAT SAMAJDAR[3]

[1]*Department of Critical Care Medicine, Institute of Post Graduate Medical Education and Research, Kolkata, West Bengal, India*

[2]*International Diabetes Federation, Brussels, Belgium*

[3]*Diabetes and Allergy-Asthma Therapeutics Speciality Clinic, Kolkata, West Bengal, India*

*Corresponding author

ABSTRACT

Diabetes mellitus (DM) is a complex condition defined by genetic, epigenetic, and environmental factors. It manifests as severe macrovascular and microvascular complications, significantly increasing mortality, blindness, renal failure, and reducing quality of life. Clinical risk factors and glycemic management alone are inadequate for forecasting vascular complications. Genetic research highlights a pronounced hereditary aspect of diabetes and its complications. Advancements in genome-wide association studies (GWAS), next-generation sequencing (NGS), and exome sequencing have identified genetic variants linked to diabetes, though these account for only a minor fraction of heritability. The pathogenesis of diabetes involves genetic, epigenetic, and environmental factors. Common variants explain only a limited portion of diabetes heritability. Aggregating identified variants for a genetic risk score lacks precision in predicting diabetes susceptibility. Consequently, the focus has shifted to rare genetic variants.

Diabetes: Novel Insights and Therapies. Anas Islam and Badruddeen (Eds)

DOI: 10.1201/9781779644596-10

Insights from epigenomics, transcriptomics, proteomics, metabolomics, and metagenomics will enhance understanding of genetic influences on diabetes. Advancements in technology, computational analysis, and collaborative research have unveiled novel genetic risk factors. The future holds promise for personalized diabetes therapies from enriched molecular genetic profiles. This chapter explores "missing heritability" in diabetes, emphasizing rare variants, gene-environment interactions, and epigenetic factors. We discuss clinical implications of recent discoveries, strategies for diabetes management, and prospective research trajectories.

7.1 INTRODUCTION

Diabetes mellitus (DM), a prevalent chronic and incapacitating ailment, pertains to a cluster of metabolic irregularities distinguished by the prolonged elevation of blood glucose levels (BGLs) stemming from deficiencies in insulin functionality and/or secretion. The prevalence of diabetes has surged notably due to alterations in sedentary habits, escalated fat consumption, an increase in obesity rates, and a progressively aging population. The International Diabetes Federation (IDF) disclosed in 2019 that diabetes affects approximately 463 million individuals globally, with projections indicating an increase to 700 million by 2040. The availability of gene expression data from microarray and whole transcriptome sequencing endeavors in vast public databases enables scientific teams to authenticate and re-evaluate data and unravel the pivotal genes implicated in chronic illnesses (Willemsen et al., 2015). The fusion of multiple data categories via sophisticated techniques in multi-omics data scrutiny has propelled the comprehension of disease biological frameworks on diverse tiers. The conversion of genetic breakthroughs into clinical management tactics for diabetes poses a substantial hurdle, with persistent efforts concentrated on harnessing genomics to refine personalized treatment methodologies. The future trajectory of diabetes care envisions a shift towards prevention and spotlighting tailored preventive approaches guided by genomic insights and molecular biomarkers. Pharmacogenomic exploration has underscored genetic variations influencing the effectiveness of diabetes therapies, such as GLP-1 receptor agonists and SGLT2 inhibitors. Personalized healthcare, steered by genetic profiling, has the potential to optimize treatment efficacy and mitigate adverse effects in diabetes care. The amalgamation of genetic data with lifestyle aspects provides a holistic stance towards personalized diabetes management, striving to boost patient outcomes and quality of life through personalized and efficient treatments (Shuldiner et al., 2011). Active research is exploring into the complex interaction between genetic variations and lifestyle components to devise personalized treatment schemes for patients with diabetes, which is of paramount importance. To achieve this objective, a comprehensive understanding of the molecular foundations of this disease is imperative. Differential expression analysis is a potent instrument for the identification of genes associated with diseases. This analytical approach has been widely employed in the examination of a diverse array of human diseases, resulting in the generation of difficult profiles detailing up- and downregulated genes (Genet et al., 2014). Notably, the abundance of gene expression data stemming from microarray and whole-transcriptome sequencing is now accessible through extensive public databases. Medical research teams leverage these datasets to authenticate and re-evaluate information through a myriad of analytical methodologies, thereby uncovering novel pivotal genes implicated in chronic illnesses. Moreover, a multitude of endeavors has been undertaken to establish connections among various data modalities by employing sophisticated techniques, aiming to construct an integrative multi-omics data analysis framework. This holistic approach holds promise for enhancing the comprehension of biological systems across multiple strata (Cho et al., 2012; Kooner et al., 2011; Steinthorsdottir et al., 2014; Voight et al., 2010,).

The persistent endeavor to identify genetic variants associated with diabetes and to clarify the fundamental pathogenic processes of the disorder has driven the application of a variety of methodologies. The extensive implementation of these approaches has resulted in the accumulation of a significant number of primary data segments. Most of these datasets are currently available in public databases, and their reassessment can provide critical insights for scholarly research (Gaulton et al., 2015; Huyghe et al., 2013; Ma et al., 2013). Consequently, intricate statistical and computational strategies are routinely employed to assess the existing medical knowledge bases. In light of the rapid expansion of the medical literature, text mining and machine learning (ML) have surfaced as two significant methodologies that have attracted considerable interest in the field of medical data analysis. Text mining constitutes a collection of systematic methodologies, including the rigorous extraction of knowledge from diverse medical textual databases, followed by the visualization and assessment of the obtained data. Text mining has been employed in medical research initiatives to investigate chronic illnesses, genetic irregularities, and the field of drug discovery. By scrutinizing genes associated with chronic ailments, text mining endeavors to unravel their biological functions and implications in disease etiology (Albrechtsen et al., 2013; Claussnitzer et al., 2014; Lohmueller et al., 2013; Manolio et al., 2009).

7.2 RECENT GENOMIC DISCOVERIES IN DIABETES MELLITUS

Recent progress in the domain of genomics has illuminated the complex genetic foundations of type 2 diabetes (T2D) and the extensive variability in glycemic characteristics among individuals, including glucose concentrations, insulin secretion, proinsulin levels, and hemoglobin A1c (HbA1c) measurements. By the end of 2011, the total number of confirmed loci (with a significance threshold of $P < 5 \times 10^{-8}$) had reached 55 for T2D and 32 for glycemic traits. Following this timeframe, the majority of newly identified loci have emerged from the analysis of common variants (with a minor allele frequency (MAF) exceeding 0.05) in increasingly larger cohorts from heterogeneous populations globally, as well as through trans-ancestry studies integrating data from various demographic groups (Kang et al., 2010; Lee et al., 2013). Notably, advancements in sequencing technologies have revealed four loci associated with either T2D or glycemic characteristics, identified through low-frequency variants ($0.005 < \text{MAF} \leq 0.05$). Furthermore, low-frequency variants with potential functional significance have been recognized in genome-wide association studies (GWAS). The cumulative count of confirmed loci has now reached approximately 88 for T2D and 83 for various glycemic traits, as documented in the scientific literature, indicating the probable presence of numerous additional loci yet to be discovered. Prospective research efforts have been made to leverage these findings by identifying additional loci and clarifying the pathogenic roles of the genetic variants and associated genes involved (Collombat et al., 2003; Kooptiwut et al., 2012).

The prevalence of type 2 diabetes (T2D) is increasing at a considerable pace, exerting a significant and escalating impact globally. Although the prevalence rates vary across demographic factors such as age, sex, and geographical location, the worldwide age-standardized prevalence of adult diabetes surpasses 9.2%, translating to approximately 347 million adults affected by diabetes. The identification of diabetes relies on parameters such as fasting blood glucose measurements, postprandial glucose concentrations following a 2-hour oral glucose tolerance test (2hGlu), and the levels of hemoglobin A1c (HbA1c), which indicates a 3-month mean BGL. A substantial proportion of individuals with T2D concurrently exhibit insulin resistance alongside conditions such as obesity, unfavorable lipid profiles, hypertension, and a proinflammatory milieu, with each of these factors likely to be subject to genetic and environmental influences. The transition to T2D is characterized by dysfunction in pancreatic islet β-cell activity and insulin resistance; nevertheless, the complex mechanisms that govern these biological phenomena are not yet fully understood. Robust evidence supports the notion that genetic factors contribute significantly to the predisposition for T2D, regulation of insulin secretion, and efficacy of insulin action. In the last 10 years, the integration of GWAS and sequencing projects has revealed genetic loci that provide valuable insights into the hereditary aspects of T2D and glycemic characteristics. These research endeavors illuminate the genetic framework of T2D, addressing elements such as the quantity, prevalence, and impact magnitudes of risk variants across various global populations while simultaneously emphasizing the polygenic characteristic of T2D, which is marked by the discovery of numerous risk variants at particular loci, indicating allelic diversity. In parallel, an expanding array of genes and variants has been associated with monogenic diabetes forms, including maturity-onset diabetes of the young (MODY) and neonatal diabetes, revealing overlap in at least five genes that are implicated in both monogenic and polygenic diabetes. A recent computational model that examined genetic architectures in relation to outcomes from T2D genetic studies highlighted the feasibility of multiple disease models, each differing in terms of locus quantity, allele frequencies, and the degree of selective pressures applied.

7.3 COMMON VARIANTS

The evolution of GWAS has catalyzed considerable progress in the detection of prevalent genetic variations (minor allele frequency [MAF] > 0.05) associated with T2D and glycemic traits. In the preliminary phases, candidate gene investigations and linkage analyses identified common genetic variations linked to T2D, specifically within PPARG, KCNJ11-ABCC8, and TCF7L2. The first five GWAS initiatives pertaining to T2D revealed six additional loci. By early 2008, a synthesis of GWAS findings and meta-analyses effectively identified 15 loci associated with T2D, with G6PC2 recognized as a locus correlated with fasting glucose concentrations. Furthermore, in 2008, the publication of the first GWAS studies conducted in non-European cohorts identified KCNQ1 as a T2D locus, with variants notably prevalent among East Asians (MAF = 0.33) while being relatively rare in Europeans (MAF ≈ 0.01). It is significant to note that the risk variants of KCNQ1 demonstrated comparable effect sizes in both population groups, highlighting the impact of allele frequencies on the detection of genetic loci.

In 2010, an extensive meta-analysis that specifically concentrated on individuals of European ancestry revealed a noteworthy second signal of genetic variants associated with T2D, which were located in proximity to the KCNQ1 gene. Interestingly, these variants exhibited a remarkably low level of linkage disequilibrium with the previously identified variants, as evidenced by a correlation coefficient of r2 being less than 0.05, thereby categorizing them as independent entities based on sophisticated conditional analyses that were conducted. As the calendar year of 2011 came to a conclusion, it became apparent that additional GWAS and subsequent meta-analyses conducted across a variety of diverse populations had successfully identified 55 distinct loci that were tied to the pathophysiology of type 2 diabetes. In parallel with these findings, by the end of 2011, the ongoing GWAS efforts had identified an aggregate of 32 loci that were associated with one or more glycemic traits, which included 17 specific loci correlated with fasting glucose levels, two loci associated with fasting insulin concentrations, five loci linked to glucose levels measured at the two-hour mark, 11 loci related to glycosylated hemoglobin (HbA1c), and nine loci connected to proinsulin, with one particular locus exclusively identified in female subjects. The observed partial overlap among the loci associated with type 2 diabetes and various glycemic traits suggests that it is indeed plausible that not all the factors that influence glucose levels in otherwise healthy individuals serve as reliable indicators of the risk for developing type 2 diabetes, and conversely, not every factor linked to type 2 diabetes risk is reflective of glycemic control in healthy populations. A significant majority of the T2D loci identified through these comprehensive studies were found to predominantly affect the functional capacity of the pancreatic islet β-cells, while a comparatively smaller number of loci were shown to exert an influence on insulin resistance mechanisms within the body. Building upon the substantial advancements achieved in this area of research, a subsequent round of GWAS meta-analysis took advantage of Metabochip, which is a specialized genotyping array meticulously designed to investigate approximately 1000 to 5000 genetic variants that are nominally linked to 23 different cardiometabolic traits and diseases, as well as to provide a detailed mapping of the 257 established loci that are associated with various diseases and traits.

The implementation of this economically viable array has provided a significant opportunity for researchers to genotype a substantially larger cohort, which in turn has greatly augmented the statistical power of subsequent meta-analyses, allowing for more robust and reliable findings. The DIAbetes genetics replication and meta-analysis (DIAGRAM) consortium has adeptly amalgamated data derived from the metabochip analysis encompassing 22,669 cases of T2D alongside 58,119 controls, integrating this with pre-existing GWAS data that included 12,171 additional T2D cases and 56,862 controls, ultimately resulting in the identification of 10 new loci that were previously unrecognized. The loci that were identified not only exhibited significant findings but also presented further compelling evidence of shared genetic associations with various other metabolic traits, notably obesity, exemplified by the gene MC4R, as well as lipid levels, with CILP2 being another notable example. Notably, CILP2 was also identified in a concurrent gene-centered study, underscoring its potential importance in the genetic landscape of metabolic disorders. Furthermore, a network analysis of genes situated in proximity to both the newly discovered and well-established T2D signals revealed a pronounced enrichment of transcription factors, with an emphasis on those that exhibit interactions with the transcriptional co-activator CREBBP, which is critically involved in the complex process of chromatin remodeling. A meticulous examination of the consistency of allelic effects across various phases of research has provided robust support for the conceptual framework, suggesting the existence of a genetic architecture that is characterized by a multitude of common causal variants, which predominantly exert relatively modest effects on the phenotypic expression of T2D. In summary, the collective findings from this comprehensive analysis not only advance our understanding of the genetic underpinnings of type 2 diabetes but also highlight the relationship between genetic factors and other metabolic traits, paving the way for future research endeavors. The implications of these discoveries are profound as they may eventually contribute to the development of targeted interventions and personalized treatment strategies for individuals affected by this complex and prevalent condition. Overall, the synergy between large-scale genetic analysis and meta-analytic methodologies has significantly propelled the field forward, offering new insights into the multifaceted nature of metabolic diseases.

7.4 STATE-OF-THE-ART GENE EDITING TECHNOLOGIES

The current global prevalence of diabetes is projected to affect an astounding 382 million individuals, a staggering statistic that underscores the profound implications of this chronic condition for the health and economic well-being of countries at all levels of development, whether they are classified as developed or developing nations. The underlying causes of T2D are thought to arise from a multifaceted and complex interaction between various genetic predispositions and a range of lifestyle factors, including dietary habits, physical activity levels, and environmental influences, which collectively contribute to the pathogenesis of this metabolic disorder. This complex relationship between genetics and lifestyle underscores the need for a comprehensive understanding of the disease mechanisms involved in T2D to inform effective prevention and intervention strategies aimed at mitigating its widespread impact on global health and economies, a theory that was initially proposed five decades ago. Lifestyle interventions have demonstrated the potential to decrease the likelihood of progressing to diabetes by 50% or more in high-risk individuals. Nevertheless, uncertainty prevails regarding whether the impact of unfavorable lifestyles varies depending on the inherent genetic predisposition to T2D. Recent developments in elucidating the genetic underpinnings of T2D and its related metabolic traits have facilitated comprehensive examination of the relationship between genetic determinants and behavioral choices regarding susceptibility to T2D. The diabetes prevention program (DPP) trial did not demonstrate any notable interactions between intervention strategies and genetic risk profiles, as determined by 34 identified T2D loci at that time. Nevertheless, the study was limited to high-risk populations and may have suffered from insufficient statistical power owing to the relatively modest sample sizes across each subgroup (947 in the placebo group, 955 in the lifestyle intervention group, and 941 in the metformin group), even within the framework of a moderately extensive intervention study. An alternative approach to investigating lifestyle interventions entails analyzing the connections between genetic susceptibility and lifestyle habits in observational cohort studies.

Nevertheless, the comprehensive investigation of such interactions has not been extensively explored in prospective cohorts, where lifestyle variables were evaluated at baseline using standardized methodologies and with adequate statistical power to derive valid conclusions. Therefore, our objective was to investigate this question through an extensive case cohort analysis conducted within the broader context of the European Prospective Investigation into Cancer and Nutrition (EPIC) study. The ethical considerations of the study were diligently addressed, with all participants providing written informed consent. The research protocol obtained endorsements from the local ethics committees of the participating nations as well as the Institutional Review Board of the International Agency for Research on Cancer. The study cohort was precisely delineated, drawing upon the comprehensive design and methodologies previously articulated in the InterAct case cohort study (InterAct Consortium, 2011), which is integrated within the EPIC cohort and involves a collaborative initiative among 29 institutions across nine European countries. The process of identifying incident cases of type 2 diabetes (T2D) was meticulous, entailing an exhaustive examination of the EPIC datasets from all participating entities, employing a multitude of information sources such as self-reported data, linkage to primary and secondary care registries, medication databases, hospital admission records, and mortality statistics. Any information acquired from subsequent follow-up assessments or external sources following the initial evaluation was considered thoroughly. To enhance the accuracy of case identification, supplementary corroborative evidence was obtained for all reported incident T2D cases originating from fewer than two independent sources, including a detailed review of individual medical records in selected centers. Importantly, cases identified in Denmark and Sweden were not based on self-reports, but were confirmed through local and national diabetes registries and pharmaceutical databases, thereby ensuring the reliability of all identified T2D cases (Oppelt et al., 2013).

The follow-up period concluded on either the date of diagnosis, December 31, 2007, or the date of death, depending on which event occurred first. Individuals exhibiting signs of diabetes at the outset of the study were excluded from the analysis. The presence of pre-existing diabetes was determined through initial self-reports of a diabetes history, physician's diagnosis, use of diabetes medication, or evidence of diabetes diagnosed post-baseline with a diagnosis date occurring prior to the baseline recruitment date. The study involved 340,234 participants of European descent who were tracked for a cumulative total of 3.99 million person-years, with an average follow-up duration of 11.7 years and a range extending from 0 to 17.5 years, resulting in the identification of 12,403 verified new cases of type 2 diabetes (T2D). Participants without stored blood samples (n = 109,625) or those with an unreported diabetes status (n = 5,821) were excluded from the study. A random, center-stratified subset of 16,835 individuals was selected. Following the exclusion of 548 individuals with pre-existing diabetes and 133 individuals with unknown diabetes status, the sub-cohort consisted of 16,154 individuals for additional analysis. The random selection method ensured that this subcohort included 778 individuals who developed T2D during the follow-up phase. The characteristics of the participants in the random sub-cohort were similar to those of all EPIC participants who satisfied the criteria for inclusion in the InterAct. Within the InterAct study, cases were monitored for an average duration of 6.9 years with a standard deviation of 3.3 years, and nearly half (49.8%) were male. The overall incidence rate of T2D in InterAct was recorded as 3.8 cases per 1000 person-years of follow-up. Anthropometric data were collected, and weight and height were measured while participants were barefoot and attired in lightweight clothing or undergarments at most research centers. Waist circumference (WC) was assessed at the narrowest region of the torso or at the midpoint between the lower ribs and iliac crest (Kozlitina et al., 2014; Mahdessian et al., 2014; Murphy et al., 2008; Thiagalingam et al., 1997).

Hip circumference was measured by performing a horizontal assessment at the site of maximal lateral extension of the hips or over the gluteal region. This metric is essential for evaluating body composition and identifying health risks associated with excessive adipose tissue accumulation in the hip region. Within a specific cohort of participants from Oxford consisting of 363 individuals, data regarding waist and hip circumferences were self-reported, thereby constraining the precision of the analyses that could be executed concerning the correlation between body measurements and health outcomes (Anderson et al., 2011; Dickson et al., 2010; Goldstein et al., 2011; Sim et al., 2011; Wray et al., 2011).

7.5 DRUGS AND GENOMICS

The propensity of an individual to manifest type 2 diabetes is influenced by the confluence of intrinsic genetic predispositions and extrinsic environmental factors. Empirical evidence has revealed a multitude of etiological origins and complex mechanisms that contribute to the pathogenesis of this condition. The escalating prevalence of type 2 diabetes on a global scale highlights the deficiencies in current preventive strategies, whereas the elevated rate of associated complications accentuates the limitations of existing therapeutic interventions. An enhanced understanding of the interactions between genetic determinants and environmental influences is essential for the formulation of more efficacious approaches to the prevention and management of type 2 diabetes (Elements, 2012; Maller et al., 2012; Mikkelsen et al., 2010; Wakefield et al., 2007).

In relation to various medical conditions, particularly prominent within the realm of rare diseases and increasingly relevant to diverse cancer types, the discipline of human genetics has produced transformative revelations concerning the fundamental biology of these disorders and has unveiled entirely novel opportunities for translational applications. Conversely, despite the significant elucidation of multiple genetic loci that influence the predisposition to type 2 diabetes, the tangible effects of these discoveries on the actual clinical management of the condition have been found to be relatively insignificant. This phenomenon is echoed across a broad spectrum of chronic diseases. The majority of ambitious efforts aimed at facilitating the incorporation of genomic medicine into standard clinical practice, such as the United Kingdom's initiative to sequence 100,000 genomes, predominantly focus on rare diseases and cancers, thereby largely neglecting the potential advantages for common chronic conditions. Consequently, some experts have concluded that the role of genetics in advancing the clinical progress of common diseases has been excessively hyped up (Gaulton et al., 2010; Parker et al., 2013; Pasquali et al., 2014).

Such feelings merge inherent impatience with a lack of understanding of the accurate timelines for translation: the majority of this scientific field is, in fact, under 10 years old. Nevertheless, they prompt a set of inquiries that must be tackled: what measures are necessary to actualize genomic medicine for prevalent complex illnesses, how would it manifest, and what consequences will it bring in the subsequent five decades (Falconer et al., 1965; Maurano et al., 2012; Pickrell et al., 2014).

7.6 GENETIC INTERPLAY IN THE PATHOPHYSIOLOGY OF TYPE 2 DIABETES MELLITUS

Recent progress in understanding the genetic foundations of type 2 diabetes and other common complex conditions can be attributed to the developments initiated in 2007. The advent of GWAS, along with the subsequent formation of a scientific and anthropological framework that enables extensive data integration, has resulted in the identification of over 100 genetic loci that are significantly associated with type 2 diabetes. Owing to the methodologies employed, the majority of the identified risk alleles have been practically applicable, displaying a widespread presence across diverse human populations. These findings collectively suggest that the origins of these type 2 diabetes risk alleles can be dated back to ancient human history, indicating a certain level of adaptability to their evolutionary consequences, which aligns with their relatively modest impact on glucose regulation. In aggregate, these 100 genetic loci account for approximately 10% of the variability in predisposition to type 2 diabetes (Agarwala et al., 2013; McClellan et al., 2010).

Most assessments of type 2 diabetes, a measure often considered fleeting by many, show significantly higher values, potentially ranging from 30% to 60%. This discrepancy has sparked considerable conjecture about the underlying nature and magnitude of the genetic factor in risk that is yet to be unveiled. However, this speculative discourse is gradually being replaced with concrete empirical findings. Accumulating evidence suggests that a substantial portion (if not the majority) of the undiscovered genetic component is situated within a long tail of common variants, each exerting increasingly modest influences. It is probable that some of the remaining variability is spread among less common alleles, which are not captured in conventional GWAS focused on common variants but are now becoming more accessible through sequencing technologies. Within this category of rarer and more recent variants, there likely exists a subset with notably significant effects on individual susceptibility to the disease. According to the data at hand, it seems that only a minor portion of the unexplored variance can be ascribed to the interactions occurring among genetic variants or between genetic elements and environmental influences (Bonnefond et al., 2012; Flannick et al., 2014; Yang et al., 2010).

7.7 THE BIOLOGY OF INTERVENTIONS

The management of type 2 diabetes is projected to experience significant changes over the course of 50 years, potentially leading to a state that is unrecognizable to current patients and healthcare providers. The current reliance on a limited array of preventive and therapeutic measures that often fail to support a sustained return to normal metabolic balance is likely to be replaced by more advanced and comprehensive strategies. Future emphasis is anticipated to shift towards safeguarding normal glucose levels in individuals identified as being at high risk, rather than reacting retroactively to the aftermath of metabolic dysfunction. These forthcoming interventions may encompass surgical procedures, cell-based therapies, and a novel class of pharmaceuticals meticulously designed to optimize effectiveness and safety profiles. In circumstances that require intervention for persons who are unable to avert the emergence of the illness, the approaches employed will directly target the underlying pathological processes, aiming to restore beta cell mass and function as well as rectify primary insulin sensitivity deficiencies, in contrast to the current focus on managing symptomatic manifestations. The future landscape of type 2 diabetes management holds promise for a paradigm shift towards more proactive, personalized, and targeted interventions that address the root causes of the disease rather than its symptoms.

Human genetics will have occupied a central position in the scientific spotlight, as the risk variants identified through population-level sequencing will shed light on specific targets and pathways that are directly involved in the onset and progression of diabetes in humans. Medications designed to target these validated human-specific factors hold the potential to offer tangible clinical benefits, thereby saving the pharmaceutical industry from the downward spiral of depending on treatments that are discovered belatedly to be effective only in mice or cell cultures. Simultaneously, a comprehensive analysis of the broader implications of diabetes-related genetic variations on overall health and disease will serve as an early indicator of the potential side effects associated with related interventions, thus enabling the prioritization of drugs that not only demonstrate safety but also confer additional positive health outcomes. This holistic approach to understanding the genetic underpinnings of diabetes and its impact on health outcomes will contribute to the selection of pharmaceutical interventions that not only address the primary condition effectively but also offer supplementary health advantages.

Currently, the fundamental principles of this strategy are discernible. The genetic makeup responsible for the objectives of sulfonylureas and thiazolidinediones contains variations linked to type 2 diabetes. Genetic variations situated both within and adjacent to the genes encoding receptors for glucose-dependent insulinotropic polypeptide and glucagon-like peptide-1 (GLP-1), which are implicated in the risk of diabetes and pertinent glycemic traits, function as a natural genetic experiment that foreshadows the clinical relevance of therapeutically modulating this pathway using GLP-1 receptor agonists and dipeptidyl peptidase-4 (DPP-4) inhibitors. A similar narrative pertains to the objectives of statins and ezetimibe, which are represented in GWAS signals related to lipid profiles. These examples provide evidence of convergence between genetic causation and therapeutic benefits. Furthermore, they illuminate the fallacy of debates surrounding the importance (or lack thereof) of modest effect sizes revealed by GWAS, and therapeutic modifications targeting the same endpoints can typically yield substantially greater outcomes.

Upon elucidating the aforementioned considerations, the most pragmatic methodology for the identification of novel genetic targets involves the detection of rare, large-effect alleles that exert substantial phenotypic consequences via sequencing techniques. The principal emphasis of this investigative approach was directed towards the PCSK9 gene. It has been approximately a decade since empirical evidence has established that loss-of-function mutations within this specific gene exert a significant influence on lipid profiles and susceptibility to coronary artery disease (CAD). Furthermore, several potent inhibitors of proprotein convertase subtilisin/Kexin type 9 (PCSK9) are being integrated into clinical therapeutics. Studies have demonstrated that individuals harboring a single functional variant of the *SLC30A8* gene exhibit a 70% reduction in the likelihood of developing diabetes, thereby underscoring the potential for innovative therapeutic strategies.

The repercussions resulting from the loss of a single (or both) copy of a specific gene are commonly observed in the extensive medical records of numerous individuals in our population. Utilizing this wealth of information poses a significant challenge in the current era and requires careful analysis and interpretation. However, achieving success in this endeavor holds the promise of yielding profound biological revelations and identifying numerous innovative targets for interventions in various medical conditions.

7.8 FROM GENETICS TO PREDICTION OF T2DM

One may observe that the provision of mechanistic insights that lead to the identification of innovative interventional targets can be perceived as knowledge acquired by collectively examining numerous human sequences. This perspective highlights the importance of analyzing a vast array of genetic data to uncover new avenues for therapeutic interventions. Additionally, there is a complementary imperative that underscores the significance of delving into how the analysis of an individual human sequence, whether it belongs to you, me, or your child, can yield valuable clinical insights. This emphasis is placed on the potential of a single genetic profile to offer pertinent information, such as the categorization of prospective disease vulnerability, delineation of particular disease classifications, or forecasting of individual reactions to an array of therapeutic alternatives.

Neonatal diabetes represents a salient example of a prospective achievement that can be realized within the discipline of medical genetics. This specific disorder is distinguished by an acute expression wherein individuals are diagnosed with diabetes within the initial six months of life. Moreover, the identification of penetrant mutations in a thoroughly characterized gene, KCNJ11, which encodes the potassium ATP (KATP) channel in beta cells, has facilitated the advancement of personalized therapeutic strategies tailored to genetic profiles. Consequently, this innovative methodology has permitted the adoption of genetically informed individualized therapy, as demonstrated by the effective administration of high-dose sulfonylureas in neonatal diabetes management.

Type 2 diabetes presents with a pronounced dichotomy in its characteristics. It is apparent from our analyses that the recognized risk variants accounted for only 10% of the variability associated with the likelihood of developing this condition. Furthermore, when evaluating the accuracy of diagnostic or prognostic measures, conventional risk factors such as age, BMI, and ethnicity significantly influence genetic testing. Although there is some evidence suggesting that the efficacy of genetic prediction may improve when performed in early life or among individuals with lower-risk profiles, it remains markedly inadequate for effective clinical implementation.

It is often a common assumption that the observed limitations in genetic discoveries are primarily due to the inadequate scope of current research endeavors, implying that broader exploration will eventually unearth new genetic variants capable of resolving the issue at hand. Nonetheless, it is crucial to acknowledge that there are two fundamental factors that will persistently hinder the extent to which genetic information alone can accurately predict risks, even if a comprehensive catalogue of predisposing genetic elements is compiled. First, the intrinsic complexity and multifactorial nature of many diseases dictate that genetic markers can only provide partial insight into the overall risk landscape, necessitating the integration of diverse data sources for a more comprehensive risk assessment. Second, the influence of environmental factors, lifestyle choices, and epigenetic modifications on disease development underscores the relationship between genetic predisposition and external influences, thereby limiting the predictive power of genetics in isolation.

Variation in genome sequences represents merely one of several determinants that influence an individual's likelihood of developing a late-onset condition, such as type 2 diabetes, which is the initial observation that is readily apparent. To gain a comprehensive understanding of the associated risk, it is imperative to not only focus on genetic predispositions, but also to integrate a multitude of other factors that affect metabolic functionality throughout an individual's lifespan. These determinants encompass early life events that may exert enduring influences via epigenetic modifications alongside the cumulative effects of environmental factors and lifestyle choices from infancy to senescence. Moreover, the stochastic nature of certain events, such as somatic mutations, contributes to this risk and warrants consideration when evaluating disease susceptibility. Consequently, an all-encompassing strategy that addresses these diverse components is essential for a more precise evaluation of an individual's risk for developing late-onset ailments, such as type 2 diabetes.

The transition of an individual from a state of wellness to an illness is profoundly influenced by the genetic, epigenetic, and environmental determinants throughout their lifetime. The insights derived from sequencing the complete genome in early life represent only a segment of the comprehensive risk profile. When we analyze the progression of an individual from a state of health to the onset of type 2 diabetes, it becomes evident that, with exhaustive and precise information, the optimal trajectory of this hypothetical individual adheres to a defined pathway represented by the blue line. Nevertheless, considering the current state of understanding, which encompasses data from GWAS, alongside restricted clinical and biochemical insights, the observable trajectory for the same individual shows poor correspondence with the actual pathway, as illustrated by the green line. By integrating more extensive information, such as acquiring the individual's genomic sequence at the age of 20 years and performing dynamic genomic profiling to establish a comprehensive molecular signature every decade, the capacity to monitor disease progression is markedly improved, as denoted by the red line. This improved monitoring capability facilitates timely intervention, as indicated by the orange arrow marking intervention at the age of 40 years, which effectively mitigates the individual's risk of developing type 2 diabetes.

In the event that it becomes feasible, through extensive research endeavors, to compile a comprehensive catalog of genetic variations that account for the majority of the presently concealed genetic diversity, the implication of these data on enhancing the accuracy of forecasting individual genetic susceptibility will not be immediate. The magnitude of the influence attributed to numerous of these genetic variations is likely to be inadequately defined to offer significant insights. The predictive power of these variants may be limited because of their lack of precision in estimating their effects, hindering their utility in risk assessment models.

In the next 50 years, we will witness the implementation of advanced strategies aimed at assessing individual risk levels for various diseases, which will involve the integration of genetic data from a wide array of risk variants along with information on the diverse environmental factors that influence risk. These cutting-edge methodologies will transcend the basic enhancements in gauging the risk determinants themselves owing to advancements in human genetics and the application of wearable sensors in conjunction with portable devices. A pivotal element of this progression is the integration of biomarkers that explicitly reflect the advancement of diseases, along with their fundamental pathophysiological characteristics. Through systematic monitoring, these biomarkers provide valuable insights into the varying levels of risk encountered by individuals throughout their lifespan. Ideally, an optimal biomarker would facilitate the refinement of imperfect evaluations of genetic susceptibilities (as delineated by genome sequencing) and exposure to risk determinants contingent upon an individual's actual journey through molecular landscapes. These trajectories will not be compared primarily against population averages, but against the individual's own historical data, akin to how authorities monitor athletes for signs of doping. For these biomarkers to effectively inform about risks throughout one's lifespan, both pre- and post-intervention, they must provide direct indications of the causal pathways involved.

The aspiration to delineate integrative, dynamic, and causal biomarkers may appear idealistic at first glance, yet a practical illustration of contemporary medical procedures can provide clarity. For instance, the utilization of cholesterol level as an assessment biomarker for CAD is based on the same criteria. This exemplifies the necessity for biomarkers to not only be indicative but also predictive and mechanistically linked to the physiological processes they aim to elucidate.

The quest for a potential biomarker corresponding to "cholesterol" in the context of type 2 diabetes prompts us to deliberate on the most suitable avenues to explore. The expanding array of genomic manifestations not only broadens our scope beyond traditional markers, but also opens up avenues for investigating molecular indicators of susceptibility, revolving around networks of genetic, transcriptomic, proteomic, and metabolomic characteristics. The availability of extensive, meticulously characterized cohorts, coupled with continuous sampling over time and integration with electronic health records (EHRs), presents the opportunity to amass extensive datasets that can be meticulously scrutinized to identify such biomarkers. The comprehensive analysis of these datasets holds the promise of unveiling novel insights into potential biomarkers for type 2 diabetes, akin to how "cholesterol" functions in cardiovascular health (Williams et al., 2014).

The complex pathophysiological diversity observed in type 2 diabetes might pose a significant challenge that could be insurmountable to unravel. An alternative perspective suggests that the integration of various forms of data over time could potentially enhance endeavors to dismantle the monolithic view of type 2 diabetes and reveal the unique mechanisms contributing to an individual's disease risk, each potentially characterized by its own distinct molecular footprint. The envisioned reclassification of type 2 diabetes is frequently oversimplified as distinct subcategories are delineated. Considering the genetic makeup and widespread nature of the relevant factors, it is probable that each individual harbors a unique array of pathophysiological predispositions to type 2 diabetes. In such a scenario, the objective should be to elucidate the specific role of each of these mechanisms in driving the progression of the disease at any given moment and customize their treatment strategies accordingly.

7.9 DIABETES CARE IN THE FUTURE

If the aforementioned scenarios materialize, the paradigm of diabetes management will have transitioned to an unrecognizable state. While affliction may not be eradicated, priority and financial resources will have shifted from therapeutic interventions to preventive measures even in affluent nations. Comprehensive, actionable, real-time insights into the risk and subtype classification of type 2 diabetes will be accessible through the amalgamation of fundamental genomic sequencing data and augmented exposure assessments, along with complex molecular biomarkers collected as a component of a universal initiative for genomic disease forecasting and monitoring. Such insights will facilitate tailored preventive approaches that utilize a considerably broader spectrum of effective therapeutic options. This will encompass advanced pharmacological agents fine-tuned for both efficacy and safety, which can be directed toward individuals based on their specific pathophysiological characteristics. If this is achieved, genomic medicine, which has already established itself as a viable approach for monogenic diabetes variants, will demonstrate similar transformative potential for more intricate manifestations of the condition.

Recent developments in the field of pharmacogenomics concerning diabetes management have revealed notable genetic heterogeneity that affects the effectiveness of GLP-1 receptor agonists and SGLT2 inhibitors in type 2 diabetes treatment. A thorough genome-wide investigation has identified particular genetic polymorphisms, including rs6923761G→A in *GLP1R* and infrequent variants in *ARRB1*, which correlate with varying glycemic responses to GLP-1 receptor agonists. This underscores the potential of personalized medicine, where genetic profiling can inform clinical decisions, optimize treatment efficacy, and minimize side effects. Concurrently, studies on SGLT2 inhibitors have shown that genetic variants in *SLC5A2* affect glucose reabsorption and treatment outcomes, although their impact on clinical practice remains unclear. Together, these insights pave the way for tailored and effective diabetes therapies, emphasizing the importance of integrating genetic information into treatment planning. By understanding how genetic factors interact with lifestyle choices, healthcare providers can offer more precise and holistic approaches to diabetes management, ultimately improving patient outcomes and quality of life. Moreover, recent studies have assessed the interplay between these genetic polymorphisms and lifestyle determinants, including dietary habits and physical exercise, with the aim of formulating comprehensive personalized therapeutic approaches for diabetic patients.

7.10 CONCLUSION

Recent genomic discoveries have significantly advanced our understanding of the complex genetic foundations of type 2 diabetes (T2D). GWAS and sequencing projects have identified numerous genetic loci associated with T2D and glycemic traits, revealing the polygenic nature of the disease. However, these identified variants only account for a small portion of the overall heritability of T2D. The pathogenesis of T2D involves a complex interplay of genetic, epigenetic, and environmental factors. Future research will focus on rare genetic variants, gene-environment interactions, and epigenetic factors to unravel the "missing heritability" in T2D. Integration of multi-omics data, including epigenomics, transcriptomics, proteomics, metabolomics, and metagenomics, will provide a more comprehensive understanding of the genetic influences on T2D. Advancements in gene editing technologies and personalized medicine approaches, such as pharmacogenomics, hold promise for developing targeted therapies based on an individual's genetic profile. The future of diabetes care is expected to shift towards prevention and personalized interventions, guided by a deeper understanding of the molecular genetic profiles of patients. Continuous advancements in technology, computational analysis, and collaborative research efforts will pave the way for more effective prevention, diagnosis, and treatment strategies for T2D.

KEYWORDS

- **diabetes mellitus**
- **epigenetics**
- **genetic variants**
- **metabolomics**
- **metagenomics**
- **molecular genetic profiles**
- **personalized medicine**
- **type 2 diabetes**

REFERENCES

Agarwala, V., Flannick, J., Sunyaev, S., & Altshuler, D. (2013). Evaluating empirical bounds on complex disease genetic architecture. *Nature Genetics, 45*(12), 1418–1427.

Albrechtsen, A., Grarup, N., Li, Y., Sparsø, T., Tian, G., Cao, H., et al. (2013). Exome sequencing-driven discovery of coding polymorphisms associated with common metabolic phenotypes. *Diabetology, 56*, 298–310.

Anderson, C. A., Soranzo, N., Zeggini, E., & Barrett, J. C. (2011). Synthetic associations are unlikely to account for many common disease genome-wide association signals. *PLoS Biology, 9*(1), e1000580.

Bonnefond, A., Clement, N., Fawcett, K., Yengo, L., Vaillant, E., Guillaume, J. L., et al. (2012). Rare *MTNR1B* variants impairing melatonin receptor 1B function contribute to type 2 diabetes. *Nature Genetics, 44*(3), 297–301.

Cho, Y. S., Chen, C. H., Hu, C., Long, J., Hee Ong, R. T., Sim, X., et al. (2012). Meta-analysis of genome-wide association studies identifies eight new loci for type 2 diabetes in East Asians. *Nature Genetics, 44*(1), 67–72.

Claussnitzer, M., Dankel, S. N., Klocke, B., Grallert, H., Glunk, V., Berulava, T., et al. (2014). Leveraging cross-species transcription factor binding site patterns: From diabetes risk loci to disease mechanisms. *Cell, 156*(1), 343–358.

Collombat, P., Mansouri, A., Hecksher-Sørensen, J., Serup, P., Krull, J., Gradwohl, G., et al. (2003). Opposing actions of *Arx* and *Pax4* in endocrine pancreas development. *Genes & Development, 17*(20), 2591–2603.

Dickson, S. P., Wang, K., Krantz, I., Hakonarson, H., & Goldstein, D. B. (2010). Rare variants create synthetic genome-wide associations. *PLoS Biology, 8*(1), e1000294.

ENCODE Project Consortium. (2012). An integrated encyclopedia of DNA elements in the human genome. *Nature, 489*(7414), 57–74.

Falconer, D. S. (1965). The inheritance of liability to certain diseases, estimated from the incidence among relatives. *Annals of Human Genetics, 29*(1), 51–76.

Flannick, J., Thorleifsson, G., Beer, N. L., Jacobs, S. B., Grarup, N., Burtt, N. P., et al. (2014). Loss-of-function mutations in *SLC30A8* protect against type 2 diabetes. *Nature Genetics, 46*(4), 357–363.

Gaulton, K. J., Ferreira, T., Lee, Y., Raimondo, A., Mägi, R., Reschen, M. E., et al. (2015). Genetic fine mapping and genomic annotation defines causal mechanisms at type 2 diabetes susceptibility loci. *Nature Genetics, 47*(12), 1415–1425.

Gaulton, K. J., Nammo, T., Pasquali, L., Simon, J. M., Giresi, P. G., Fogarty, M. P., et al. (2010). A map of open chromatin in human pancreatic islets. *Nature Genetics, 42*(3), 255–259.

Genet, N. (2014). Genome-wide trans-ancestry meta-analysis provides insight into the genetic architecture of type 2 diabetes susceptibility. *Nature Genetics, 46*(3), 234–244.

Goldstein, D. B. (2011). The importance of synthetic associations will only be resolved empirically. *PLoS Biology, 9*(1), e1001008.

Huyghe, J. R., Jackson, A. U., Fogarty, M. P., Buchkovich, M. L., Stančáková, A., Stringham, H. M., et al. (2013). Exome array analysis identifies new loci and low-frequency variants influencing insulin processing and secretion. *Nature Genetics, 45*(2), 197–201.

InterAct Consortium. (2011). Design and cohort description of the InterAct Project: An examination of the interaction of genetic and lifestyle factors on the incidence of type 2 diabetes in the EPIC Study. *Diabetology, 54*, 2272–2282.

Kang, H. M., Sul, J. H., Service, S. K., Zaitlen, N. A., Kong, S. Y., Freimer, N. B., et al. (2010). Variance component model to account for sample structure in genome-wide association studies. *Nature Genetics, 42*(4), 348–354.

Kooner, J. S., Saleheen, D., Sim, X., Sehmi, J., Zhang, W., Frossard, P., et al. (2011). Genome-wide association study in people of South Asian ancestry identifies six novel susceptibility loci for type 2 diabetes. *Nature Genetics, 43*(10), 984.

Kooptiwut, S., Plengvidhya, N., Chukijrungroat, T., Sujjitjoon, J., Semprasert, N., Furuta, H., et al. (2012). Defective *PAX4* R192H transcriptional repressor activities associated with maturity onset diabetes of the young and early onset-age of type 2 diabetes. *Journal of Diabetes and Its Complications, 26*(4), 343–347.

Kozlitina, J., Smagris, E., Stender, S., Nordestgaard, B. G., Zhou, H. H., Tybjærg-Hansen, A., et al. (2014). Exome-wide association study identifies a *TM6SF2* variant that confers susceptibility to nonalcoholic fatty liver disease. *Nature Genetics, 46*(4), 352–356.

Lee, S., Teslovich, T. M., Boehnke, M., & Lin, X. (2013). General framework for meta-analysis of rare variants in sequencing association studies. *The American Journal of Human Genetics, 93*(1), 42–53.

Lohmueller, K. E., Sparsø, T., Li, Q., Andersson, E., Korneliussen, T., Albrechtsen, A., et al. (2013). Whole-exome sequencing of 2,000 Danish individuals and the role of rare coding variants in type 2 diabetes. *The American Journal of Human Genetics, 93*(6), 1072–1086.

Ma, R. C. W., Hu, C., Tam, C. H., Zhang, R., Kwan, P., Leung, T. F., et al. (2013). Genome-wide association study in a Chinese population identifies a susceptibility locus for type 2 diabetes at 7q32 near *PAX4*. *Diabetology, 56*, 1291–1305.

Mahdessian, H., Taxiarchis, A., Popov, S., Silveira, A., Franco-Cereceda, A., Hamsten, A., et al. (2014). *TM6SF2* is a regulator of liver fat metabolism influencing triglyceride secretion and hepatic lipid droplet content. *Proceedings of the National Academy of Sciences, 111*(24), 8913–8918.

Maller, J. B., McVean, G., Byrnes, J., Vukcevic, D., Palin, K., Su, Z., et al. (2012). Bayesian refinement of association signals for 14 loci in 3 common diseases. *Nature Genetics, 44*(12), 1294–1301.

Manolio, T. A., Collins, F. S., Cox, N. J., Goldstein, D. B., Hindorff, L. A., Hunter, D. J., et al. (2009). Finding the missing heritability of complex diseases. *Nature, 461*(7265), 747–753.

Maurano, M. T., Humbert, R., Rynes, E., Thurman, R. E., Haugen, E., Wang, H., et al. (2012). Systematic localization of common disease-associated variation in regulatory DNA. *Science, 337*(6099), 1190–1195.

McClellan, J., & King, M. C. (2010). Genetic heterogeneity in human disease. *Cell, 141*(2), 210–217.

Mikkelsen, T. S., Xu, Z., Zhang, X., Wang, L., Gimble, J. M., Lander, E. S., et al. (2010). Comparative epigenomic analysis of murine and human adipogenesis. *Cell, 143*(1), 156–169.

Morris, A. P., Voight, B. F., Teslovich, T. M., Ferreira, T., Segrè, A. V., Steinthorsdottir, V., et al. (2012). Large-scale association analysis provides insights into the genetic architecture and pathophysiology of type 2 diabetes. *Nature Genetics, 44*(9), 981–990.

Murphy, R., Ellard, S., & Hattersley, A. T. (2008). Clinical implications of a molecular genetic classification of monogenic β-cell diabetes. *Nature Clinical Practice Endocrinology & Metabolism, 4*(4), 200–213.

Oppelt, A., Lobert, V. H., Haglund, K., Mackey, A. M., Rameh, L. E., Liestøl, K., et al. (2013). Production of phosphatidylinositol 5-phosphate via *PIKfyve* and *MTMR3* regulates cell migration. *EMBO Reports, 14*(1), 57–64.

Parker, S. C., Stitzel, M. L., Taylor, D. L., Orozco, J. M., Erdos, M. R., Akiyama, J. A., et al. (2013). Chromatin stretch enhancer states drive cell-specific gene regulation and harbor human disease risk variants. *Proceedings of the National Academy of Sciences, 110*(44), 17921–17926.

Pasquali, L., Gaulton, K. J., Rodríguez-Seguí, S. A., Mularoni, L., Miguel-Escalada, I., Akerman, I., et al. (2014). Pancreatic islet enhancer clusters enriched in type 2 diabetes risk-associated variants. *Nature Genetics, 46*(2), 136–143.

Pickrell, J. K. (2014). Joint analysis of functional genomic data and genome-wide association studies of 18 human traits. *The American Journal of Human Genetics, 94*(4), 559–573.

Sim, X., Ong, R. T. H., Suo, C., Tay, W. T., Liu, J., Ng, D. P. K., et al. (2011). Transferability of type 2 diabetes implicated loci in multi-ethnic cohorts from Southeast Asia. *PLoS Genetics, 7*(4), e1001363.

Steinthorsdottir, V., Thorleifsson, G., Sulem, P., Helgason, H., Grarup, N., Sigurdsson, A., et al. (2014). Identification of low-frequency and rare sequence variants associated with elevated or reduced risk of type 2 diabetes. *Nature Genetics, 46*(3), 294–298.

Thiagalingam, A., Lengauer, C., Baylin, S. B., & Nelkin, B. D. (1997). *RREB1*, a *ras* responsive element binding protein, maps to human chromosome 6p25. *Genomics, 45*(3), 630–632.

Voight, B. F., Scott, L. J., Steinthorsdottir, V., Morris, A. P., Dina, C., Welch, R. P., et al. (2010). Twelve type 2 diabetes susceptibility loci identified through large-scale association analysis. *Nature Genetics, 42*(7), 579–589.

Wakefield, J. (2007). A Bayesian measure of the probability of false discovery in genetic epidemiology studies. *The American Journal of Human Genetics, 81*(2), 208–227.

Willemsen, G., Ward, K. J., Bell, C. G., Christensen, K., Bowden, J., Dalgård, C., et al. (2015). The concordance and heritability of type 2 diabetes in 34,166 twin pairs from international twin registers: The discordant twin (DISCOTWIN) consortium. *Twin Research and Human Genetics, 18*(6), 762–771.

Williams, A. L., Jacobs, S. B., Moreno-Macías, H., Huerta-Chagoya, A., Churchhouse, C., Márquez-Luna, C., et al. (2014). Sequence variants in *SLC16A11* are a common risk factor for type 2 diabetes in Mexico. *Nature, 506*(7486), 97–101.

Wray, N. R., Purcell, S. M., & Visscher, P. M. (2011). Synthetic associations created by rare variants do not explain most GWAS results. *PLoS Biology, 9*(1), e1000579.

Yang, J., Benyamin, B., McEvoy, B. P., Gordon, S., Henders, A. K., Nyholt, D. R., et al. (2010). Common SNPs explain a large proportion of the heritability for human height. *Nature Genetics, 42*(7), 565–569.

PART IV
Advanced Scientific Insights

CHAPTER 8

Proteomics in Diabetes: Unveiling the Complexities of the Proteomic Landscape

MUHAMMAD MUZAMMAL,[1] SANA FATIMA,[1]
HAMNA BATOOL HASHMI,[1] MARIA SHAFIQ,[2] and ARSHAD FARID[1,*]

[1]*Gomal Center of Biochemistry and Biotechnology, Gomal University, Dera Ismail Khan, Khyber Pakhtunkhwa, Pakistan*

[2]*Gomal Medical College, Dera Ismail Khan, Khyber Pakhtunkhwa, Pakistan*

*Corresponding author

ABSTRACT

Proteomics deals with protein analysis and modifications forming a system at cellular, tissue, or organism levels. Techniques in proteomics screen protein samples to analyze altered expression quantitatively and qualitatively. This characteristic allows proteomics to be used for molecular analysis of disease-related proteins, drug production, and treatment effects. Diabetes is a heterogeneous disorder caused by alterations in genes and their products. While a mutated gene can cause diabetes, not every transcriptional alteration affects protein, making it crucial to study mRNA expression and protein level changes. Many proteomics techniques can be applied for such analysis. For diabetic patients, these techniques help analyze healthy tissues and disease pathophysiology. Proteomic techniques also assess diabetes treatment outcomes based on patients' protein levels. Results from these techniques provide a list of elevated or lowered protein levels directly related to a patient's diabetic state. However, these results

Diabetes: Novel Insights and Therapies. Anas Islam and Badruddeen (Eds)

DOI: 10.1201/9781779644596-12

must categorize proteins by location and function to overview their pathophysiology. The proteomic approach is more effective when analyzing the interaction of resultant protein levels with interacting proteins. Proteomics has identified many proteins involved in diabetes pathogenesis.

8.1 INTRODUCTION

Homeostasis between glucose levels is described as a balance in the ingested glucose along with the manufacture of glucose within the body, the utilization of glucose, and the uptake of glucose. There are various organs that regulate this balance, along with the involvement of various hormones, such as insulin, that stimulate the uptake/utilization of glucose and glucagon, growth hormones, glucagon, and catecholamines that work to increase the concentrations of body glucose.

When the balance in glucose levels is disturbed within the body, it leads to a diseased condition. When this lack of balance is due to lowered insulin levels or, in severe cases, the absence of insulin, the disease is called diabetes mellitus (DM) (Donath and Halban, 2004). There are two types of DM, named DM type I and type II. In the case of type I (DMT1), the beta cells of the pancreas are lost as a consequence of an autoimmune attack where immune cells such as WBCs and macrophages attack the cells of the islets of Langerhans. DMT1 is also known as insulitis (Jörns et al., 2005). During the attack, pro-inflammatory cytokines are released; in response, beta cells release iNOS, which in turn elevates the production levels of nitric oxide, which acts as a trigger to activate apoptosis in the beta cells (Eizirik and Mandrup-Poulsen, 2001). Due to apoptosis in beta cells, the mass of pancreatic cells depletes, which can be observed at the time of diagnosis of DMT1 (Muralidhara and Srikanta, 2015).

In the case of diabetes mellitus type II (DMT2), beta cell function deterioration remains imminent over time. Recently, the rate of this deterioration has been quantified. It is observed that in patients with a lessened glucose tolerance, there is a decline in glucose-stimulated insulin secretion (GSIS) of 1.4%–2.2% per year, whereas in normal people, this rate was slower, as it is not possible to study the mass of a patient's pancreas over time. It is difficult to describe whether this rate of lowered functionality is due to the lowered mass of the beta cells of the pancreas or the deteriorated function of these cells affecting the patients with DMT2 (Kanat et al., 2012). However, post-mortem studies (post-mortem) have shown that there is, in fact, a loss of mass of beta cells that is caused by the apoptosis of these cells (Roefs et al., 2017).

These results for apoptotic beta cells in DMT2 are also supported by the presence of elevated levels of apoptotic proteins belonging to the caspase family in the beta cells of patients.

Both types of DM are complex in nature and are caused by the altered expression of various genetic factors (Lin et al., 2023). Therefore, it is very important to analyze variations in the expression of various proteins simultaneously. There are many techniques that can be utilized for such analysis, such as microarrays. mRNA array is a very useful technique, as it is extremely specific and can immediately identify the differential expression of genes. Additionally, this technique can also be utilized to answer specific questions by designing specific arrays that can measure variations in genes that are present in a single pathway. However, the limitation of this technique is that it is unable to analyze any post-translational variations, which are an important factor in the functioning of a protein (Andrikopoulos, 2016).

Usually, there is a mutual relationship between the mRNA level and the consequent protein formation, but sometimes this may not be the case. For instance, in the pancreatic cells of rats, there was no effect of the levels of mRNA of GLUT2 on the production of dexamethasone, but elevated degradation in pancreatic cells decreased the level of GLUT2 proteins (Karbaschi and Zardooz, 2023). In another analysis, 19 proteins from the liver of humans were analyzed, and the results showed a positive mutual relationship between proteins and their mRNA levels (Kadota et al., 2006). Other analyses did not show any significant differences in this relationship. However, some studies conducted in yeast cells showed that the level of mRNA did not affect some genes, but the proteins of these genes showed a 20-fold variation (Gygi et al., 1999). All of these studies show that this mutual relationship is not sufficient to provide data on protein expression. Therefore, it is necessary to understand cellular functionality and implement techniques that measure protein levels directly.

Proteomic studies aim to simultaneously measure the levels of these proteins across various samples. The data obtained via this analysis are consequently utilized in various molecular studies in the field of medicine. In the case of diabetes, various studies have used proteomic techniques.

8.2 DIABETES MELLITUS (DM)

DM is a metabolic disease characterized by hyperglycemia and is classified into two types: DMT1 and DMT2. DMT1 is an autoimmune disorder that produces insufficiency of insulin secretion permanently; however, DMT2 is considered mainly lowered insulin secretion, usually followed by resistance towards insulin. The total percentage of individuals suffering from DM continues to rise worldwide, with 425 million patients suffering from DM in 2017, and the number of cases is expected to surge to 629 million by the end of 2045 (Cho, 2017). As DM is linked with macro- and microvascular difficulties, enhanced health care charges and optimum strategies to overcome this disease are required as soon as possible (Khaw et al., 2004).

DMT2 is a major problem, and people come across it globally. It is a metabolic syndrome that occurs due to deficiencies in insulin emission or peripheral insulin resistance, and the inability of insulin cells to respond to insulin. The increasing burden of DMT2 is a major concern for health-care systems worldwide, with 1 in 11 people presently diagnosed with diabetes, and ~90% of them have this disorder (Khan et al., 2020). DMT2 is the outcome of various interactions among epigenetic, genetic, and environmental factors. Deficiencies in beta-cells for a long time can affect the levels of insulin and may cause extreme glucotoxicity in pancreatic cells, causing decreased insulin secretion. Release of insulin and its action on cells have to accurately meet metabolic needs; thus, the molecular mechanisms responsible for the production and secretion of insulin and its reaction in targeted issues may be tightly regulated. Therefore, problems or defects in any of the mechanisms listed above can cause a metabolic imbalance that leads to the pathogenesis of DMT2 (Cho et al., 2018).

DMT2 has become one of the most severe health problems in this century. Since the 1980s, more or less all of the globe has suffered a sudden rise in the pervasiveness of DMT2. Although type 3 diabetes was initially thought to be a disease that only affected middle-aged as well as elderly individuals, since the 2000s, the relative surge in the cases and prevalence of DMT2 has been perceived in young people (aged < 40 years), adolescents, and children (Stumvoll et al., 2005).

8.3 EPIDEMIOLOGY

According to WHO guidelines, DM is a lingering, metabolic sickness characterized by raised BGLs, leading to harm to the heart, eyes, nerves, kidneys, vasculature, and nerves. In diabetes mellitus, over 90% of the reports describe DMT2, a condition manifested by low release of insulin via the pancreas, insulin resistance in tissues, and a scant insulin secretion response (Rosengren and Dikaiou, 2023). Advancement of this disorder causes insulin to sustain glucose homeostasis, which is the source of hyperglycemia. Individuals suffering from DMT2 are mainly categorized as obese with elevated body fat, mainly in the abdominal region of a person. Under such conditions, adipose tissue facilitates insulin resistance through various inflammatory pathways. The main factors that contribute to DMT2 are a sedentary lifestyle, global obesity increase, population aging, and high caloric diets, which doubles the occurrence and pervasiveness of DMT2 (Zhou et al., 2016). Advancement of the disease (diabetes type 2) causes secretion of insulin, which makes it difficult to sustain homeostasis of glucose, leading to hyperglycemia.

Organs, including the pancreas, skeletal cells, kidney, intestine, liver, brain, and adipose cells, are mainly implicated in the progression of DMT2. Other important pathophysiological factors that contribute to the onset of DMT2 have also emerged, and progressive data suggest their roles (Schwartz et al., 2016).

8.4 RISK FACTORS

The risk constituents for DMT2 involve a multifarious combination of metabolic, genetic, and environmental aspects that intermingle with each other, facilitating its prevalence. Although non-variable risk factors of DMT2 (culture and family background/genetic inclination) have a solid genetic basis, data suggest that various reports of DMT2 can be reduced by perfecting the key risk elements responsible (obesity, unhealthy diet, and reduced physical activity) for the disease (Blüher, 2019).

The complex phenomenon of DMT2 can be affected by different factors, such as genetics, lifestyle, and environmental factors. Some of the key risk factors, along with references to recent research, are as follows (Figure 8.1):

1. **Obesity and Body Composition:** Elevated body fat, specifically around the abdomen, is strongly associated with an elevated risk of DMT2. Research suggests that dysfunction in adipose tissue and pro-inflammatory cytokine secretion contributes to insulin resistance (Klimek-Tulwin et al., 2019).
2. **Unhealthy Diet**: Consumption of a diet with a high content of processed food, saturated fats, and refined sugars is mainly linked

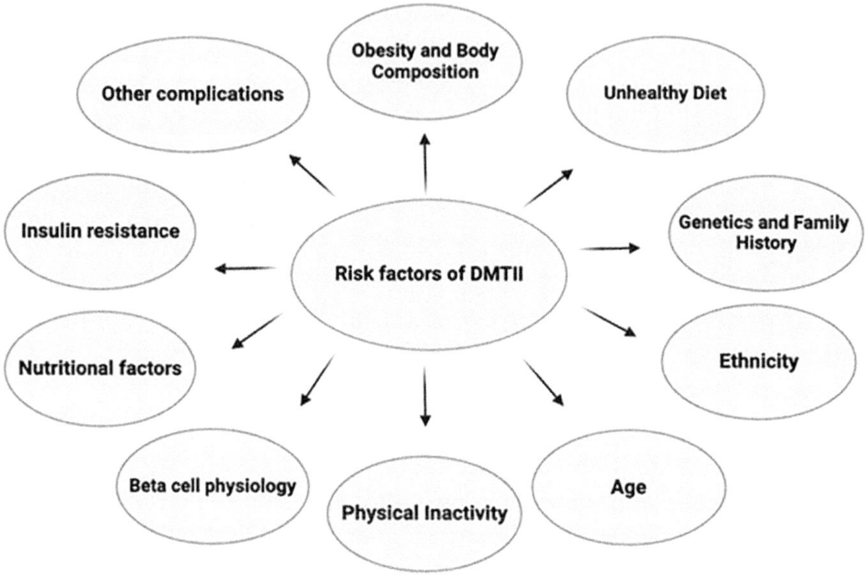

FIGURE 8.1 Risk factors of diabetes mellitus.

with an increased risk of DMT2. However, diets supplemented with fruit, whole grains, vegetables, and lean proteins have been shown to reduce the risk of disease (Ley et al., 2014).

3. **Genetics and Family History**: A family background of DMT2 is a greater risk for individuals, indicating genetic predisposition. Recent studies have identified various genetic variants that are associated with an elevated risk of DMT2 (Sesti et al., 2018).

4. **Ethnicity**: Certain ethnic factions, such as Hispanics, African Americans, Pacific Islanders, and Native Americans, have a greater incidence of DMT2 than Caucasians (Egede and Walker, 2020). Genetic diversity plays a key role in DMT2 progression. In the last 10 years, various genome-wide studies involving DMT2 have presented the complex polygenic quality of the disease, in which several of these loci enhance the chance of diabetes type 2 via initial consequences on insulin release and a secondary effect by reduction of insulin action (Fuchsberger et al., 2016). DMT2 is a complex disease with many genes that contribute to its development, including obesity, insulin resistance, and environmental

factors. Insulin resistance in DMT2 leads to increased glucose production in the liver, along with lowered glucose absorption in muscle and adipose cells at a constant insulin level. Additionally, malfunctioning β cells cause insufficient insulin release to sustain normal glucose levels (Asmat et al., 2016).

5. **Age**: The chance of acquiring DMT2 surges with age, especially after the age of 45. This could be attributed to age-associated variations in metabolism and reduced physical activity. The sum of adults with DMT2 is increasing rapidly worldwide, principally owing to better life expectancy associated with longstanding prior experience with cardiometabolic risk factors, particularly excess skeletal muscle shrinkage, adiposity, and decreased physical dosing (Dunning et al., 2014). From 2017 to 2045, the population of adults aged ≥65 years globally with DM is forecasted to expand to 253 million, while the population aged 65–99 years is anticipated to increase to 1.42 billion (Weinstein et al., 2004). DM prevalence levels off in older persons, which most likely represents a balance between the rising prevalence in this age group and greater mortality among those detected with DMT2 earlier in life.

6. **Physical Inactivity**: A sedentary lifestyle has been associated with a greater risk of DMT2. Regular physical activity boosts insulin sensitivity and aids in maintaining a healthy body weight. A sedentary routine is an added risk element for DMT2, which showed a 34% and 56% decrease in the risk of developing DMT2 in partakers walking 2–3 hours every week or no less than 40 minutes per week, respectively (Vetrivel et al., 2013). Physical activities provide three key values for impeding the start of DMT2. Physical activity also lowers the levels of disreputable intra-abdominal lipids, a recognized risk factor for IR (Strasser, 2013). Finally, moderate-power exercise has been proven to enhance the absorption of glucose by 40%. Physical actions enhance glucose uptake and insulin sensitivity and can ameliorate or even reverse inflammation along with oxidative stress, both of which are predisposing factors for DMT2 (Bunney et al., 2017).

7. **Beta Cell Physiology:** Insulin is produced by β-cells and is primarily synthesized as pre-proinsulin. To produce proinsulin,

preproinsulin undergoes conformational alterations in the endoplasmic reticulum (ER) with the help of many proteins. Proinsulin then travels from the ER to the Golgi apparatus (GA), where it flows into immature secretory vesicles and is fragmented into C-peptide along with insulin (Ross, 2003). Historically, malfunction of β-cells has been linked to mortality. Recent research suggests that the malfunctioning of β-cells in DMT2 may be related to an intricate system of exchanges between the external environment and numerous biochemical procedures implicated in cell biology. Hyperglycemia and hyperlipidemia are mutually associated in an undue dietary condition, analogous to that found in obesity, which favors IR and chronic inflammation. β-cells may lose islet integrity due to genetic sensitivity to toxic stresses, such as metabolic/oxidative stress, inflammatory stress, inflammation, amyloid stress, and ER stress (Hermida and Balligand, 2014).

8. **Nutritional Factors:** A diet that raises blood glucose along with traveling very-low-density lipoproteins, chylomicrons, and their remnants, all of which are high in triglycerides, causes a surge in ROS levels, which can cause anomalous production of inflammatory molecules. Given that inflammation is a known stimulant of oxidative stress, the two progressions interact synergistically after a heavy meal, amplifying the harmful postprandial effects. The prolonged and considerable increase in steady-state ROS levels contributes significantly to the pathophysiology of DMT2 and IR (Malik and Hu, 2019). Diets high in sugar, particularly refined sugars and sugary beverages, have been linked to a surge in the risk of DMT2. Excessive sugar intake can cause insulin resistance and obesity. Similarly, intake of a diet rich in saturated and trans lipids can also be related to insulin resistance, which in turn can cause DMT2 in many young adults (Reynolds et al., 2019). A low-fiber diet, that is, a diet with a low intake of fruits, grains, and vegetables, can also be related to an enhanced risk of DMT2. The intake of a fiber-rich diet helps in the regulation of sugar in the blood and improves insulin sensitivity. The intake of highly processed food, which usually has a high concentration of sugars and fats along with poor nutritional value, can also lead to the development of DMT2 (Ripsin et al., 2009).

9. **Insulin Resistance (IR):** It is a chronic condition in which cells lose their ability to sense insulin and become insensitive to it. Insulin resistance reduces the synthesis of glycogen as well as catabolism of protein in muscle cells, whereas it stops lipoprotein lipase action in adipose cells, raising FFA and inflammatory marker cytokines. Increased cytokine flow alters insulin sensitivity and interrupts glucose metabolism (Czech, 2017). Insulin resistance also refers to the metabolic reaction of insulin-responsive cells to insulin, or, at a systematic level, a lowered reaction to moving insulin by levels of glucose. Insulin resistance or insulin-deficient conditions fall into three main categories: (i) weakened insulin release; (ii) insulin competitors; and (iii) weakened insulin response in the recipient tissues. The last category includes three major organs other than the pancreatic insulin-susceptible organs that play important roles. The faulty action of insulin in these organs is frequently accompanied by the onset of systemic IR, gradually leading to DMT2 (Haffner et al., 1998).
10. **DMT2 Outcomes/Complications:** DMT2 enhances the death toll in adults via CVD as well as stroke by 2–4× and is linked to micro- and macrovascular problems, the latter of which include advanced atherosclerosis resulting in severe peripheral vascular disease, along with an enhanced risk of cerebrovascular disease (Nesto, 2004). These factors contribute to DMT2's status as an important risk variable for CVD, most likely due to the association between many molecular procedures and pathophysiological pathways. These comprise involvement of IR in atherosclerosis, oxidative stress, vascular function, and hypertension, vascular performance, macrophage accumulation, as well as inflammation. Other complications, such as CVDs, nephropathy, retinopathy, and neuropathy, develop as a result of prolonged DMT2 (Nesto, 2004) (Figure 8.2).

8.5 RELATIONSHIP BETWEEN OBESITY AND T2DM

8.5.1 ADIPOSE TISSUE

Adipose tissue acts as the body's primary fuel store, providing a crucial transportable energy source required for existence when food is short. Triglycerides are a 5x better source of energy than glycogen because of

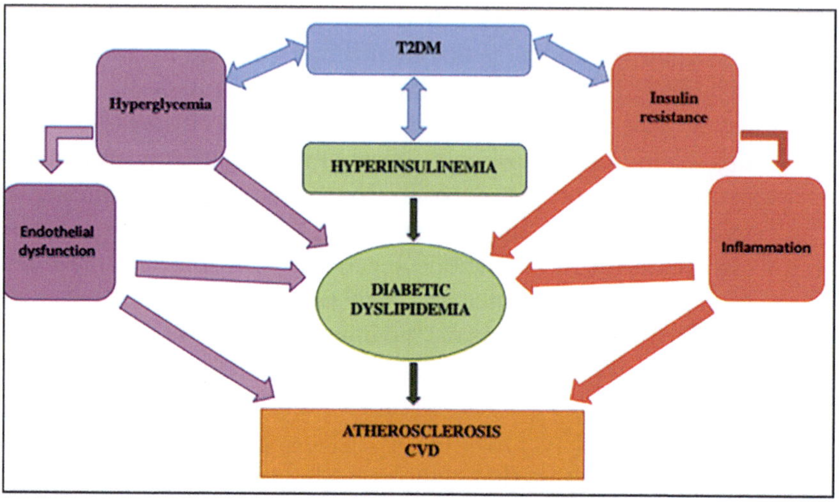

FIGURE 8.2 Complications of diabetes mellitus type 2 (T2DM).

their enhanced energy density and hydrophobicity. Adipose tissue also manufactures and releases adipokines and exosomes, which regulate critical physiological functions such as hunger, reproductive performance, and insulin action (Funcke and Scherer, 2019). Excess body fat causes a number of metabolic aberrations and disorders, such as resistance to insulin, atherogenic dyslipidemia, beta cell dysfunction, prediabetes, and DMT2. Obesity, which alters both insulin action and beta cell function, is most likely to be responsible for the recent rise in the prevalence of DMT2 worldwide (Klein et al., 2022).

Adipose tissue must be metabolically flexible to deal with the substantial and quick changes in energy balance that occur during the duration of feeding as well as fasting during the course of the day, and to react to changes in energy equilibrium that result in adipose tissue development or decrease. Adipose tissue mass increases with chronic positive energy balance owing to triglyceride buildup in adipocytes, resulting in greater adipocyte size and structural reorganization to supply the scaffolding required to maintain a larger adipocyte mass (Smith et al., 2020).

8.5.2 OBESITY AND T2DM

Obesity is a well-established risk factor for the development of DMT-II. Excess body fat, especially in abdominal adipose cells, can contribute to the development of insulin resistance along with abnormalities in glucose metabolism, which can lead to the development of DMT2. If the adipose tissue is not functioning properly, there can be a release of adipokines and pro-inflammatory cytokines that can lead to aggravation of insulin resistance, which can lead to DMT2. Environmental and genetic factors influence the progression of DMT2 and obesity. Previous research has identified various genetic factors that cause DMT2 as well as obesity, which show a relationship between the two (Qatanani and Lazar, 2007).

To lower the risk of DMT2, there is a dire need to change diet along with an increase in physical exercise. Such interventions can produce enhanced sensitivity towards insulin and can lead to better metabolic health. Bariatric surgery, that is, gastric bypass, is another applicable treatment option for serious obesity and can cause substantial weight loss and improvement in metabolic parameters, involving glycemic control in patients with DMT2 (Bellou et al., 2018). Obesity is a major risk factor for DMT2 and is related to metabolic changes that cause IR. There was a correlation between BMI and age at the time of diagnosis of DMT2. The specific processes by which obesity promotes DMT2 and IR are still unknown; nevertheless, multiple factors have been shown to be essential in the progression of this serious condition, requiring both cell-autonomous pathways as well as inter-organ communication (Hillier and Pedula, 2003).

Finally, moderate strenuous activity can upregulate glucose absorption. Exercise not only enhances the absorption of glucose and insulin sensitivity but can also reduce or even eliminate inflammation as well as oxidative stress. According to previous studies, beta-cell mass is reduced prior to the commencement of DMT2. However, in the case of obesity, beta-cell mass is expected to grow because plasma levels in obese people rise to compensate for insulin resistance, a phenomenon called hyperinsulinemia (Candler et al., 2018). Obesity is more frequent in young-onset DMT2 than in late-onset DMT2 patients. Some studies have shown that over 80% of youngsters with DMT2 have obesity upon presentation, compared to ~50% of those with later-onset DMT2. Young persons with DMT2 appear to have larger amounts of fat in their muscles and liver than older adults with DMT2 (~3 times greater). Other proposed obesity-related processes include elevated circulating fatty acid levels and chronic inflammation (Cotten, 2020) (Figure 8.3).

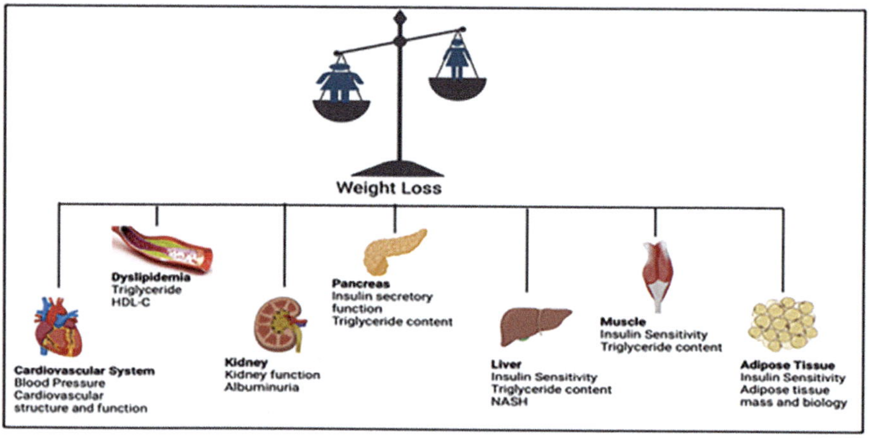

FIGURE 8.3 Relationship between DMT2 and obesity.

8.6 PANCREAS AND ISLETS OF LANGERHANS

Its main role is to produce digestive enzymes and hormones that regulate blood sugar levels (BSLs).

8.6.1 EXOCRINE FUNCTION

The pancreas releases enzymes that are digestive in nature, such as amylase, proteases, and lipases, in the small intestine that can help in the digestive process of carbs, proteins, and fats. Abnormalities in exocrine function of the pancreas can cause pancreatic insufficiency (Rorsman and Ashcroft, 2018).

8.6.2 ENDOCRINE FUNCTION

The Langerhans islets are involved in the release of various hormones into the blood. Insulin is one of the primary hormones of the pancreas and is involved in sugar uptake from the blood. The other hormone is glucagon, which stimulates the liver to release sugars by converting glycogen into glucose (Inagaki, 2019).

8.6.3 BLOOD GLUCOSE REGULATION

The pancreas is also involved in the regulation of glucose concentration in the blood so that the cells of the body can function properly. Both glucagon and insulin are involved in regulating the blood sugar concentration. If the hormones are not properly working, the balance of the hormones is lost, which can lead to the development of DM (Henquin, 2009).

8.6.4 REGULATION OF PANCREATIC HORMONE SECRETION

There are various factors that are related to maintaining the release of pancreatic hormones, such as the level of glucose, feedback mechanisms, and neuronal signals. Once these factors are disturbed, the hormonal balance is disturbed, leading to DM (Da Silva Xavier, 2018).

8.6.5 ISLETS OF LANGERHANS

Islets of Langerhans have been investigated for DM, as they are significant in the regulation of glucose homeostasis. Langerhans' islets are micro-organs that play a vital role in glucose homeostasis by controlling the release of hormones. PP cells release pancreatic polypeptide, a hormone thought to primarily affect the exocrine pancreas as well as the liver. A human pancreas has between 3.2 and 14.8 million islets, with a total islet volume ranging from 0.5 to 2.0 cm^3 (Da Silva Xavier, 2018).

8.7 CELLULAR COMPOSITION

The cellular architecture and organization of pancreatic islets varies between and within species. Inter-species variation has already been linked to functional distinctions (Briant et al., 2018). Insulin and glucagon are hormones that affect the entire body, whereas δ-cell somatostatin acts exclusively locally because of its short circulation time (<1 min). Among the two main isoforms (14 and 28 amino acids long), pancreatic δ-cells release the somatostatin-14 variant, which is 14 amino acids long, via Ca^{2+}-dependent exocytosis. These three major secretory products, as well as additional transmitters, play critical signaling roles in islets. The role of pancreatic polypeptides in islet cell communication is unclear. Insulin levels track in opposition to glucagon levels across the physiological blood glucose range, and their subsequent activities are almost entirely opposite to each other. Insulin production is inhibited during hypoglycemia, whereas high glucagon levels enhance the hepatic glucose output. As glucose levels rise, glucagon production is significantly reduced, and insulin levels rise. Somatostatin, released by δ-cells, regulates both hormones. Type 1 and type 2 cause dysregulation of all three secretory dynamics. The success of insulin in the treatment of diabetes has shifted the focus to β-cell research (Ng et al., 2021).

8.8 COMMUNICATION PATHWAYS IN THE ISLET

There are three types of communication mechanisms: electrical synapses that travel through cell gap junctions; chemical synapses or paracrine signaling between adjacent or close cells; and juxtacrine signaling that occurs directly between cells. Islet cells use all these pathways, some of which are well understood.

8.8.1 β-CELLS

There are three types of communication mechanisms: electrical synapses that travel through cell gap junctions; chemical synapses or paracrine signaling between adjacent or close cells; and juxtacrine signaling that occurs directly between cells. Islet cells use all these pathways, some of which are well-understood. Beta cells are the most important type of cells studied among the islets of Langerhans. Insulin is bundled into secretory granules at a concentration of approximately 100 mM as a complex with zinc and is secreted in response to elevated glucose (and other nutrients) concentrations and neurotransmitter stimulation caused by meals. β-cells are the sole insulin-secreting cell type in the body, and the multistep mechanism of glucose-stimulated insulin secretion (GSIS) is well understood. The conventional GSIS model includes proximal activities, such as glucose transport, intermediate metabolism, and phosphorylation. Insulin is the predominant hormone released by cells. Defects in insulin secretion cause diabetes, although aberrant production of islet glucagon and somatostatin does not appear to have substantial physiological consequences on their own. Diabetes is caused by aberrant pancreatic insulin synthesis. However, many aspects of insulin manufacturing in pancreatic islet beta cells remain unknown. Evidence suggests that abnormalities in insulin production contribute to the etiology of type 1 and DMT2, including monogenetic variants (Vasiljević et al., 2020).

8.8.2 PROTEOMICS OF PANCREATIC ISLETS ALONG WITH BETA-CELLS

The key aim of protein profiling is to characterize the expression of various proteins that are detected in various tissues, such as islets of Langerhans, which (Ortsäter and Bergsten, 2006) enables the mapping of proteins and their expression in various tissues. Primarily, the proteomic reference map of the islets of Langerhans was constructed by Sanchez et al. (2001). Researchers extracted proteins from the pancreas of mice and displayed a 2-dimensional gel electrophoresis (2DGE) map. This study identified 63 spots on a map belonging to 44 proteins. In a similar study, Nicolls et al. (2003) extracted proteins from the islets of Langerhans of mice and performed 2DGE and MALDI-TOFMS. This analysis identified 150 spots that belonged to 87 proteins. Of these 87 proteins, 50% of the 44 spots from an earlier study were also observed. Both studies provided similar results regarding the cellular localization of proteins. Most of the proteins found belonged to the cytosol, mitochondria, and endoplasmic reticulum. As far as the function of these proteins is concerned, all of them either have metabolic functions or function as chaperones.

These results show that for the islets to function, both the metabolic and chaperone proteins are important, which is why they are abundantly expressed here, as 2DGE techniques can also detect the abundant proteins (Gygi et al., 2000).

A smaller portion (approximately 2–5%) belonged to the signaling function in these studies. These results can be justified as signaling proteins are short-lived and thus are not abundant; thus, they were not observed during the protein analysis.

In proteomic analysis, there was no similarity in the classification of proteins. Different bioinformatics tools, such as Swiss-Prot and ontology databases, can be used for the classification of proteins according to their function and cellular localization. However, these sites are free for use, but not all proteins are annotated, and it does not identify whether some proteins have more than one function or localization.

In another study, protein profiling was performed on human islets of Langerhans using 2DGE and MALDI-TOF MS profiling (Ahmed et al., 2005). In this study, 130 spots belonging to 66 proteins were identified. Upon comparison, the protein profiles of mice and humans were found to be similar, which shows that the protein profiles remained the same across the species. For example, in all 3 studies, glucose-regulated protein (GRP) and protein disulfide isomerase (PDI), which act as chaperones in the ER, were found. Although these studies-initiated protein profiling, the results showed that only a small portion was analyzed. To increase coverage, another study used 2D LC/MS/MS to profile the proteins of human islets. This study detected 29,000 spots belonging to 3365 proteins, which is the most comprehensive study for protein profiling of human islets (Metz et al., 2006). In this study, the ingenuity pathways application was employed, through which proteins were profiled according to their related pathways.

To increase the coverage of proteomic analysis, subcellular fractions can be obtained prior to the analysis. To make this technique successful, stringent control must be taken to ensure organelle purity in the fractions. In a previous study, Brunner et al. (2007) performed proteomic analysis on granules from islets that secreted insulin, taken from a clonal cell line of rats. In this study, these granules were primarily obtained through two-step enrichment via centrifugation. The obtained fraction was positive for both insulin and beta-granin, which act as markers for insulin-secreting granules, whereas the fraction was negative for calreticulin, which acts as a marker for proteins that are localized in mitochondria. A total of 130 proteins were detected in this fraction, which was more than the analyzed proteins in the total cell lysate. These identified proteins comprised intravesicular proteins (44%) and membrane proteins (45%). The proteins belonging to the intra-vesicular class are secretory proteins from the beta cells of the pancreas, such as insulin, whereas some of these proteins were identified to have hydrolase action, which is related to lysosomal proteins. These results show that it might be possible that during fractionation, granules and lysosomal proteins co-migrated, or that during insulin degradation via crinophagy, secretory granules fuse to lysosomes, which is why both types of proteins were present in the same fraction. On the other hand, the results also support the hypothesis of "sorting by retention," which postulates that upon maturation, all secretory granules change into mature granules or into lysosomes (Sandberg and Borg, 2006).

8.9 PROTEOMIC TECHNIQUES AND DIABETES

Various studies have described defects in the action or secretion of insulin, release of hepatic glucose, or the functioning of adipocytes that consequently cause DMT2. In recent years, there has been a focus on the genetic factors that may be mutated to cause the disease. Additionally, there has been a focus on other tools, such as genome analysis or positional cloning techniques, to identify other pathways that may be involved in the pathogenesis of DMT2. For instance, in a study conducted on Mexican Americans, SNP mutations were found in *calpain 10* gene using a positional cloning technique. The gene is located at 2q37. In addition, another locus was also found on chromosome 15, which was observed to subsequently increase the chances of the mutation in calpain 10, which is related to DMT2. Another study also showed the association of this mutation with decreased activity of the β3-adrenergic receptor, which sheds light on the pathogenesis of DMT2 with complex gene interactions (Salih et al., 2021).

These studies show the importance of proteomic techniques for the analysis of protein expression in various tissues in normal people in comparison to the patients of DMT2, so that the role of various proteins in causing resistance to insulin, production of adipo-cytokines, dysfunction of beta cells of the islets, disturbed release of hepatic glucose, and increased damage susceptibility of the end organs can be understood. To date, various studies have been conducted on diabetic animal models or cell lines using proteomic techniques. It is also possible to employ these techniques on various tissues and/or sera obtained from patients with diabetes. For instance, due to defects in mitochondrial genes, some patients suffer from DMT2, which shows a maternal inheritance pattern and are inherently deaf. As proteomic analysis of mitochondrial genes has become possible, it has also become important to check for mitochondrial mutations in patients suffering from diabetes (Maassen, 2002) (Figure 8.4).

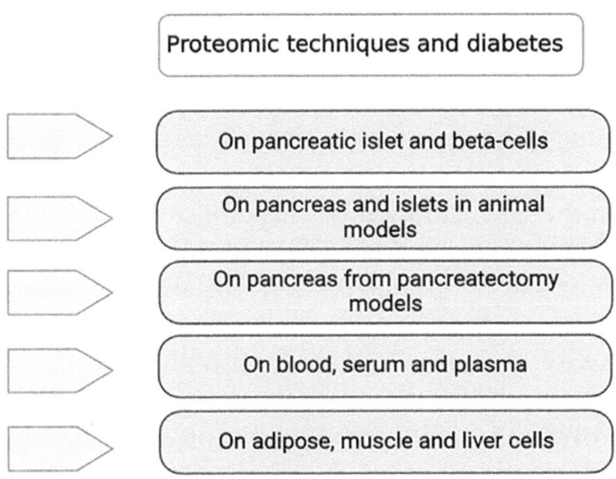

FIGURE 8.4 Proteomic techniques and diabetes.

8.9.1 PROTEOMIC ANALYSIS OF GLUCOSE INDUCED CHANGES IN PANCREATIC ISLET AND BETA-CELLS

Glucose is a trigger for the secretion of insulin and thus can produce sustained secretion of insulin. When these carbohydrates enter the body, they undergo glycolysis primarily, followed by the Krebs cycle and the electron transport chain (ETC) that sequentially produce ATPs. ATP production causes the closing of KATP channels present in the membrane, causing membrane depolarization, and an influx of calcium takes place along with the exocytosis of insulin (Rutter, 2001).

Pyruvate carboxylase is an enzyme abundantly expressed in pancreatic beta cells. About 40% of the released pyruvate then, as a result, is changed into oxaloacetate. According to some studies, glucose metabolism can generate ROS in both *in vitro* and *in vivo* experiments. It is thus deduced that if there is prolonged exposure of beta cells to glucose, their functioning might be impaired, and it may also induce apoptosis, which is called glucotoxicity (Wang et al., 2005).

A comparative analysis was performed on the changing protein profiles and measuring the effect of glucose on beta clonal cells and islets of Langerhans. When the islets obtained from rat models were exposed to different concentrations of glucose, proteins formed in the islets were separated and produced as a result of the exposure by utilizing this approach, and it was observed that the levels of various proteins were altered (Kolesar et al., 2012). Glucospondins respond to elevated glucose levels; however, they have not been observed. In one study, a rise in glucose concentration consequently stimulated the production of 10 to 20-fold of 10 proteins localized in the islet. The other proteins were stimulated for two to four-fold production (Guest et al., 1991).

Another study showed similar results in isolated islets from mice that were cultured in the presence of glucose for a day. 2DGE showed an increase in the concentration of chaperones like GRP58 and GRP94, which implicate an increased need for the synthesis capacity of cellular proteins (Ahmed and Bergsten, 2005). It was also observed that there was an increase in the levels of proteins that support the maturation and movement of secretory granules. This study also showed increased levels of antioxidants and heat shock proteins. These results show that an increase in the levels of glucose will consequently increase the capacity of beta cells to produce insulin. In addition, with increased capacity, an increase in the cell mass of beta cells can also be observed as an adaptation to insulin resistance.

In another study, Fernandez et al. (2008) performed both proteomic and metabolomic analyses when isolated beta cells were exposed to different concentrations of glucose for 2 days. At relatively high concentrations of glucose, glucotoxicity was observed, which in turn reduced the secretion of insulin. Metabolic analysis was performed by spectrometry and chromatography. The results showed that the beta cells under such conditions had more Krebs cycle intermediates along with the presence of nine amino acids. Proteomic analysis was also performed via 2DGE, which showed approximately 800 spots, of which 305 spots were different compared to cells cultured at lower glucose levels. 75 of these 305 spots were found to be unique. The results showed a correlation between the levels of the metabolites and their respective proteins. This observation indicates that the availability of substrate and regulation of allosteric enzymes is more significant for determination of the levels of metabolites in comparison to the levels of actual enzymes.

Proteomic studies have also shown that one protein can be observed at different spots with varying intensities. Such results are more commonly seen in the representation of post-translational modifications of proteins. These results show that it is not necessary for glucose to change the expression of proteins, which might change the characteristics of the protein during modifications (Wu et al., 2005).

8.9.2 PROTEOMIC OF PANCREAS AND ISLETS OF OBESITY AND DMT2 IN ANIMAL MODELS

Resistance to insulin consequently causes beta cells to respond by increasing insulin secretion to maintain normal glucose levels. Animal models such as Zucker fatty (ZF) rats and Zucker diabetic fatty (ZDF) rats have been used to study obesity and diabetes, respectively. ZDFs were developed via inbreeding of ZFs. ZFs had a maintained glucose level as they had an increased beta cell mass, which increased the secretion of glucose, even though they had developed resistance to insulin. The data showed that if the beta cell mass needs to be increased, undifferentiated progenitor cells can form new beta cells (Topp et al., 2007).

A study was performed using 2DGE from pancreases obtained from mice that were fed a high-fat diet and were diabetic. The results showed enhanced regenerating protein 1 (REG1) and REG2 in the islets during the early development of diabetes. With the progression of diabetes, lower levels of glutathione peroxidase (GPx) were also observed, indicating oxidative stress. To analyze the mechanism caused by changes induced by obesity on the proteome of the islets, we compared normal mice with fatty mice. A mutation in the leptin hormone gene caused normal mice to become obese. Insulin resistance was observed in obese mice. In response to insulin resistance, increased insulin secretion was observed in obese mice, and these mice developed beta cell hypertrophy (Sanchez et al., 2002).

A comparison of 2DGE of islet maps was performed for normal and obese mice, and the results showed varying expression of nine proteins that were involved in the organization of the actin cytoskeleton. Actin cytoskeleton variation is important, as it occurs during exocytosis and the movement of secretory granules of insulin. In another study, insulin-resistant mice were treated with insulin-sensitizing agents, which restored the alteration formed in obese mice (Lu et al., 2008).

In muscle IGF receptor (MKR) mice that are resistant to insulin, beta cell hypertrophy was observed. Mutations in these mice producing this resistance are observed in the insulin-like growth factor-1 receptor that is targeted to the skeletal muscles; thus, these mice do not have a direct defect in the beta cells. These mice are highly resistant to insulin and thus have increased levels of insulin observed at the age of only 14 days, and their tolerance towards glucose is impaired, which can be observed at the age of 5 weeks (Fernández et al., 2001).

Another study was performed on MKR mice that were 10 weeks of age, and their islets were compared to those of normal mice. In this study, 590 unique proteins were identified, along with more than 1000 proteins that were expressed differentially. As there is an increased demand for insulin, it was observed that in MKR mice, there is an increased level of molecular chaperones. Along with these proteins, there is also an enhanced level of ER-associated protein degradation, as reported by Lu et al. (2008).

All these results show that there is increased folding of proteins in the islets, which in turn produces substances that are cytotoxic. In the later stages of diabetes in MKR mice, cytotoxicity can occur in beta cells. In comparison, there have been observations of increased biosynthesis of proteins, protein degradation and folding, and increased levels of proteins that are involved in the production of insulin, along with proteins involved in insulin processing as well as exocytosis. It was also observed that these mice had lower levels of glucose metabloc proteins. These findings show how GSIS was reduced in these mice (Lu et al., 2008).

8.9.3 PROTEOMICS OF PANCREATECTOMY MODELS OF THE PANCREAS

Partial pancreas removal has been widely used to study the regeneration of pancreatic cells. It was observed that protein expression changes in the rat models that had regenerated pancreases after 120 h and 60% pancreatectomy and 180 h after 90% pancreatectomy. These models were analyzed using 2DGE and mass spectrometry. No significant differences were observed between the two models. Nonetheless, the studies showed similar proteins to those found in pancreatectomy models. The identified proteins were metabolic proteins of glucose, amino acids, and lipids, along with proteins involved in signal transduction, protein synthesis, and apoptosis (Yang et al., 2006).

8.9.4 PROTEIN PROFILING OF BLOOD, SERUM, AND PLASMA

Diabetes affects various organs of the patient, and as the blood is always in contact with every organ, it is likely that the secreted proteins can be seen in the circulating blood. When the plasma obtained from the blood of a normal individual and a diabetic patient was compared, various proteins were different. For example, visfatin, resistin, adiponectin, leptin, and interleukin-6 were observed to be different. Furthermore, various circulatory proteins have been implicated in the pathogenesis of diabetes via various mechanisms. To identify the stage of DMT2, the insulin concentration was measured to reflect the changes in beta cells. In addition, as blood is very easy to access, it also makes it fascinating to study any changes in other blood-related diseases (Norata et al., 2007).

Recently, various techniques have been developed that enable the measurement of proteins on a large scale in biological samples, along with proteomic analysis of blood for various diseases (Laronga et al., 2003). While performing protein profiling of the blood, it is important to consider that a huge chunk of this composition will be common proteins, such as immunoglobulins or albumin. Thus, to detect proteins that are not present in abundance in the plasma or blood, the abundant proteins must be depleted first via various techniques. In contrast, there is also a risk that while performing these fractionations, along with the bulk of the abundant proteins, other proteins might also be lost (Gong et al., 2006).

Primarily, a blood profiling study on DMT2 was performed by Jiang et al. (2003), in which they focused on various proteins in the cell membranes of RBCs in patients with DMT2. The results showed a total of 27 proteins that were present in increased concentrations, whereas 15 were present in lower concentrations when compared with the control. Two of the proteins with higher concentrations were arginase and flotillin-1, whereas one with lower concentrations was syntaxin 1C. These results led to further research in which the interaction between the two upregulated proteins was analyzed. The results showed that flotillin-1 is a membrane protein in RBCs, whereas arginase is a soluble protein that interacts with flotillin-1. Owing to this interaction between the two proteins, arginase activity was significantly upregulated in patients with DMT2.

Another study was performed on plasma obtained from human blood, and proteomic analysis was performed on patients with DMT2 or insulin resistance. In this study, to analyze protein I, low abundance fractionation was done primarily, and the samples obtained were analyzed via surface-enhanced laser desorption/ionization time-of-flight spectrometry (SELDI TOF-MS). The protein haptoglobin was found to be upregulated in the plasma of patients compared to controls. Furthermore, various other proteins, such as fibrinogen and C3 and C1 inhibitors, which are involved in the inflammatory response, were altered in the plasma of patients in comparison to the control. The proteins identified in this study were associated with DMT2 and its development. The aim of this study was to analyze the variations in plasma protein levels in both types of patients, that is, DMT2 and insulin resistance, in comparison to controls. In addition, early insulin response (EIR) was analyzed, and the results were compared to those of individuals with normal glucose tolerance (NGT) (Zhang et al., 2004).

The differences in EIR among the three groups of individuals were profiled, and nine plasma proteins were found to have varied concentrations. Most of these nine proteins reflected varied concentrations in a comparison of DMT2 and NGT, irrespective of any changes in EIR. Compared to NGT, individuals suffering from DMT2 with enhanced EIR had downregulated apolipoprotein H (ApoH) in the blood plasma. On the other hand, in comparison to NGT, when EIR was reduced, there was no reduction in the level of ApoH. This difference in EIR was comparable as the glycemic level of both groups was kept constant; thus, any difference in EIR was reflected as changes in the genetic data of the groups. In the present study, there was not a single protein whose difference can be implicated in EIR, which reinforces the polygenic nature of DMT2. Variations in plasma proteins can be implicated as a disease manifestation rather than the cause of the disease. These results are in line with those of another study in which the diabetic environment was compared to the genetic factors during failure of beta cell development (Sundsten et al., 2008).

Protein profiles in the serum of NGT patients were compared to those of newly diagnosed DMT2 patients to check for differences in the function of beta cells along with a family history of diabetes (FHD). 13 proteins were present at different concentrations in the groups. Five of these 13 proteins were downregulated, whereas eight were upregulated in the serum obtained from the DMT2 group. On the other hand, a comparison was made among individuals with lowered function of beta cells as well as FHD and the other group with lowered function of beta cells but no FHD. In this comparison, three of the already found proteins were observed again and were implicated as a genetic consequence, whereas the other 10 proteins were not observed again, indicating that they were not related to FHD but because of variation in the diabetic environment.

Apolipoprotein CIII (ApoCIII), albumin, and an unidentified protein were observed as a result of various genetic factors. In contrast, there were 10 proteins like TTR, which varied as a consequence of the diabetic environment.

All these studies that were performed on the plasma obtained from human subjects identified many proteins that were already implicated in diabetes. For example, ApoCIII was found at elevated concentrations in patients with DMT2, and it has already been measured in patients with DMT1 serum, along with its relation to cardiovascular risk factors (Sundsten et al., 2008).

Similarly, TTR was observed to be lowered in the plasma of DMT2, and a similar result was observed in another study that reported lowered levels of TTR in rat models when treated with streptozotocin (STZ) (Kim et al., 2006; Sundsten et al., 2007, 2008b). There is also an observation of lowered levels of TTR in DMT1 as well as during inflammation (Johnson et al., 2007).

Another protein, C-reactive protein, is elevated in the serum of patients with DMT2 and in patients with severe insulin resistance. The elevated levels are implicated in inflammation in the patient's body, which can also be interpreted as lower levels of TTR in the blood serum of patients with DMT2 (Sjöholm and Nyström, 2006).

Lower levels of other proteins, such as albumin and ApoH, have also been reported to be a variation observed in diabetic patients as a result of inflammation. Both proteins are produced in response to inflammation and are responsible for DMT2 pathogenesis. This has been reported in both animal and human models. As this study considered newly diagnosed patients with DMT2, there were no reports of kidney problems; thus, it seems unlikely that lowered levels of albumin in the blood serum can be reflected in increased levels of albumin during urinary excretion. Additionally, albumin levels were lower in DMT2 patients than in NGT patients, but a similar result was observed in a comparison of NGT patients with and without FHD. Nonetheless, albumin levels are increased in urinary excretion in patients with normoalbuminuric DMT2 (Narita et al., 2006). For further insights into the molecular variations that are implicated in DM, protein levels in the serum of both normal and STZ-treated rats were compared, and it was found that there was an increased expression of eight proteins in diabetic rats. Of these eight, one protein was identified as C-reactive protein. Although this protein has also been observed in previous studies to be present in abundance in diabetic subjects and is a predictor of the progression of diabetes in human subjects, it is still not an acute phase reactant protein in rats (Pradhan et al., 2001).

Protein levels have also been checked by utilizing various antidiabetic drugs obtained from plants/fungi and observing their effects in many studies. Tsuneki et al. (2004) observed the effect of green tea leaves on the serum proteins of mice and reported seven proteins that showed reduced levels of more than 3-folds, whereas seven proteins were found to be 3-folds elevated in concentration after treatment when a comparison was made between diabetic and control mice. A comparison of these two sets of results showed that one of these proteins was specific to DMT2 and showed sensitivity towards green tea leaves. This protein was not identified and had a mass of 4212 Da, which was found to be lowered significantly in diabetic type II subjects as well as in subjects treated with green tea leaves.

In another study, the effect of a treatment obtained via polysaccharides from a fungus was observed against hyperglycemia. The levels of proteins were compared between control mice and STZ-induced diabetic mice. The results of this study showed that there were 50 differentially regulated proteins and 20 spots that were identified as diabetes-related proteins. The protein patterns were examined and compared between the two groups and were found to be different. Nine proteins (apolipoprotein A1, haptoglobin, albumin, vitronectin, apolipoprotein E, transthyretin monomer, immunoglobulin kappa-chain, kallikrein binding protein, and transthyretin tetramer) were found to vary significantly in diabetic subjects, whereas the normal concentration of all of these proteins was restored once the subjects received treatment. On the other hand, seven proteins—apolipoprotein AIV, 1-inhibitor III, ceruloplasmin, hemopexin, transferrin, fetuin, and serine protease inhibitor—varied in diabetic subjects, but their concentrations were not restored to healthy levels after treatment (Kim et al., 2006).

8.9.5 PROTEIN PROFILING OF FAT, MUSCLE, AND LIVER

BGLs are regulated by the action of insulin on three targets in the body: muscle, liver, and adipose tissue. Primarily, through the action of insulin, glucose in the blood is absorbed and used in muscle cells and adipose tissue. Glucose is utilized and converted into glycogen mainly in the liver and muscle cells, whereas the breakdown of glucose is simultaneously reduced at the same time by the action of insulin, which results in a net gain of glycogen storage. Glucogenetic pathways suppress glucose release via other inhibitory enzymes. In contrast, in the fasting state, the opposite reaction takes place, during which glycogen is broken down into glucose and the level of insulin is reduced. To increase the levels of glucose in the blood under such conditions, the processes of glycogenolysis (glycogen breakdown) and gluconeogenesis (glucose synthesis) in the liver are enhanced. Simultaneously, the production of glycogen is reduced along with a reduction in the uptake of glucose in tissues that are sensitive to insulin, which results in elevated levels of glucose in the blood. In diseased conditions, that is, DMT2, glucose homeostasis is disturbed; thus, it is important to study the effects of protein patterns in the beta cells of the pancreas or blood, as well as the protein pattern in other parts that are involved in maintaining a normal level of glucose in the body. All three of the major targets of insulin, that is, adipocyte tissue, liver, and muscle cells, show a relationship with DMT2, as well as resistance to insulin. For this purpose, Schmid et al. (2004) used 2DGE to detect specific markers of a diet with high fat content, as well as insulin resistance. For this study, both white and brown adipose tissue were collected, along with liver and muscle cells, from mice fed a high-fat diet (obese) as well as from mice fed a normal diet (lean). A comparison of the tissues between these groups revealed various proteins that were differentially expressed. More than half of these proteins were detected in brown adipose tissue. Most of the proteins detected were related to stress and redox proteins. Additionally, mitochondrial proteins that belonged to Krebs cycle as well as respiratory chain reactions were also found to be expressed differently in obese mice. Proteomic analysis of the obese mice showed that as these mice were fed a high-fat diet, they had an excess of energy in comparison to the expenditure of energy; thus, to defend against it, mice gained weight, and the energy was dissipated by the regulation of the proteome of brown adipose tissue. Obesity is closely associated with DMT2 if it is present as a fat mass, whereas visceral obesity is associated with insulin resistance (Wilding, 2007).

The storage/release of energy is mainly involved in the white adipose tissue, which is also an endocrine organ. Various bioactive molecules such as adipokines are secreted from these tissues. Studies suggest that a disturbance in the production of these secretions may lead to resistance to insulin as well as DMT2, along with other cardiovascular problems (McPherson and Jones, 2003).

One of the mechanisms that can couple obesity (visceral) to other metabolic problems is low-grade inflammation, which leads to DMT2. Tissue proteomic analysis of white adipose tissue was performed via 2DGE in both mice and humans. Nonetheless, in associating adipose cells with diabetes, analysis of adipose cell secretion is also important. In a previous study, the secreted proteins in human tissues were analyzed for proteomic analysis using various mechanisms. The results of the study identified 300 proteins, of which 70 were identified as secreted proteins from adipose tissue. To analyze the association between adipose secretion proteins and DMT2, characterization of fatty tissue along with a comparison of secretion between patients with DMT2 and healthy individuals is important. A previous study suggested that if adipose cells fail to differentiate, it can consequently lead to the development of DMT2 (Danforth, 2000).

When analyzed in humans via 2DGE, 175 proteins were detected, of which 40 were involved in the formation of adipose cells. Various proteins belonging to various functional families have been found to be involved in the genesis of adipocytes. In addition, various proteins that belonged to heat shock proteins have been identified as the cause of DMT2 (DeLany et al., 2005).

In maintaining glucose homeostasis, skeletal muscles also play an important role by taking up and using glucose, independent of the presence of glucose. Disturbance of this balance can also contribute to the pathogenesis of DMT2 or obesity. In one study, proteomic analysis was performed on the proteins of skeletal muscle in a comparison of obese and lean subjects. The results of this study showed that proteins like glyceraldehyde-3-phosphate dehydrogenase, adenylate kinase, and aldolase A were elevated in obese subjects compared to those in lean subjects (Hittel et al., 2005).

Proteomic analysis of human muscles is an important approach for gaining insights into the biochemical basis of normal and diseased subjects. In a previous study, proteomic analysis was performed on skeletal muscles taken from healthy individuals via 1DGE and HPLC spectrometry. The results showed over 1000 proteins in healthy subjects. Many of these proteins are contractile proteins, whereas others are related to metabolic pathways for glucose and lipids. 22% of these proteins were identified as mitochondrial proteins. Additionally, proteins belonging to cell-cell signaling and the calcium homeostasis pathway were also detected (Højlund et al., 2008).

To investigate the pathophysiological mechanisms of DMT2, similar approaches are needed to characterize subjects with diabetes. Insulin resistance in the liver, along with the overproduction of lipoproteins, has been reported in subjects with insulin resistance. Proteomic analysis of the liver was performed to determine liver insulin resistance in hamsters with insulin resistance. To analyze any mechanism that links the development of liver insulin resistance to the overproduction of lipoproteins, proteomic analysis was performed on hepatic ER via 2DGE. The results of this analysis showed 34 proteins that were expressed differentially. Various proteins, that is, ERp46, ER60, ERp29, TAP1, and glutamate dehydrogenase, were reduced, whereas P-glycoprotein, alpha-glucosidase, PDI, fibrinogen, apolipoprotein E, and GRP94 were elevated in insulin-resistant hamsters (Morand et al., 2005).

8.10 CONCLUSION

Proteomic studies aim to measure various proteins in biological samples. The data obtained from these studies are then analyzed to determine various mechanisms involved in the health of the subject at a molecular level. The general approach of proteomic studies is to primarily characterize the sample and then identify the changes in the proteins that, in turn, will change the phenotype.

In the case of DM, many studies have aimed to characterize the pattern of protein expression in all tissues that may be associated with the pathophysiology of the disease. However, the results obtained to date are limited to identifying the levels of proteins that might be upregulated or downregulated in healthy and diseased subjects. Other studies have classified these proteins based on their localization within cells and their functions. However, all studies lacked consensus in classifying these proteins. In conclusion, proteomic studies provide insights into the disease at a molecular level, but new technologies are needed with regard to this technique, along with better strategies that can provide data that are in consensus for various studies.

ACKNOWLEDGMENT

We are thankful to all members of the Laboratory of Human Molecular Genetics at the Gomal Centre of Biochemistry and Biotechnology, Gomal University, Dera Ismail Khan, for their help in finding suitable literature.

CONFLICT OF INTEREST

None

FUNDING

None

DATA AVAILABILITY STATEMENT

Data are available on the password-protected laptops of M. M. and S. F. and will be available on request.

ETHICAL APPROVAL

Not Applicable

KEYWORDS

- **biomarker discovery**
- **diabetes mellitus**
- **disease pathophysiology**
- **homeostasis**
- **insulin resistance**
- **lipoproteins**
- **protein expression profiling**
- **protein–protein interactions**
- **proteomics**

REFERENCES

Ahmed, M., & Bergsten, P. (2005). Glucose-induced changes of multiple mouse islet proteins analyzed by two-dimensional gel electrophoresis and mass spectrometry. *Diabetology, 48*(3). https://doi.org/10.1007/s00125-004-1661-7 (accessed on 2nd February 2026).

Ahmed, M., Forsberg, J., & Bergsten, P. (2005). Protein profiling of human pancreatic islets by two-dimensional gel electrophoresis and mass spectrometry. *Journal of Proteome Research, 4*(3). https://doi.org/10.1021/pr050024a (accessed on 2nd February 2026).

Andrikopoulos, S. (2016). Genetic causes of impaired insulin secretion in DMT2. *Endocrine Abstracts.* https://doi.org/10.1530/endoabs.44.s11.1 (accessed on 2nd February 2026).

Asmat, U., Abad, K., & Ismail, K. (2016). Diabetes mellitus and oxidative stress—A concise review. *Saudi Pharmaceutical Journal, 24*(5). https://doi.org/10.1016/j.jsps.2015.03.013 (accessed on 2nd February 2026).

Bellou, V., Belbasis, L., Tzoulaki, I., & Evangelou, E. (2018). Risk factors for DMT2 mellitus: An exposure-wide umbrella review of meta-analyses. *PLoS ONE, 13*(3). https://doi.org/10.1371/journal.pone.0194127 (accessed on 2nd February 2026).

Blüher, M. (2019). Obesity: Global epidemiology and pathogenesis. *Nature Reviews Endocrinology, 15*(5). https://doi.org/10.1038/s41574-019-0176-8 (accessed on 2nd February 2026).

Briant, L. J. B., Reinbothe, T. M., Spiliotis, I., Miranda, C., Rodriguez, B., & Rorsman, P. (2018). δ-cells and β-cells are electrically coupled and regulate α-cell activity via somatostatin. *Journal of Physiology, 596*(2). https://doi.org/10.1113/JP274581 (accessed on 2nd February 2026).

Brunner, Y., Couté, Y., Iezzi, M., Foti, M., Fukuda, M., Hochstrasser, D. F., et al. (2007). Proteomics analysis of insulin secretory granules. *Molecular and Cellular Proteomics, 6*(6). https://doi.org/10.1074/mcp.M600443-MCP200 (accessed on 2nd February 2026).

Bunney, P. E., Zink, A. N., Holm, A. A., Billington, C. J., & Kotz, C. M. (2017). Orexin activation counteracts decreases in nonexercised activity thermogenesis (NEAT) caused by high-fat diet. *Physiology and Behavior, 176.* https://doi.org/10.1016/j.physbeh.2017.03.040 (accessed on 2nd February 2026).

Candler, T. P., Mahmoud, O., Lynn, R. M., Majbar, A. A., Barrett, T. G., & Shield, J. P. H. (2018). Continuing rise of DMT2 incidence in children and young people in the UK. *Diabetic Medicine, 35*(6). https://doi.org/10.1111/dme.13609 (accessed on 2nd February 2026).

Cho, N. H. (2017). *IDF Diabetes Atlas, 8th Edition.* International Diabetes Federation.

Cho, N. H., Shaw, J. E., Karuranga, S., Huang, Y., da Rocha Fernandes, J. D., Ohlrogge, A. W., et al. (2018). *IDF Diabetes Atlas: Global estimates of diabetes prevalence for 2017 and projections for 2045. Diabetes Research and Clinical Practice, 138, 271–281.* https://doi.org/10.1016/j.diabres.2018.02.023 (accessed on 2nd February 2026).

Cotten, S. W. (2020). Evaluation of exocrine pancreatic function. In *Contemporary Practice in Clinical Chemistry.* https://doi.org/10.1016/b978-0-12-815499-1.00033-8 (accessed on 2nd February 2026).

Czech, M. P. (2017). Insulin action and resistance in obesity and DMT2. *Nature Medicine, 23*(7). https://doi.org/10.1038/nm.4350 (accessed on 2nd February 2026).

Da Silva Xavier, G. (2018). The cells of the islets of Langerhans. *Journal of Clinical Medicine, 7*(3). https://doi.org/10.3390/jcm7030054 (accessed on 2nd February 2026).

Danforth, E. J. (2000). Failure of adipocyte differentiation causes type II diabetes mellitus? [1]. *Nature Genetics, 26*(1). https://doi.org/10.1038/79111 (accessed on 2nd February 2026).

Defronzo, R. A. (2009). From the triumvirate to the ominous octet: A new paradigm for the treatment of DMT2 mellitus. *Diabetes, 58*(4). https://doi.org/10.2337/db09-9028 (accessed on 2nd February 2026).

DeLany, J. P., Floyd, Z. E., Zvonic, S., Smith, A., Gravois, A., Reiners, E., et al. (2005). Proteomic analysis of primary cultures of human adipose-derived stem cells. *Molecular and Cellular Proteomics, 4*(6). https://doi.org/10.1074/mcp.M400198-MCP200 (accessed on 2nd February 2026).

Donath, M. Y., & Halban, P. A. (2004). Decreased beta-cell mass in diabetes: Significance, mechanisms and therapeutic implications. *Diabetology, 47*(3). https://doi.org/10.1007/s00125-004-1336-4 (accessed on 2nd February 2026).

Dunning, T., Sinclair, A., & Colagiuri, S. (2014). New IDF guideline for managing DMT2 in older people. *Diabetes Research and Clinical Practice, 103*(3). https://doi.org/10.1016/j.diabres.2014.03.005 (accessed on 2nd February 2026).

Egede, L. E., & Walker, R. J. (2020). Structural racism, social risk factors, and COVID-19–A dangerous convergence for Black Americans. *New England Journal of Medicine, 383*(12). https://doi.org/10.1056/nejmp2023616 (accessed on 2nd February 2026).

Eizirik, D. L., & Mandrup-Poulsen, T. (2001). A choice of death–The signal-transduction of immune-mediated beta-cell apoptosis. *Diabetology, 44*(12). https://doi.org/10.1007/s001250100021 (accessed on 2nd February 2026).

Fernández, A. M., Kim, J. K., Yakar, S., Dupont, J., Hernandez-Sanchez, C., Castle, A. L., et al. (2001). Functional inactivation of the *IGF-I* and insulin receptors in skeletal muscle causes DMT2. *Genes and Development, 15*(15). https://doi.org/10.1101/gad.908001 (accessed on 2nd February 2026).

Fernandez, C., Fransson, U., Hallgard, E., Spégel, P., Holm, C., Krogh, M., et al. (2008). Metabolomic and proteomic analysis of a clonal insulin-producing β-cell line (*INS-1 832/13*). *Journal of Proteome Research, 7*(1). https://doi.org/10.1021/pr070547d (accessed on 2nd February 2026).

Fuchsberger, C., Flannick, J., Teslovich, T. M., Mahajan, A., Agarwala, V., Gaulton, K. J., et al. (2016). The genetic architecture of DMT2. *Nature, 536*(7614). https://doi.org/10.1038/nature18642 (accessed on 2nd February 2026).

Funcke, J. B., & Scherer, P. E. (2019). Beyond adiponectin and leptin: Adipose tissue-derived mediators of inter-organ communication. *Journal of Lipid Research, 60*(10). https://doi.org/10.1194/jlr.R094060 (accessed on 2nd February 2026).

Gong, Y., Li, X., Yang, B., Ying, W., Li, B., Zhang, Y., et al. (2006). Different immunoaffinity fractionation strategies to characterize the human plasma proteome. *Journal of Proteome Research, 5*(6). https://doi.org/10.1021/pr0600024 (accessed on 2nd February 2026).

Guest, P. C., Bailyes, E. M., Rutherford, N. G., & Hutton, J. C. (1991). Insulin secretory granule biogenesis. Co-ordinate regulation of the biosynthesis of the majority of constituent proteins. *Biochemical Journal, 274*(1). https://doi.org/10.1042/bj2740073 (accessed on 2nd February 2026).

Gygi, S. P., Corthals, G. L., Zhang, Y., Rochon, Y., & Aebersold, R. (2000). Evaluation of two-dimensional gel electrophoresis-based proteome analysis technology. *Proceedings of the National Academy of Sciences of the United States of America, 97*(17). https://doi.org/10.1073/pnas.160270797 (accessed on 2nd February 2026).

Gygi, S. P., Rochon, Y., Franza, B. R., & Aebersold, R. (1999). Correlation between protein and mRNA abundance in yeast. *Molecular and Cellular Biology, 19*(3). https://doi.org/10.1128/mcb.19.3.1720 (accessed on 2nd February 2026).

Haffner, S. M., Lehto, S., Rönnemaa, T., Pyörälä, K., & Laakso, M. (1998). Mortality from coronary heart disease in subjects with DMT2 and in nondiabetic subjects with and without prior myocardial infarction. *New England Journal of Medicine, 339*(4). https://doi.org/10.1056/nejm199807233390404 (accessed on 2nd February 2026).

Henquin, J. C. (2009). Regulation of insulin secretion: A matter of phase control and amplitude modulation. *Diabetology, 52*(5). https://doi.org/10.1007/s00125-009-1314-y (accessed on 2nd February 2026).

Hermida, N., & Balligand, J. L. (2014). Low-density lipoprotein-cholesterol-induced endothelial dysfunction and oxidative stress: The role of statins. *Antioxidants and Redox Signaling, 20*(8). https://doi.org/10.1089/ars.2013.5537 (accessed on 2nd February 2026).

Hillier, T. A., & Pedula, K. L. (2003). Complications in young adults with early-onset DMT2: Losing the relative protection of youth. *Diabetes Care, 26*(11). https://doi.org/10.2337/diacare.26.11.2999 (accessed on 2nd February 2026).

Hittel, D. S., Hathout, Y., Huffman, E. P., & Houmard, J. A. (2005). Proteome analysis of skeletal muscle from obese and morbidly obese women. *Diabetes, 54*(5). https://doi.org/10.2337/diabetes.54.5.1283 (accessed on 2nd February 2026).

Højlund, K., Yi, Z., Hwang, H., Bowen, B., Lefort, N., Flynn, C. R., et al. (2008). Characterization of the human skeletal muscle proteome by one-dimensional gel electrophoresis and HPLC-ESI-MS/MS. *Molecular and Cellular Proteomics, 7*(2). https://doi.org/10.1074/mcp.M700304-MCP200 (accessed on 2nd February 2026).

Inagaki, N. (2019). 4. Entero-pancreatic endocrine function and diabetes. *Nihon Naika Gakkai Zasshi, 108*(9). https://doi.org/10.2169/naika.108.1713 (accessed on 2nd February 2026).

Jiang, M., Jia, L., Jiang, W., Hu, X., Zhou, H., Gao, X., et al. (2003). Protein dysregulation in red blood cell membranes of type 2 diabetic patients. *Biochemical and Biophysical Research Communications, 309*(1). https://doi.org/10.1016/S0006-291X(03)01559-6 (accessed on 2nd February 2026).

Johnson, A. M., Merlini, G., Sheldon, J., Ichihara, K., & Johnson, A. M. (2007). Clinical indications for plasma protein assays: Transthyretin (prealbumin) in inflammation and malnutrition. *Clinical Chemistry and Laboratory Medicine, 45*(3).

Jörns, A., Günther, A., Hedrich, H. J., Wedekind, D., Tiedge, M., & Lenzen, S. (2005). Immune cell infiltration, cytokine expression, and β-cell apoptosis during the development of type 1 diabetes in the spontaneously diabetic LEW.1AR1/Ztm-iddm rat. *Diabetes, 54*(7). https://doi.org/10.2337/diabetes.54.7.2041 (accessed on 2nd February 2026).

Kadota, K., Tominaga, D., Asai, R., & Takahashi, K. (2006). Correlation analysis of mRNA and protein abundances in human tissues. *Genome Letters, 2*(4). https://doi.org/10.1166/gl.2003.033 (accessed on 2nd February 2026).

Kanat, M., Mari, A., Norton, L., Winnier, D., DeFronzo, R. A., Jenkinson, C., et al. (2012). Distinct β-cell defects in impaired fasting glucose and impaired glucose tolerance. *Diabetes, 61*(2). https://doi.org/10.2337/db11-0995 (accessed on 2nd February 2026).

Karbaschi, R., & Zardooz, H. (2023). Pancreatic *GLUT2* protein expression and isolated islets insulin secretion decreased in high-fat fed rat dams. *Journal of Diabetes and Metabolic Disorders, 22*(2). https://doi.org/10.1007/s40200-023-01274-6 (accessed on 2nd February 2026).

Khan, M. A. B., Hashim, M. J., King, J. K., Govender, R. D., Mustafa, H., & Al Kaabi, J. (2020). Epidemiology of DMT2–Global burden of disease and forecasted trends. *Journal of Epidemiology and Global Health, 10*(1). https://doi.org/10.2991/JEGH.K.191028.001 (accessed on 2nd February 2026).

Khaw, K. T., Wareham, N., Bingham, S., Luben, R., Welch, A., & Day, N. (2004). Association of hemoglobin A1c with cardiovascular disease and mortality in adults: The European prospective investigation into cancer in Norfolk. *Annals of Internal Medicine, 141*(6). https://doi.org/10.7326/0003-4819-141-6-200409210-00006 (accessed on 2nd February 2026).

Kim, S. W., Hwang, H. J., Kim, H. M., Lee, M. C., Lee, M. S., Choi, J. W., et al. (2006). Effect of fungal polysaccharides on the modulation of plasma proteins in streptozotocin-induced diabetic rats. *Proteomics, 6*(19). https://doi.org/10.1002/pmic.200500933 (accessed on 2nd February 2026).

Klein, S., Gastaldelli, A., Yki-Järvinen, H., & Scherer, P. E. (2022). Why does obesity cause diabetes? *Cell Metabolism, 34*(1). https://doi.org/10.1016/j.cmet.2021.12.012 (accessed on 2nd February 2026).

Klimek-Tulwin, M., Knap, J., Reda, M., & Masternak, M. (2019). Physical activity in prevention and treatment of DMT2 mellitus. *Journal of Education, Health and Sport, 9*(9).

Kolesar, J. E., Taguchi, Y. V., Cramer, R. L., Wang, C., Chou, S. H., Soleimanpour, S. A., et al. (2012). Evidence for mitochondrial adaptation to chronic glucose exposure in beta cells. *Mitochondrion, 12*(5). https://doi.org/10.1016/j.mito.2012.07.095 (accessed on 2nd February 2026).

Ley, S. H., Hamdy, O., Mohan, V., & Hu, F. B. (2014). Prevention and management of DMT2: Dietary components and nutritional strategies. *The Lancet, 383*(9933). https://doi.org/10.1016/S0140-6736(14)60613-9 (accessed on 2nd February 2026).

Lin, J., Moradi, E., Salenius, K., Lehtipuro, S., Häkkinen, T., Laiho, J. E., et al. (2023). Distinct transcriptomic profiles in children prior to the appearance of type 1 diabetes-linked islet autoantibodies and following enterovirus infection. *Nature Communications, 14*(1). https://doi.org/10.1038/s41467-023-42763-9 (accessed on 2nd February 2026).

Lu, H., Yang, Y., Allister, E. M., Wijesekara, N., & Wheeler, M. B. (2008). The identification of potential factors associated with the development of DMT2: A quantitative proteomics approach. *Molecular and Cellular Proteomics, 7*(8). https://doi.org/10.1074/mcp.M700478-MCP200 (accessed on 2nd February 2026).

Maassen, J. A. (2002). Mitochondrial diabetes: Pathophysiology, clinical presentation, and genetic analysis. *American Journal of Medical Genetics–Seminars in Medical Genetics, 115*(1). https://doi.org/10.1002/ajmg.10346 (accessed on 2nd February 2026).

Malik, V. S., & Hu, F. B. (2019). Sugar-sweetened beverages and cardiometabolic health: An update of the evidence. *Nutrients, 11*(8). https://doi.org/10.3390/nu11081840 (accessed on 2nd February 2026).

McPherson, R., & Jones, P. H. (2003). The metabolic syndrome and DMT2: Role of the adipocyte: Editorial review. *Current Opinion in Lipidology, 14*(6). https://doi.org/10.1097/00041433-200312000-00001 (accessed on 2nd February 2026).

Metz, T. O., Jacobs, J. M., Gritsenko, M. A., Fontès, G., Qian, W. J., Camp, D. G., et al. (2006). Characterization of the human pancreatic islet proteome by two-dimensional LC/MS/MS. *Journal of Proteome Research, 5*(12). https://doi.org/10.1021/pr060322n (accessed on 2nd February 2026).

Morand, J. P. F., Macri, J., & Adeli, K. (2005). Proteomic profiling of hepatic endoplasmic reticulum-associated proteins in an animal model of insulin resistance and metabolic dyslipidemia. *Journal of Biological Chemistry, 280*(18). https://doi.org/10.1074/jbc.M413343200 (accessed on 2nd February 2026).

Muralidhara Krishna, C. S., & Srikanta, S. (2015). Type 1 diabetes pathogenesis—Prevention? *Indian Journal of Endocrinology and Metabolism, 19*(7). https://doi.org/10.4103/2230-8210.155404 (accessed on 2nd February 2026).

Nesto, R. W. (2004). Correlation between cardiovascular disease and diabetes mellitus: Current concepts. *American Journal of Medicine, 116*(5 SUPPL. 1). https://doi.org/10.1016/j.amjmed.2003.10.016 (accessed on 2nd February 2026).

Ng, X. W., Chung, Y. H., & Piston, D. W. (2021). Intercellular communication in the islet of Langerhans in health and disease. *Comprehensive Physiology, 11*(3). https://doi.org/10.1002/cphy.c200026 (accessed on 2nd February 2026).

Norata, G. D., Ongari, M., Garlaschelli, K., Raselli, S., Grigore, L., & Catapano, A. L. (2007). Plasma resistin levels correlate with determinants of the metabolic syndrome. *European Journal of Endocrinology, 156*(2). https://doi.org/10.1530/eje.1.02338 (accessed on 2nd February 2026).

Ortsäter, H., & Bergsten, P. (2006). Protein profiling of pancreatic islets. *Expert Review of Proteomics, 3*(6). https://doi.org/10.1586/14789450.3.6.665 (accessed on 2nd February 2026).

Pradhan, A. D., Manson, J. E., Rifai, N., Buring, J. E., & Ridker, P. M. (2001). C-reactive protein, interleukin 6, and risk of developing DMT2 mellitus. *Journal of the American Medical Association, 286*(3). https://doi.org/10.1001/jama.286.3.327 (accessed on 2nd February 2026).

Qatanani, M., & Lazar, M. A. (2007). Mechanisms of obesity-associated insulin resistance: Many choices on the menu. *Genes and Development, 21*(12). https://doi.org/10.1101/gad.1550907 (accessed on 2nd February 2026).

Reynolds, A., Mann, J., Cummings, J., Winter, N., Mete, E., & Te Morenga, L. (2019). Carbohydrate quality and human health: A series of systematic reviews and meta-analyses. *The Lancet, 393*(10170). https://doi.org/10.1016/S0140-6736(18)31809-9 (accessed on 2nd February 2026).

Ripsin, C. M., Kang, H., & Urban, R. J. (2009). Management of blood glucose in DMT2 mellitus. *American Family Physician, 79*(1).

Roefs, M. M., Carlotti, F., Jones, K., Wills, H., Hamilton, A., Verschoor, M., et al. (2017). Increased vimentin in human α- and β-cells in DMT2. *Journal of Endocrinology, 233*(3). https://doi.org/10.1530/JOE-16-0588 (accessed on 2nd February 2026).

Rorsman, P., & Ashcroft, F. M. (2018). Pancreatic β-cell electrical activity and insulin secretion: Of mice and men. *Physiological Reviews, 98*(1). https://doi.org/10.1152/physrev.00008.2017 (accessed on 2nd February 2026).

Rosengren, A., & Dikaiou, P. (2023). Cardiovascular outcomes in type 1 and DMT2. *Diabetology, 66*(3). https://doi.org/10.1007/s00125-022-05857-5 (accessed on 2nd February 2026).

Ross, R. (2003). Does exercise without weight loss improve insulin sensitivity? *Diabetes Care, 26*(3). https://doi.org/10.2337/diacare.26.3.944 (accessed on 2nd February 2026).

Rutter, G. A. (2001). Nutrient-secretion coupling in the pancreatic islet β-cell: Recent advances. *Molecular Aspects of Medicine, 22*(6). https://doi.org/10.1016/S0098-2997(01)00013-9 (accessed on 2nd February 2026).

Salih, A. M., Gattia, K. J., & Jabbar, A. D. (2021). The correlation between the gene that encoding Calpain-10 and DMT2 mellitus in Wasit Province. *Annals of Tropical Medicine & Public Health, 24*(05). https://doi.org/10.36295/asro.2021.24504 (accessed on 2nd February 2026).

Sanchez, J. C., Chiappe, D., Verset, V. C., Hoogland, C., Binz, P. A., Paesano, S., et al. (2001). The mouse SWISS-2D PAGE database: A tool for proteomics study of diabetes and obesity. *Proteomics, 1*(1). https://doi.org/10.1002/1615-9861(200101)1:1<136::AID-PROT136>3.0.CO;2-1 (accessed on 2nd February 2026).

Sanchez, J. C., Converset, V., Nolan, A., Schmid, G., Wang, S., Heller, M., et al. (2002). Effect of rosiglitazone on the differential expression of diabetes-associated proteins in pancreatic islets of C57Bl/6 lep/lep mice. *Molecular & Cellular Proteomics: MCP, 1*(7). https://doi.org/10.1074/mcp.M200033-MCP200 (accessed on 2nd February 2026).

Sandberg, M., & Borg, L. A. H. (2006). Intracellular degradation of insulin and crinophagy are maintained by nitric oxide and cyclo-oxygenase 2 activity in isolated pancreatic islets. *Biology of the Cell, 98*(5). https://doi.org/10.1042/bc20050085 (accessed on 2nd February 2026).

Schmid, G. M., Converset, V., Walter, N., Sennitt, M. V., Leung, K. Y., Byers, H., et al. (2004). Effect of high-fat diet on the expression of proteins in muscle, adipose tissues, and liver of C57BL/6 mice. *Proteomics, 4*(8). https://doi.org/10.1002/pmic.200300810 (accessed on 2nd February 2026).

Schwartz, S. S., Epstein, S., Corkey, B. E., Grant, S. F. A., Gavin, J. R., & Aguilar, R. B. (2016). The time is right for a new classification system for diabetes: Rationale and implications of the β-cell-centric classification schema. *Diabetes Care, 39*(2). https://doi.org/10.2337/dc15-1585 (accessed on 2nd February 2026).

Sesti, G., Antonelli Incalzi, R., Bonora, E., Consoli, A., Giaccari, A., Maggi, S., et al. (2018). Management of diabetes in older adults. *Nutrition, Metabolism and Cardiovascular Diseases, 28*(3). https://doi.org/10.1016/j.numecd.2017.11.007 (accessed on 2nd February 2026).

Sjöholm, Å., & Nyström, T. (2006). Inflammation and the etiology of DMT2. *Diabetes/Metabolism Research and Reviews, 22*(1). https://doi.org/10.1002/dmrr.568 (accessed on 2nd February 2026).

Smith, G. I., Polidori, D. C., Yoshino, M., Kearney, M. L., Patterson, B. W., Mittendorfer, B., et al. (2020). Influence of adiposity, insulin resistance, and intrahepatic triglyceride content on insulin kinetics. *Journal of Clinical Investigation, 130*(6). https://doi.org/10.1172/JCI136756 (accessed on 2nd February 2026).

Strasser, B. (2013). Physical activity in obesity and metabolic syndrome. *Annals of the New York Academy of Sciences, 1281*(1). https://doi.org/10.1111/j.1749-6632.2012.06785.x (accessed on 2nd February 2026).

Stumvoll, M., Goldstein, B. J., & Van Haeften, T. W. (2005). DMT2: Principles of pathogenesis and therapy. *Lancet, 365*(9467). https://doi.org/10.1016/S0140-6736(05)61032-X (accessed on 2nd February 2026).

Sundsten, T., Östenson, C. G., & Bergsten, P. (2008). Serum protein patterns in newly diagnosed DMT2 mellitus–Influence of diabetic environment and family history of diabetes. *Diabetes/Metabolism Research and Reviews, 24*(2). https://doi.org/10.1002/dmrr.789 (accessed on 2nd February 2026).

Sundsten, T., Zethelius, B., Berne, C., & Bergsten, P. (2008). Plasma proteome changes in subjects with DMT2 mellitus with a low or high early insulin response. *Clinical Science, 114*(7, 8). https://doi.org/10.1042/CS20070323 (accessed on 2nd February 2026).

Topp, B. G., Atkinson, L. L., & Finegood, D. T. (2007). Dynamics of insulin sensitivity, β-cell function, and β-cell mass during the development of diabetes in *fa/fa* rats. *American Journal of Physiology–Endocrinology and Metabolism, 293*(6). https://doi.org/10.1152/ajpendo.00572.2007 (accessed on 2nd February 2026).

Tsuneki, H., Ishizuka, M., Terasawa, M., Wu, J. B., Sasaoka, T., & Kimura, I. (2004). Effect of green tea on blood glucose levels and serum proteomic patterns in diabetic (*db/db*) mice and on glucose metabolism in healthy humans. *BMC Pharmacology, 4*. https://doi.org/10.1186/1471-2210-4-18 (accessed on 2nd February 2026).

Vasiljević, J., Torkko, J. M., Knoch, K. P., & Solimena, M. (2020). The making of insulin in health and disease. *Diabetology, 63*(10). https://doi.org/10.1007/s00125-020-05192-7 (accessed on 2nd February 2026).

Vetrivel Venkatasamy, V., Pericherla, S., Manthuruthil, S., Mishra, S., & Hanno, R. (2013). Effect of physical activity on insulin resistance, inflammation and oxidative stress in diabetes mellitus. *Journal of Clinical and Diagnostic Research, 7*(8). https://doi.org/10.7860/JCDR/2013/6518.3306 (accessed on 2nd February 2026).

Wang, H., Kouri, G., & Wollheim, C. B. (2005). *ER* stress and *SREBP-1* activation are implicated in β-cell glucolipotoxicity. *Journal of Cell Science, 118*(17). https://doi.org/10.1242/jcs.02513 (accessed on 2nd February 2026).

Weinstein, A. R., Sesso, H. D., Lee, I. M., Cook, N. R., Manson, J. A. E., Buring, J. E., et al. (2004). Relationship of physical activity vs body mass index with DMT2 in women. *JAMA, 292*(10). https://doi.org/10.1001/jama.292.10.1188 (accessed on 2nd February 2026).

Wilding, J. P. H. (2007). The importance of free fatty acids in the development of DMT2. *Diabetic Medicine, 24*(9). https://doi.org/10.1111/j.1464-5491.2007.02186.x (accessed on 2nd February 2026).

Wu, J., Lenchik, N. J., Pabst, M. J., Solomon, S. S., Shull, J., & Gerling, I. C. (2005). Functional characterization of two-dimensional gel-separated proteins using sequential staining. *Electrophoresis, 26*(1). https://doi.org/10.1002/elps.200406176 (accessed on 2nd February 2026).

Yang, M., Liu, W., Wang, C. Y., Liu, T., Zhou, F., Tao, J., et al. (2006). Proteomic analysis of differential protein expression in early process of pancreatic regeneration in pancreatectomized rats. *Acta Pharmacological Sinica, 27*(5). https://doi.org/10.1111/j.1745-7254.2006.00317.x (accessed on 2nd February 2026).

Zhang, R., Barker, L., Pinchev, D., Marshall, J., Rasamoelisolo, M., Smith, C., et al. (2004). Mining biomarkers in human sera using proteomic tools. *Proteomics, 4*(1). https://doi.org/10.1002/pmic.200300495 (accessed on 2nd February 2026).

Zhou, B., Lu, Y., Hajifathalian, K., Bentham, J., Di Cesare, M., Danaei, G., et al. (2016). Worldwide trends in diabetes since 1980: A pooled analysis of 751 population-based studies with 4.4 million participants. *The Lancet, 387*(10027). https://doi.org/10.1016/S0140-6736(16)00618-8 (accessed on 2nd February 2026).

CHAPTER 9

Immunomodulation in Diabetes: The Dynamic Role of the Immune System

AMIT ANAND,[1] AKSHANSH KUMAR,[2] S. N. MANJULA,[3]
NEERAJ KUMAR FULORIA,[4] and KENGANORA MRUTHUNJAYA[1,*]

[1]*Department of Pharmacognosy, JSS College of Pharmacy, JSS Academy of Higher Education and Research, Mysuru, Karnataka, India*

[2]*Department of Pharmaceutical Biotechnology, JSS College of Pharmacy, JSS Academy of Higher Education and Research, Mysuru, Karnataka, India*

[3]*Department of Pharmacology, JSS College of Pharmacy, JSS Academy of Higher Education and Research, Mysuru, Karnataka, India*

[4]*Department of Pharmaceutical Chemistry, Faculty of Pharmacy, AIMST University, Semeling Campus, Bedong, Kedah, Malaysia*

*Corresponding author

ABSTRACT

Diabetes and the immune system interact dynamically with complex cellular connections and immunomodulatory processes. This chapter examines the interaction between the immune system and diabetes, clarifying immunomodulation mechanisms in both types. Type 1 diabetes, an autoimmune disease, is characterized by abnormal immune responses destroying pancreatic β-cells, causing insulin deficiency. It explains how autoreactive T cells, B cells, and cytokines coordinate pancreatic inflammation and β cell death, covering novel immunotherapy strategies to maintain β-cell activity and build immunological tolerance. Persistent

Diabetes: Novel Insights and Therapies. Anas Islam and Badruddeen (Eds)

DOI: 10.1201/9781779644596-13

low-grade inflammation in T2DM worsens insulin resistance and impairs beta cell function. The chapter examines interactions among immune cells, fat tissues, and metabolic pathways, highlighting proinflammatory cytokines, adipokines, and macrophage polarization in driving insulin resistance and systemic inflammation. It investigates how immunomodulatory medications may enhance insulin resistance and metabolic outcomes in type 2 diabetes. The chapter covers the immunometabolism paradigm, emphasizing the relationship between metabolic control and immune cell function, exploring how metabolic signals influence immune cell polarization and activation. Overall, this chapter summarizes diabetes-related immunomodulation, emphasizing the interaction between the immune system and metabolic abnormalities. Insights into these pathways can lead to innovative immunotherapeutic approaches for treating diabetes and its effects.

9.1 INTRODUCTION

9.1.1 *OVERVIEW OF DIABETES MELLITUS*

Over the past 50 years, rapid globalization and shifts in lifestyle have led to significant transformations in politics, society, the environment, and human behavior. Diabetes is becoming much more common in both affluent and less-affluent countries; it mostly affects disadvantaged communities and indigenous populations. Diabetes mellitus (DM) is a chronic condition characterized by faulty protein and fat metabolism and elevated blood glucose levels (BGLs) (Zimmet et al., 2014). BGLs rise because the cells cannot metabolize glucose because of inadequate insulin secretion by the pancreas or ineffective cellular use of the generated insulin. Diabetes mellitus is mostly seen in three forms: type 1 diabetes is brought on by the body and produces insufficient insulin. This condition is known as "insulin-dependent diabetes mellitus (IDDM)" or "juvenile diabetes" (Tao et al., 2015). Anomalies in the metabolism of proteins, fats, and carbohydrates are the primary features of type 2 diabetes mellitus (T2DM). This condition may result from insulin resistance, insufficient insulin production, or a combination of both. Approximately 90% of all diabetes cases are T2DM, which is far more frequent than gestational or type 1 diabetes mellitus. Our understanding of the genesis and course of type 2 diabetes has significantly advanced in recent years. T2DM primarily arises from a progressive reduction in insulin production by pancreatic beta cells, often coupled with pre-existing insulin resistance in the skeletal muscle, liver, and adipose tissue (Plows et al., 2018). Globally, 14% of pregnancies are affected by GDM, according to the most recent data available from the International Diabetes Federation (IDF) (2017). The development and progression of T2DM has significantly enhanced the condition and is primarily driven by a gradual decline in insulin production from pancreatic beta cells, often accompanied by pre-existing insulin resistance in the skeletal muscle, liver, and adipose tissue. Gestational diabetes mellitus (GDM) is a common pregnancy complication that is characterized by the onset of spontaneous hyperglycemia. Globally, 14% of pregnancies are affected by GDM, according to the most recent data available from the IDF (Nicholson, 2016).

9.1.2 UNDERSTANDING THE IMMUNE SYSTEM

The problems that mammalian immune systems address are not exclusive to higher animals; they affect all living species and are ignored by none. The force of natural selection is ever present and unending. Emerging infectious illnesses may influence human history in the same way as epidemics and pandemics (Cooper, 2010). Understanding how to effectively utilize our highly evolved immune system for human health is essential to address this threat. Numerous biological components, including mast cells, dendritic cells, eosinophils, neutrophils, basophils, lymphocytes, and macrophages, constitute the immune system. Numerous cell types are transient inhabitants of distinct anatomical locations. Lymphocytes and blood are recycled via lymphatic circulation (Sharma and Sharma, 2022). The human body has two different types of immunity. These two types of immunity are innate and adaptive. Innate immunity serves as the initial line of defense against infection. To the best of our knowledge, microorganisms and all living organisms have continual interactions. One of its unique characteristics is that innate immunity exists before microbial encounters occur. Microbes promptly elicit innate immune responses and precede the development of adaptive immune responses. The innate immune system recognizes a smaller range of antigens, most of which are fundamental structural components specific to microbes (Kiboneka, 2021). The evolution of the adaptive immune system has been fueled by the vast diversity of antigenic structures and the ability of infections to change to elude host identification (Rai et al., 2021). The cells that comprise the adaptive immune system include B lymphocytes originating from the bone marrow, which create antibodies, and T lymphocytes, which develop in the thymus and are effectors of the cellular immunological responses. The lymphocytes are continuously in motion. After developing in the thymus and bone marrow, cells from primary lymphoid organs migrate to secondary lymphoid organs such as the spleen and lymph nodes (Abós et al., 2022). These organs are responsible for capturing circulating antigens from the blood and lymph, respectively. Adaptive immune responses initiate at these sites, often as a result of innate immune system signals from circulating pathogens, either directly or through pathogen-activated cutaneous or antigen-presenting cells (APCs) in the mucosa that migrate to the secondary organs of lymphoid tissue. After leaving the lymph nodes and spleen, lymphocytes can travel to different parts of the body to perform their effector roles (Leadbetter and Karlsson, 2021).

9.2 IMMUNOPATHOGENESIS OF DIABETES

9.2.1 DIABETES MELLITUS (T1DM)

The thymus, spleen, and peripheral nodes are essential components of both the innate and adaptive immune systems, widely distributed in animals, and they play crucial roles in the pathophysiology of type 1 diabetes mellitus. The innate immune system mounts the immune response against various infections. According to recent research using a non-obese diabetic (NOD) mouse model, gut bacterial interactions with the innate immune system may play a crucial epigenetic role in altering susceptibility to type 1 diabetes (T1D). The innate system does not change in response to repeated inputs, whereas the adaptive system increases and improves. When an external stimulus (such as an infection) activates APCs and subsequently engages the autoantigens, the innate system triggers the adaptive system (Atkinson and Mirmira, 2023). Cells such as platelets, T and B lymphocytes, mono- and polynuclear phagocytes, and basophils make up the two arms of the immune system. The results of immune responses are influenced by humoral and cellular responses between the innate and adaptive systems (Starska-Kowarska, 2023). A brief description of the mechanism of the occurrence of diabetes is depicted in Figure 9.1.

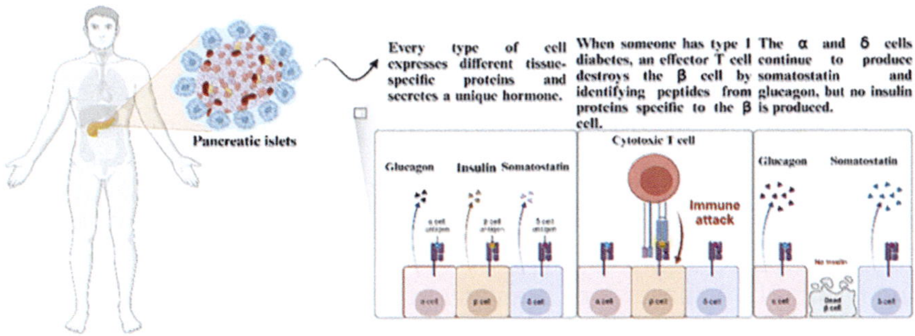

FIGURE 9.1 Mechanism involved in type 1 diabetes mellitus.

9.2.1.1 AUTOIMMUNE DESTRUCTION OF BETA CELLS

The confidence around total B-cell death or ablation in T1D has improved, as evidenced by a number of recent clinical investigations demonstrating that individuals with long-standing T1D have considerable residual B-cell activity. This implies that B cell regeneration occurs in many individuals, or that B cell death ceases. Evidence suggests that T1DM is an autoimmune disease in which the beta cells are targeted by themselves (Wilcox et al., 2016). The variability of immune infiltrates within a single pancreas, the expression by beta cells of multiple gene variants that impact islet inflammation and are susceptible to type 1 diabetes, increased endoplasmic reticulum (ER) stress, metabolic biomarkers that precede the earliest signs of autoimmunity, and impaired proinsulin processing that affects stressed beta cells, which may further enhance ER stress, and HLA Class I (HLA-I) presentation of proinsulin peptides are among the observations that have been made. The capacity of beta cells to trigger autoimmune activation and islet inflammation triggers protective responses that may later turn detrimental (Mallone and Eizirik, 2020). Endocrine cells are defined as hormone-secreting cells organized in glands without a ductal system owing to their significant vascularization. These cells immediately release their products into circulation. Several facets of this concept may aid in explaining beta-cell vulnerability (Rosol et al., 2024). Type 1 diabetes is caused by the progressive destruction of insulin-producing pancreatic cells. Despite much research on the origin of autoimmune diabetes, the mechanisms underlying early-stage cell death remain unexplained. Studies have shown the toxicity of type I and proinflammatory cytokines, such as IL-1, TNF-α, and IFN-γ, in human islet cells, particularly in B cells. An increasing body of evidence indicates that apoptosis may be the primary mechanism resulting in cell death and is a significant factor in T1DM (Dettmer et al., 2022).

9.2.1.2 ROLE OF T CELLS AND AUTOANTIBODIES

Islet cell autoantibodies (ICA) are the primary antibodies linked to the development of type 1 diabetes. Antibodies against protein tyrosine phosphatase (IA2 or ICA512), glutamic acid decarboxylase (GAA or GAD), and insulin (IAA) have since been identified. The presence of many persistently positive antibodies is highly associated with the development of type 1 diabetes, and these antibodies may persist for years prior to the onset of clinically severe hyperglycemia (Kawasaki, 2023). Indirect immunofluorescence was used to identify islet cell autoantibodies (ICAs), which were first found in T1DM patients with and autoimmune endocrine illness. All endocrine islet cells in animals are reactive to these antibodies. These are called islet cell cytoplasmic antibodies because of their reaction to islet intracellular components (Winter et al., 2022). Patients with T1DM also have a cytoplasmic ICA. Numerous studies from different nations have demonstrated the importance of IAA in the prediction of diabetes. Anti-insulin autoantibodies seem unique in that the age at which type 1 diabetes manifests is strongly and negatively correlated with the levels of these antibodies. At the time of T1D diagnosis, IAA was discovered to be mostly composed of IgG1, with smaller amounts of IgG4 and IgG2 (Jia and Yu, 2023). Table 9.1 summarizes the roles of different T cells in type 1 diabetes.

TABLE 9.1 Role of Different T cells in T1DM

Types of T Cell	Role of T Cell in T1D	References
CD8+ T	Effect β-cell cytotoxicity and contribute to islet inflammation	Tsai et al. (2008)
CD4 T	When exposed to *in vitro* re-stimulation, CD4 T cells from T1D patients generate more IL-21 than T cells from non-diabetic people	Walker and von Herrath (2015)
Follicular helper T (Tfh) cells	Pathogenesis of T1D	Varela-Calvino et al. (2017a)
CD8+ T	Firstly, the production of cytotoxic T lymphocytes that are specific to islets seems to be a significant effector mechanism that results in the beta cells being destroyed. By differentiating into memory-like autoregulatory T cells, a differentiation pathway that may be induced with nanoparticle vaccines, the same cells may be crucial in halting the onset of clinical signs	Roep et al. (2021)

TABLE 9.1 *(Continued)*

Types of T Cell	Role of T Cell in T1D	References
CD57+, CD8+ T cells	The study conducted by the authors demonstrated that changes in the makeup of peripheral CD57+CD8+ T cells occur over the course of T1D, taking advantage of the disease's distinct peri-remission period	Varela-Calvino et al. (2017b)

9.2.2 *TYPE 2 DIABETES MELLITUS (T2DM)*

According to the World Health Organization (WHO), diabetes mellitus is a long-term metabolic disorder characterized by high BGLs that can lead to damage to the kidneys, heart, blood vessels, eyes, and nerves over time. T2DM represents more than 90% of all diabetes cases and is characterized by insulin resistance in body tissues, insufficient insulin secretion by pancreatic islet β-cells, and an inadequate compensatory insulin secretory response. As the disease worsens, insulin secretion is unable to maintain glucose homeostasis (Mukhtar et al., 2020). In this disease, adipose tissue employs a number of inflammatory processes, including dysregulation of adipokines and increased production of free fatty acids (FFAs), to create insulin resistance (IR). The aging population, high-calorie meals, sedentary lifestyles, and global increase in obesity are the major causes of the T2DM epidemic, which has increased the incidence and prevalence of T2DM (Chait and den Hartigh, 2020).

9.2.2.1 *CHRONIC INFLAMMATION AND INSULIN RESISTANCE*

Given that obesity and metabolic syndrome, affected by lifestyle choices, are major risk factors for type 2 diabetes, chronic inflammation has been proposed as an underlying cause of disease progression. Furthermore, dysregulation of the innate immune system caused by hyperglycemia results in elevated levels of circulating inflammatory proteins known as cytokines, which may lead to chronic inflammation in type 2 diabetes. Furthermore, current studies suggest that the interplay between genetic and environmental variables, such as nutrition and lifestyle, may affect the control of chronic inflammation. Type 2 diabetes and related problems may arise from this condition. The natural progression of type 2 diabetes is associated with inflammation (Naidoo et al., 2018). Numerous cross-sectional studies have demonstrated a favorable correlation between the characteristics of diabetes-related insulin resistance syndrome and inflammatory markers, such as CRP, TNF-α, and interleukin-6 (IL-6). Insulin resistance and reduced insulin production are the hallmarks of type 2 diabetes. It is well accepted that the accumulation of fatty acids in metabolically active (non-adipose) tissues, such as the liver and muscles, is one of the primary causes of insulin resistance. Consequently, many studies have been conducted to determine the processes through which excess lipids reduce the effects of insulin. Adipose tissue is the primary source of circulating fatty acids (Zozulinska and Wierusz-Wysocka, 2006).

9.2.2.2 MACROPHAGE INFILTRATION IN ADIPOSE TISSUE

Adipocyte hyperplasia and hypertrophy assist in the growth of adipose tissue (AT), and hypertrophy appears to be more frequent in adults. Larger adipocytes are linked to an increase in insulin resistance and diabetes. For both humans and animals, adipocyte size is a potent and reliable indicator of macrophage accumulation in the adipose tissue. Given the number of studies on macrophages in the field of general immunology, it would be beneficial to review some of their general characteristics. One subtype of myeloid cells, called macrophages, is produced by the hematopoietic stem cells (HSCs) present in the bone marrow (Bourlier and Bouloumie, 2009). Following their generation, HSCs first give rise to monocytes, followed by common myeloid progenitors or CMPs. Monocytes in the bloodstream move into nearby inflammatory areas when they detect danger signals. Chemo-attractants played a major role in mediating this movement. Subsequently, these cells develop into DCs or macrophages (Lee, 2013). AT growth is stimulated by both adipocyte hyperplasia and hypertrophy; however, hypertrophy appears to be more common in adults. Significant findings regarding the effects of macrophage infiltration into the AT were obtained. First, both studies demonstrated that macrophages, not adipocytes, were the primary source of inflammatory cytokines, including TNF-α and macrophage inflammatory protein (MIP)-1α in AT (Surmi and Hasty, 2008).

9.3 IMMUNOMODULATORY MECHANISMS

9.3.1 REGULATORY T CELLS (TREGS)

Several functional and genetic studies have been conducted on regulatory T cells (Tregs) from individuals with type 1 diabetes, indicating that the pathophysiology of the condition is partially influenced by the dysfunction of these cells. Peripheral blood Treg numbers are usually unaffected by type 1 diabetes; nevertheless, they can alter the expression profile of signature genes and reduce the suppressive action of these cells. Tregs from individuals with type 1 diabetes exhibit increased expression of protein tyrosine phosphatase (PTPN2), a negative regulator of IL-2 signaling. This is accompanied by decreased phosphorylation of signal transducer and activator of transcription 5, a key downstream signaling component, in response to IL-2 (Zi et al., 2022). These alterations most likely stem from Tregs compromising IL-2 signaling. Additionally, SNPs in epigenetic regulatory regions critical for Treg identity have been linked to type 1 diabetes. Treg dysfunction and type 1 diabetes are directly connected, according to studies on immune dysregulation and polyendocrinopathy enteropathy X-linked (IPEX) syndrome, where FOXP3 mutations produce varying degrees of Treg dysfunction and multi-organ autoimmunity, which frequently includes type 1 diabetes (Park et al., 2020). Compelling evidence connecting Treg dysfunction to type 1 diabetes, along with their capacity to suppress immune responses in various conditions, has prompted multiple efforts to enhance Treg function through autologous cell therapy approaches. Importantly, *ex vivo* IL-2 expression appears to counterattack the reduction in IL-2 induced STAT 5 activation, implying improved function of patient-derived infused cells. With the completion of phase I clinical studies, autologous Treg administration in patients with recent-onset type 1 diabetes was tested. No serious side effects were noted, suggesting that this medication is safe and avoided. Likewise, the results showed no significant effects of combining intraportal allogeneic islet transplantation with autologous Treg injections (Ben-Skowronek et al., 2021). Encouraging evidence shows that, compared to a matched control group, children who underwent regulatory T cell (Treg) therapy retained higher C-peptide levels and required less insulin one year after treatment. (Zieliński et al., 2024). Similarly, Bluestone et al. (2021) discovered that while there were no appreciable changes in disease severity, some patients' C-peptide levels were sustained for more than two years following therapy, despite the fact that the trial was not intended to evaluate effectiveness. Crucially, within weeks of infusion, both studies found a sharp drop in the number of circulating Tregs. Apart from the first sharp decrease, Bluestone et al. (2021) also noted a biphasic exponential reduction, with the longer-lived Treg subgroup accounting for approximately 10–25% of the infused cells during the second phase. The primary phenotype of these cells, which remained visible for up to a year following infusion, was naïve or memory stem-like, as shown by the expression of CD45RA and CCR7, as opposed to the central memory-like phenotype, which was identified as CCR7+CD45RA−CD45RO+ prior to infusion (Bluestone et al., 2021). Consequently, it is evident that long-lived cells exist even in the setting of polyclonal Treg treatment, and they may be crucial for preserving long-term effectiveness over the long run. Nonetheless, the generally poor effectiveness of existing polyclonal Treg treatments indicates the need for novel approaches to improve Treg survival, function, and proliferation *in vivo*. In patients with type 1 diabetes, adding low-dose IL-2 medication to Treg therapy can boost the number of Treg cells; nevertheless, this approach is not optimal because it may lead to the proliferation of inflammatory cell subsets (Bluestone et al., 2023). When taken as a whole, these outcomes have safety and unclear efficacy are comparable to those of several previous trials evaluating polyclonal Treg cell treatment in other disease situations. To improve effectiveness by focusing on Treg phenotype, antigen specificity, and survival, a number of novel genetic engineering techniques have been developed. It is hoped that these advancements will allow Tregs to reach their maximum potential (Eggenhuizen et al., 2020).

9.3.2 CYTOKINES AND CHEMOKINES

Cytokines are prospective targets for immunotherapy, as they are important players in the intricate multicellular interactions that lead to type 1 diabetes (T1D) between immune cells and pancreatic β cells. It is believed that cytokines that promote regulatory activities, such as IL-10, TGF-β, and IL-33, can prevent β-cell destruction and restore immunological tolerance. In contrast, cytokines such as TNF, IL-6, IL-17, and IL-21, which encourage the development and activity of diabetogenic immune cells, cause the establishment and progression of type 1 diabetes. However, because cytokines that induce β-cell death have context-dependent pro- or anti-inflammatory properties, addressing these dysregulated cytokine networks does not necessarily have consistent benefits. As only a few studies have been published to date, the functions of IL-5 and IL-9 in T1D remain inadequately understood (Velikova et al., 2021a). The proliferation of CD19+, IgM^{+}, and B cells in mice is facilitated by IL-5, which also encourages B cells to secrete IL-10, which has a strong suppressive effect on the pathophysiology of diabetes. Patients with T1D have elevated blood levels of IL-9 expression, which is associated with the size of the Th9 effector subpopulations and predicts HbA1c values. However, the exact function of IL-9 in T1D remains unclear (Lu et al., 2020). Numerous studies have shown the impact of cytokines IL-4 and IL-13, which are encoded by nearby genes and transduce signals via a largely shared receptor (IL-4Rα) in T1D. Type-2 cytokines have been shown to stimulate type-2 immune responses and have the potential to inhibit autoimmune illnesses caused by type 1. Patients with T1D have elevated blood levels of IL-9 expression, which is associated with the size of the Th9 effector subpopulations and predicts HbA1c values. However, the exact function of IL-9 in T1D remains unclear (Ramponi et al., 2022a). Numerous studies have shown the impact of cytokines IL-4 and IL-13, which are encoded by nearby genes and transduce signals via a largely shared receptor (IL-4Rα) in T1D. According to earlier research, chemokines may be crucial for the development and management of immunological microenvironments in individuals with T1DM (Ramponi et al., 2022b). Furthermore, studies have shown that chemokines have emerged as significant signaling molecules that regulate the pathophysiological processes of type 2 diabetes. Chemokines are the four subfamilies that constitute the largest family of cytokines. Chemokines function as signaling molecules in the inflammatory response, triggering a spectrum of pro-inflammatory mediators and inflammatory factors. These inflammatory substances activate cytokine-signaling proteins. Consequently, insulin signaling receptor activation by pancreatic cells is inhibited, enhancing insulin resistance and the eventual development of type 2 diabetes and prediabetes (Varra et al., 2024). Chemokines are involved with 23 distinct receptors. Chemokines that differ in their concentration in PDM and T2DM patients and are considered as possible novel biomarkers are unknown. A comprehensive study or meta-analysis of the function of chemokines in the development of PDM and T2DM has not yet been conducted. The representation of chemokine signal transduction pathways in the pathophysiology of PDM and T2DM may offer new targets and strategies for the prevention, diagnosis, and treatment of these conditions (Ramessur et al., 2022).

9.3.2.1 TGF-B AND INTERLEUKIN-10 (IL-10)

As a two-edged sword, anti-inflammatory cytokines can reduce inflammation and weaken immunity. The role of these cytokines in individuals with latent tuberculosis infection (LTBI) varies according to their level of glucose intolerance (Khdair et al., 2023). The LTB-PDM group had substantially higher serum levels of IL-27, IL-10, and IL-1Ra than the LTB-NGT group did. The LTB-NDM group had higher levels of IL-27 and IL-10, whereas TGF-β levels were lower than those in the LTB-NGT group. Comparing the LTB-KDM and LTB-NGT groups, lower serum levels of IL-27 and higher levels of IL-1Ra and TGF-β were observed. In LTB+ patients in the NGT, PDM, and NDM groups, but not in the KDM group, TB antigens caused the production of IL-1Ra. These cytokine levels showed diabetes stage–specific regulation due to comorbidity with LTBI (Fan et al., 2022). Significant abnormalities in anti-inflammatory cytokine levels and recall secretion, as observed in LTB+KDM individuals, may promote DM–TB synergy. The common pathogenic trait shared by all types of diabetes mellitus is the destruction of beta cells or their improper functioning. Resolving the underlying process may help in diabetes therapy by protecting the β cell population and function. Numerous roles for TGF-β signaling exist in the growth, operation, division, death, and dedifferentiation of β cells. During development, the β cell lineage expands when TGF-β signaling is inhibited. Nevertheless, Tgfbr1 deletion eliminates inflammation-induced β cell proliferation but had no effect on insulin demand-induced β cell proliferation (dos Santos Haber et al., 2023). The primary traditional TGF-β signaling repressor of β-cell proliferation in response to systemic insulin demand is Smad3, but not Smad2. Smad3 is a crucial mediator and an excellent target for type 2 diabetes therapy because it concurrently enhances β-cell activity and apoptosis, insulin resistance, and systemic insulin resistance in diabetic animal models, resulting in the elimination of overt diabetes. Nevertheless, in investigations conducted on animal studies, Smad7 has debatable effects on β cell proliferation and glucose homeostasis. In contrast, Tgfb1 overexpression shields β-cells against autoimmune destruction without compromising their ability to function (Xie et al., 2022).

9.3.2.2 TNF-A AND IL-6

At least four distinct chemical alterations have the potential to disrupt insulin signaling, some of which have been shown to occur when TNF-α is added to cell cultures. The initial modification identified was the serine phosphorylation of IRS-1. As a result of this modification, IRS-1 is now resistant to tyrosine phosphorylation triggered by insulin. As a result, insulin-stimulated glucose transport is impaired, and PI-3 kinase docking decreases. It has been demonstrated that TNF-α causes this alteration in cell types that are most relevant to insulin resistance: C2C12 muscle cells, rat hepatoma cells, and mouse adipocytes (Fadaei et al., 2020). Tumor necrosis factor (TNF)-mediated serine phosphorylation of IRS-1 in 3T3-L1 adipocytes requires the mitogen-activated protein (MAP) kinase pathway. The second effect of adding TNF to rat hepatoma cells is that it phosphorylates and activates SH-PTPase, a protein tyrosine phosphatase that quickly removes tyrosine phosphate groups from IRS-1 and FAK, thereby stopping the action of insulin. Third, protein phosphate PP-1 is phosphorylated at position 2 by TNF-α, rendering it inactive. Insulin stimulates glucose storage by phosphorylating and activating PP-1 at site 1 (Nikolic et al., 2020). Activated PP-1 activates glycogen synthase and inhibits phosphorylase. The mechanism of action of TNF-α has been established in rabbit skeletal muscle and L6 muscle cells. Lastly, compared to insulin receptors (IRs) isolated from the muscle of insulin-responsive participants, IRs from insulin-resistant subjects' muscles are serine/threonine phosphorylated and have reduced intrinsic tyrosine kinase activity. The capacity of IRs to phosphorylate IRS-1 and autophosphorylate may be inhibited by serine/threonine phosphorylation (López-Gambero et al., 2020). It has been demonstrated that phorbol esters can reduce tyrosine kinase activity in IRs isolated from healthy tissue, and that alkaline phosphatase can restore tyrosine kinase activity in IRs isolated from insulin-resistant muscle *in vitro.* According to available data, protein kinase C (PKC)-theta mediates serine/threonine phosphorylation of inhibitory receptors (IRs). There is no evidence linking TNF-α expression to the latter mechanism (Goltermann et al., 2021). TNF-α treatment of Fao hepatoma cells has been shown to increase IRS-1 serine phosphorylation and decrease PI3K docking, while having no effect on the tyrosine kinase activity of isolated IRs. The pleiotropic cytokine interleukin (IL)-6 plays a major role in immunoregulation and non-immune processes in most cell types and tissues that are not part of the immune system (Bluemel et al., 2020). Numerous *in vivo* and *in vitro* studies, including epidemiological, genetic, rodent, and human studies, have examined the potential involvement of IL-6 in the pathogenesis of obesity, insulin resistance, β-cell death, T1DM, and T2DM. These investigations point to the IL-6's pathogenetic and preventive effects in diabetes (Lim et al., 2024).

9.3.3 INNATE IMMUNE CELLS

In the early critical hours and days of life, the innate immune system protects against foreign invaders and environmental hazards as the first line of defense. For the host to survive, it must be able to recognize harmful microbes and launch appropriate defense mechanisms to eliminate them (Liaskou et al., 2014). Tissue-resident or circulating leukocytes, mainly phagocytic macrophages and neutrophils, together with dendritic cells and natural killer (NK) cells, as well as epithelial barriers that keep microbes out of the body, function to coordinate innate immunity. The main role of the innate immune system is to mediate inflammation, which is the act of delivering blood and plasma components to regions where tissue homeostasis has been compromised, including following infection or injury (Costa et al., 2021). The effects of diabetes on various innate immune cells are summarized in Table 9.2.

TABLE 9.2 Impact of Diabetes on Innate Immune Cells

Types of Cells	Role of Cells	Effects on Diabetes	References
Macrophages (M1)	Involved in proinflammatory responses	Increased production of TNF-α, M1, and IL-6	Wang et al. (2014)
Macrophages (M2)	Antagonize M1 responses and provide anti-inflammatory responses	Decreased production of M2 and IL-10	Abumaree et al. (2013)
Natural killer cells	Act as a defense mechanism	Enhanced production of IL-8, TNF-α, and IL-22	Kucuksezer et al. (2021)
Dendritic cells	Help in the initiation of active immune responses and activation of T cells	Increased TNF-α, IL-6, IL-12, and IL-23	Chandrasekharan et al. (2022)
Neutrophils	Help in providing acute inflammatory responses	Increased production of neutrophils, TNF-α, IL-6, and IL-8	Chan et al. (2021)
NKT cells (natural killer T cells)	Regulation of T cells	Increased IFN-γ and decreased production of IL-10 and IL-4	Vallerskog et al. (2010)

9.3.3.1 MACROPHAGES AND DENDRITIC CELLS

Macrophages are phagocytes that have undergone evolutionary conservation and evolved over 500 million years ago. Ilya Metchnikoff made their initial discovery around the end of the 1800s (2014). One of the key roles of macrophages in both areas is to support the immune system by removing and destroying pathogenic cells through phagocytosis and the release of cytokines. In addition to their role in acute inflammation, macrophages are recognized as key regulators of chronic inflammation (Thornley et al., 2016). Most chronic illnesses, including type 2 diabetes and atherosclerosis, are caused by macrophages, which facilitate the production of chemokines that attract more immune cells to the site of inflammation (Meshkani and Vakili, 2016). Because of their unique appearance, which distinguishes them from macrophages, DCs were first discovered in the spleens of mice by Steinman and Cohn. They were then shown to be the most effective inducers of the mixed lymphocyte response. This finding sets the stage for several studies conducted over the course of several decades that have demonstrated the critical role DCs play in inducing adaptive immune responses (Khan et al., 2022). Specialized accessory cells known as dendritic cells (DCs) were first identified in adherent mononuclear cell preparations derived from mouse spleen. These cells have a distinct appearance that may help differentiate them from other adherent cells, such as monocytes and macrophages (Liu and Nussenzweig, 2010). Several studies have searched for blood samples from T1D patients who have been diagnosed with dendritic cell complications. The decrease in the number of cDC1s and NKT cells during diagnosis was correlated with decreased residual β-cell function after a year in a longitudinal analysis of immunological features in newly diagnosed T1D children. Reduction in cDCs and pDCs, as well as reduced expression of CCR2 in these cells, was seen in another study that included freshly diagnosed pediatric patients with T1D (Mbongue et al., 2017).

9.3.3.2 NATURAL KILLER (NK) CELLS

More than 30 years ago, NK cells were discovered to serve as cytotoxic effectors in the innate immune system. Later research revealed that NK cells are a unique group of large granular lymphocytes present in peripheral tissues that are not lymphoid or lymphoid organs. The circulation and a number of organs, including the bone marrow, spleen, lymph nodes, liver, lung, omentum, gut, and placenta, contain natural killer (NK) cells (Vivier et al., 2008). It is well known that NK cells grow primarily in the bone marrow, similar to B and myeloid cells (Mandal and Viswanathan, 2015). NK cells play a protective role in both therapeutic and preventive approaches against the development of T1DM. In NOD mice undergoing full Freund's adjuvant therapy, NK cells mediate protective benefits against autoimmune diabetes by secreting IFN-γ and downregulating auto-reactive cytotoxic T lymphocytes specific to beta cells. Additionally, NK cells with an NK3-like phenotype in NOD mice administered polyinosinic-polycytidylic acid promote Th2 bias in immunological responses, which helps to reduce the development of diabetes (Nekoua et al., 2020). Figure 9.2 depicts the mechanism of action of natural killer cells in type-1 diabetes.

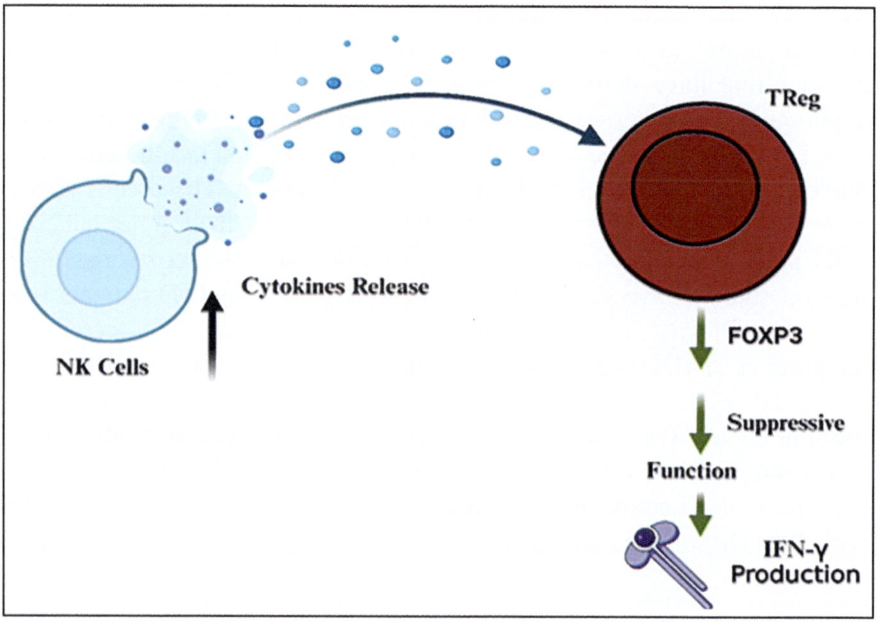

FIGURE 9.2 Mechanism of action of NK cells in T1D.

9.4 THERAPEUTIC APPLICATIONS

9.4.1 IMMUNOTHERAPY APPROACHES

9.4.1.1 BIOLOGICS TARGETING CYTOKINES

In the past 10 years, there has been a growing number of novel biological entities, also known as biologics, that are connected to cytokines. Biologics include decoy receptors that target cytokines, antibodies that neutralize or block the receptors of inflammatory cytokines, and recombinant proteins that act as receptor agonists or antagonists to occupy and inhibit receptor binding (Velikova et al., 2021b). A broad class of cellular messenger molecules, known as cytokines, control pro- and anti-inflammatory signals, which in turn control inflammatory responses. Anti-cytokine medicines are frequently prescribed as disease-modifying drugs to individuals with rheumatoid arthritis. Various cytokines are now being targeted for biological therapy of inflammatory and autoimmune illnesses. Moreover, several cytokines influence glucose metabolism (Velikova et al., 2024). Anakinra, a naturally occurring IL-1 receptor antagonist, has been shown to improve type 2 diabetes treatment results, despite the absence of evidence connecting the disease to an autoimmune etiology. The results of the trial are in line with those from models of type 1 diabetes, indicating that enhanced metabolic control was not caused by insulin resistance, which is also thought to be mediated through IL-1β, but rather by direct protective effects on β-cells. After treatment, elevated C-peptide responses persisted for up to 39 weeks. Anakinra is thought to obstruct immune cells' and pancreatic islet cells' pro-inflammatory signals. This prevents beta cell death induced by IL-1, a hallmark of both type-1 and type-2 diabetes (Ke et al., 2021).

9.4.1.2 IMMUNE CHECKPOINT INHIBITORS

Immune checkpoints have a significant potential to trigger autoimmune disorders, such as diabetes mellitus, by dysregulating host immunity. Because they prevent immune cells from attacking body cells at random and promote self-tolerance, inhibitory immunological checkpoints are a crucial part of the immune system (Youssef et al., 2021). Several inhibitory immunological checkpoints were identified in our system, such as T-cell immunoglobulin mucin protein-3 and lymphocyte activation genes. This, in turn, activates downstream protein tyrosine phosphatases (also known as "Src homology region 2 domain-containing phosphatase-1/2," or "SHP1/2"). This is because PD-1 and TCR are closely related in the immunological synapse. Moreover, PD-1 can stop T cell activation by severing the link between B7.1 and CD28 costimulatory signals (Quandt et al., 2020). The primary players in this PD-1 regulatory system are the PD-1 receptor (*Pdcd1*) and its associated ligands PD-L1 (B7-H1 or CD274) and PD-L2. Because it has been shown that these immune inhibitory receptors, which belong to the CD28/B7 family, are either soluble or membrane-attached, studying this pathway is difficult. PD-1 and PD-L1 strongly support immunological tolerance via several mechanisms. Researchers have found that blocking PD-1 or PD-L1 impairs immune tolerance by causing T cells to migrate more slowly, exposing them to dendritic cells for longer periods, producing more cytokines, and enhancing T cell receptor signaling, all of which are linked to autoimmunity. It has been shown that in response to interferon-γ, T, B, and dendritic cells constitutively generate PD-L1. Nevertheless, recent studies have demonstrated that PD-L2 expression may be generated in a diverse array of immune and non-immune cells contingent upon microenvironmental cues (Yang et al., 2020). It was previously thought that APCs are the only cells that express PD-L2. Remarkably, because PD-L2 has 2–4 times higher affinity for PD-1 than PD-L1, it can compete with PD-L1 for PD-1 binding. However, the precise function of PD-L2 in modifying immune responses in cancer therapy is still under debate and is a subject of much research (Khan and Gerber, 2020). The primary mechanism by which peripheral tissues exhibit autoantigen tolerance is elimination of highly autoreactive T and B cells during lymphocyte maturation. Some peripheral processes, such as T cell depletion, senescence, or immunological checkpoints, occur if autoreactive cells manage to evade this elimination phase. One of these checkpoints, PD-1/PD-L1, is crucial for suppressing excessive immune response. Immunity is an important factor in the pathophysiology of diabetes. An inappropriate host immune response supports both T1D and T2D. Because of T cell-mediated death, inappropriate insulin production by pancreatic β-cells causes T1D. B cells, the second arm of the immune system, also participate in this process by secreting autoantibodies. The devastation of β-cells and onset of T1D are mostly caused by four autoantibodies: IA-2A, glutamic acid decarboxylase (GAD-65), insulin autoantibody (IAA), and islet cell antibody (ICA). IA-2A targets protein tyrosine phosphatase, whereas ICA targets cytoplasmic proteins in beta cells. The interaction between T cells and autoantibodies ultimately leads to the lysis of β cells, which reduces the host's capacity to release insulin and causes type 1 diabetes (Kong and Flynn, 2014). The potential use of secreted autoantibodies as T1D indicators has been previously studied. Those who test positive for at least two islet cell autoantibodies are thought to have a 50% risk of developing type 1 diabetes. However, clinical trials have demonstrated that B cell depletion with rituximab, a chimeric monoclonal antibody against CD20, which is mostly present on the surface of immune system B cells, can stop the advancement of type 1 diabetes. The pathophysiology of type 2 diabetes (T2D) is associated with an aberrant immune response, although β-cell death by the immune system is not a predisposing factor. Although extremely unlikely, T2D might have a negative impact on the CPI; nevertheless, it is possible (Chye et al., 2022). Combining immune checkpoint inhibitors can increase their anti-cancer effect; nevertheless, this will increase the likelihood of developing autoimmune diabetes. Although hyperglycemia is an uncommon side effect of CPI monotherapy, the frequency of this adverse event increases with the use of CPIs in combination (Wang et al., 2023). Furthermore, understanding the processes behind the development of diabetes as a result of these therapeutic interventions is crucial for understanding the mechanisms underlying the development of classical diabetes. This will direct scientists in their quest to avoid PD-1/PD-L1 inhibitor-induced autoimmune side effects while maintaining the anticancer efficacy of the drugs. To date, a number of immune checkpoints have been identified; however, more studies are still needed to identify other immune checkpoints that may be activating or inhibiting, but have not been found (Zhai et al., 2021). In addition, it would be very beneficial to attempt to block additional immune checkpoints such as TIM-3, LAG3, and others, and to link each one to the emergence of immune-related adverse outcomes. Notably, determining the $CD4^+$ T cell activation state before initiating immune checkpoint inhibitors may be valuable in predicting the efficacy of treatment and the likelihood of developing autoimmune side effects as a result of the medication (Gianchecchi and Fierabracci, 2018).

9.4.1.3 TOLEROGENIC VACCINES

Unlike immunogenic vaccinations, which induce an immunological response against a pathogen, these vaccines attempt to reduce the pathogenic immune response to both allergens and autoantigens. Tregs are essential for regulating immune responses. They consist of natural Treg (nTreg) cells, which differentiate in the thymus and mostly recognize autoantigens, and induced Treg (iTreg) cells, which develop from various effector Th cell types in the periphery. Tregs disrupt metabolism, affect the development and function of dendritic cells (DCs), and produce cytokines including TGF-β and IL-10, which reduce inflammation (Ogra et al., 2001). Decreased Treg levels and impaired function have been linked to various autoimmune and inflammatory disorders (Cappellano et al., 2019). People with T1D are becoming far more frequent, especially young infants. This has prompted intensive research efforts centered on the development of self-antigen-specific (such as insulin-specific) immunotherapies as a safe and targeted means of preventing type 1 diabetes (T1D). In fact, treatments that target certain self-antigens have advanced (Serr et al., 2014). T1D still has no recognized treatment, and utilizing dipilizab has not always prevented or reduced disease progression to stage 3 or insulin-requiring diabetes in those with the condition. Thus, the search for a more comprehensive and long-lasting treatment is ongoing. More recent information is available, demonstrating that tDCs act to strengthen, rebuild, and reinforce at least three tightly entangled networks of immunoregulatory and suppressive leukocytes. Expert opinions and prior good evaluations have already been released. tDC may be considered the command center of a multi-level, multi-dimensional defensive network because no other T1D therapy has yet to achieve what it has (Giannoukakis, 2023).

9.4.2 ROLE OF LIFESTYLE INTERVENTIONS

9.4.2.1 DIET AND EXERCISE

A crucial tactic for promoting weight reduction and lifestyle adjustment is included in the majority of programs. Behavioral lifestyle therapies often combine measures aimed at encouraging food and physical activity improvements with behavioral components (Gostoli et al., 2024). The advent of cutting-edge medical technologies has opened new possibilities for better diabetic care. This is particularly important given the intricacy of the condition and the need for constant monitoring and adjustments to the treatment plan. They include advanced glucose monitoring equipment and patient data tracking and analysis software. Artificial intelligence (AI) is a tool that improves patient outcomes and care by analyzing vast datasets to forecast risks, precisely interpreting test findings, and creating personalized treatment regimens. When AI is incorporated into the health care system, it has the potential to significantly reduce the burden of controlling diabetes and shift the field toward a more proactive and targeted approach. Along with identifying knowledge gaps and offering recommendations for future studies, it assesses AI's readiness for incorporation into healthcare (Khalifa and Albadawy, 2024). Some people prefer a high-carbohydrate, low-fat (HCLF) diet. However, successful energy restriction and carbohydrate meal planning are key components of metabolic management and weight loss. Studies indicate that the majority of high-carbohydrate items in HCLF diets should come from whole grains and other forms of high-fiber, complex carbohydrates, particularly those with a low glycemic index. The HCLF diet was not the only available choice. All healthy diets that vary greatly in their macronutrient balances aid in weight loss, provided that an energy deficit is maintained; nevertheless, the differences between the diets become more apparent when they are followed. Consequently, diets may be tailored to the preferences of individual clients. The two alternative strategies discussed below are high-protein diets and diets of the Mediterranean style (Walker et al., 2010a). An increasing amount of data from short-term dietary experiments suggests that typical low-fat, high-carbohydrate diets are not as effective for weight loss as low-carbohydrate, high-protein diets. Studies have shown that when weight is reduced, proteins help retain lean body mass, decrease hunger, and increase thermogenesis. Regardless of weight fluctuations, high-protein diets may help individuals with type 2 diabetes by improving insulin sensitivity and glycemic management, as well as by reducing the chance of developing the disease. However, due to concomitant increases in fat consumption, faster deterioration in renal function, and greater calcium loss that may result in kidney stones and osteoporosis, there are concerns that high-protein diets might lead to dyslipidemia (Walker et al., 2010b). Based on studies of the dietary customs of several Mediterranean cultures, Ancel keys originally described the Mediterranean diet in the 1960s. The Mediterranean diet is a plant-based diet that places heavy emphasis on whole grains, monounsaturated fats, fresh, in-season produce, and fruits as a traditional dessert. This also calls for a reduction in the consumption of red and processed meat. Olive oil is the major source of fat. It is commonly known that the Mediterranean diet improves glucose management and lowers the risk of heart related diseases in persons with T2D. However, there is a dearth of scientific research on the relationship between Mediterranean diet and glycemic management in individuals with T1DM, particularly in younger individuals. When children with T1D ate more cereals and fish for breakfast and less candy and sweets, they showed a favorable link between a lower mean glucose level and improved HbA1c level (Larsen et al., 2011).

9.4.3 STRESS MANAGEMENT

Stress is thought to have two different effects on glycemic control: directly through a physiological mechanism and indirectly by getting in the way of usual self-care practices. Cortisol and catecholamines are released as a result of physiological arousal, which is associated with stress and hyperglycemic response. Stress can also affect diabetes management by interfering with medication administration, physical activity, and dietary maintenance (Soo and Lam, 2009). Increasing the provider's understanding of the potential for diabetes is the first step in addressing its discomfort. When asked with specific questions or given the opportunity to self-evaluate using a structured screening instrument, the majority of patients may not even be aware that they are experiencing discomfort. Several tools are available to assess emotional discomfort associated with diabetes mellitus. These validated scales can be used in clinical settings (Tareen and Tareen, 2017).

9.5 CLINICAL CHALLENGES AND FUTURE DIRECTIONS

9.5.1 PERSONALIZED IMMUNOMODULATORY THERAPIES

The inability of individual treatments to stop or reverse the course of the illness thus far (teplizumab just postponing clinical progression) may be due to the intricacy of the immunological networks underlying type 1 diabetes. Therefore, it may be necessary to target several routes to provide long-lasting control, ultimately providing a multi-pronged therapy that can be tailored (Deligne et al., 2022). Few immunomodulatory drugs with comparable modes of action have been successfully combined into preclinical models to create clinical trials. In a phase 1 experiment, combined medication was evaluated in type 1 diabetes patients in an effort to promote Treg proliferation and function. This medication impaired C-peptide secretion despite the predicted increase in Tregs, suggesting that the adverse effects of rapamycin on β-cell survival and function offset the tolerance-inducing effect of combination therapy. In contrast, ATG therapy alone was comparable, supporting the ongoing phase 2 study (NCT04509791). Overall, these experiments were not successful, and they might have performed better. For aAb+ at-risk individuals, clinical investigations suggesting combinations of immunotherapies are underway. One such study is a phase II experiment utilizing rituximab and abatacept (NCT03929601). One may hypothesize that the ideal place to start would be to combine antigen-specific immunotherapy with general targeted immunotherapy to selectively and synergistically decrease autoreactive T cell responses while enhancing antigen-specific tolerogenic processes

(Linsley et al., 2021). To date, few studies have examined microbiota-based therapeutics, despite strong evidence linking gut dysbiosis to type 1 diabetes. Most of these trials have focused on fecal transplants, prebiotic/postbiotic therapies, or short-chain fatty acid (SCFA) injections, all of which contribute to the beneficial effects of a healthy microbiota. Further research is needed to determine how these therapies mediate their immunomodulatory effects. Although appealing, the therapeutic effect of autologous polyclonal Treg infusion in T1D patients is minimal; nevertheless, Treg survival and function may be improved by immunomodulatory drugs. Tregs may play a significant role in combination therapies. Patients receiving treatment showed increases in the numbers of infused and endogenous Tregs, but they also showed a significant increase in the growth and activation of cytotoxic CD8+ T cells and NK cells (Li et al., 2020). Utilizing Tregs specific to β-cell antigens based on the medical record of the patient would be an additional and most likely safer way to increase the effectiveness and specificity of this type of cell treatment. This may involve two main approaches: first, using anti-CD3 or anti-CD20 mAbs to block immune responses and related inflammation, and second, enhancing regulatory mechanisms. Anti-CD3 treatment resulted in diabetes remission when BDC2. Autoantigen-specific Tregs were infused, but polyclonal Tregs were not, according to a preclinical study conducted in NOD mice. The B-cell compartment undergoes substantial alterations throughout the progression of T1D due to the presence of autoantibodies that cause the disease. These changes include variations in the frequency of transitional and anergic B cells, along with their responsiveness to IL-21 and B-cell receptor signaling, which are distinct at each stage. This suggests that the timing of interventions targeting B cells is crucial (Serr et al., 2021). Additionally, patients who responded well to rituximab therapy showed higher BCR signaling. Combinatory strategies that consider the phenotype and functions of B cells at particular stages of T1D development may steer patients toward tolerance. Combining immunomodulatory medications with those that aid in restoring the quantity and/or function of damaged β-cells is another strategy for customized combination treatments that may be appropriate for individuals with more severe conditions. For recent-onset T1D patients, ligarglutide, an analog of glucagon-like peptide-1 (GLP-1) that may enhance β-cell mass and function, was coupled with an anti-IL-21 neutralizing mAb, resulting in modest preservation of β cells (Jacobsen et al., 2018). Additionally, liraglutide-related clinical studies using *ex vivo* expanded Tregs are ongoing. The replacement of pancreatic β-cells with modified β-cells derived from induced pluripotent stem cells (iPSCs) is gaining momentum and has the potential to be used in conjunction with certain immunotherapies to treat patients who are obviously diabetic (stage 3 and beyond). In conclusion, every clinical study, including patients with stage 3 T1D, suggests a combination treatment consisting of the selected drug plus daily subcutaneous insulin delivery. This may contribute to some degree to insulin antigen-specific effects. All things considered, combination therapies necessitate considering the right ratio of medications and treatment orders that produce synergistic or complementary effects, in addition to choosing patients who will respond best to the treatment at the right stage of their illness (Ma et al., 2021).

9.5.2 BIOMARKERS FOR TREATMENT RESPONSE

A biomarker is defined as a trait that may indicate pathogenic processes, common biological processes, or pharmacological responses to treatment. Traditional and innovative biomarkers are two categories in which the biomarkers are separated. While the latter, like miRNAs and other proteomic markers, are less often utilized in clinical care, the former, such as HbA1c, are well characterized in research and clinical medicine. To identify new topics for additional experimental research, we concentrated on diagnostic molecular biomarkers, such as proteomics and microRNAs implicated in T1DM and T2DM. Pyridoxal phosphate (PLP) is a cofactor used by this enzyme. Furthermore, two different isoforms of GAD, GAD1 and GAD2, are found in mammals; only GAD2 is expressed in the pancreas. Autoantibodies against GAD1 and GAD2 were produced in T1DM patients. Patients with type 1 diabetes may also exhibit abnormal protein levels (Pearson, 2016). As a glycoprotein, IGRP is exclusive to islet cells and is a member of the glucose-6-phosphatase family. The G6Pase family includes the well-known members, G6Pase-β and G6Pase-α, of which G6Pase-β is widely expressed. IGRP binds to the endoplasmic reticulum (ER) membrane via many helices. IGRP is an essential component in gluconeogenesis and glycogenolysis. Moreover, it has been established that IGRP plays a part in maintaining blood glucose homeostasis (Bundy and Krischer, 2020). Given that the IGRP locus contains the T1D susceptibility region, IDDM7, IGRP may be a potential gene for T1DM. Recent research on T1D has indicated that autoantibodies are generated against IGRP; hence, autoantibody expression levels may be a useful biomarker for the diagnosis of T1D. IA-2 is a 979-residue inactive enzyme belonging to the transmembrane protein tyrosine phosphatase family. Residues 379, 24, and 576 correspond to its intracellular, transmembrane, and extracellular domains, respectively. Recent research has indicated that IA-2 is a crucial component of secretory granules in neuroendocrine cells. IA2 is located at location 35 on the long arm of chromosome 2. The IA-2 gene contains 16 exons and covers more than 20 kb of the genomic DNA. Furthermore, it is thought to be an important autoantigen in T1D. As autoantibodies to IA-2 develop years before T1D clinical manifestations, they can be utilized as predictive biomarkers to determine the likelihood of developing T1D (Jarchum et al., 2008).

9.6 CHALLENGES AND FUTURE PERSPECTIVES

Diabetes, especially type 2 diabetes, presents significant challenges and opportunities for immune regulation. An autoimmune disease called T1D causes insulin insufficiency by attacking pancreatic beta cells. Traditional medicine focuses on blood glucose management rather than on addressing the underlying autoimmune response. Accurately targeting autoimmune responses during therapy without impairing the overall immune function is difficult. Furthermore, the diversity of patient demographics, sickness stages, and genetic backgrounds make it difficult to find a single medicine that is effective for everyone. Although one form of modern immunomodulatory treatment that has shown promise is monoclonal antibodies that target specific immune cells, there are still difficulties, including unfavorable side responses and limited long-term efficacy (Eizirik et al., 2020). Teplizumab, an anti-CD3, can delay the onset of type 1 diabetes; however, it carries the risk of infections and other immune-related complications, and its benefits may gradually diminish over time (Andrade, 2009). Future prospects include the development of more targeted and customized immunotherapies. Advances in genetics and biomarker studies may make it simpler to identify patients who could benefit from certain treatments. Combining immunomodulation with regenerative medicine methods, such as beta-cell replacement or regeneration, may yield more comprehensive solutions. Additionally, state-of-the-art methods, such as delivery systems based on nanoparticles and immunotherapies specific to certain antigens, have the potential to reduce side effects while increasing specificity. To achieve long-term disease modification and improve patient outcomes, successful immunomodulation in diabetes will likely require a multimodal approach that combines state-of-the-art technologies with personalized medicine (Goswami et al., 2022).

9.7 CONCLUSION

The chapter concludes by summarizing the complex interplay between immunological systems and the etiology of diabetes and emphasizing the possibility of therapeutic intervention. Numerous immune cells, including T cells, B cells, and macrophages, along with the complex interactions between cytokines and other inflammatory mediators, are responsible for this autoimmune attack. Understanding these immunological pathways will aid in the development of novel immunomodulatory therapies. Current approaches to restoring immunological homeostasis and shielding β-cells from autoimmune assault include immune tolerance induction, regulatory T-cell treatment, and cytokine modulation. Biotechnology breakthroughs have made it easier to create more focused and tailored treatments, which may lessen the side effects of broad-spectrum immunosuppression. Furthermore, the immune system plays a role in conditions other than type 1 diabetes. Immune cell infiltration in metabolic organs and chronic inflammation contribute to insulin resistance and β-cell function in type 2 diabetes. Immunomodulation has two benefits: first, it reduces inflammation to enhance insulin sensitivity while maintaining β-cell function.

ACKNOWLEDGMENT

The authors express heartfelt gratitude toward the leadership and management of the JSS College of Pharmacy, JSS Academy of Higher Education and Research (JSS AHER), Mysuru, Karnataka, India.

COMPETING INTEREST STATEMENT

The authors declare no conflict of interest.

DISCLAIMER

None

FUNDING

Not applicable

KEYWORDS

- **autoimmunity**
- **chronic inflammation**
- **diabetes mellitus**
- **immunometabolism**
- **immunomodulation**
- **β-cell dysfunction**

REFERENCES

Abós, B., Bailey, C., & Tafalla, C. (2022). Adaptive immunity. In *Principles of Fish Immunology* (pp. 105–140). Springer International Publishing. https://doi.org/10.1007/978-3-030-85420-1_3 (accessed on 2nd February 2026).

Abumaree, M. H., Al Jumah, M. A., Kalionis, B., Jawdat, D., Al Khaldi, A., Abomaray, F. M., et al. (2013). Human placental mesenchymal stem cells (pMSCs) play a role as immune suppressive cells by shifting macrophage differentiation from inflammatory M1 to anti-inflammatory M2 macrophages. *Stem Cell Reviews and Reports, 9*(5), 620–641. https://doi.org/10.1007/s12015-013-9455-2 (accessed on 2nd February 2026).

Andrade, L. E. C. (2009). Future perspective for diagnosis in autoimmune diseases. *Anais da Academia Brasileira de Ciências, 81*(3), 367–380. https://doi.org/10.1590/S0001-37652009000300004 (accessed on 2nd February 2026).

Atkinson, M. A., & Mirmira, R. G. (2023). The pathogenic "symphony" in type 1 diabetes: A disorder of the immune system, β cells, and exocrine pancreas. *Cell Metabolism, 35*(9), 1500–1518. https://doi.org/10.1016/j.cmet.2023.06.018 (accessed on 2nd February 2026).

Ben-Skowronek, I., Sieniawska, J., Pach, E., Wrobel, W., Skowronek, A., Tomczyk, Z., et al. (2021). Potential therapeutic application of regulatory T cells in diabetes mellitus type 1. *International Journal of Molecular Sciences, 23*(1), 390. https://doi.org/10.3390/ijms23010390 (accessed on 2nd February 2026).

Bluemel, S., Wang, Y., Lee, S., & Schnabl, B. (2020). Tumor necrosis factor alpha receptor 1 deficiency in hepatocytes does not protect from non-alcoholic steatohepatitis, but attenuates insulin resistance in mice. *World Journal of Gastroenterology, 26*(33), 4933–4944. https://doi.org/10.3748/wjg.v26.i33.4933 (accessed on 2nd February 2026).

Bluestone, J. A., Buckner, J. H., & Herold, K. C. (2021). Immunotherapy: Building a bridge to a cure for type 1 diabetes. *Science, 373*(6554), 510–516. https://doi.org/10.1126/science.abh1654 (accessed on 2nd February 2026).

Bluestone, J. A., McKenzie, B. S., Beilke, J., & Ramsdell, F. (2023). Opportunities for Treg cell therapy for the treatment of human disease. *Frontiers in Immunology, 14.* https://doi.org/10.3389/fimmu.2023.1166135 (accessed on 2nd February 2026).

Bourlier, V., & Bouloumie, A. (2009). Role of macrophage tissue infiltration in obesity and insulin resistance. *Diabetes & Metabolism, 35*(4), 251–260. https://doi.org/10.1016/j.diabet.2009.05.001 (accessed on 2nd February 2026).

Bundy, B. N., & Krischer, J. P. (2020). A quantitative measure of treatment response in recent-onset type 1 diabetes. *Endocrinology, Diabetes & Metabolism, 3*(3). https://doi.org/10.1002/edm2.143 (accessed on 2nd February 2026).

Cappellano, G., Comi, C., Chiocchetti, A., & Dianzani, U. (2019). Exploiting PLGA-based biocompatible nanoparticles for next-generation tolerogenic vaccines against autoimmune disease. *International Journal of Molecular Sciences, 20*(1), 204. https://doi.org/10.3390/ijms20010204 (accessed on 2nd February 2026).

Chait, A., & den Hartigh, L. J. (2020). Adipose tissue distribution, inflammation and its metabolic consequences, including diabetes and cardiovascular disease. *Frontiers in Cardiovascular Medicine, 7.* https://doi.org/10.3389/fcvm.2020.00022 (accessed on 2nd February 2026).

Chan, L., Karimi, N., Morovati, S., Alizadeh, K., Kakish, J. E., Vanderkamp, S., et al. (2021). The roles of neutrophils in cytokine storms. *Viruses, 13*(11), 2318. https://doi.org/10.3390/v13112318 (accessed on 2nd February 2026).

Chandrasekharan, U. M., Kaur, R., Harvey, J. E., Braley, C., Rai, V., Lee, M., et al. (2022). TNFR2 depletion reduces psoriatic inflammation in mice by downregulating specific dendritic cell populations in lymph nodes and inhibiting IL-23/IL-17 pathways. *Journal of Investigative Dermatology, 142*(8), 2159–2172.e9. https://doi.org/10.1016/j.jid.2021.12.036 (accessed on 2nd February 2026).

Chye, A., Allen, I., Barnet, M., & Burnett, D. L. (2022). Insights into the host contribution of endocrine-associated immune-related adverse events to immune checkpoint inhibition therapy. *Frontiers in Oncology, 12.* https://doi.org/10.3389/fonc.2022.894015 (accessed on 2nd February 2026).

Cooper, E. L. (2010). Evolution of immune systems from self/not self to danger to artificial immune systems (AIS). *Physics of Life Reviews, 7*(1), 55–78. https://doi.org/10.1016/j.plrev.2009.12.001 (accessed on 2nd February 2026).

Costa, F. R. C., Leite, J. A., Rassi, D. M., da Silva, J. F., Elias-Oliveira, J., Guimarães, J. B., et al. (2021). NLRP1 acts as a negative regulator of Th17 cell programming in mice and humans with autoimmune diabetes. *Cell Reports, 35*(8), 109176. https://doi.org/10.1016/j.celrep.2021.109176 (accessed on 2nd February 2026).

Deligne, C., You, S., & Mallone, R. (2022). Personalized immunotherapies for type 1 diabetes: Who, what, when, and how? *Journal of Personalized Medicine, 12*(4), 542. https://doi.org/10.3390/jpm12040542 (accessed on 2nd February 2026).

Dettmer, R., Niwolik, I., Cirksena, K., Yoshimoto, T., Tang, Y., Mehmeti, I., et al. (2022). Proinflammatory cytokines induce rapid, NO-independent apoptosis, expression of chemotactic mediators and interleukin-32 secretion in human pluripotent stem cell-derived beta cells. *Diabetology, 65*(5), 829–843. https://doi.org/10.1007/s00125-022-05654-0 (accessed on 2nd February 2026).

dos Santos Haber, J. F., Barbalho, S. M., Sgarbi, J. A., de Argollo Haber, R. S., de Labio, R. W., Laurindo, L. F., et al. (2023). The relationship between type 1 diabetes mellitus,

TNF-α, and IL-10 gene expression. *Biomedicines, 11*(4), 1120. https://doi.org/10.3390/biomedicines11041120 (accessed on 2nd February 2026).

Eggenhuizen, P. J., Ng, B. H., & Ooi, J. D. (2020). Treg enhancing therapies to treat autoimmune diseases. *International Journal of Molecular Sciences, 21*(19), 7015. https://doi.org/10.3390/ijms21197015 (accessed on 2nd February 2026).

Eizirik, D. L., Pasquali, L., & Cnop, M. (2020). Pancreatic β-cells in type 1 and type 2 diabetes mellitus: Different pathways to failure. *Nature Reviews Endocrinology, 16*(7), 349–362. https://doi.org/10.1038/s41574-020-0355-7 (accessed on 2nd February 2026).

Fadaei, R., Bagheri, N., Heidarian, E., Nouri, A., Hesari, Z., Moradi, N., et al. (2020). Serum levels of IL-32 in patients with type 2 diabetes mellitus and its relationship with TNF-α and IL-6. *Cytokine, 125*, 154832. https://doi.org/10.1016/j.cyto.2019.154832 (accessed on 2nd February 2026).

Fan, X., Zhang, X., Liu, L. C., Kim, A. Y., Curley, S. P., Chen, X., et al. (2022). Interleukin-10 attenuates renal injury after myocardial infarction in diabetes. *Journal of Investigative Medicine, 70*(5), 1233–1242. https://doi.org/10.1136/jim-2021-002008 (accessed on 2nd February 2026).

Gianchecchi, E., & Fierabracci, A. (2018). Inhibitory receptors and pathways of lymphocytes: The role of PD-1 in Treg development and their involvement in autoimmunity onset and cancer progression. *Frontiers in Immunology, 9*. https://doi.org/10.3389/fimmu.2018.02374 (accessed on 2nd February 2026).

Giannoukakis, N. (2023). Tolerogenic dendritic cells in type 1 diabetes: No longer a concept. *Frontiers in Immunology, 14*. https://doi.org/10.3389/fimmu.2023.1212641 (accessed on 2nd February 2026).

Goltermann, J., Repple, J., Redlich, R., Dohm, K., Flint, C., Grotegerd, D., et al. (2021). Apolipoprotein E homozygous ε4 allele status: Effects on cortical structure and white matter integrity in young to mid-age sample. *European Neuropsychopharmacology, 46*, 93–104. https://doi.org/10.1016/j.euroneuro.2021.02.006 (accessed on 2nd February 2026).

Gostoli, S., Raimondi, G., Popa, A. P., Giovannini, M., Benasi, G., & Rafanelli, C. (2024). Behavioral lifestyle interventions for weight loss in overweight or obese patients with type 2 diabetes: A systematic review of the literature. *Current Obesity Reports, 13*(2), 224–241. https://doi.org/10.1007/s13679-024-00552-5 (accessed on 2nd February 2026).

Goswami, T. K., Singh, M., Dhawan, M., Mitra, S., Emran, T. B, Rabaan, A. A., et al. (2022). Regulatory T cells (Tregs) and their therapeutic potential against autoimmune disorders–Advances and challenges. *Human Vaccines & Immunotherapeutics, 18*(1). https://doi.org/10.1080/21645515.2022.2035117 (accessed on 2nd February 2026).

Jacobsen, L. M., Newby, B. N., Perry, D. J., Posgai, A. L., Haller, M. J., & Brusko, T. M. (2018). Immune mechanisms and pathways targeted in type 1 diabetes. *Current Diabetes Reports, 18*(10), 90. https://doi.org/10.1007/s11892-018-1066-5 (accessed on 2nd February 2026).

Jarchum, I., Nichol, L., Trucco, M., Santamaria, P., & DiLorenzo, T. P. (2008). Identification of novel IGRP epitopes targeted in type 1 diabetes patients. *Clinical Immunology, 127*(3), 359–365. https://doi.org/10.1016/j.clim.2008.01.015 (accessed on 2nd February 2026).

Jia, X., & Yu, L. (2023). Understanding islet autoantibodies in prediction of type 1 diabetes. *Journal of the Endocrine Society, 8*(1). https://doi.org/10.1210/jendso/bvad160 (accessed on 2nd February 2026).

Kawasaki, E. (2023). Anti-islet autoantibodies in type 1 diabetes. *International Journal of Molecular Sciences, 24*(12), 10012. https://doi.org/10.3390/ijms241210012 (accessed on 2nd February 2026).

Ke, Q., Kroger, C. J., Clark, M., & Tisch, R. M. (2021). Evolving antibody therapies for the treatment of type 1 diabetes. *Frontiers in Immunology, 11.* https://doi.org/10.3389/fimmu.2020.624568 (accessed on 2nd February 2026).

Khalifa, M., & Albadawy, M. (2024). Artificial intelligence for diabetes: Enhancing prevention, diagnosis, and effective management. *Computer Methods and Programs in Biomedicine Update, 5,* 100141. https://doi.org/10.1016/j.cmpbup.2024.100141 (accessed on 2nd February 2026).

Khan, F. U., Khongorzul, P., Raki, A. A., Rajasekaran, A., Gris, D., & Amrani, A. (2022). Dendritic cells and their immunotherapeutic potential for treating type 1 diabetes. *International Journal of Molecular Sciences, 23*(9), 4885. https://doi.org/10.3390/ijms23094885 (accessed on 2nd February 2026).

Khan, S., & Gerber, D. E. (2020). Autoimmunity, checkpoint inhibitor therapy and immune-related adverse events: A review. *Seminars in Cancer Biology, 64,* 93–101. https://doi.org/10.1016/j.semcancer.2019.06.012 (accessed on 2nd February 2026).

Khdair, S. I., Al-Naimat, O. S., Jarrar, W., Al-Qerem, W., & Khudeir, F. A. (2023). The influence of TNF-α, IL-6, TGF-β1, IFN-γ, IL-10 polymorphisms on predisposition to diabetes mellitus among Jordanian patients. *Endocrine, Metabolic & Immune Disorders–Drug Targets, 23*(5), 681–691. https://doi.org/10.2174/1871530322666220827143530 (accessed on 2nd February 2026).

Kiboneka, A. (2021). Principals of innate and adaptive immunity. Immunity to microbes & fundamental concepts in immunology. *World Journal of Advanced Research and Reviews, 10*(3), 188–197. https://doi.org/10.30574/wjarr.2021.10.3.0271 (accessed on 2nd February 2026).

Kong, Y. M., & Flynn, J. C. (2014). Opportunistic autoimmune disorders potentiated by immune-checkpoint inhibitors anti-CTLA-4 and anti-PD-1. *Frontiers in Immunology, 5.* https://doi.org/10.3389/fimmu.2014.00206 (accessed on 2nd February 2026).

Kucuksezer, U. C., Aktas Cetin, E., Esen, F., Tahrali, I., Akdeniz, N., Gelmez, M. Y., et al. (2021). The role of natural killer cells in autoimmune diseases. *Frontiers in Immunology, 12.* https://doi.org/10.3389/fimmu.2021.622306 (accessed on 2nd February 2026).

Larsen, R. N., Mann, N. J., Maclean, E., & Shaw, J. E. (2011). The effect of high-protein, low-carbohydrate diets in the treatment of type 2 diabetes: A 12-month randomized controlled trial. *Diabetology, 54*(4), 731–740. https://doi.org/10.1007/s00125-010-2027-y (accessed on 2nd February 2026).

Leadbetter, E. A., & Karlsson, M. C. I. (2021). Invariant natural killer T cells balance B cell immunity. *Immunological Reviews, 299*(1), 93–107. https://doi.org/10.1111/imr.12938 (accessed on 2nd February 2026).

Lee, J. (2013). Adipose tissue macrophages in the development of obesity-induced inflammation, insulin resistance and type 2 diabetes. *Archives of Pharmacal Research, 36*(2), 208–222. https://doi.org/10.1007/s12272-013-0023-8 (accessed on 2nd February 2026).

Li, C., Jiang, P., Wei, S., Xu, X., & Wang, J. (2020). Regulatory T cells in tumor microenvironment: New mechanisms, potential therapeutic strategies and future prospects. *Molecular Cancer, 19*(1), 116. https://doi.org/10.1186/s12943-020-01234-1 (accessed on 2nd February 2026).

Liaskou, E., Jeffery, L. E., Trivedi, P. J., Reynolds, G. M., Suresh, S., Bruns, T., et al. (2014). Loss of CD28 expression by liver-infiltrating T cells contributes to pathogenesis of primary sclerosing cholangitis. *Gastroenterology, 147*(1), 221–232.e7. https://doi.org/10.1053/j.gastro.2014.04.003 (accessed on 2nd February 2026).

Lim, W. S., Teoh, S. E., Tang, A. S. P., Tan, B. J. M., Lee, J. Y., Yau, C. E., et al. (2024). The effects of anti-TNF-α biologics on insulin resistance and insulin sensitivity in patients with rheumatoid arthritis: An updated systematic review and meta-analysis. *Diabetes & Metabolic Syndrome: Clinical Research & Reviews, 18*(4), 103001. https://doi.org/10.1016/j.dsx.2024.103001 (accessed on 2nd February 2026).

Linsley, P. S., Greenbaum, C. J., & Nepom, G. T. (2021). Uncovering pathways to personalized therapies in type 1 diabetes. *Diabetes, 70*(4), 831–841. https://doi.org/10.2337/db20-1185 (accessed on 2nd February 2026).

Liu, K., & Nussenzweig, M. C. (2010). Origin and development of dendritic cells. *Immunological Reviews, 234*(1), 45–54. https://doi.org/10.1111/j.0105-2896.2009.00879.x (accessed on 2nd February 2026).

López-Gambero, A. J., Sanjuan, C., Serrano-Castro, P. J., Suárez, J., & Rodríguez de Fonseca, F. (2020). The biomedical uses of inositols: A nutraceutical approach to metabolic dysfunction in aging and neurodegenerative diseases. *Biomedicines, 8*(9), 295. https://doi.org/10.3390/biomedicines8090295 (accessed on 2nd February 2026).

Lu, J., Liu, J., Li, L., Lan, Y., & Liang, Y. (2020). Cytokines in type 1 diabetes: Mechanisms of action and immunotherapeutic targets. *Clinical & Translational Immunology, 9*(3). https://doi.org/10.1002/cti2.1122 (accessed on 2nd February 2026).

Ma, X., Liu, Z., Ilyas, I., Little, P. J., Kamato, D., Sahebka, A., et al. (2021). GLP-1 receptor agonists (GLP-1RAs): Cardiovascular actions and therapeutic potential. *International Journal of Biological Sciences, 17*(8), 2050–2068. https://doi.org/10.7150/ijbs.59965 (accessed on 2nd February 2026).

Mallone, R., & Eizirik, D. L. (2020). Presumption of innocence for beta cells: Why are they vulnerable autoimmune targets in type 1 diabetes? *Diabetology, 63*(10), 1999–2006. https://doi.org/10.1007/s00125-020-05176-7 (accessed on 2nd February 2026).

Mandal, A., & Viswanathan, C. (2015). Natural killer cells: In health and disease. *Hematology/Oncology and Stem Cell Therapy, 8*(2), 47–55. https://doi.org/10.1016/j.hemonc.2014.11.006 (accessed on 2nd February 2026).

Mbongue, J. C., Nieves, H. A., Torrez, T. W., & Langridge, W. H. R. (2017). The role of dendritic cell maturation in the induction of insulin-dependent diabetes mellitus. *Frontiers in Immunology, 8.* https://doi.org/10.3389/fimmu.2017.00327 (accessed on 2nd February 2026).

Meshkani, R., & Vakili, S. (2016). Tissue resident macrophages: Key players in the pathogenesis of type 2 diabetes and its complications. *Clinica Chemical Acta, 462*, 77–89. https://doi.org/10.1016/j.cca.2016.08.015 (accessed on 2nd February 2026).

Mukhtar, Y., Galalain, A., & Yunusa, U. (2020). A modern overview on diabetes mellitus: A chronic endocrine disorder. *European Journal of Biology, 5*(2), 1–14. https://doi.org/10.47672/ejb.409 (accessed on 2nd February 2026).

Naidoo, V., Naidoo, M., & Ghai, M. (2018). Cell- and tissue-specific epigenetic changes associated with chronic inflammation in insulin resistance and type 2 diabetes mellitus. *Scandinavian Journal of Immunology, 88*(6). https://doi.org/10.1111/sji.12723 (accessed on 2nd February 2026).

Nekoua, M. P., Dechaumes, A., Sane, F., Alidjinou, E. K., Moutairou, K., Yessoufou, A., et al. (2020). Enteroviral pathogenesis of type 1 diabetes: The role of natural killer cells. *Microorganisms, 8*(7), 989. https://doi.org/10.3390/microorganisms8070989 (accessed on 2nd February 2026).

Nicholson, L. B. (2016). The immune system. *Essays in Biochemistry, 60*(3), 275–301. https://doi.org/10.1042/EBC20160017 (accessed on 2nd February 2026).

Nikolic, I., Leiva, M., & Sabio, G. (2020). The role of stress kinases in metabolic disease. *Nature Reviews Endocrinology, 16*(12), 697–716. https://doi.org/10.1038/s41574-020-00418-5 (accessed on 2nd February 2026).

Ogra, P. L., Faden, H., & Welliver, R. C. (2001). Vaccination strategies for mucosal immune responses. *Clinical Microbiology Reviews, 14*(2), 430–445. https://doi.org/10.1128/CMR.14.2.430-445.2001 (accessed on 2nd February 2026).

Park, J. H., Lee, K. H., Jeon, B., Ochs, H. D., Lee, J. S., Gee, H. Y., et al. (2020). Immune dysregulation, polyendocrinopathy, enteropathy, X-linked (IPEX) syndrome: A systematic review. *Autoimmunity Reviews, 19*(6), 102526. https://doi.org/10.1016/j.autrev.2020.102526 (accessed on 2nd February 2026).

Pearson, E. R. (2016). Personalized medicine in diabetes: The role of 'omics' and biomarkers. *Diabetic Medicine, 33*(6), 712–717. https://doi.org/10.1111/dme.13075 (accessed on 2nd February 2026).

Plows, J. F., Stanley, J. L., Baker, P. N., Reynolds, C. M., & Vickers, M. H. (2018). The pathophysiology of gestational diabetes mellitus. *International Journal of Molecular Sciences, 19*(11), 3342. https://doi.org/10.3390/ijms19113342 (accessed on 2nd February 2026).

Quandt, Z., Young, A., & Anderson, M. (2020). Immune checkpoint inhibitor diabetes mellitus: A novel form of autoimmune diabetes. *Clinical and Experimental Immunology, 200*(2), 131–140. https://doi.org/10.1111/cei.13424 (accessed on 2nd February 2026).

Rai, K. R., Shrestha, P., Yang, B., Chen, Y., Liu, S., Maarouf, M., et al. (2021). Acute infection of viral pathogens and their innate immune escape. *Frontiers in Microbiology, 12*. https://doi.org/10.3389/fmicb.2021.672026 (accessed on 2nd February 2026).

Ramessur, R., Corbett, M., Marshall, D., Acencio, M. L., Barbosa, I. A., Dand, N., et al. (2022). Biomarkers of disease progression in people with psoriasis: A scoping review. *British Journal of Dermatology, 187*(4), 481–493. https://doi.org/10.1111/bjd.21627 (accessed on 2nd February 2026).

Ramponi, G., Brunetta, E., & Folci, M. (2022a). Role of Th1 and Th2 in autoimmunity. In *Translational Autoimmunity* (pp. 61–92). Elsevier. https://doi.org/10.1016/B978-0-12-822564-6.00020-3 (accessed on 2nd February 2026).

Roep, B. O., Thomaidou, S., van Tienhoven, R., & Zaldumbide, A. (2021). Type 1 diabetes mellitus as a disease of the β-cell (do not blame the immune system?). *Nature Reviews Endocrinology, 17*(3), 150–161. https://doi.org/10.1038/s41574-020-00443-4 (accessed on 2nd February 2026).

Rosol, T. J., Brändli-Baiocco, A., Hoenerhoff, M. J., & Vahle, J. L. (2024). Endocrine system. In *Haschek and Rousseaux's Handbook of Toxicologic Pathology* (pp. 517–631). Elsevier. https://doi.org/10.1016/B978-0-12-821046-8.00002-5 (accessed on 2nd February 2026).

Serr, I., Drost, F., Schubert, B., & Daniel, C. (2021). Antigen-specific Treg therapy in type 1 diabetes–Challenges and opportunities. *Frontiers in Immunology, 12.* https://doi.org/10.3389/fimmu.2021.712870 (accessed on 2nd February 2026).

Serr, I., Weigmann, B., Franke, R. K., & Daniel, C. (2014). Treg vaccination in autoimmune type 1 diabetes. *Bio Drugs, 28*(1), 7–16. https://doi.org/10.1007/s40259-013-0060-3 (accessed on 2nd February 2026).

Sharma, S. R., & Sharma, B. (2022). Immunity: A step-by-step overview. *Homeopathic Links, 35*(01), 048–055. https://doi.org/10.1055/s-0042-1745813 (accessed on 2nd February 2026).

Soo, H., & Lam, S. (2009). Stress management training in diabetes mellitus. *Journal of Health Psychology, 14*(7), 933–943. https://doi.org/10.1177/1359105309341146 (accessed on 2nd February 2026).

Starska-Kowarska, K. (2023). The role of different immunocompetent cell populations in the pathogenesis of head and neck cancer—Regulatory mechanisms of pro- and anti-cancer activity and their impact on immunotherapy. *Cancers (Basel), 15*(6), 1642. https://doi.org/10.3390/cancers15061642 (accessed on 2nd February 2026).

Surmi, B., & Hasty, A. (2008). Macrophage infiltration into adipose tissue: Initiation, propagation and remodeling. *Future Lipidology, 3*(5), 545–556. https://doi.org/10.2217/17460875.3.5.545 (accessed on 2nd February 2026).

Tao, Z., Shi, A., & Zhao, J. (2015). Epidemiological perspectives of diabetes. *Cell Biochemistry and Biophysics, 73*(1), 181–185. https://doi.org/10.1007/s12013-015-0598-4 (accessed on 2nd February 2026).

Tareen, R. S., & Tareen, K. (2017). Psychosocial aspects of diabetes management: Dilemma of diabetes distress. *Translational Pediatrics, 6*(4), 383–396. https://doi.org/10.21037/tp.2017.10.04 (accessed on 2nd February 2026).

Thornley, T. B., Agarwal, K. A., Kyriazis, P., Ma, L., Chipashvili, V., Aker, J. E., et al. (2016). Contrasting roles of islet resident immunoregulatory macrophages and dendritic cells in experimental autoimmune type 1 diabetes. *PLoS One, 11*(3), e0150792. https://doi.org/10.1371/journal.pone.0150792 (accessed on 2nd February 2026).

Tsai, S., Shameli, A., & Santamaria, P. (2008). Chapter 4: CD8+ T cells in type 1 diabetes. *Advances in Immunology, 100*, 79–124. https://doi.org/10.1016/S0065-2776(08)00804-3 (accessed on 2nd February 2026).

Vallerskog, T., Martens, G. W., & Kornfeld, H. (2010). Diabetic mice display a delayed adaptive immune response to *Mycobacterium tuberculosis*. *The Journal of Immunology, 184*(11), 6275–6282. https://doi.org/10.4049/jimmunol.1000304 (accessed on 2nd February 2026).

Varela-Calviño, R., Calviño-Sampedro, C., Gómez-Touriño, I., & Cordero, O. J. (2017a). Apportioning blame: Autoreactive CD4+ and CD8+ T cells in type 1 diabetes. *Archives of Immunology and Therapy Experimentalis (Warsz), 65*(4), 275–284. https://doi.org/10.1007/s00005-016-0452-4 (accessed on 2nd February 2026).

Varra, F. N., Varras, M., Varra, V. K., & Theodosis Nobelos, P. (2024). Molecular and pathophysiological relationship between obesity and chronic inflammation in the manifestation of metabolic dysfunctions and their inflammation mediating treatment options (Review). *Molecular Medicine Reports, 29*(6), 95. https://doi.org/10.3892/mmr.2024.13219 (accessed on 2nd February 2026).

Velikova, T. V., Kabakchieva, P. P., Assyov, Y. S., & Georgiev, T. A. (2021a). Targeting inflammatory cytokines to improve type 2 diabetes control. *BioMed Research International, 2021*, 1–12. https://doi.org/10.1155/2021/7297419 (accessed on 2nd February 2026).

Velikova, T., Valkov, H., Aleksandrova, A., Peshevska-Sekulovska, M., Sekulovski, M., & Shumnalieva, R. (2024). Harnessing immunity: Immunomodulatory therapies in COVID-19. *World Journal of Virology, 13*(2). https://doi.org/10.5501/wjv.v13.i2.92521 (accessed on 2nd February 2026).

Vivier, E., Tomasello, E., Baratin, M., Walzer, T., & Ugolini, S. (2008). Functions of natural killer cells. *Nature Immunology, 9*(5), 503–510. https://doi.org/10.1038/ni1582 (accessed on 2nd February 2026).

Walker, K. Z., O'Dea, K., Gomez, M., Girgis, S., & Colagiuri, R. (2010a). Diet and exercise in the prevention of diabetes. *Journal of Human Nutrition and Dietetics, 23*(4), 344–352. https://doi.org/10.1111/j.1365-277X.2010.01061.x (accessed on 2nd February 2026).

Walker, L. S. K., & von Herrath, M. (2015). CD4 T cell differentiation in type 1 diabetes. *Clinical and Experimental Immunology, 183*(1), 16–29. https://doi.org/10.1111/cei.12672 (accessed on 2nd February 2026).

Wang, N., Liang, H., & Zen, K. (2014). Molecular mechanisms that influence the macrophage M1–M2 polarization balance. *Frontiers in Immunology, 5*. https://doi.org/10.3389/fimmu.2014.00614 (accessed on 2nd February 2026).

Wang, S. J., Dougan, S. K., & Dougan, M. (2023). Immune mechanisms of toxicity from checkpoint inhibitors. *Trends in Cancer, 9*(7), 543–553. https://doi.org/10.1016/j.trecan.2023.04.002 (accessed on 2nd February 2026).

Wilcox, N. S., Rui, J., Hebrok, M., & Herold, K. C. (2016). Life and death of β cells in type 1 diabetes: A comprehensive review. *Journal of Autoimmunity, 71*, 51–58. https://doi.org/10.1016/j.jaut.2016.02.001 (accessed on 2nd February 2026).

Winter, W. E., Pittman, D. L., & Jialal, I. (2022). Practical clinical applications of islet autoantibody testing in type 1 diabetes. *Journal of Applied Laboratory Medicine, 7*(1), 197–205. https://doi.org/10.1093/jalm/jfab113 (accessed on 2nd February 2026).

Xie, F., Teng, L., Lu, J., Xu, J., Zhang, C., Yang, L., et al. (2022). Interleukin-10-modified adipose-derived mesenchymal stem cells prevent hypertrophic scar formation via regulating the biological characteristics of fibroblasts and inflammation. *Mediators of Inflammation, 2022*, 1–16. https://doi.org/10.1155/2022/6368311 (accessed on 2nd February 2026).

Yang, H., Yao, Z., Zhou, X., Zhang, W., Zhang, X., & Zhang, F. (2020). Immune-related adverse events of checkpoint inhibitors: Insights into immunological dysregulation. *Clinical Immunology, 213*, 108377. https://doi.org/10.1016/j.clim.2020.108377 (accessed on 2nd February 2026).

Youssef, N., Noureldein, M., Daoud, G., & Eid, A. A. (2021). Immune checkpoint inhibitors and diabetes: Mechanisms and predictors. *Diabetes & Metabolism, 47*(3), 101193. https://doi.org/10.1016/j.diabet.2020.09.003 (accessed on 2nd February 2026).

Zhai, Y., Moosavi, R., & Chen, M. (2021). Immune checkpoints, a novel class of therapeutic targets for autoimmune diseases. *Frontiers in Immunology, 12*. https://doi.org/10.3389/fimmu.2021.645699 (accessed on 2nd February 2026).

Zi, C., He, L., Yao, H., Ren, Y., He, T., & Gao, Y. (2022). Changes of Th17 cells, regulatory T cells, Treg/Th17, IL-17 and IL-10 in patients with type 2 diabetes mellitus: A systematic review and meta-analysis. *Endocrine, 76*(2), 263–272. https://doi.org/10.1007/s12020-022-03043-6 (accessed on 2nd February 2026).

Zieliński, M., Sakowska, J., Iwaszkiewicz-Grześ, D., Gliwiński, M., Hennig, M., Żalińska, M., et al. (2024). PD-1 receptor (+) T cells are associated with the efficacy of the combined treatment with regulatory T cells and rituximab in type 1 diabetes children via regulatory T cells suppressive activity amelioration. *International Immunopharmacology, 132*, 111919. https://doi.org/10.1016/j.intimp.2024.111919 (accessed on 2nd February 2026).

Zimmet, P. Z., Magliano, D. J., Herman, W. H., & Shaw, J. E. (2014). Diabetes: A 21st century challenge. *The Lancet Diabetes & Endocrinology, 2*(1), 56–64. https://doi.org/10.1016/S2213-8587(13)70112-8 (accessed on 2nd February 2026).

Zozulińska, D., & Wierusz-Wysocka, B. (2006). Type 2 diabetes mellitus as inflammatory disease. *Diabetes Research and Clinical Practice, 74*(2), S12–S16. https://doi.org/10.1016/j.diabres.2006.06.007 (accessed on 2nd February 2026).

CHAPTER 10

Synthetic Innovations: Engineering Solutions in Diabetes

WAN NURHIDAYAH WAN HANAFFI,[1,2] NAZISH NASEEM,[3] USAMA AHMAD,[3,*] ANAS ISLAM,[3] and MOHD. MUAZZAM KHAN[3]

[1]*Laboratoire de Chimie Physique Macromoléculaire, Université de Lorraine, CNRS, Nancy, France*

[2]*Department of Immunology, School of Medical Sciences, Universiti Sains Malaysia, Kelantan, Malaysia*

[3]*Faculty of Pharmacy, Integral University, Lucknow, Uttar Pradesh, India*

*Corresponding author

ABSTRACT

The global increase in diabetes incidence necessitates the investigation of innovative management strategies for this chronic illness. Advances in synthetic innovations are crucial to address the complexities of diabetes treatment. The convergence of synthetic biology and engineered biological systems has fostered novel therapeutic methods, particularly for insulin administration and glucose management. Key innovations include engineered cells, encapsulation techniques, and biohybrid devices that enhance diabetes management while minimizing the frequency of insulin injection. These synthetic advancements are transforming diabetes care by designing biological systems for specific functions, such as insulin release in response to glucose levels. This domain has the capacity to develop advanced therapies that replicate natural glucose regulation by pancreatic β-cells, thereby offering an alternative to conventional treatment methods.

Diabetes: Novel Insights and Therapies. Anas Islam and Badruddeen (Eds)

DOI: 10.1201/9781779644596-14

Significant progress has been made in glucose-responsive synthetic systems and nanomedicines that regulate insulin release according to glucose elevation, emulating β-cell functionality. These novel approaches promise to enhance the quality of life of patients with diabetes by facilitating natural glucose control.

10.1 INTRODUCTION: THE STORY OF DIABETES

The historical chronology of diabetes can be delineated over a span exceeding 3500 years, originating in ancient Egypt, where the earliest documented reference to this ailment was inscribed on the Ebers Papyrus circa 1550 BCE. This manuscript elucidates the condition characterized by polyuria; a clinical manifestation presently acknowledged as indicative of diabetes mellitus (Carpenter et al., 2006). Ancient Indian medical practitioners observed the sweetness present in the urine of individuals with diabetes, calling it "madhumeha," which translates to "honey urine" (Lakhtakia, 2013).

The word "diabetes" originates from the Greek word "siphon," introduced by the Greek physician Aretaeus of Cappadocia in the 2nd century CE to describe a condition in which patients appeared to "pass water like a siphon" (Retief and Cilliers, 2009). The term "mellitus," meaning "honey-sweet," was later added by British surgeon Thomas Willis in the 17th century to differentiate this condition from diabetes insipidus, which does not involve sugar metabolism (Willis, 1674).

During the Middle Ages, diabetes was widely misunderstood and believed to be a disorder of the kidneys or other organs. Treatments were basic and generally ineffective, consisting of dietary restrictions, herbal remedies, and bloodletting (Tattersall, 2009).

Significant advances in the understanding and management of diabetes began in the 19th century. In 1869, Paul Langerhans, a German medical student, identified clusters of cells in the pancreas, later named the Islets of Langerhans. These cells produce insulin, a hormone essential for regulating glucose (Tepperman, 1988).

The most crucial advancements in the history of diabetes occurred in the early 20th century. In 1921, Canadian researchers Frederick Banting and Charles Best, with the assistance of John Macleod and James Collip, successfully isolated insulin and demonstrated its effectiveness in reducing blood glucose levels (BGLs) in diabetic dogs. The first successful insulin treatment of a human patient, a 14-year-old boy named Leonard Thompson, occurred in 1922, ushering in a new era of diabetes management (Bliss, 1997).

Insulin therapy has changed diabetes from a deadly disease to a manageable chronic condition. In the ensuing decades, improvements in insulin production, such as the creation of long-acting and synthetic insulins, have significantly enhanced patient outcomes (Banting et al., 1922). By the mid-20th century, the introduction of oral hypoglycemic agents offered new ways to manage type 2 diabetes (Alhadramy, 2016).

The late 20th and early 21st centuries witnessed significant progress in diabetes research and treatment. Innovations, such as continuous glucose monitors (CGMs), insulin pumps, and advancements in synthetic biology and bioengineering, including glucose-responsive insulin (GRI) and islet cell transplantation, have emerged. These developments aim to improve diabetes management by closely replicating natural glucose regulation and reducing the daily burden of disease management (Jarosinski et al., 2021).

Currently, despite diabetes persisting as a considerable global health dilemma, continuous investigative efforts and technological innovations are progressively improving the quality of life for millions across the globe, instilling optimism for more efficacious therapeutic interventions and the possibility of a future remedy (Zimmet et al., 2001). A brief history of its development is illustrated in Figure 10.1.

10.1.1 GLOBAL PREVALENCE AND CHALLENGES

Diabetes mellitus (DM) has rapidly become a major global health issue. By the year 2023, it is projected that more than 540 million individuals worldwide will be affected by diabetes, and this number is expected to rise to 783 million by 2045 (Sun et al., 2022; WHO, 2023). The escalating incidence is driven by an array of determinants, including demographic transitions towards older age groups, the progressive movement towards urban living, alterations in nutritional practices, and the worldwide increase in rates of obesity (McLachlan et al., 2016; Zimmet et al., 2014). The fight against this growing public health emergency demands concerted efforts to promote health, improve access to healthcare, and ongoing research to create more effective preventative and treatment strategies.

An estimated 529–537 million adults worldwide between the ages of 20 and 79 years were predicted to have diabetes in 2021, with an estimated prevalence of 6.1% to 10.5% (Forouhi and Wareham, 2022; Ong

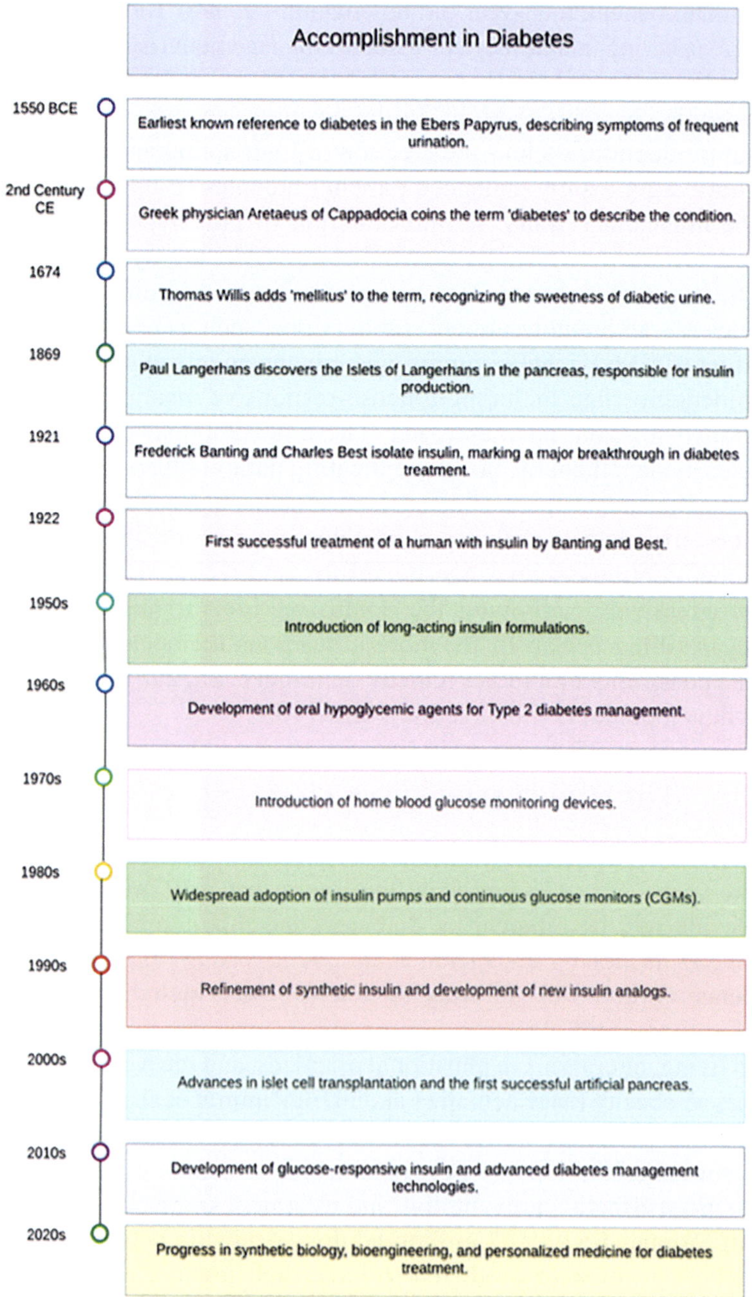

FIGURE 10.1 Developments in diabetes.

et al., 2023; Sun et al., 2022). According to Sun et al. (2022), there is a significant difference in prevalence between urban areas (12.1%) and rural areas (8.3%), as well as between high-income countries (11.1%) and low-income countries (5.5%). Type 2 diabetes accounts for over 90% of all diabetes cases, and its prevalence is driven by factors such as obesity, poor diet, and physical inactivity (Greg and Bracco, 2019).

The highest age-standardized prevalence rates in 2021 were observed in North Africa, the Middle East (9.3%), and Oceania (12.3%) (Ong et al., 2023). In contrast, regions like Northeastern Europe reported lower prevalence rates of approximately 6% (Greg and Bracco, 2019). Nations such as Qatar have extraordinarily high age-specific prevalence rates of 76.1% for those aged 75–79 years (Ong et al., 2023).

Globally, diabetes is expected to affect 783 million people by 2045, accounting for 12.2% of the population. With a predicted growth rate of 21.1%, middle-income nations are predicted to experience the largest increases (Sun et al., 2022). It is projected that 1.31 billion people worldwide will develop diabetes by 2050, with prevalence rates above 10% in various areas, especially Latin America, the Middle East, and North Africa (Ong et al., 2023).

High body mass index (BMI) is a major risk factor, accounting for over half of the global type 2 diabetes burden (Ong et al., 2023). Environmental factors, such as PM2.5, and socioeconomic factors, such as GDP per capita, also influence the prevalence (Li et al., 2020). The rise in diabetes prevalence is closely linked to the increasing rates of obesity, urbanization, and aging populations (Li et al., 2020).

10.1.2 CURRENT TREATMENT MODALITIES

Diabetes mellitus (DM) imposes substantial challenges on individuals, families, communities, and nations. Timely identification and management of diabetes is critical for mitigating disease progression and complications. Although type 1 diabetes mellitus (T1DM) presents greater prevention challenges, type 2 diabetes mellitus (T2DM) is often preventable via lifestyle modifications, including nutritious diets, consistent physical activity, and weight management. Nonadherence constitutes the primary barrier to effective diabetes treatment (Liu et al., 2015). Historically, diverse plants have been utilized worldwide as dietary supplements and traditional remedies for various health problems. Many plant-based medicines, traditionally believed to be effective, have been evaluated for their therapeutic potential in the treatment of diabetes, with some showing promising therapeutic effects. One study investigated the role of herbal extracts in glucose reduction and highlighted mechanisms such as insulin mimicry, β-cell regeneration, and glucose uptake enhancement (Elhassaneen et al., 2022). Plants used for diabetes self-management include *Aloe vera*, bitterbark, cinnamon, coconut, ginger, lime, mango, fever grass, and neem. These plants have been noted for their efficacy in reducing BGLs and mitigating T2DM symptoms. Lifestyle adjustments, specifically dietary changes and exercise, are essential nondrug aspects of T2DM management. Exercise is highly encouraged for those at risk, diagnosed, or seeking diabetes prevention (Jain et al., 2023).

Current diabetes treatments involve various pharmacological options that are customized for patients. Metformin has been established as the primary medication for T2DM because of its efficacy in reducing blood sugar levels (BSLs). Sulfonylureas are also used to enhance insulin secretion from the pancreas under these conditions. Insulin therapy is fundamental for the effective management of BGLs in patients with T1DM. The use of a pharmacological management system, including sensors and monitors, can improve diabetes care by providing real-time feedback on the effects of medication. A review of current medications emphasizes the necessity of comprehending the variability in treatment efficacy among individuals, which informs innovative therapeutic strategies and pharmacy interventions. A holistic approach to diabetes management encompasses these strategies, along with lifestyle changes, such as diet and exercise (ADA, 2021).

10.1.3 NEED FOR INNOVATIVE APPROACHES

The necessity for novel diabetes treatment methodologies arises from the deficiencies of current therapies, which inadequately replicate physiological processes and impose a patient burden. Progress in synthetic biology and bioengineering presents potential remedies by creating systems that closely resemble glucose regulation in the body. These advancements seek to enhance treatment effectiveness and alleviate the patient burden by addressing the issues inherent in existing diabetes management approaches.

Current diabetes therapies, including insulin and hypoglycemic agents, require ongoing monitoring and modification, posing challenges for patients. This is especially relevant for hypoglycemia prevention, a prevalent complication associated with heightened cardiovascular events and mortality risk (Svetlova and Gurieva, 2023).

Current type 2 diabetes mellitus (T2DM) therapies focus on enzymatic inhibition but lack curative potential and may worsen health issues (Rasouli et al., 2023). The absence of extensive longitudinal studies and models representative of human diabetes complications constrains the current treatment efficacy (Martín-Carro et al., 2023).

10.1.4 SIGNIFICANCE OF SYNTHETIC INNOVATIONS IN DIABETES MANAGEMENT

Synthetic advancements in diabetes management have markedly improved the treatment and control of type 1 and 2 diabetes. These advancements include various technologies and synthetic compounds that optimize glucose monitoring, insulin delivery, and therapeutic approaches. The incorporation of these technologies into diabetes care may revolutionize management strategies and enhance efficiency and personalization.

1. **Synthetic Molecules and Receptors:** Selective synthetic receptors: The creation of synthetic receptors for selective glucose interactions is a significant advancement in diabetes management. These receptors can be designed to improve glucose binding via hydrophilic and hydrophobic interactions, which may enhance glucose regulation (Shirinfar and Ahmed, 2019).

2. **Synthetic Beta Cells:** Genetically engineered synthetic beta cells replicate natural insulin production during hyperglycemia. These cells detect glucose concentrations and trigger insulin synthesis and secretion, presenting an innovative strategy for diabetes management that closely resembles the physiological mechanisms (Liu et al., 2022).

3. **Advances in Type 2 Diabetes Treatment:** Research on synthetic molecules has revealed compounds that target pathways in T2DM. These advancements suggest the possibility of more precise treatments, accommodating the complex nature of DM-2 and facilitating personalized medicine (de Lima et al., 2020).

While synthetic innovations present advantages, issues such as expenses, accessibility, and patient education persist. However, the continuous development of synthetic innovations suggests the potential for enhanced and individualized diabetes management.

10.2 SYNTHETIC INNOVATIONS IN DIABETES TREATMENT

10.2.1 OVERVIEW OF SYNTHETIC BIOLOGY AND ENGINEERING

Synthetic biology is an interdisciplinary field that combines biology, chemistry, engineering, and computer science to create new biological entities or to redesign current biological systems. In the context of diabetes therapy, synthetic biology seeks to develop artificial systems capable of performing certain functions, such as insulin generation and release, in response to glucose levels. Engineering, particularly bioengineering, is critical for transforming synthetic systems into useful applications. Fueled by the synergy between these disciplines, the development of innovative therapeutic techniques has the potential to transform diabetes treatments. Building on this essential multidisciplinary approach, engineered biology is driving a revolutionary age in diabetes treatment innovation by developing novel therapeutic approaches (Zhao et al., 2023). Advanced systems that self-regulate insulin production and release it based on glucose concentration have been established through interdisciplinary integration (Deepa et al., 2023).

The progression of innovations in diabetes therapy has led to a significant shift from conventional insulin administration techniques to the formulation of highly advanced closed-loop systems, known as artificial pancreas systems. Based on live glucose readings, the artificial pancreas operates by constantly monitoring BGLs by adjusting the insulin fusion rates and regulating insulin delivery to ensure optimal glycemic levels. This adjustment is important to ensure glycemic stability and could reduce the risk of hyperglycemia and hypoglycemia among patients (Moon et al., 2021; Nwokolo and Hovorka, 2023; Pinnaro and Tansey, 2021).

Aligned with these innovations, recent progress in synthetic biology, which aims to produce insulin, has further progressed through the development of glucose-responsive synthetic systems and bioengineered cellular entities. These innovative systems are meticulously designed to respond to hyperglycemic conditions by producing and releasing insulin, which could potentially replace the daily regimen of conventional insulin injections. A prominent example is the encapsulation technology development of β-cells, which are designed to function as synthetic insulin-producing cells (IPCs), thus potentially reducing the daily burdens of diabetes management and enhancing patient adherence (Rege et al., 2017).

These innovations aim to improve patient care by providing a more convenient approach to ensure optimal blood glucose regulation. This approach not only improves clinical outcomes but also reduces the long-term complications of diabetes. It has been predicted that innovations in synthetic biology will become crucial to overcoming the current shortcomings in diabetes care by providing non-invasive and more effective alternatives. Recent research and developments hold the promise of improving the diabetes treatment landscape, ultimately leading to better patient outcomes and a reduction in the cost of healthcare.

10.2.2 EVOLUTION OF ENGINEERING SOLUTIONS IN DIABETES

Over the past few decades, there have been significant breakthroughs in diabetes engineering innovations. Initially, efforts were focused on improving insulin delivery apparatuses, such as insulin pumps and pens, in terms of both the design and operating efficiency. However, more recent developments have led toward the development of more complex systems that can independently control BGLs. These developments include closed-loop insulin administration devices, known as artificial pancreas systems, which continuously monitor BGLs, adjust insulin dosage, and optimize insulin delivery in real time.

The implementation of synthetic biology has further broadened the possibilities, permitting the development of engineered cells and tissues, as well as glucose-responsive systems, which represent the next wave of diabetes treatment. Diabetic engineering solutions have radically improved patient care by combining technical advances with novel treatment techniques. These advancements have not only improved glycemic management but also the quality of life of patients with diabetes. This development may be observed in many crucial areas, including breakthroughs in glucose monitoring, changes in insulin delivery systems, and the introduction of new therapeutic approaches.

Continuous glucose monitoring (CGM) systems are among the most significant developments in the treatment of diabetes. Since its launch in 1999, CGM systems have been considered the gold standard of care for people with type 1 and type 2 diabetes who require insulin therapy (Bode et al., 2021; ElSayed et al., 2023).

In contrast to traditional fingerstick techniques, CGM provides real-time glucose level data, allowing patients to make timely and educated decisions regarding their nutritional intake, physical activity, and insulin requirements. This immediate monitoring provides patients with a better understanding of their glucose changes, reducing the risk of both hyperglycemia and hypoglycemia. According to previous research, using CGM significantly enhances HbA1c levels, which is a crucial sign of long-term glycemic control (Miller, 2020).

The integration of CGM with automated insulin administration systems has resulted in the development of hybrid closed-loop systems, also known as artificial pancreas systems. These devices can automatically adjust the insulin dosage based on real-time glucose readings, which eliminates the need for patients to monitor their health manually. These hybrid closed-loop systems represent a big step forward toward fully autonomous diabetes care by significantly minimizing the possibility of human errors and improving glycemic stability (Moon et al., 2021).

The evolution of insulin administration strategies reflects progress in glucose monitoring technologies. Conventional insulin delivery methods that allow for continuous subcutaneous insulin infusion have evolved into advanced hybrid systems that closely mimic the physiological insulin response of the pancreas. When integrated with CGM devices, these modern insulin pumps allow for precise insulin administration based on real-time glucose measurements, reducing the incidence of both hyperglycemia and hypoglycemia complications and ultimately improving patients' long-term health outcomes (Berget et al., 2019; Zahid et al., 2023).

A noteworthy advancement in this field is the development of smart insulin pens and patch pumps. Insulin pens are precisely designed to monitor and document insulin dosages, providing crucial data that supports both patients and healthcare providers in improving diabetes management. Patients who require multiple daily injections find that patch pumps, which offer a discrete and user-centric insulin delivery system, are particularly helpful. According to Kompala and Neinstein (2022) and Sy et al. (2022), these developments improve patient compliance and satisfaction while also increasing accessibility to insulin therapy.

Innovative therapeutic strategies extend beyond glucose monitoring and insulin delivery, addressing a larger range of diabetes-related issues. The introduction of GLP-1 receptor agonists and SGLT2 inhibitors has signified a significant leap in diabetes therapy. These medications not only help lower BSLs, but also offer critical protection for renal and cardiovascular health, reducing the long-term risks associated with diabetes. Their crucial function in the treatment of diabetes is highlighted by their dual therapeutic potential (Liakos et al., 2023; Olanrewaju et al., 2023).

Simultaneously, innovative technologies are being explored as novel approaches for managing diabetes. For instance, electrochemical methods that convert excess glucose into energy offer a promising substitute that might eventually supplement or replace existing therapeutic approaches. These developments are examples of unwavering efforts to enhance diabetes care and reduce the daily effects of the disease on patients' lives (Dhankhar et al., 2023; Sugandh et al., 2023).

The advancement of engineering solutions in the context of diabetes management has resulted in substantial improvements in patient care, including real-time glucose monitoring, advanced insulin delivery systems, and ground-breaking therapies. Although these developments have significantly improved diabetes control, concerns regarding the accessibility and affordability of technology persist. Continuous research and development are required to address these problems and to improve the effectiveness and accessibility of diabetes treatment options. As discipline improves, it holds the prospect of making even larger changes in the lives of those affected by diabetes. Among the breakthroughs leading to this progress, synthetic inventions have emerged as a vital area of focus in diabetes care. Key milestones in advancements in diabetes care are summarized in Table 10.1.

TABLE 10.1 Key Milestones in Advancements in Diabetes Care

Milestone	Description	Significance	Year
Foundational concepts in synthetic biology	Integration of biology, chemistry, engineering, and computer science to design and construct new biological systems	Established the groundwork for innovative therapeutic solutions in diabetes care	Early 2000s
Continuous glucose monitoring (CGM) systems	Introduction of CGM systems that provide real-time data on glucose levels	Revolutionized glucose monitoring, enabling better management decisions and improved HbA1c levels	1999 (initial introduction), 2010s (extensive use)
Development of artificial pancreas systems	Creation of closed-loop systems that continuously monitor glucose levels and adjust insulin delivery	Enhanced glycemic control by automating insulin delivery, reducing manual management of diabetes	2000s–2010s

TABLE 10.1 *(Continued)*

Milestone	Description	Significance	Year
Gene editing technologies (e.g., CRISPR)	Development of gene-editing tools to modify genes involved in insulin production	Enabled precise genetic modifications to improve insulin production and function	2010s
Introduction of encapsulated β-cells	Engineering of encapsulated β-cells designed to produce insulin in response to glucose levels	Provided a potential alternative to daily insulin injections, aiming to improve patient adherence	Mid-2010s
Emergence of hybrid closed-loop systems	Integration of CGM with insulin delivery systems for autonomous glucose regulation	Marked a significant step toward fully autonomous diabetes management by improving glycemic stability	2010s–2020s
Advancement of smart insulin pens and patch pumps	Development of smart insulin pens and patch pumps that enhance insulin delivery and tracking	Improved insulin management and patient adherence through more user-friendly and discreet options	2020s
Development of electrochemical approaches	Exploration of technologies that convert excess glucose into energy	Offered potential new methods for diabetes management, complementing or replacing traditional therapies	Emerging
Introduction of GLP-1 receptor agonists and SGLT2 inhibitors	Launch of medications that lower blood glucose and offer cardiovascular and renal protection	Addressed both glycemic control and long-term complications, providing dual therapeutic benefits	Recent years
Advances in cellular reprogramming	Reprogramming of non–β-cells to function like insulin-producing β-cells	Paved the way for new strategies in diabetes treatment by creating alternative sources of insulin	2020s
Synthetic insulin production systems	Development of engineered systems for *in vitro* synthesis of insulin	Provided a more scalable and potentially cost-effective method for insulin production	Recent years

10.2.3 ROLE OF SYNTHETIC INNOVATIONS IN DIABETES MANAGEMENT

With the continuous advancement of diabetes management, artificial technologies have become increasingly important for meeting unmet needs in this field. These innovations are meticulously designed to mimic the normal functions of the pancreas to achieve more precise and physiologically relevant regulation of blood glucose concentrations. The need for regular insulin injections may be significantly reduced or eliminated by producing cells that release insulin in response to changes in blood glucose. Furthermore, glucose-sensitive synthetic systems are designed to administer insulin in a manner that closely mimics the body's regulatory mechanisms, reducing the risks associated with hyperglycemia and hypoglycemia. Such technologies not only provide the possibility of improving patient outcomes but also reduce the burden of disease management, making diabetes care both more effective and less invasive (Sugandh et al., 2023).

Advances in synthetic innovations have played a major role in the development of bioengineered insulin delivery systems, making it possible to manage glucose levels more effectively. For example, insulin delivery systems that are sensitive to glucose levels can be carefully engineered to respond to variations in BGLs on their own and release insulin as needed. These advancements allow for more precise control of BSLs, which reduces the risk of both hyperglycemia and hypoglycemia. Concurrently, improvements in the wearable systems and synthetic design of insulin delivery devices have improved the portability and ease of treatment, thereby helping diabetics control their condition better on their own. The increasing demand for these artificial technologies reflects a greater understanding of their benefits for patients and medical professionals, supported by policies that support patient access to cutting-edge care options. Advancements in synthetic innovation are expected to further tailor therapeutic approaches and improve clinical outcomes (Chen et al., 2017; Kovatchev, 2019).

Artificial technologies continue to drive progressive changes in the field of diabetes treatment by transforming the treatment approaches. The development of glucose-sensitive insulin patches, a wearable, noninvasive insulin administration alternative, is a well-known example of this process. These patches have the potential to respond on their own to fluctuations in BGLs, which can lead to more precise insulin administration and reduce the need for patients to administer manual injections. Furthermore, synthetic systems designed to interface with real-time glucose-monitoring sensors significantly improve the performance of these wearable devices by ensuring adequate insulin release at appropriate intervals. These technological developments not only improve adherence to treatment procedures but also allow patients to control their condition with ease and assurance (Domingo-Lopez et al., 2022; Mansour et al., 2024).

Advances in omics technologies have further unveiled novel avenues for personalized diabetes care, providing more tailored treatments for an individual's distinct biological profile. These synthetic developments in omics have enabled the evaluation of large datasets to improve diabetic therapies, resulting in more effective interventions. Artificial intelligence (AI) enhances these improvements by scrutinizing intricate datasets to create prediction models, thereby driving the evolution of precision medicine in diabetic care. These artificial innovations highlight the critical role that innovation plays in improving the health outcomes of those with diabetes (Guan et al., 2023; Kang, 2024). The roles of synthetic biology and engineering in diabetes management are illustrated in Figure 10.2.

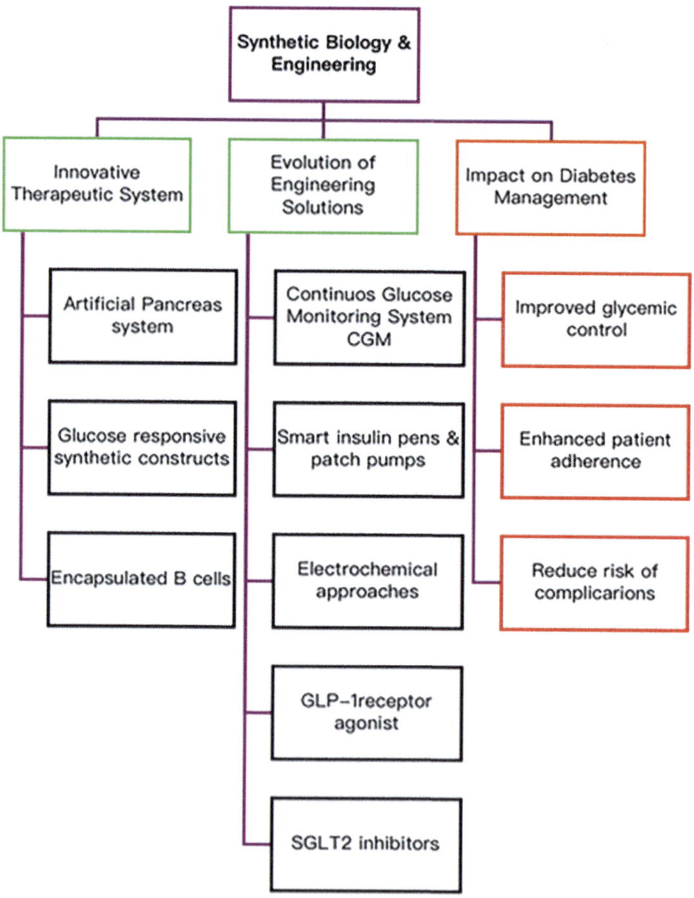

FIGURE 10.2 Synthetic biology and engineering and their role in diabetes management.

10.3 ENGINEERED CELLS AND TISSUES

10.3.1 UTILIZATION IN DIABETES TREATMENT

The use of engineered cells and tissues in diabetes treatment is a cutting-edge approach that aims to restore or replace the function of damaged pancreatic β-cells. These engineered cells are designed to produce and secrete insulin in response to BGLs, thereby mimicking the natural function of the pancreas (Arutyunyan et al., 2020; Shahjalalet al., 2018). Tissue engineering, on the other hand, involves the development of bioengineered tissues that can be implanted into the body to restore the function of damaged organs. In the context of diabetes, tissue engineering has the potential to create pancreatic tissue that can produce insulin and regulate BGLs, offering a long-term solution for patients with insulin-dependent diabetes (Siehler et al., 2021).

10.3.2 ADVANCES IN ENGINEERED CELLS FOR INSULIN PRODUCTION

Significant advances have been made in the development of cells designed to produce insulin. Numerous cell types, including fibroblasts and stem cells, have been successfully genetically modified by researchers to produce insulin in response to glucose levels. These cells are encapsulated in biocompatible materials to protect them from the immune system and genetically altered to express the insulin gene. Encapsulation allows insulin to be released under controlled conditions and ensures that the glucose levels are maintained within a specific range. To replace insulin injections and provide a more physiological approach to diabetes care, the ultimate goal of this research was to construct a bioartificial pancreas that can be implanted into patients.

Given these advancements, islet cell transplantation has been explored as an alternative in response to the persistent challenges faced by whole organ pancreatic transplantation, including organ rejection, vascular complications, limited organ availability, and the burden of lifelong immunosuppression. However, this approach encountered difficulties due to donor availability and side effects of immunosuppression.

Consequently, recent research has shifted toward stem cell-based therapies, which hold promise for reconstituting immune tolerance and preserving β-cell function. Notably, a novel therapy called VX-880 was developed to grow insulin-producing beta cells from allogeneic stem cells, with clinical trials beginning in 2021, following FDA approval. Another approach, VX-264, uses encapsulation to avoid immunosuppression but requires surgical implantation (Raoufinia et al., 2024).

In 2023, the FDA approved Lantidra, the first allogeneic pancreatic islet cell therapy, for adults with type 1 diabetes who experience severe hypoglycemia. This groundbreaking treatment showed that 21–30% of participants no longer required insulin one-year post-treatment, with benefits lasting over five years in some cases. However, the therapy is associated with mild-to-serious adverse events linked to the treatment dose and methods of islet cell infusion.

10.3.3 TISSUE ENGINEERING APPROACHES FOR DIABETES

The development of bioengineered pancreatic tissue that can release insulin in response to glucose levels is a key component of tissue-engineering solutions for diabetes management. This strategy may offer individuals with type 1 diabetes who lack functional pancreatic β-cells a long-term solution. Researchers are exploring various approaches to produce bioengineered tissues, such as differentiating stem cells into β-cells that produce insulin and using 3D bioprinting to construct pancreatic tissue. By integration with the host tissue after transplantation, these bioengineered tissues can return normal insulin production to the body. Although this method is still in its early stages, it has potential for the management of diabetes in the future (Amer et al., 2014; Salg et al., 2019).

Tissue engineering has made it possible to create novel therapies for diabetes, particularly type 1 diabetes (T1D). Differentiating induced pluripotent stem cells (iPSCs) or embryonic stem cells (ESCs) into IPCs, which respond well to glucose levels, is a promising approach. The differentiation process must be carefully regulated to ensure the production of functional IPCs and to lower the chance of undifferentiated cells, which may eventually result in cancer. Another approach is to create 3D structures called pancreatic organoids, which mimic the composition and operation of the pancreas. These organoids increase the effectiveness of beta-cell replacement treatment and establish a more physiologically suitable environment for insulin production by enhancing IPC survival and functionality (Ghoneim et al., 2024; Silva et al., 2022; Wan et al., 2022).

In addition, scaffolds and devices are being developed to assist in the transplantation of tailored IPCs by providing structural support, increasing cell adhesion, and facilitating nutrition exchange while preserving cells from the host immune response. Encapsulation techniques shield IPCs from immunological rejection by forming a physical barrier around the cells; however, comprehensive physiological glucose regulation remains difficult to achieve. Researchers are investigating the synthesis of universal stem cells via genetic alteration to reduce immunological rejection, and suicide gene technology is being used as a safety mechanism to destroy potentially hazardous cells (Jeyagaran et al., 2022; Zhou et al., 2023). Identifying suitable implantation sites such as the omentum is crucial for supporting cell survival and function. Collectively, these tissue engineering approaches aim to create functional, safe, and translatable solutions for beta cell replacement therapy in diabetes management, thereby addressing the limitations of traditional islet transplantation (Abadpour et al., 2021).

Another interesting tissue engineering strategy is the creation of bioartificial pancreases that incorporate IPCs into a supporting scaffold to mimic pancreatic function. This strategy seeks to address the limitations of current treatments such as insulin therapy and islet transplantation by potentially restoring normal insulin production and glucose regulation (Jeyagaran et al., 2022; Zhou et al., 2023).

Furthermore, 3D bioprinting technology employs specialized printers to layer biomaterials and cells, resulting in tissue-like structures with precise spatial layouts. This approach enables patient-specific customization by increasing cell survival and function by replicating the intricate architecture of pancreatic tissue. Successful bioprinting requires the careful selection of appropriate cells, such as β-cells, and biomaterials, such as hydrogels. Current research aims to identify biomaterials that promote cell development and imitate the pancreatic microenvironment, with alginate being a popular choice owing to its immunological isolation features, despite significant drawbacks (Bishop et al., 2017; Persaud et al., 2022).

Nonetheless, vascularization remains a major challenge because establishing a functioning blood supply is critical for nutrient and oxygen delivery. To overcome this issue, researchers are investigating microfluidic devices and enhanced bioprinting techniques to create vascular networks within bioprinted structures. Furthermore, post-bioprinting maturation in bioreactors is essential because it improves cell connections and tissue development, guaranteeing that the created tissues can respond to physiological cues and release insulin efficiently. Finally, well-designed clinical trials are required to determine the safety and efficacy of bioprinted pancreatic tissues in humans (Ghosh et al., 2024; Nwokoye and Abilez, 2024).

Ongoing research is focused on refining bioprinting methods, discovering new biomaterials, and improving the *in vivo* performance of engineered tissues, with advances in immunoisolation techniques and hybrid encapsulation systems that improve the integration and functionality of these constructs. Thus, advances in tissue engineering are a significant step forward in the development of successful type 1 diabetes therapeutics (Ghosh et al., 2023).

Furthermore, Baranova et al. (2024) highlighted the development of cell-engineered pancreatic constructs (CEPCs), which are formed by combining islets of Langerhans with a biocompatible matrix carrier to mimic the native pancreatic tissue environment, thus providing a potential treatment for type 1 diabetes mellitus (T1D). This study emphasizes the importance of biocompatible scaffolds, notably tissue-specific scaffolds created by decellularizing human pancreatic fragments, in preserving the viability and functionality of islets after transplantation.

To directly compare the effectiveness of CEPCs and isolated islets of Langerhans in regulating BGLs, the study included a comparative trial in which rats with experimental T1D were administered these organ transplants peritoneally. These results demonstrate that CEPCs have a more potent antidiabetic effect, resulting in a greater reduction in BGLs, indicating a possible potential for improvement in long-term diabetes control. Over a 10-week follow-up period, CEPCs continued to maintain decreased BGLs, suggesting that this tissue-engineering approach may offer a long-term diabetic therapy solution. The study concluded by highlighting the potential of bioartificial structures to improve pancreatic islet performance using biocompatible scaffolds and efficient delivery systems, thereby improving treatment results for individuals with T1D.

Lewis and Wells (2021) studied the use of innovative methods to generate functional pancreatic β-cells. A challenge to effective diabetes treatment is the production of immature β-cells with poor activity from traditional two-dimensional (2D) monolayer preparations. However, by offering a more physiologically appropriate environment, moving to three-dimensional (3D) spheroid cultures has been shown to increase the maturity and efficiency of these cells. Cell–cell and cell-extracellular matrix interactions are improved by using 3D culture systems, which are essential for β-cell development. Compared with 2D methods, this method produces more functioning cells. While scaffold-free approaches enable cells to self-assemble into 3D structures that closely mimic the natural tissue architecture, scaffold-based techniques are used in tissue engineering to provide structural support for cell growth and organization.

Collectively, these approaches improve the physiological relevance and functionality of tissues. Bioreactor systems enable β-cell growth and maturation by maintaining ideal culture conditions, providing a consistent supply of nutrients and oxygen, and eliminating waste. Integrating gene editing technologies, such as CRISPR, improves differentiation by targeting specific signaling pathways and transcription factors, resulting in more mature and responsive IPCs. The utilization of 3D culture systems, scaffold-based and scaffold-free approaches, bioreactors, and gene editing represents a dramatic leap in tissue engineering, enabling considerable advances in the generation of functional β cells for diabetes treatment (Lewis and Wells, 2021).

One important approach is to develop IPCs, such as HEK-293-β cells. These cells are designed to detect BGLs and produce insulin in response, demonstrating the ability to maintain glucose homeostasis for more than three weeks and effectively correct diabetic hyperglycemia in type 1 diabetes (T1D) mice within three days of implantation. Synthetic biology advances these efforts by creating genetic constructs that regulate cell processes, allowing the created cells to respond to specific indicators such as glucose levels and release therapeutic drugs in a controlled manner. Overexpression of specific genes or transcription factors can direct stem cells to become functional IPCs, creating a renewable source for diabetes treatment (Yan et al., 2023).

Advanced approaches, such as CRISPR/dCas9 bio switches, are also being investigated to precisely control gene expression in modified cells, addressing issues such as nutritional overconsumption and cell toxicity (Cai et al., 2023; Cheng et al., 2013). Engineered human cells, such as HEK-293-β, may be manufactured cost-effectively while conforming to pharmaceutical requirements, making them promising for clinical applications. These cells aim to provide high-purity and stable products for the treatment of diabetes. Collectively, these novel tissue engineering technologies are opening the door to more effective and tailored diabetic treatments (Yan et al., 2023).

10.4 GLUCOSE-RESPONSIVE SYNTHETIC SYSTEMS

10.4.1 CONCEPT AND DEVELOPMENT

Insulin therapy is limited by the risk of hypoglycemia and insufficient glycemic control, despite advances in maintaining exact blood insulin levels. Individuals with insulin-dependent diabetes, including type 1 and advanced type 2, require careful and continuous insulin administration, including mealtimes and overnight, to maintain tight glucose control and avoid severe hypoglycemic episodes. These dangers limit the full potential of insulin therapy (Yu et al., 2016).

To overcome these obstacles, a smart therapeutic system that mimics the endogenous glucose-responsive release of insulin is critical for optimal diabetes treatment, while avoiding hypoglycemia. Such technology would be a step forward in precision medicine, adapting medication in real time to an individual's glucose levels, thereby increasing efficacy and lowering negative effects. Integrating glucose-responsive components into insulin molecules or delivery systems is a promising strategy for mimicking the dynamic insulin production of pancreatic β-cells through advanced alterations in pharmacokinetics and pharmacodynamics (Sun et al., 2017).

In this context, glucose-responsive synthetic systems have significantly improved diabetes treatments. These systems are intended to release insulin or other antidiabetic drugs in response to changes in BGLs, resulting in a more natural and precise manner of glucose regulation. The creation of glucose-responsive systems requires synthetic biology, materials science, and engineering to design systems that can sense glucose levels and release insulin in a controlled manner. This strategy attempts to mimic the normal function of the pancreas while reducing the need for frequent blood glucose monitoring and insulin administration (Olanrewaju et al., 2023).

Glucose-responsive synthetic systems have significantly improved the treatment of diabetes. These systems are intended to release insulin or other antidiabetic drugs in response to changes in BGLs, resulting in a more natural and precise manner of glucose regulation. The creation of glucose-responsive systems requires synthetic biology, materials science, and engineering to design systems that can sense glucose levels and release insulin in a controlled manner. This strategy attempts to mimic the normal function of the pancreas, while reducing the need for frequent blood glucose monitoring and insulin administration (Bercea and Lupu, 2024; Rege et al., 2017).

Glucose-responsive synthetic systems are designed to adapt to glucose levels in a controlled manner, providing significant advantages in biological applications, such as drug delivery and diabetes treatment. These systems undergo conformational changes or chemical reactions in response to glucose. Glucose specifically interacts with particular polymers, altering their solubility and triggering the release of encapsulated drugs. Alternatively, other systems use glucose-specific enzymes to alter the characteristics of the system, thereby allowing medication release. Development tactics include choosing appropriate materials, such as amphiphilic glycomacromolecules with functional groups designed to interact with glucose, and using advanced synthesis processes, such as solid-phase polymer synthesis, to achieve precise control over the properties (Wang et al., 2021; Webber and Anderson, 2015).

There are numerous applications, including controlled drug delivery for insulin and other drugs, improved therapeutic results for diabetic patients, and increased efficacy of antiviral and antibacterial therapies by optimizing drug release timing and location. Despite these developments, obstacles remain, such as ensuring material stability and biocompatibility, and meeting regulatory standards. Addressing these problems is critical for developing glucose-responsive systems that have the potential to greatly improve health outcomes, notably in diabetes control and tailored medicine delivery (Jäck et al., 2024).

Expanding on these ideas, glucose-responsive synthetic systems are enhanced drug delivery platforms that release therapeutic molecules, such as insulin, in response to glucose levels in the body. They are vital for diabetes management because maintaining good blood glucose control is critical for patient health. The underlying method involves monitoring glucose concentrations and releasing insulin as needed. When glucose levels rise, insulin is released to lower BSLs, replicating the natural function of the pancreas. Recent advances have resulted in the creation of smart hydrogels, such as those based on silk fibroin and functionalized with phenylboronic acid (PBA), to interact with glucose (Mansoor et al., 2021).

These hydrogels are intended to self-assemble, cross-link, and encapsulate glucose-sensing components and insulin. Their injectability is a major characteristic because dynamic bonding allows for facile injection with a needle, making them suitable for clinical applications. Insulin and glucose sensors are also long-term stable, owing to their hydrogel nature. According to *in vivo* tests using diabetic rat models, during hyperglycemic settings, the hydrogel breaks down because of oxidative cleavage of hydrogen peroxide generated by the glucose-sensing element. This effectively lowers BGLs over time and allows controlled insulin release. As it customizes drug administration to patient glucose levels, this strategy has significant implications for personalized medicine and may enhance diabetes control and quality of life. In summary, glucose-responsive synthetic systems have marked significant advancements in drug delivery technology, and new materials, such as silk fibroin, show promise as efficient, self-regulating treatment options (Maity et al., 2023).

In addition to these advancements, improved insulin analogs known as glucose-responsive insulins (GRIs) react instantly to changes in the plasma glucose levels. By minimizing the risk of hypoglycemia associated with conventional insulin therapy, these devices can either activate a stronger type of insulin or facilitate its release into the bloodstream based on glucose levels. GRIs release insulin in response to glucose, intrinsic GRIs alter their activity based on glucose levels, and GRIs use technology to monitor glucose levels and release insulin, as needed. Pharmaceutical kinetic models, such as PAMERAH, which mimic the glucoregulatory systems of rats and humans, are widely used in the development of these systems. To evaluate and improve the GRI designs for clinical applications, this model is essential (Yang et al., 2020).

However, adapting these designs from rodent models to human applications presents substantial problems because changes in parameter spaces across species must be considered when predicting the therapeutic efficacy in humans. Future research will focus on quantitative analysis and computational frameworks to guide innovations in insulin delivery, with the goal of improving diabetes care. In conclusion, glucose-responsive synthetic systems represent a promising improvement in diabetes management, with ongoing research refining their design and clinical efficacy. Computational models are essential for this research process, opening a path for more effective and safer insulin therapy (Yuan et al., 2014).

This progress in glucose-responsive technology has resulted in the development of systems designed to detect and respond to glucose levels in the body. When glucose levels rise, these systems can release therapeutic drugs such as insulin in a controlled manner, similar to the normal pancreatic response. The dual response to glucose and pH improves medication delivery control by ensuring that insulin is delivered only when needed, thus reducing the risk of hypoglycemia. Synthetic systems have been developed using glucose-responsive polymersomes that encapsulate pharmaceuticals and allow for permeability changes in response to glucose levels. Researchers have added glucose-sensitive components to polymersomes, such as polymers that swell or shrink in response to glucose concentration, influencing insulin release rates (Yang and Cao, 2017).

Additionally, the incorporation of pH sensitivity improved these systems. For example, in acidic environments, such as those found in specific tissues, polymersomes can release insulin more easily, resulting in a dual regulatory mechanism. The principal use of these systems is in insulin delivery for diabetes control. These systems help maintain blood sugar within a healthy range by ensuring that insulin is released in response to high glucose levels, enhancing therapeutic efficacy and patient compliance by reducing injection frequency and the negative effects associated with inappropriate doses. Future research should focus on enhancing system performance, particularly responsiveness and stability under physiological settings, in order to develop a completely automated insulin administration system for real-time glucose management. In conclusion, glucose-responsive synthetic systems represent a substantial improvement in drug delivery technology, particularly for diabetes treatment. Their ability to respond to changes in glucose and pH provides a controlled and effective therapeutic technique that promises better health outcomes for patients (Zhou et al., 2021).

Upon these innovations, glucose-responsive synthetic systems have been designed to respond to changes in glucose levels, making them especially helpful in biological applications, including drug administration and glucose monitoring. These systems are designed to change their features or behavior in response to glucose concentrations by incorporating specific chemical groups such as PBA, which forms reversible complexes with glucose molecules. The fundamental process includes glucose binding to PBA, resulting in a conformational shift in the polymer structure that can cause the release of encapsulated pharmaceuticals or adjust the capsule's permeability, allowing for regulated drug administration depending on glucose levels (Ma and Shi, 2014; Yang and Cao, 2017).

Common materials utilized include polymers, such as poly(lysine) and alginate, which are chosen for their biocompatibility and capacity to produce hydrogels that contain therapeutic medicines. The development process is divided into several stages, including the synthesis of polymers containing PBA groups, creation of capsules that can encapsulate drugs while maintaining glucose responsiveness, and testing and optimization of these capsules *in vitro* and *in vivo* to ensure appropriate responses to glucose fluctuations. These systems have tremendous potential in diabetes care because they can provide insulin in response to rising BGLs, thereby improving therapeutic outcomes while reducing the side effects associated with standard drug delivery methods (Mohanty et al., 2022).

Ongoing research aims to increase the sensitivity and specificity of these systems by investigating new materials and mechanisms and merging them with wearable technologies for real-time monitoring and medicine delivery. In conclusion, glucose-responsive synthetic systems represent a state-of-the-art method of drug delivery. They combine material science, chemistry, and biomedical engineering to enable novel healthcare solutions while utilizing natural glucose fluctuations to maximize therapeutic interventions (Mansour et al., 2019). Table 10.2 provides a comparative overview of the use of tissue engineering and modified cells in the treatment of diabetes.

10.4.2 NANOMEDICINES FOR INSULIN MODULATION

Nanomedicines have emerged as a promising domain in the regulation of insulin for the management of diabetes, presenting innovative alternatives to conventional insulin therapies. These advancements aspire to enhance patient adherence, optimize insulin delivery efficacy, and mitigate the complications associated with diabetes treatment. The incorporation of nanotechnology within insulin delivery frameworks has culminated in the creation of diverse nanocarriers that facilitate the controlled release, targeted delivery, and augmented bioavailability of insulin. This discourse investigates the contemporary landscape of nanomedicine in insulin modulation, emphasizing various nanocarrier systems, their operational mechanisms, and their prospective advantages.

Insulin administration with nanocarriers shows promise in improving diabetes control. Insulin and other therapeutic peptides, such as cathelicidin-derived peptides, have been delivered to target β-cells via polymeric nanoparticles such as poly(lactic-co-glycolic acid) (PLGA) nanoparticles. These nanoparticles significantly augment insulin functionality and facilitate pancreatic regeneration, as evidenced in type 1 diabetic rat models, which exhibit notable enhancements in glucose tolerance and β-cell mass (Cristelo et al., 2023). The development of several nanocarrier systems has also made efficient use of chitosan and other natural polymers. Chitosan nanoparticles are being investigated for their biocompatibility and potential to improve the absorption of insulin in the gastrointestinal tract in conjunction with other naturally occurring polymers such as dextran and alginate. These carriers constitute integral components of advanced nanocarrier systems designed for the effective oral and pulmonary administration of insulin (Sabu and Pramod, 2020; Sharma et al., 2015).

In addition to polymeric nanocarrier systems, lipid-based nanocarriers have been widely studied for active drug delivery in the control of diabetes. Lipid-based vesicular systems such as solid lipid nanoparticles (SLNs) and liposomes have been used for oral insulin delivery because they provide prolonged and regulated release. These carriers enhance insulin bioavailability and replicate the natural insulin route, overcoming hurdles, such as first-pass metabolism (Kaklotar et al., 2016; Sabu and Pramod, 2020).

Nanomedicines are currently undergoing extensive investigation and advancement to strategically target particular receptors, including GLP-1 receptors on β-cells, with the aim of augmenting the accuracy of insulin administration. This methodology not only optimizes insulin efficacy but also contributes to pancreatic tissue regeneration (Cristelo et al., 2023).

Stimuli-responsive nanoformulations, exemplified by insulin-conjugated quantum dots enveloped in chitosan/glucose polymers, have been meticulously engineered to react with changes in pH and the presence of glucosidase enzymes, thereby facilitating the release of insulin in accordance with physiological requirements. This innovative formulation has demonstrated encouraging efficacy in the attenuation of BGLs, while simultaneously averting the incidence of hypoglycemia in various animal models (Hunt et al., 2024).

10.4.3 IMPLICATIONS FOR DIABETES CONTROL

The advancement of glucose-responsive synthetic systems and nanomedicines has led to substantial ramifications in the management of diabetes. These pioneering developments possess the capacity to enhance the effectiveness of diabetes therapies, mitigate the likelihood of complications, and elevate the overall quality of life of affected individuals. By facilitating a more organic and integrated approach to glucose regulation, these systems can alleviate challenges associated with disease management and foster greater patient compliance with therapeutic protocols. Furthermore, the ability to regulate insulin secretion in accordance with glucose concentrations may aid in the prevention of hyperglycemic and hypoglycemic episodes, which frequently arise as complications of diabetes treatment. As scholarly inquiry into this domain continues to progress, these innovations are anticipated to play a pivotal role in the forthcoming landscape of diabetes care.

Insulin-dendrimer nanocomplexes offer a novel strategy for diabetes management via GRI delivery. These complexes integrate insulin with dendrimers, facilitating a system that responds to BGLs and potentially enhancing the efficacy and safety of insulin therapy. This approach mitigates current insulin therapy challenges, including the risk of hypoglycemia and frequent administration requirements. Insulin-dendrimer nanocomplexes employ electrostatic and dynamic-covalent interactions to stabilize a complex formed by a synthetic dendrimer carrier and insulin analog. The design of this complex allows for glucose responsiveness, releasing insulin in response to elevated glucose levels, thereby emulating pancreatic insulin secretion. The dendrimer enhances both the solubility and stability of insulin, enabling controlled extended release. This was accomplished by incorporating a high-affinity glucose-binding motif that triggers insulin release upon glucose elevation (Xian et al., 2024). A principal benefit of insulin-dendrimer nanocomplexes is their glucose-responsive characteristic, which minimizes the risk of hypoglycemia by ensuring timely insulin release. This aspect is especially advantageous for patients who have difficulty stabilizing BGLs. Furthermore, the prolonged action duration, potentially allowing weeklong glucose management from a single dose, significantly improves convenience and adherence relative to daily insulin injections (Xian et al., 2024).

Bioinspired fatty-acid-modified nanoparticles offer a novel approach to diabetes therapy by utilizing the beneficial characteristics of fatty acids to improve drug delivery. These nanoparticles are designed to enhance the delivery of insulin and other therapeutics through fatty acid surface modifications, which increases stability, bioavailability, and targeting precision. This method is especially advantageous for diabetes treatment, in which accurate and effective insulin delivery is vital. A study focused on fatty acid-modified chitosan nanoparticles aimed at optimizing insulin delivery to the liver, which is a key site for insulin action. By attaching lauric and oleic acids to chitosan, these nanoparticles demonstrated superior insulin loading efficiency and liver targeting, leading to significantly enhanced antidiabetic effectiveness compared to unmodified insulin (Li et al., 2018).

In an alternative investigation, calcium phosphate nanoparticles conjugated with lauric acid and encapsulated in alginate have demonstrated the capability to facilitate pH-dependent, sustained release of insulin. This formulation preserves the stability of insulin while providing a non-toxic delivery mechanism, rendering it appropriate for oral administration (Paul and Sharma, 2010). In a separate examination, it was noted that the self-assembly of fatty acid conjugates, including the lisofyllin-linoleic acid conjugate, into micellar structures significantly enhanced cellular uptake and prolonged the half-life of therapeutic compounds. Such outcomes contribute to improved bioavailability and a reduction in dosing frequency, which are beneficial for patient adherence and overall efficacy of treatment in the management of diabetes (Italiya et al., 2019).

Fatty acid-modified nanoparticles can be specifically engineered for targeted therapeutic interventions, particularly for addressing fatty acid metabolic pathways associated with diabetic cardiomyopathy. For example, research has demonstrated that astragalus polysaccharide liposome nanoparticles can modulate the expression of fatty acid translocase, thereby enhancing fatty acid metabolism and diminishing myocardial tissue metabolism under diabetic conditions (Ji et al., 2023). The adaptability of fatty acid-modified nanoparticles also encompasses their prospective application in the fabrication of composites with metal-organic frameworks, which have the potential to significantly augment their functional attributes for drug delivery purposes.

Glucose-responsive synthetic systems, such as konjac glucomannan/concanavalin A nanoparticles, present a significant opportunity for the oral administration of insulin in the management of diabetes mellitus. These nanomedicinal formulations can respond to variations in glucose concentrations, thereby facilitating the release of insulin in accordance with physiological demands, which may enhance the regulation of glycemic levels. Through the application of glucose-responsive technologies, these systems are poised to augment the efficacy and accuracy of insulin delivery, ultimately contributing to improved diabetes management outcomes. Advancements in glucose-sensitive synthetic systems and nanomedicines have profound implications for the progression of diabetes therapies by enabling targeted and adaptive mechanisms for insulin delivery (Xu et al., 2022).

One study examined a novel insulin delivery system utilizing enzyme-based nanoparticles that were responsive to BGLs. Nanoparticles made from hyaluronic acid and 2-nitroimidazole with insulin and glucose oxidase were synthesized via ionic gelation. The stability assessments revealed that the nanoparticles were stable for up to 30 days at 4°C. *In vitro* analyses indicated that insulin release from these nanoparticles was significantly heightened under hyperglycemic conditions (400 mg/dL) within 10 min, whereas minimal release occurred under normoglycemic conditions (100 mg/dL), highlighting their potential for diabetes management by emulating physiological glucose regulation. The study concluded that these enzyme-based nanoparticles demonstrate rapid and efficacious responsiveness to elevated glucose levels, indicating their viability as a biomimetic system for sustained insulin release under hyperglycemic conditions. This innovation may address the shortcomings of prior electronic insulin delivery systems and enhance diabetes management through a more responsive and targeted insulin delivery mechanism that promptly adjusts to fluctuating glucose levels (Jana et al., 2020).

Nanomedicines have been used in insulin replacement therapy. This therapy necessitates multiple injections and carries the risk of hypoglycemia due to the narrow therapeutic index of insulin, impacting BGL control. To mitigate these issues, GRI delivery systems have been developed to emulate β-cell functionality, enhance blood glucose control, and reduce the injection frequency. These systems aim to tightly regulate BGLs and diminish the risk of hypoglycemia. The current study involved glucose-responsive materials integrated with three primary glucose-sensing elements: glucose oxidase (GOx), PBA, and glucose-binding molecules. These materials are engineered to detect fluctuations in glucose concentration or associated signals, such as pH, H_2O_2 levels, and O_2 concentration, and adjust their properties accordingly. Building on these glucose-responsive materials, various carriers such as hydrogels, micro/nanoparticles, liposomes, complexes, cell–drug conjugates, and microneedle (MN) array patches have been developed by other research groups. These delivery systems can facilitate insulin release through glucose-stimulated mechanisms including swelling/contraction, dissolution, pore size alteration, charge reversal, and polymer degradation (Yao et al., 2022).

The implementation of molecular docking methodologies in the design of glucose-responsive nanoparticles has significantly enhanced the development process, facilitating the effective screening and optimization of functional materials. This approach has been extensively utilized in the fabrication of insulin-delivering nanoparticles that exhibit enhanced performance and biocompatibility (Shen et al., 2022).

Although glucose-responsive synthetic systems and nanomedicines signify considerable progress, their translation into clinical practice continues to encounter challenges. Consistency across diverse physiological conditions is paramount. Furthermore, the prolonged safety and adverse effects associated with these novel materials necessitate a thorough investigation. Nonetheless, ongoing research in this field is positioned to revolutionize diabetes management, potentially resulting in more efficacious and patient-oriented therapeutic approaches.

10.5 FUTURE DIRECTIONS AND CHALLENGES

Prospective developments in synthetic innovations for diabetes management exhibit considerable promise, as advancements in synthetic biology and nanotechnology have established a foundation for increasingly personalized

TABLE 10.2 Comparative Summary of Engineered Cells and Tissue Engineering Utilized in Diabetes Management

Approach	Description	Advantages	Challenges	Examples	Cell Types & Sources	Encapsulation Materials	Clinical Trial Status	Immunoisolation Techniques	Vascularization Solutions	Gene Editing Technologies	References
Engineered cells	Cells genetically modified to produce insulin in response to glucose. Encapsulated in biocompatible materials to protect from immune response and control release.	• Potential to create a bioartificial pancreas • Reduces need for insulin injections • Controlled insulin release	• Immune system response • Encapsulation challenges • Need for surgical implantation • Long-term stability	VX-880, VX-264, Lantidra	Stem cells, fibroblasts	Alginate, hydrogel	VX-880 (phase 1), Lantidra (FDA approved)	Encapsulation	Microfluidic systems, advanced bioprinting	CRISPR, dCas9	Raoufinia et al. (2024); Yan et al. (2023)
Tissue engineering	Development of bioengineered pancreatic tissues using methods such as 3D bioprinting and stem cell differentiation to replace functional β-cells.	• Potential for a long-term diabetes solution • Can create personalized tissues • Mimics natural pancreatic function	• Vascularization issues • Risk of immune rejection • Complexity of tissue integration • Tumorigenicity of undifferentiated cells	3D bioprinted tissues, pancreatic organoids	Embryonic stem cells (ESCs), iPSCs	Alginate, hydrogels	Early-stage research	Immunoisolation barriers	Microfluidic systems, vascular networks	CRISPR, gene editing	Abadpour et al. (2021); Ghosh et al. (2023)
Bioartificial pancreas	Integration of insulin-producing cells into supportive scaffolds to replicate pancreatic function, addressing limitations of current treatments.	• Restores normal insulin production • May overcome limitations of insulin therapy and islet transplantation • Customizable	• Vascularization remains a challenge • Biocompatibility of scaffolds • Surgical implantation	Bioartificial pancreases	β-cells, stem cells	Alginate, collagen	Preclinical trials	Immunoisolation	Microfluidic systems, bioreactors	CRISPR, gene editing	Baranova et al. (2024); Ghosh et al. (2023)
Cell-engineered pancreatic constructs (CEPCs)	Combining islets of Langerhans with biocompatible matrix carriers to mimic native pancreatic tissue, improving management of type 1 diabetes.	• More potent antidiabetic effects • Better long-term management • Improved function compared to isolated islets	• Effective scaffold development needed • Long-term safety and efficacy • Challenges in carrier administration	CEPCs	Islets of Langerhans	Biocompatible matrices	Comparative study (animal models)	Biocompatible scaffolds	Not applicable	Not applicable	Baranova et al. (2024)
3D culture systems	Use of 3D spheroid cultures to improve the functionality and maturity of β-cells, enhancing their effectiveness for diabetes therapy.	• Improves cell functionality • Mimics natural tissue environment • Enhances β-cell maturation and efficiency	• Complexity of maintaining 3D cultures • Need for optimized bioreactor conditions • Limited scalability	3D spheroid cultures	β-cells	Not applicable	Not applicable	Not applicable	Not applicable	CRISPR, gene editing	Lewis and Wells (2021)
HEK-293-β cells	HEK-293 cells engineered to produce insulin in response to glucose, capable of maintaining glucose homeostasis and correcting hyperglycemia in animal models.	• Effective in managing hyperglycemia • Promising cost-effective production • Responsive to glucose levels	• Requires further development for human use • Production cost and regulatory hurdles • Long-term stability	HEK-293-β cells	HEK-293 cells	Not applicable	Preclinical trials	Not applicable	Not applicable	CRISPR/dCas9	Cai et al. (2023); Yan et al. (2023)

and efficacious therapeutic interventions. Nevertheless, these innovations also give rise to substantial challenges, including ethical dilemmas and the imperative for comprehensive regulatory frameworks. The incorporation of these technologies into diabetes treatment has the capacity to fundamentally transform therapeutic approaches; however, meticulous attention to the accompanying challenges is essential for their effective deployment.

Synthetic biology is advancing the creation of functional islet-like tissues, which may yield a reliable source of GRI-secreting cells for the management of diabetes (Saxena et al., 2020). Genetically engineered synthetic beta cells have been designed to replicate the natural insulin synthesis mechanism, presenting a promising strategy to enhance clinical results in diabetes management (Liu et al., 2022). Nonetheless, obstacles such as the assurance of prolonged functionality, safety, and resolution of manufacturing challenges continue to exist within the domain of synthetic biology (Saxena et al., 2020).

Nanomedicines have distinctive characteristics with the potential to significantly improve therapeutic efficacy in the management of diabetes. They facilitate the emergence of personalized therapeutic approaches; however, obstacles to commercialization, including large-scale manufacturing and rigorous clinical assessments, persist. The development of synthetic molecules and receptors that exhibit selective interactions with glucose represents another domain of innovation, which may contribute to the development of more precise diabetes management methodologies (Shirinfar and Ahmed, 2019).

Although advancements in synthetic innovations pertaining to diabetes management present considerable potential, they simultaneously engender apprehensions regarding data privacy, ethical dilemmas, and the imperative for comprehensive regulatory frameworks. The trajectory of diabetes care is anticipated to incorporate a synthesis of technological progress along with human supervision to ascertain the provision of safe and efficacious treatment modalities. The emergence of novel therapeutic approaches, including implantable drug delivery systems and automated closed-loop systems, is poised to further augment diabetes management. However, the hurdles associated with commercialization and practical application must be systematically addressed to actualize their complete efficacy (Kerr et al., 2018).

10.6 CONCLUSION

Synthetic innovations signify a paradigm shift in the management of diabetes, presenting renewed optimism for countless individuals afflicted with this enduring condition. Through the utilization of synthetic biology and engineering principles, it is feasible to devise sophisticated therapeutic methodologies that more accurately replicate the physiological mechanisms of the human body, thus enhancing patient outcomes and the overall quality of life. These advancements, encompassing engineered cellular structures and tissues, glucose-responsive synthetic systems, and nanomedicines, have the capacity to revolutionize the domain of diabetes management. Nonetheless, the effective deployment of these innovative technologies necessitates meticulous examination of ethical, technological, and regulatory obstacles. As scholarly inquiry into this domain progresses, synthetic innovations are strategically positioned to assume a pivotal role in the forthcoming landscape of diabetes therapy, facilitating the emergence of more efficacious, less invasive, and patient-centric treatment modalities.

KEYWORDS

- **bioreactor**
- **closed-loop systems**
- **diabetes mellitus**
- **drug delivery systems**
- **glucose-responsive systems**
- **insulin delivery**
- **nanomedicine**
- **synthetic biology**

REFERENCES

Alhadramy, M. S. (2016). Diabetes and oral therapies: A review of oral therapies for diabetes mellitus. *Journal of Taibah University Medical Sciences, 11*(4), 317–329.

American Diabetes Association. (2021). 9. Pharmacologic approaches to glycemic treatment: Standards of Medical Care in Diabetes—2021. *Diabetes Care, 44*(Supplement_1), S111–S124.

Baghbantaraghdari, Z., Galardo, F., & Torino, E. (2023). Glucose-responsive materials: Properties, design, and applications. In *Stimuli-Responsive Materials for Biomedical Applications* (Vol. 1436, pp. 231–249). American Chemical Society.

Banting, F. G., Best, C. H., Collip, J. B., Campbell, W. R., & Fletcher, A. A. (1922). Pancreatic extracts in the treatment of diabetes mellitus. *Canadian Medical Association Journal, 12*(3), 141.

Berget, C., Messer, L. H., & Forlenza, G. P. (2019). A clinical overview of insulin pump therapy for the management of diabetes: Past, present, and future of intensive therapy. *Diabetes Spectrum, 32*(3), 194–204.

Bliss, M. (1997). The discovery of insulin: The inside story. *Publications of the American Institute of the History of Pharmacy, 16*, 93–99.

Bode, B., King, A., Russell-Jones, D., & Billings, L. K. (2021). Leveraging advances in diabetes technologies in primary care: A narrative review. *Annals of Medicine, 53*(1), 805–816.

Cai, R., Lv, R., Shi, X., Yang, G., & Jin, J. (2023). CRISPR/dCas9 tools: Epigenetic mechanism and application in gene transcriptional regulation. *International Journal of Molecular Sciences, 24*(19).

Carpenter, S., Rigaud, M., Barile, M., Priest, T. J., Perez, L., & Ferguson, J. B. (2006). *The Ebers Papyrus* (p. 3). Bard College.

Chen, C., Zhao, X. L., Li, Z. H., Zhu, Z. G., Qian, S. H., & Flewitt, A. J. (2017). Current and emerging technology for continuous glucose monitoring. *Sensors, 17*(1), 182.

Cheng, A. W., Wang, H., Yang, H., Shi, L., Katz, Y., Theunissen, T. W., et al. (2013). Multiplexed activation of endogenous genes by CRISPR-on, an RNA-guided transcriptional activator system. *Cell Research, 23*(10), 1163–1171.

Cristelo, C., Nunes, R., Pinto, S., Marques, J. M., Gama, F. M., & Sarmento, B. (2023). Targeting β cells with cathelicidin nanomedicines improves insulin function and pancreas regeneration in type 1 diabetic rats. *ACS Pharmacology & Translational Science, 6*(10), 1544–1560.

de Lima, J. A. L., de Sá, R. A. Q. C., Ramos, V., Bandeira, F. H. D. S., de Assunção, M. A. S., dos Anjos, F. B. R., et al. (2020). Synthetic molecules applied in the treatment of type 2 diabetes. *Metabolism, 3*, 14.

Deepa Maheshvare, M., Raha, S., König, M., & Pal, D. (2023). A pathway model of glucose-stimulated insulin secretion in the pancreatic β-cell. *Frontiers in Endocrinology, 14*.

Dhankhar, S., Chauhan, S., Mehta, D. K., Saini, K., Saini, M., & Gautam, V. (2023). Novel targets for potential therapeutic use in diabetes mellitus. *Diabetology & Metabolic Syndrome, 15*(1), 17.

Domingo-Lopez, D. A., Lattanzi, G., Schreiber, L. H. J., Wallace, E. J., Wylie, R., O'Sullivan, J., et al. (2022). Medical devices, smart drug delivery, wearables and technology for the treatment of diabetes mellitus. *Advanced Drug Delivery Reviews, 185*, 114280.

Elhassaneen, Y., Nasef, A., & Elkerdasy, A. (2022). Studying the bioactive compounds content, antioxidant activities in barley and their relationship with diabetes in rats. *Journal of Home Economics-Menofia University, 32*(2), 80–98.

ElSayed, N. A., Aleppo, G., Aroda, V. R., Bannuru, R. R., Brown, F. M., Bruemmer, D., et al. (2023). 7. Diabetes technology: Standards of care in diabetes—2023. *Diabetes Care, 46*(Supplement_1), S111–S127.

Forouhi, N. G., & Wareham, N. J. (2010). Epidemiology of diabetes. *Medicine, 38*(11), 602–606.

Gregg, E. W., & Bracco, P. (2019). The dynamics of diabetes prevalence, morbidity, and mortality. In *The Diabetes Textbook: Clinical Principles, Patient Management and Public Health Issues* (pp. 11–21).

Guan, Z., Li, H., Liu, R., Cai, C., Liu, Y., Li, J., et al. (2023). Artificial intelligence in diabetes management: Advancements, opportunities, and challenges. *Cell Reports Medicine, 4*(10), 101213.

Hodgkinson, C. P., Gomez, J. A., Mirotsou, M., & Dzau, V. J. (2010). Genetic engineering of mesenchymal stem cells and its application in human disease therapy. *Human Gene Therapy, 21*(11), 1513–1526.

Hoffman, T., Antovski, P., Tebon, P., Xu, C., Ashammakhi, N., Ahadian, S., et al. (2020). Synthetic biology and tissue engineering: Toward fabrication of complex and smart cellular constructs. *Advanced Functional Materials, 30*(26), 1909882.

Hunt, N. J., Lockwood, G. P., Heffernan, S. J., Daymond, J., Ngu, M., Narayanan, R. K., et al. (2024). Oral nanotherapeutic formulation of insulin with reduced episodes of hypoglycemia. *Nature Nanotechnology, 19*(4), 534–544.

Italiya, K. S., Mazumdar, S., Sharma, S., Chitkara, D., Mahato, R. I., & Mittal, A. (2019). Self-assembling lisofylline-fatty acid conjugate for effective treatment of diabetes mellitus. *Nanomedicine: Nanotechnology, Biology and Medicine, 15*(1), 175–187.

Jäck, N., Hemming, A., & Hartmann, L. (2024). Synthesis of dual-responsive amphiphilic glycomacromolecules: Controlled release of glycan ligands via pH and UV stimuli. *Macromolecular Rapid Communications*, 2400439.

Jain, D., Singla, N., & Kumar, R. (2023). Anti-diabetic potential of natural plant sources: An assessment of awareness and consumption among diabetics. *Indian Journal of Nutrition and Dietetics, 60*(4).

Jana, B. A., Shinde, U., & Wadhwani, A. (2020). Synthetic enzyme-based nanoparticles act as smart catalyst for glucose responsive release of insulin. *Journal of Biotechnology, 324*, 1–6.

Jarosinski, M. A., Dhayalan, B., Rege, N., Chatterjee, D., & Weiss, M. A. (2021). 'Smart' insulin-delivery technologies and intrinsic glucose-responsive insulin analogues. *Diabetology, 64*, 1016–1029.

Ji, Y., Zhu, D., Qin, S., & Yang, Y. (2023). Astragalus polysaccharide liposome nanoparticles mediate fatty acid translocase (FAT)/CD36 to improve fatty acid metabolism and regulate glucocorticoid receptor levels in diabetic cardiomyopathy. *Materials Express, 13*(11), 1848–1854.

Kaklotar, D., Agrawal, P., Abdulla, A., Singh, R. P., Mehata, A. K., & Muthu, M. S. (2016). Transition from passive to active targeting of oral insulin nanomedicines: Enhancement in bioavailability and glycemic control in diabetes. *Nanomedicine, 11*(11), 1465–1486.

Kang, S. (2024). Technological innovations transforming diabetes care in practice. *The Journal of Korean Diabetes, 25*(2), 57–61.

Kerr, D., Axelrod, C., Hoppe, C., & Klonoff, D. C. (2018). Diabetes and technology in 2030: A utopian or dystopian future? *Diabetic Medicine, 35*(4), 498–503.

Kompala, T., & Neinstein, A. B. (2022). Smart insulin pens: Advancing digital transformation and a connected diabetes care ecosystem. *Journal of Diabetes Science and Technology, 16*(3), 596–604.

Kovatchev, B. (2019). A century of diabetes technology: Signals, models, and artificial pancreas control. *Trends in Endocrinology & Metabolism, 30*(7), 432–444.

Lakhtakia, R. (2013). The history of diabetes mellitus. *Sultan Qaboos University Medical Journal, 13*(3), 368.

Li, H., Zhang, Z., Bao, X., Xu, G., & Yao, P. (2018). Fatty acid and quaternary ammonium modified chitosan nanoparticles for insulin delivery. *Colloids and Surfaces B: Bio Interfaces, 170*, 136–143.

Li, J., Wang, S., Han, X., Zhang, G., Zhao, M., & Ma, L. (2020). Spatiotemporal trends and influence factors of global diabetes prevalence in recent years. *Social Science & Medicine, 256*, 113062.

Liakos, A., Karagiannis, T., Avgerinos, I., Malandris, K., Tsapas, A., & Bekiari, E. (2023). Management of type 2 diabetes in the new era. *Hormones, 22*(4), 677–684.

Liu, H., Cao, M. M., Wang, Y., Li, L. C., Zhu, L. B., Xie, G. Y., et al. (2015). Endoplasmic reticulum stress is involved in the connection between inflammation and autophagy in type 2 diabetes. *General and Comparative Endocrinology, 210*, 124–129.

Liu, J., Xue, J., Fu, L., Xu, J., Lord, M. S., & Liang, K. (2022). Genetically encoded synthetic beta cells for insulin biosynthesis and release under hyperglycemic conditions. *Advanced Functional Materials, 32*(18), 2111271.

Maity, B., Moorthy, H., & Govindaraju, T. (2023). Glucose-responsive self-regulated injectable silk fibroin hydrogel for controlled insulin delivery. *ACS Applied Materials & Interfaces, 15*(43), 49953–49963.

Mansour, M., Saeed Darweesh, M., & Soltan, A. (2024). Wearable devices for glucose monitoring: A review of state-of-the-art technologies and emerging trends. *Alexandria Engineering Journal, 89*, 224–243.

Martín-Carro, B., Donate-Correa, J., Fernández-Villabrille, S., Martín-Vírgala, J., Panizo, S., Carrillo-López, N., et al. (2023). Experimental models to study diabetes mellitus and its complications: Limitations and new opportunities. *International Journal of Molecular Sciences, 24*(12), 10309. https://doi.org/10.3390/ijms241210309

McLachlan, S., et al. (2016). Worldwide trends in diabetes since 1980: Pooled analysis of 751 population-based measurement studies with over 4.4 million participants. *The Lancet, 387*(10027).

Miller, E. M. (2020). Using continuous glucose monitoring in clinical practice. *Clinical Diabetes, 38*(5), 429–438.

Moon, S. J., Jung, I., & Park, C. Y. (2021). Current advances of artificial pancreas systems: A comprehensive review of the clinical evidence. *Diabetes & Metabolism Journal, 45*(6), 813–839.

Nwokolo, M., & Hovorka, R. (2023). The artificial pancreas and type 1 diabetes. *The Journal of Clinical Endocrinology & Metabolism, 108*(7), 1614–1623.

Olanrewaju, O. A., Sheeba, F., Kumar, A., Ahmad, S., Blank, N., Kumari, R., et al. (2023). Novel therapies in diabetes: A comprehensive narrative review of GLP-1 receptor agonists, SGLT2 inhibitors, and beyond. *Cureus, 15*(12), e51151.

Ong, K. L., Stafford, L. K., McLaughlin, S. A., Boyko, E. J., Vollset, S. E., Smith, A. E., et al. (2023). Global, regional, and national burden of diabetes from 1990 to 2021, with projections of prevalence to 2050: A systematic analysis for the Global Burden of Disease Study 2021. *The Lancet, 402*(10397), 203–234.

Paul, W., & Sharma, C. P. (2010). Fatty acid conjugated calcium phosphate nanoparticles for protein delivery. *International Journal of Applied Ceramic Technology, 7*(2), 129–138.

Pinnaro, C. T., & Tansey, M. J. (2021). The evolution of insulin administration in Type 1 diabetes. *J Diabetes Mellitus, 11*(5), 249–277.

Raoufinia, R., Rahimi, H. R., Saburi, E., & Moghbeli, M. (2024). Advances and challenges of the cell-based therapies among diabetic patients. *J Transl Med, 22*(1), 435.

Rasouli, H., Ramalho, T. C., Popović-Djordjević, J. B., & Devkota, H. P. (2023). Editorial: New opportunities in drug design for the management and treatment of type 2 diabetes. *Frontiers in Pharmacology, 14.* https://doi.org/10.3389/fphar.2023.1187057 (accessed on 2nd February 2026).

Retief, F., & Cilliers, L. (2009). Aretaeus of Cappadocia: The forgotten physician. *Acta Academica, 41*(4), 23–39.

Sabu, C., & Pramod, K. (2020). Advanced nanostructures for oral insulin delivery. *Nanoscience in Medicine, 1*, 187–212.

Saxena, P., Bojar, D., Zulewski, H., & Fussenegger, M. (2020). Synthetic biology technologies for beta cell generation. In *Transplantation, Bioengineering, and Regeneration of the Endocrine Pancreas* (pp. 407–420). Academic Press.

Sharma, G., Sharma, A. R., Nam, J. S., Doss, G. P. C., Lee, S. S., & Chakraborty, C. (2015). Nanoparticle-based insulin delivery system: The next generation efficient therapy for Type 1 diabetes. *Journal of Nanobiotechnology, 13*, 1–13.

Shen, D., Yu, H., Wang, L., Feng, J., Zhang, Q., Pan, J., et al. (2022). Glucose-responsive nanoparticles designed via a molecular-docking-driven method for insulin delivery. *Journal of Controlled Release, 352*, 527–539.

Shirinfar, B., & Ahmed, N. (2019). Diabetes treatment: Selective synthetic receptor for glucose. *Chemistry Open, 8*(1), 84–86. http://dx.doi.org/10.1002/open.201800279 (accessed on 2nd February 2026).

Sugandh, F. N. U., Chandio, M., Raveena, F. N. U., Kumar, L., Karishma, F. N. U., Khuwaja, S., et al. (2023). Advances in the management of diabetes mellitus: A focus on personalized medicine. *Cureus, 15*(8).

Sun, H., Saeedi, P., Karuranga, S., Pinkepank, M., Ogurtsova, K., Duncan, B. B., et al. (2022). IDF Diabetes Atlas: Global, regional and country-level diabetes prevalence estimates for 2021 and projections for 2045. *Diabetes Research and Clinical Practice, 183*, 109119.

Sun, W., Hu, Q., Ji, W., Wright, G., & Gu, Z. (2017). Leveraging physiology for precision drug delivery. *Physiological Reviews, 97*(1), 189–225.

Svetlova, O. V., & Gurieva, I. V. (2023). Innovative technologies in the management of diabetes mellitus: Prevention of hypoglycemia. *Medical Council, 17*(9), 89–95. https://doi.org/10.21518/ms2023-167 (accessed on 2nd February 2026).

Sy, S. L., Munshi, M. M., & Toschi, E. (2022). Can smart pens help improve diabetes management? *J Diabetes Sci Technol, 16*(3), 628–634.

Tattersall, R. (2009). *Diabetes: The Biography*. Oxford University Press.

Tepperman, J. (1988). A view of the history of biology from an islet of Langerhans. In *Endocrinology: People and Ideas* (pp. 285–333).

Wang, J., Wang, Z., Yu, J., Kahkoska, A. R., Buse, J. B., & Gu, Z. (2020). Glucose-responsive insulin and delivery systems: Innovation and translation. *Adv Mater, 32*(13), 1902004.

Willis, T. (1674). *Pharmaceutice rationalis: Or, An Exercitation of The Operations of Medicines in Humane Bodies*. Dring, Harper, Leigh.

World Health Organization. (2023). Diabetes. https://www.who.int/news-room/fact-sheets/detail/diabetes (accessed on 2nd February 2026).

Xian, S., Xiang, Y., Liu, D., Fan, B., Mitrová, K., Ollier, R. C., et al. (2024). Insulin–dendrimer nanocomplex for multi-day glucose-responsive therapy in mice and swine. *Advanced Materials, 36*(5), 2308965.

Xu, M., Huang, J., Jiang, S., He, J., Wang, Z., Qin, H., et al. (2022). Glucose sensitive konjac glucomannan/concanavalin A nanoparticles as oral insulin delivery system. *International Journal of Biological Macromolecules, 202*, 296–308.

Yan, X., Liu, X., Zhao, C., & Chen, G. Q. (2023). Applications of synthetic biology in medical and pharmaceutical fields. *Signal Trans Duct Target Ther, 8*(1), 199.

Yao, Y., Ji, K., Wang, Y., Gu, Z., & Wang, J. (2022). Materials and carriers' development for glucose-responsive insulin. *Accounts of Materials Research, 3*(9), 960–970.

Yu, J., Zhang, Y., Bomba, H., & Gu, Z. (2016). Stimuli-responsive delivery of therapeutics for diabetes treatment. *Accounts of Chemical Research, 1*(3), 323–337.

Zahid, M., Dowlatshahi, S., Kansara, A. H., & Sadhu, A. R. (2023). The evolution of diabetes technology–options toward personalized care. *Endocrine Practice, 29*(8), 653–662.

Zhao, N., Song, Y., Xie, X., Zhu, Z., Duan, C., Nong, C., et al. (2023). Synthetic biology-inspired cell engineering in diagnosis, treatment, and drug development. *Signal Transduction and Targeted Therapy, 8*(1), 112.

Zimmet, P., Alberti, K. G. M. M., & Shaw, J. (2001). Global and societal implications of the diabetes epidemic. *Nature, 414*(6865), 782–787.

Zimmet, P., Alberti, K. G., Magliano, D. J., & Bennett, P. H. (2016). Diabetes mellitus statistics on prevalence and mortality: Facts and fallacies. *Nature Reviews Endocrinology, 12*(10), 616–622.

PART V
Personalized and Regenerative Medicine

CHAPTER 11

Personalized Medicine Strategies Tailored to Diabetes Management

FAROGH AHSAN,[1,*] SHAHZADI BANO,[2] TARIQUE MAHMOOD,[1] ABDUL RAHMAN KHAN,[3] and MOHD. MASIH UZZAMAN KHAN[4]

[1]*Department of Pharmacy, Integral University, Dasauli, Lucknow, Uttar Pradesh, India*

[2]*Department of Applied Sciences, Jahangirabad Institute of Technology, Jahangirabad Fort, Barabanki, Uttar Pradesh, India*

[3]*Department of Chemistry, Integral University, Dasauli, Lucknow, Uttar Pradesh, India*

[4]*Department of Pharmaceutical Chemistry and Pharmacognosy, Unaizah College of Pharmacy, Qassim University, Unaizah, Al-Qassim, Saudi Arabia*

*Corresponding author

ABSTRACT

Personalized medicine is a promising approach for optimizing diabetes treatment by customizing care based on patient characteristics, including genetics and lifestyle. This section provides an overview of personalized diabetes management strategies, emphasizing recent developments, challenges, and future pathways. It begins by discussing the concept of customized medicine and its relevance to diabetes, highlighting the importance of individualized treatment in improving outcomes and minimizing complications. It examines factors influencing diabetes management, such as genetic predisposition, metabolic profiles, and environmental influences, and their integration into personalized treatment plans. The chapter explores methodologies and technologies in personalized diabetes care,

Diabetes: Novel Insights and Therapies. Anas Islam and Badruddeen (Eds)

DOI: 10.1201/9781779644596-16

including genetic testing, biomarker evaluation, and digital health tools. It discusses predictive modeling and machine learning (ML) algorithms to forecast disease progression and treatment outcomes, enabling healthcare providers to make individualized treatment decisions. Additionally, the chapter addresses challenges in implementing personalized medicine in diabetes care, such as ethical considerations, data privacy concerns, and resource access. It explores solutions to these challenges and emphasizes interdisciplinary collaboration and patient engagement. Finally, the chapter outlines future prospects for advancing personalized diabetes management, focusing on omics data, wearable technologies, and AI algorithms, concluding with the significant potential of personalized medicine to transform diabetes care and enhance patient outcomes.

11.1 INTRODUCTION

Diabetes is a multifaceted metabolic disorder characterized by high blood sugar levels (BSLs) due to inadequate insulin secretion, the body's resistance to insulin, or both (Dilworth et al., 2021). Diabetes poses a major global health challenge, with increasing prevalence and varying clinical presentations. Personalized medicine has gained attention as a promising strategy to enhance diabetes management by adapting treatments based on an individual's unique traits, genetic profile, and environmental influences. Personalized medicine, often referred to as precision medicine, is a healthcare approach that considers individual differences in genetics, the environment, and lifestyle. The goal is to tailor prevention, diagnosis, and treatment strategies to the distinctive characteristics of each patient, marking a significant shift from the conventional one-size-fits-all approach, recognizing that individuals respond differently to disease and therapeutic interventions (Ginsburg et al., 2009).

Personalized medicine has immense potential to transform diabetes management. Given the heterogeneity of diabetes, personalized approaches can enhance the precision of diagnosis, predict disease progression, optimize treatment efficacy, and minimize adverse effects (Chan et al., 2011). By leveraging individual genetic predispositions and metabolic profiles and by considering environmental factors, clinicians can customize interventions to achieve better outcomes, including glycemic management, prevention of complications, and improved quality of life (Nicholson, 2006).

Genetics plays a critical role in the susceptibility and progression of diabetes. Variations in specific genes can influence insulin production, glucose metabolism, and response to medications. Understanding an individual's genetic predisposition enables targeted interventions such as early screening for at-risk populations and personalized pharmacotherapy (Prasad and Groop, 2015). Metabolic profiling provides insights into an individual's unique metabolic fingerprints, including glucose tolerance, lipid metabolism, and hormonal regulation. This information helps identify personalized dietary recommendations, exercise plans, and medication regimens tailored to optimize metabolic control. Environmental influences such as food, exercise, stress, and exposure to pollutants significantly impact diabetes risk and management (Morais et al., 2021). Personalized medicine considers these factors when developing tailored lifestyle interventions and behavioral modifications that complement medical treatments. Advancements in genomic technologies have facilitated genetic testing of diabetes-related variants. Genome-wide association studies (GWAS) have helped identify genetic markers associated with diabetes risk and treatment response (Imamura and Maeda, 2011). Genetic testing enables risk stratification, the diagnosis of monogenic forms of diabetes, and the prediction of complications. Biomarkers, including glycated hemoglobin (HbA1c), C-peptide, and lipid profiles, serve as indicators of disease status and treatment responses (Addissouky et al., 2023). Personalized medicine utilizes biomarker analysis to monitor disease progression, adjust therapeutic regimens, and assess individualized risk profiles. Digital health tools, such as mobile apps, wearable devices, and telemedicine platforms, facilitate real-time tracking of glucose levels, physical activity, and medication adherence. These platforms integrate data to provide personalized feedback, support self-management, and enable remote consultation with healthcare providers (Shan et al., 2019).

Predictive analysis methods, such as machine learning (ML) algorithms, examine various datasets to forecast diabetes progression. By incorporating genetic, clinical, and lifestyle data, these models can identify individuals at high risk for targeted interventions and personalized monitoring. ML algorithms forecast individual responses to antidiabetic medications based on genetic and clinical profiles. These predictive tools optimize treatment selection, dosage adjustments, and therapeutic outcomes while minimizing adverse reactions (Venkatachalapathy et al., 2021).

Ethical challenges arise concerning genetic privacy, informed consent, and equitable access to personalized interventions. Clinicians must navigate the ethical dilemmas associated with genetic testing, data sharing, and patient autonomy in personalized diabetes management. Data safety and confidentiality concerns are high priorities in personalized medicine, given the sensitivity of genetic and health-related information. Robust data governance frameworks are necessary to safeguard patient confidentiality and mitigate privacy risk. The implementation of personalized medicine requires adequate resources, including specialized training, infrastructure for genetic testing, and reimbursement models. Disparities in access to personalized interventions pose challenges to equitable healthcare delivery (Parker, 2024).

The effective implementation of personalized medicine in diabetes management necessitates interdisciplinary collaboration among clinicians, geneticists, bioinformaticians, and behavioral scientists. Collaborative efforts optimize data interpretation, care coordination, and patient-centered decision-making. Active patient engagement is essential for successful adoption of personalized medicine. Empowering individuals with diabetes through education, shared decision making, and self-management support promotes treatment adherence and long-term health outcomes (Cordeiro, 2014).

Combining data from genomics, transcriptomics, proteomics, and metabolomics offers potential for thorough disease profiling and tailored treatment strategies. Multi-omics approaches enable a holistic understanding of the diabetes pathophysiology and inform targeted interventions. Advancements in wearable technologies have enabled the continuous observation of glucose levels, workouts, and vital signs. The incorporation of wearable devices with machine-learning algorithms enhances real-time data analytics and personalized feedback for diabetes management (Witt et al., 2019). Artificial intelligence (AI) algorithms, including deep learning and neural networks, have revolutionized diabetes care by predicting outcomes, optimizing treatment algorithms, and facilitating precision medicine. AI-powered decision support systems provide clinicians with a personalized vision for effective patient management (Guan et al., 2023).

Personalized medical strategies tailored for diabetes management harness the power of genetics, metabolic profiling, and environmental influences to optimize care delivery. Despite challenges in implementation, innovative methodologies and technologies pave the way for precision-based interventions, fostering interdisciplinary collaboration, patient engagement, and the future integration of omics data and AI. Embracing personalized medicine in diabetes management promises to revolutionize healthcare delivery, offering tailored solutions that improve the consequences and standards of life for individuals living with diabetes.

11.1.1 PERSONALIZED MEDICINE

Personalized medicine, often referred to as precision medicine, represents a groundbreaking approach to healthcare that focuses on customizing medical care and interventions based on individual traits, including genetics, lifestyle, and environmental influences. The fundamental idea is to shift from the ordinary one-size-fits-all model to targeted and effective therapies. This field leverages advancements in genomics, biomarker research, and data analytics to gain deeper insights into the distinct characteristics of each patient's disease and their response to treatment (Anaya et al., 2016).

A crucial component of precision medicine is the use of genetic information to inform medical decisions. Advances in genome sequencing allow quick and thorough analysis of an individual's genetic code, providing valuable insights into disease susceptibility, drug breakdown, and potential responses to treatment (Cordero and Ashley, 2012). By identifying genetic variations related to particular diseases, clinicians can categorize patients into subgroups that may respond differently to certain therapies. In addition to genomics, personalized medicine incorporates other 'omics' data—such as transcriptomics, proteomics, and metabolomics—to offer a holistic view of disease procedure and treatment responses (Olivier et al., 2019). Biomarkers derived from these analyses serve as indicators of disease, disease progression, or therapeutic outcomes. For instance, circulating tumor DNA in the bloodstream can reveal real-time information about a cancer's genetic makeup, aiding treatment monitoring and adaptation (Corcoran, 2019).

Another key aspect of personalized medicine involves leveraging clinical data and health records to customize treatment plans. Electronic health records (EHRs) and machine-learning algorithms assist in the examination of vast datasets to identify patterns associated with patient outcomes. By combining clinical data with genetic information and lifestyle factors, healthcare workers can optimize treatment strategies to maximize their efficacy and minimize adverse effects (Shickel et al., 2017).

The impact of personalized medicine extends beyond oncology to various fields such as cardiology, neurology, and infectious diseases. For example, in cardiology, inherent testing can identify patients at a greater risk of adverse drug reactions to certain heart medications. Understanding host genetics in infectious diseases can elucidate why individuals respond differently to pathogens and vaccines (Chan and Ginsburg, 2011).

Ethical, legal, and societal implications (ELSI) are critical considerations in the implementation of personalized medicine. Issues such as patient privacy, informed consent for genetic testing, and unbiased access to advanced diagnostics and therapies must be addressed. Furthermore, the affordability and scalability of personalized medicine technologies pose challenges for their widespread adoption in diverse healthcare settings (Alvarez et al., 2022).

Thus, personalized medicine signifies a transformative shift towards more precise and effective healthcare delivery. It integrates cutting-edge technologies, including genomics, 'omics' sciences, and data analytics, to modify medical interventions to specific patients. While significant progress has been made, further research and investment are needed to address scientific, regulatory, and ethical challenges, and to fully leverage personalized medicine to improve patient outcomes (Figure 11.1).

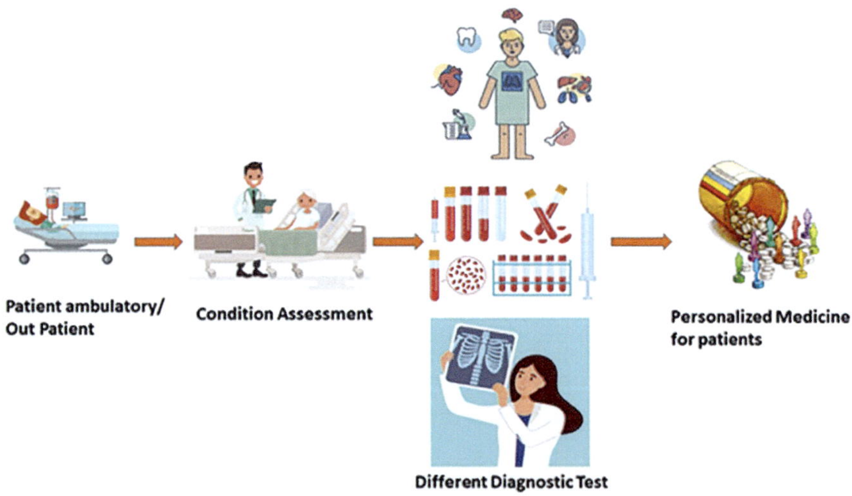

FIGURE 11.1 Graphical representation of personalized medicine.

11.1.2 RELEVANCE TO DIABETES MANAGEMENT

Diabetes mellitus (DM) is a complex metabolic disorder characterized by elevated blood glucose levels (BGLs), primarily due to insulin resistance and/or inadequate insulin production by the pancreas. This chronic condition affects millions of people worldwide and presents a significant challenge owing to its heterogeneity in presentation, progression, and response to treatment (Yadav et al., 2024).

Personalized medicine for diabetes mellitus is a revolutionary approach that customizes treatment strategies for each patient, considering their unique genetic, environmental, and clinical factors. Personalized medicine in diabetes highlights the importance of shifting away from a one-size-fits-all strategy towards targeted therapies that consider the heterogeneity of the disease and the variability in treatment responses among individuals (Sugandh et al., 2023).

The concept of personalized medicine for diabetes involves leveraging advancements in genetic and molecular profiling to stratify patients into distinct subtypes with specific treatment responses and risks. For instance, recent research has identified different genetic variants linked to type 1 and 2 diabetes, influencing disease susceptibility and replying to different medications. By examining a person's genetic profile, clinicians can assess their risk of developing diabetes, their response to particular medications, and identify personalized prevention strategies (Fitipaldi et al., 2018).

One promising area of personalized medicine for diabetes is the development of tailored insulin treatment. Continuous glucose monitoring (CGM) paired with advanced algorithms delivers real-time data on glucose levels, allowing the customization of insulin doses to meet individual needs. Additionally, genetic testing can help to identify patients who are likely to benefit from specific insulin formulations or complementary therapies. This approach can improve treatment outcomes and reduce the risk of adverse effects such as hypoglycemia (Rodbard et al., 2017). In clinical practice, the implementation of personalized medicine requires interdisciplinary collaboration among endocrinologists, geneticists, pharmacologists, and informatics experts. Integrated EHRs and bioinformatics tools are essential for aggregating and analyzing large datasets, enabling the conversion of genetic insights into practical clinical decisions. Additionally, patient education and engagement are critical in promoting adherence to personalized treatment plans and lifestyle modifications (Abul-Husn and Kenny, 2019).

Despite its potential, several challenges remain in the widespread adoption of personalized medicine for diabetes. Challenges include the expensive nature of genetic testing, lack of access to specialized expertise, and ethical concerns regarding data privacy and informed consent. Nonetheless, continuous research and technological innovations are gradually addressing these obstacles and facilitating personalized and effective diabetes care.

11.2 FACTORS INFLUENCING DIABETES MANAGEMENT: A FOCUS ON GENETIC PREDISPOSITION

Diabetes mellitus is a persistent metabolic condition characterized by elevated BGLs, which arise from insufficient insulin production or inability of the body to utilize insulin effectively. This intricate disorder is influenced by various genetic and environmental factors, and genetic susceptibility plays a crucial role in determining an individual's likelihood of developing diabetes and affecting disease management.

11.2.1 UNDERSTANDING GENETIC PREDISPOSITION TO DIABETES

Type 1 and type 2 diabetes represent the two main categories of diabetes, each of which is characterized by unique genetic factors.

1. **Type 1 Diabetes (T1D):** This is an autoimmune disorder characterized by the attack of the immune system and destruction of insulin-secreting beta cells located in the pancreas. Although the precise etiology of T1D is not fully understood, a genetic predisposition is a key factor. Specific human leukocyte antigen (HLA) genes, particularly those located within the HLA complex on chromosome 6, are associated with an elevated risk of developing T1D. Variations in genes, such as HLA-DR3-DQ2 and HLA-DR4-DQ8, significantly contribute to the autoimmune response leading to T1D (Klak et al., 2020).
2. **Type 2 Diabetes (T2D):** This is a multifactorial condition characterized by insulin resistance and relative insulin deficiency. Genetic factors play a crucial role in the development of T2D, with heritability estimates between 20% and 80%. Numerous genetic variants have been associated with an elevated risk of T2D, including those that affect insulin secretion (e.g., TCF7L2 and KCNJ11) and insulin action (e.g., PPARG and IRS1). These variants interact with environmental factors, including diet, physical activity, and obesity, to affect the susceptibility to T2D (Stančáková et al., 2016).

11.2.1.1 IMPACT OF GENETIC PREDISPOSITION ON DIABETES MANAGEMENT

Genetic predisposition influences various aspects of diabetes management, including:

1. **Risk Assessment:** Genetic testing can help identify individuals who are at an increased risk of developing diabetes. For example, individuals carrying specific HLA genotypes associated with T1D or T2D-related genetic variants can be informed of their increased risk, prompting early monitoring and preventive measures (Tsunoda, 2019).
2. **Treatment Personalization:** Thus, genetic information can guide personalized treatment approaches. For instance, in T2D, knowledge of certain genetic variants (e.g., TCF7L2) can influence medication choices. Individuals with specific variants may respond better to certain oral antidiabetic drugs (e.g., sulfonylureas) than others (Ordelheide et al., 2018).
3. **Glycemic Control:** Genetic factors contribute to variations in the glycemic response and insulin sensitivity among individuals with diabetes. Understanding these genetic determinants can aid in optimizing glucose-lowering therapies and achieving better glycemic control (Shaham et al., 2008).
4. **Complication Risk Prediction:** Certain genetic markers are associated with an increased risk of diabetes-related complications such as kidney disease (nephropathy), eye damage (retinopathy), and heart disease. Genetic testing can help to identify individuals who may benefit from enhanced monitoring and early intervention to mitigate the risk of these complications (Ma, 2016).

11.2.1.2 CHALLENGES AND CONSIDERATIONS

Although genetic predisposition is integral to diabetes management, several challenges and considerations must be acknowledged.

1. **Polygenic Nature:** Diabetes susceptibility is influenced by multiple genetic variants of the genome. The polygenic nature of diabetes necessitates a comprehensive genetic profiling to capture the full spectrum of genetic risk factors (Udler et al., 2019).

2. **Gene-Environment Interactions:** Genetic predisposition interacts with environmental factors (e.g., diet, physical activity, and obesity) to modulate the risk of diabetes. Strategies for diabetes management must consider gene-environment interactions (Tremblay and Hamet, 2019).

3. **Ethical and Psychological Implications:** Genetic testing for diabetes risk raises ethical concerns regarding privacy, confidentiality, and potential psychological impacts (e.g., anxiety and stigma). Genetic counseling and education are essential to address these concerns (Andrews and Zuiker, 2002).

4. **Limited Predictive Power:** Although genetic testing can identify individuals at a higher risk of diabetes, it does not offer absolute predictions. Many people with an elevated genetic risk may never develop the disease, emphasizing the need to consider genetic data alongside clinical assessments and lifestyle factors (Prasad and Groop, 2015).

Genetic predisposition significantly influences diabetes management by affecting risk assessment, treatment personalization, glycemic control, and complication risk prediction (Sirdah and Reading, 2020). Understanding the genetic basis of diabetes enables personalized approaches for its prevention, diagnosis, and treatment. However, challenges such as the polygenic nature of diabetes and gene-environment interactions underscore the complexity of the genetic contributions to diabetes. Future research and clinical efforts should focus on integrating genetic information into comprehensive diabetes management strategies, while addressing ethical and practical considerations.

11.2.2 UNDERSTANDING THE METABOLIC PROFILE

Diabetes management involves a complex array of processes that are affected by numerous factors, one of which is the individual's metabolic profile. A person's metabolic profile encompasses a range of physiological parameters that affect how the body processes glucose and regulates insulin levels. Understanding these factors is crucial for optimizing diabetes care and achieving better health outcomes. This study explored the key elements of the metabolic profile and their implications for diabetes management.

11.2.2.1 *INSULIN RESISTANCE*

Insulin resistance is a defining characteristic of type 2 diabetes and plays a crucial role in its management. It is characterized by diminished responsiveness of cells to insulin, which results in a decreased ability to absorb glucose from the bloodstream. Those who experience insulin resistance typically require elevated amounts of insulin to sustain normal BGLs, which can put considerable pressure on the pancreas. Various factors that contribute to insulin resistance encompass obesity, lack of physical activity, genetic factors, and the influence of specific medications.

Managing insulin resistance requires implementing lifestyle changes, including weight reduction, consistent physical activity, and adjustments to dietary habits. Furthermore, pharmacological treatments such as metformin and insulin sensitizers may enhance insulin sensitivity and assist in achieving better glycemic control in patients with diabetes (Czech, 2017).

11.2.2.2 *BETA-CELL FUNCTION*

β-cells located in the pancreas are responsible for the production and secretion of insulin in response to elevated BGLs. In diabetes, beta cell dysfunction can lead to inadequate insulin secretion, resulting in persistent hyperglycemia. Factors influencing beta cell function include genetic factors, autoimmune destruction (as seen in type 1 diabetes), and chronic hyperglycemia.

Preservation of beta cell function is crucial for diabetes management. Early intervention with medications that support beta cell health, such as incretin-based therapies (e.g., GLP-1 receptor agonists), can help maintain insulin production and improve glycemic control (Meloni et al., 2013).

11.2.2.3 *BODY COMPOSITION AND ADIPOSE TISSUE*

Body composition, particularly the distribution of adipose tissue (fat), plays a crucial role in managing diabetes. Excess visceral fat, commonly associated with obesity, is associated with insulin resistance and chronic inflammation, which are factors that play a significant role in the development and progression of type 2 diabetes. Additionally, adipose tissue releases hormones and cytokines (adipokines), which affect insulin sensitivity and glucose metabolism (Wondmkun, 2020).

Weight management through calorie restriction, increased physical activity, and possibly bariatric surgery in severe cases can help reduce adipose tissue and improve metabolic health in individuals with diabetes (Bays, 2023).

11.2.2.4 DIETARY FACTORS

Dietary choices significantly affect glycemic control and overall metabolic health. A diet high in refined carbohydrates, sugars, and saturated fats can worsen insulin resistance and lead to weight gain. Conversely, a diet abundant in fiber, whole grains, lean proteins, and healthy fats helps to maintain stable BGLs and enhances metabolic health.

Nutritional counseling and education are essential components of diabetes management. Dietitians can help individuals develop personalized meal plans that optimize glycemic control while meeting their nutritional needs (O'Keefe et al., 2008).

11.2.2.5 PHYSICAL ACTIVITY

Insulin sensitivity is improved by regular physical activity, which enhances glucose uptake by muscles and promotes overall cardiovascular health. A sedentary lifestyle is associated with increased insulin resistance and a higher risk of obesity and type 2 diabetes. Conversely, engaging in aerobic and resistance exercises can aid in regulating BGLs and reducing the need for diabetes medication.

Healthcare providers should encourage regular physical activity tailored to individual capabilities and preferences as part of their diabetes management strategies (Imierska et al., 2020).

11.2.2.6 MEDICATIONS AND TREATMENT APPROACHES

Individuals with diabetes frequently require pharmacological treatments to maintain the target level of sugar in the blood and reduce the risk of complications. The choice of medication is prejudiced by factors such as the length of time since diagnosis, existing comorbidities, and patient preferences. Commonly prescribed drugs include metformin, sulfonylureas, insulin, SGLT-2 inhibitors, GLP-1 receptor agonists, and DPP-4 inhibitors (Taylor et al., 2021).

Personalized treatment plans that consider metabolic profiles are essential for optimizing diabetes management and minimizing adverse effects. Diabetes management is influenced by various factors related to an individual's metabolic profile. Understanding and addressing these factors through personalized interventions is crucial for optimizing glycemic management, averting complications, and improving the overall quality of life of those living with diabetes.

11.2.3 ENVIRONMENTAL INFLUENCES

Effective management of diabetes requires consideration of a range of factors that extend beyond individual behaviors and medical treatments. Environmental influences play a substantial role in determining how people with diabetes cope with their conditions. These influences can affect access to resources, social support networks, lifestyle choices, and overall health outcomes (Hill-Briggs et al., 2021). Understanding these factors is the key to developing comprehensive strategies for effective diabetes management.

One key environmental factor influencing diabetes management is access to health care amenities. People residing in areas with limited healthcare facilities or health professionals may face challenges in obtaining regular check-ups, medications, or specialized care for diabetes. Lack of access can hinder proper management and lead to complications. Studies have shown that individuals in underserved communities or rural areas often experience disparities in diabetes outcomes owing to healthcare access issues (Dendup et al., 2018). Social and economic factors also play critical roles. Socioeconomic status influences the availability of nutritious food, secure housing, and opportunities for physical exercise, all of which are crucial for effective diabetes management. Lower-income individuals may struggle to afford nutritious foods or diabetes medications, leading to poorer glycemic control and health outcomes (Huang et al., 2014). Additionally, social support networks, including family and community resources, can significantly affect diabetes management. Strong support systems can provide encouragement, help with lifestyle changes, and reduce stress, whereas a lack of support may lead to feelings of isolation and difficulty in effectively managing the condition (Hill-Briggs et al., 2021).

Environmental factors such as the surroundings also play a significant role in diabetes management. Neighborhoods that lack safe areas for physical activity or access to fresh produce can lead to sedentary lifestyles and poor dietary choices, thereby increasing the risk of diabetes. Urban planning that promotes walkability, bicycle ability, and access to parks can encourage physical activity and healthier lifestyles, ultimately supporting better diabetes management outcomes (Aarthi et al., 2022). Cultural influences are another important factor. Cultural beliefs and practices regarding food, exercise, and health-seeking behaviors can impact diabetes management approaches. For instance, traditional diets high in carbohydrates or cultural norms surrounding portion sizes may affect blood sugar control. Healthcare providers need to be culturally competent, understand, and respect diverse cultural practices to effectively tailor diabetes management plans (Deol et al., 2022).

Environmental stressors such as pollution and exposure to environmental toxins can also influence diabetes management. Studies have suggested that air pollution and chemical exposure may be responsible for insulin resistance and diabetes risks (Bodin et al., 2015). Addressing these environmental factors through policy interventions and public health measures is crucial for developing comprehensive diabetes management strategies.

Diabetes management is profoundly influenced by environmental factors that extend beyond individual control. Access to healthcare services, socioeconomic status, social support networks, built environment characteristics, cultural considerations, and environmental stressors all contribute to the complexity of diabetes management. Recognizing and addressing these environmental influences are essential for developing holistic approaches to diabetes care that promote better health outcomes and reduce disparities among individuals with diabetes (Brown, 2013). Public health initiatives and policy interventions designed to improve these environmental factors are crucial to support effective diabetes management across all populations (Table 11.1).

11.3 THE METHODOLOGIES AND TECHNOLOGIES IN PERSONALIZED MEDICINE

11.3.1 GENETIC TESTING

Genetic testing is essential in the realm of personalized medicine, as it provides critical information about a person's genetic makeup and associated risks for various diseases. This essay explores the methodologies and technologies employed in genetic testing for personalized medicine, highlighting its significance in modern healthcare.

TABLE 11.1 Different Factors Having an Impact on Diabetes Management

Factor	Description	Impact on Diabetes Management
Genetic predisposition	Refers to inherited genetic variations that influence susceptibility to diabetes.	• Determines the likelihood of developing type 1 or type 2 diabetes. • Affects response to specific treatments and medications. • Guides personalized screening and monitoring protocols for at-risk individuals.
Metabolic profile	Encompasses individual characteristics related to glucose metabolism, lipid levels, and body weight.	• Influences insulin sensitivity and secretion. • Dictates dietary and lifestyle recommendations based on glycemic control goals. • Shapes the choice of pharmacological interventions such as insulin or oral hypoglycemic agents.
Environmental influences	Includes lifestyle factors, dietary habits, physical activity levels, and socioeconomic conditions.	• Impacts overall glycemic control and disease progression. • Determines the need for personalized diabetes education and behavioral interventions. • Affects the likelihood of developing diabetes-related complications, such as cardiovascular disease and neuropathy.

11.3.1.1 METHODOLOGIES IN GENETIC TESTING

Genetic testing involves examining an individual's DNA to detect variations linked to disease susceptibility, drug reactions, and other health-related factors (Franceschini et al., 2018). Genetic testing methodologies have advanced remarkably in recent years, propelled by breakthroughs in genomics and bioinformatic research.

1. **Sequencing Technologies:** The core methodology in genetic testing is DNA sequencing, which identifies the exact nucleotide sequence in an individual's DNA. Next-generation sequencing (NGS) technologies, such as those used in Illumina platforms, have transformed genetic testing by making it faster and more affordable for sequencing entire genomes or specific gene panels. NGS enables the detection of genetic mutations associated with diseases, facilitating a more accurate analysis and personalized treatment plans (Xuan et al., 2013).
2. **Genome-Wide Association Studies (GWAS):** These examine the genomes of extensive populations to identify genetic variants

associated with particular traits or diseases. This approach has played a crucial role in uncovering the genetic foundations of complex conditions such as diabetes, heart disease, and cancer. The results of GWAS aid in personalized medicine by identifying genetic markers that inform risk evaluation and treatment choices (Cano-Gamez and Trynka, 2020).

3. **Polygenic Risk Scores (PRS):** These estimate a person's genetic risk for specific diseases by examining various genetic variants throughout the genome. By integrating data from large-scale genetic studies, the PRS provides personalized risk assessments that can inform preventive strategies and targeted interventions (Lewis and Vassos, 2020).
4. **Pharmacogenomics:** This studies the impact of genetic differences on how individuals respond to drugs, thereby allowing for more tailored and effective treatment options. This methodology guides personalized drug selection and dosage optimization, minimizes adverse effects, and improves the treatment outcomes. For instance, genetic testing can identify patients with specific CYP2D6 variants who are at risk of poor response to certain antidepressants (Malsagova et al., 2020).

11.3.1.2 TECHNOLOGIES DRIVING PERSONALIZED MEDICINE

Advancements in technologies underpin the application of genetic testing in personalized medicine:

1. **Bioinformatics:** These tools and databases are essential for interpreting genetic data. Algorithms are employed to analyze sequencing results, identify genetic variants, and predict their functional impact on genes and proteins.
2. **ML and AI Algorithms:** These were employed to uncover patterns in large genetic datasets, assisting in disease classification, patient stratification, and treatment prediction.
3. **Single-Cell Sequencing:** This new technology allows the examination of individual cells, offering valuable insights into the diversity of cells within tissues and tumors. Single-cell sequencing is essential for understanding disease mechanisms and developing targeted treatments (Levy et al., 2022; Vadapalli et al., 2022).

11.3.1.3 SIGNIFICANCE AND CHALLENGES

Genetic testing has transformed healthcare by enabling precise diagnostics and tailored treatments. It facilitates early disease detection, guides personalized prevention strategies, and optimizes therapeutic interventions. Challenges such as data privacy, regulatory concerns, and ethical issues related to genetic information must be addressed to guarantee the responsible application of personalized medicine (Manolio et al., 2013).

Genetic testing is essential for personalized medicine, as it offers unique insights into a person's genetic profile and the risk of developing diseases. Progress in sequencing technologies, bioinformatics, and data analytics is accelerating the incorporation of genetic testing into clinical settings and transforming healthcare delivery. Research is increasingly revealing the complex connections between genetics and diseases, and personalized medicine holds great promise for improving patient outcomes and advancing precision healthcare (Figure 11.2).

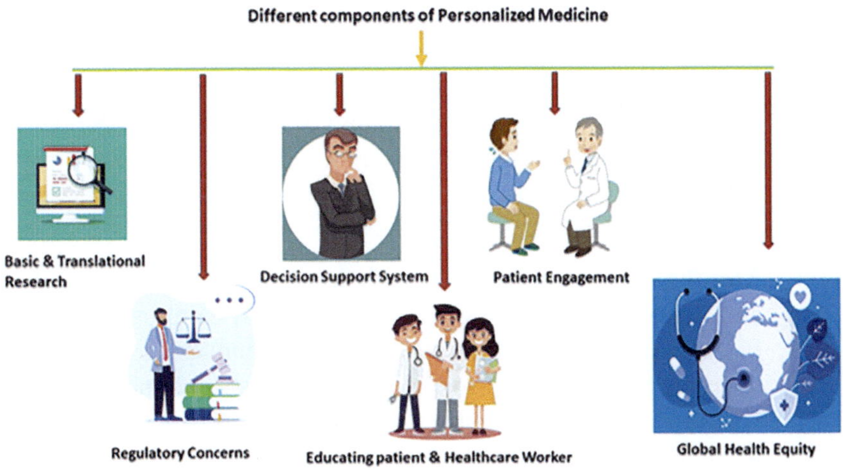

FIGURE 11.2 Different components of personalized medicine.

11.3.2 BIOMARKER ANALYSIS

Biomarkers are quantifiable indicators that help assess normal biological functions, track disease development, or gauge the effectiveness of medical treatments. This paradigm shift is made possible through the integration of advanced technologies and methodologies, particularly biomarker analysis (Landeck et al., 2016). Biomarkers are essential for enabling personalized medicine as they assist in disease diagnosis, prognosis, and treatment selection.

11.3.2.1 BIOMARKER TYPES AND ANALYSIS METHODOLOGIES

1. **Genomic Biomarkers:** Genetic biomarkers, such as single nucleotide polymorphisms (SNPs), gene mutations, and gene expression profiles, play a crucial role in personalized medicine. Advanced technologies, such as NGS, enable detailed genomic profiling, which helps identify genetic variations associated with disease risk, progression, and treatment effectiveness. For instance, pharmacogenomics uses these genomic markers to predict how individuals respond to specific medications, enhancing drug selection and dosage for improved therapeutic outcomes (Ziegler et al., 2012).
2. **Proteomic Biomarkers**: Proteomic analysis involves studying proteins and their modifications to identify disease-specific biomarkers. Mass spectrometry (MS) and immunoassays are commonly employed techniques for proteomic biomarker discovery and validation. These biomarkers can provide insights into disease mechanisms and assist in the development of targeted therapies (Hudler et al., 2014).
3. **Metabolic Biomarkers**: Metabolomics focuses on profiling small molecules (metabolites) in biological samples. Metabolic biomarkers can reflect the physiological changes associated with diseases or drug responses. Nuclear magnetic resonance (NMR) spectroscopy and mass spectrometry are the principal tools used in metabolomics for biomarker identification (Jacob et al., 2019).
4. **Imaging Biomarkers**: Medical imaging techniques, such as magnetic resonance imaging (MRI), computed tomography (CT), and positron emission tomography (PET), offer noninvasive methods to observe physiological functions and disease traits. Biomarkers obtained from these imaging methods support early diagnosis, staging, and tracking of diseases (Mitterhauser et al., 2014).

11.3.2.2 TECHNOLOGIES ENABLING BIOMARKER ANALYSIS

1. **Next-Generation Sequencing (NGS)**: These technologies allow for quick and affordable sequencing of complete genomes, making it easier to identify genetic variations linked to diseases and responses to medications.
2. **Mass Spectrometry (MS)**: It is a versatile investigative technique used in proteomics and metabolomics for biomarker discovery and quantification.
3. **Microarray Analysis**: Microarray platforms allow for rapid analysis of gene expression patterns, making it easier to discover gene signatures that are specific to certain diseases.
4. **Digital PCR (dPCR)**: This offers precise quantification of nucleic acids, enhancing the sensitivity and accuracy of genetic biomarker detection.
5. **High-Content Screening (HCS)**: This conglomerates automated microscopy with image study to screen large libraries of compounds and assess their effects on cellular pathways, aiding in drug discovery and personalized treatment development (Sorbini et al., 2024).

11.3.2.3 CLINICAL APPLICATIONS OF BIOMARKER ANALYSIS IN PERSONALIZED MEDICINE

1. **Cancer:** Biomarkers play a critical role in cancer diagnosis (e.g., HER2 in breast cancer), prognosis (e.g., BRCA mutations), and treatment selection (e.g., EGFR mutations guiding targeted therapies).
2. **Cardiovascular Diseases**: Biomarkers such as troponin and B-type natriuretic peptide (BNP) are used for detecting and checking heart conditions.
3. **Neurological Disorders**: Biomarkers such as amyloid beta and tau proteins assist in the early detection and tracking of disease progression in Alzheimer's disease (AD).

Methodologies and technologies for biomarker analysis are fundamental to the advancement of personalized medicine (Wishart et al., 2016).

Healthcare professionals can leverage genomic, proteomic, metabolic, and imaging biomarkers to make informed decisions based on individual patient profiles. This approach optimizes treatment effectiveness, reduces adverse effects, and improves patient outcomes. As technology progresses, biomarker-driven strategies will continue to transform healthcare delivery, leading to more precise, effective, and personalized treatment options.

11.3.3 DIGITAL HEALTH PLATFORMS

Digital health platforms are vital in advancing personalized medicine as they combine technology with healthcare to customize treatments and interventions for individual patients. These platforms leverage various digital tools and data analytics to gather, process, and interpret large volumes of patient-specific information, ultimately enabling more accurate and effective medical care (Johnson et al., 2021). The key components of digital health platforms in personalized medicine include the following:

1. **Data Collection and Integration:** Digital health platforms gather a variety of datasets, together with EHRs, genomics, wearable device data (such as from fitness trackers), lifestyle information, and patient-reported outcomes. These integrated data help build an inclusive profile of each patient's health status and needs.
2. **Advanced Analytics and AI**: ML algorithms and AI are used to examine extensive datasets, recognize patterns, and produce insights that guide tailored treatment choices. For example, AI-driven platforms can predict patient responses to specific medications by considering genetic markers and previous treatment outcomes.
3. **Clinical Decision Support**: Digital platforms provide clinicians with real-time decision support tools that incorporate personalized data and evidence-based guidelines to optimize treatment plans. This can include alerts for potential drug interactions, tailored dosage recommendations, and reminders for preventive screening.
4. **Remote Monitoring and Telemedicine**: Digital health platforms facilitate continuous monitoring of patients beyond traditional healthcare settings through remote sensors and telemedicine. This ability enables prompt identification of health problems and swift actions to address them, thereby enhancing personalized care delivery.

5. **Patient Engagement and Education**: Many platforms incorporate patient engagement features, such as mobile apps or patient portals that provide personalized health information, educational resources, and tools for self-management. This promotes active patient participation in care (Kasoju et al., 2023).

Examples of digital health platforms driving personalized medicine include IBM Watson Health, which uses AI to investigate medical data for precision oncology, and 23andMe, a direct-to-consumer genetic testing service that offers personalized health insights based on genetic information (Obermeyer and Emanuel, 2016).

These platforms are transforming healthcare by empowering clinicians with actionable insights and engaging patients in health management. However, challenges persist, including interoperability issues, data privacy concerns, and the necessity for the robust validation of AI-driven clinical tools.

11.4 PREDICTIVE MODELING AND MACHINE LEARNING

11.4.1 DISEASE PROGRESSION

Predicting disease progression and personalized treatment for diabetes using modeling and ML methods is a rapidly developing field of study that offers significant potential for enhancing patient outcomes. By leveraging large-scale datasets, advanced algorithms, and personalized patient information, researchers and clinicians can develop predictive models to anticipate disease trajectories and accordingly tailor interventions (Kasula et al., 2023). The following is an overview of how this is applied:

1. **Predictive Modeling for Diabetes Progression**: ML models can utilize EHR, lifestyle factors, clinical biomarkers, and genetic data to predict the progression of diabetes. For instance, predictive models have been developed to forecast the transition from prediabetes to diabetes based on various risk factors and individual profiles (e.g., obesity, family history, and glucose levels) (Smith et al., 2018).
2. **Personalized Treatment Recommendations**: ML algorithms can analyze patient-specific data to recommend tailored treatment strategies. This includes optimizing insulin dosages, suggesting dietary modifications, or identifying ideal times for

physical activity based on individual responses and health status (Kavakiotis et al., 2017).

3. **Early Detection and Intervention**: ML models can identify subtle trends in patient data that indicate the early stages of diabetes progression, allowing for timely interventions to prevent complications (Zhou et al., 2018).
4. **Precision Medicine Approaches**: Researchers can uncover genetic markers that affect diabetes risk and treatment responses by combining ML with genetic data, facilitating precision medicine in diabetes management (Mahajan et al., 2018).

11.4.2 TREATMENT RESPONSE

Predictive treatment response modeling using ML is a key factor in promoting tailored treatment approaches for diabetes. Diabetes management is inherently complex owing to variations in disease progression and individual responses to treatment. The ability to predict treatment outcomes based on patient-specific characteristics is instrumental for optimizing therapy and improving patient outcomes.

Diabetes is a long-term metabolic condition characterized by irregular BSLs. Managing diabetes usually involves lifestyle changes, medication, and sometimes, insulin therapy. However, treatment responses can vary significantly among individuals, making it challenging to achieve optimal glycemic control and prevent complications. Predictive modeling employs data-based techniques to recognize trends and anticipate how specific patients may react to various treatments (Galindo et al., 2023).

ML, which falls under the umbrella of AI, is particularly useful here, as it can process extensive datasets and reveal intricate connections among variables. By utilizing various data sources, such as genetic data, medical records, lifestyle choices, and biomarkers, ML algorithms can be used to develop tailored predictive models. These models can predict treatment responses based on individual patient characteristics, thereby enabling clinicians to tailor interventions accordingly (Javaid et al., 2022).

A key application of predictive modeling in diabetes treatment is the prediction of medication efficacy and adverse effects. For example, ML algorithms can analyze patient facts to forecast which oral antidiabetic drugs are most likely to achieve the target glucose levels with minimal side effects for a specific patient. This personalized approach improves treatment adherence and reduces the risk of complications associated with ineffective or poorly tolerated medications.

Another area where predictive modeling excels is insulin therapy optimization. Insulin dosing requirements can vary significantly among individuals, making it challenging to achieve stable glycemic control. ML models can analyze CGM data, meal patterns, physical activity levels, and other factors to predict optimal insulin dosages tailored to individual patient needs. This approach minimizes the risk of hypoglycemia and hyperglycemia episodes and improves overall diabetes management (Bell et al., 2020). Furthermore, predictive modeling contributes to the development of risk stratification tools for diabetic complications. By analyzing longitudinal patient data, ML can identify individuals at a high risk for cardiovascular events, kidney disease, or retinopathy. This enables proactive intervention and targeted monitoring to prevent or delay complications, resulting in better patient outcomes and lower healthcare expenses.

Predictive treatment response modeling using ML offers significant potential for advancing personalized treatment strategies for diabetes care. By controlling data and AI, clinicians can make informed decisions tailored to the unique features and needs of individual patients. However, it is essential to emphasize the significance of data features, model interpretability, and validation when developing reliable predictive models for clinical use (Derevitskii et al., 2020).

11.5 CHALLENGES IN IMPLEMENTING PERSONALIZED MEDICINE

11.5.1 ETHICAL CONSIDERATIONS

Ethical dilemmas in personalized medicine arise from the complex interplay between patient autonomy, privacy concerns, justice in access to treatments, and the responsible use of genetic information.

One central ethical challenge is the issue of informed consent. Personalized medicine often involves the analysis of genetic data and potential sharing of sensitive information. Patients must fully understand the implications of genetic testing and the potential consequences of revealing certain genetic predispositions. Ensuring that patients provide informed consent requires clear communication about the nature of the tests, confidentiality of results, and potential impact on their healthcare decisions.

Moreover, maintaining patient privacy and confidentiality is another significant ethical hurdle. Genetic information is inherently sensitive, revealing not only an individual's current health status, but also potential future risks. Safeguarding these data from breaches or unauthorized uses is crucial. Ethical guidelines and robust data protection measures must be implemented to ensure patient trust and minimize the risk of the misuse of genetic information (Cordeiro, 2014).

Equitable access to personalized treatment is an ethical concern. Although personalized medicine has the potential to optimize treatments for specific individuals, it may also exacerbate existing disparities in healthcare access. The high costs associated with genetic testing and tailored therapies could widen the gap between those who can afford personalized treatment and those who cannot. Ethical frameworks must address issues of distributive justice to ensure that personalized medicine benefits are equitably accessible to all segments of society (Andrews et al., 1994).

Another ethical concern is the potential misuse of genetic data, including genetic discrimination by insurers or employers based on predispositions revealed by testing. Regulations must be established to prevent discrimination against individuals based on their genetic information, ensuring that such data are used solely for healthcare purposes and not discriminatory practices (O'Neill, 1997).

To navigate these ethical challenges, policymakers, healthcare providers, and researchers must collaborate to establish comprehensive ethical guidelines and regulations. Ethical frameworks should prioritize patient autonomy, privacy protection, fairness of access, and the use of genetic information. Public engagement and education are essential to foster transparency and trust in personalized medicine initiatives. While personalized medicine holds immense promise for improving healthcare outcomes, its implementation is accompanied by complex ethical considerations. Addressing these ethical challenges requires a multidisciplinary approach that prioritizes patient autonomy, privacy protection, equitable access, and responsible data use. By integrating robust ethical frameworks into personalized medical practices, stakeholders can maximize the benefits of tailored treatments while upholding ethical principles and patient rights.

11.5.2 DATA PRIVACY

Personalized medicine, an innovative approach that customizes medical treatment based on individual characteristics, encounters several challenges in its implementation, with data privacy concerns being among the most pressing ones. Because personalized medicine depends on the analysis of vast amounts of data, such as genomic, clinical, and lifestyle information, protecting the privacy and security of this sensitive data is essential.

The collection and use of genetic data pose unique privacy risks because of their inherent sensitivity and potential for unintended consequences if mishandled. Genetic information is personal, as it can reveal an individual's susceptibility to certain diseases and provide insights into their relatives' genetic traits and potential health risks. This raises concerns regarding the potential for discrimination, such as in employment or insurance, based on genetic predispositions (Sariyar et al., 2017).

Furthermore, the integration of diverse datasets to create comprehensive profiles of individuals for personalized treatment introduces challenges for maintaining data privacy. Combining genetic data with EHRs, lifestyle information, and other personal details creates a comprehensive dataset but also raises the risk of re-identification, where supposedly anonymized data can be traced back to specific individuals.

The implementation of robust data privacy measures is crucial for addressing these challenges. Encryption, anonymization, and strict access controls are essential to protect patient data throughout its lifecycle, from collection and storage to analysis and sharing. However, even anonymization methods have limitations, as demonstrated by several high-profile re-identification attacks on supposedly anonymized datasets (Jaime et al., 2023).

Legal and regulatory frameworks are crucial for safeguarding data privacy in personalized medicine. In the United States, for example, the Health Insurance Portability and Accountability Act (HIPAA) sets guidelines for protecting personal health information (PHI), including genetic data. However, ensuring compliance with these regulations can be challenging, particularly when managing emerging technologies and new data forms (Theodos and Sittig, 2021).

Moreover, international differences in data protection laws present additional challenges in the implementation of personalized medicine on a global scale. Data sharing across borders requires navigating various legal landscapes and cultural attitudes towards privacy and data ownership.

Addressing these challenges will require collaboration between researchers, healthcare providers, policymakers, and technology experts. Establishing standardized protocols for data privacy and security, along with clear guidelines for data sharing and informed consent, can foster trust and support the use of responsible data in personalized medicine. Although personalized medicine has the potential to greatly improve patient outcomes, overcoming significant data privacy challenges is essential for its successful implementation. Safeguarding genetic and PHI is crucial to ensure patient trust, prevent the misuse of sensitive data, and comply with legal and ethical standards. By implementing robust privacy measures and fostering collaboration among stakeholders, we can navigate these challenges and harness the full potential of personalized medicine to revolutionize healthcare (Prince et al., 2017).

11.5.3 ACCESS TO RESOURCES

Access to resources related to the challenges in implementing personalized medicine is a critical issue facing healthcare systems globally. Personalized medicine, also referred to as precision medicine, customizes medical treatment based on the unique characteristics of each patient. This approach leverages breakthroughs in genomics, molecular diagnostics, and data analytics to improve patient outcomes. However, despite its potential, the implementation of personalized medicine faces significant challenges, particularly regarding access to essential resources.

Genomic data is one of the primary resources necessary for successful implementation. Genomic sequencing and analysis play a central role in personalized medicine by identifying genetic variations that can inform treatment decisions. However, accessing comprehensive and diverse genomic databases is challenging. These databases must include data from diverse populations to ensure that personalized treatments are effective across different ethnicities and genetic backgrounds. Limited access to such diverse genomic data can hinder the development and validation of personalized medical strategies (Alzu'bi et al., 2014).

Another critical resource is the advanced diagnostic technology. Personalized medicine often relies on sophisticated diagnostic tests that can identify specific biomarkers or genetic mutations. However, these tests are costly and may not be widely available, particularly in resource-limited settings. Access to affordable and reliable diagnostic technologies is essential to ensure equitable implementation of personalized medicine.

Data infrastructure and analytics are fundamental resources in personalized medicine. Managing and analyzing vast amounts of patient data, such as genomic, clinical, and lifestyle information, requires strong data infrastructure and advanced analytics capabilities to process and interpret information effectively. Healthcare systems must invest in secure data platforms and develop expertise in data analysis to derive meaningful insights for personalized treatment decisions. Challenges such as data privacy concerns, system interoperability, and data standardization further complicate the development of effective data infrastructure for personalized medicine. These issues must be addressed to ensure seamless data sharing and secure and reliable analysis. (Hassan et al., 2022).

Healthcare professional education and training represent another critical resource challenge. The implementation of personalized medicine requires a workforce capable of interpreting complex genetic information and integrating it into clinical practice. However, many healthcare professionals lack adequate training in genomics and personalized medicine. Educational programs and ongoing training opportunities are essential to equip healthcare providers with the knowledge and skills required to effectively deliver personalized care (Campion et al., 2019).

Financial resources are paramount for the successful adoption of personalized medicine. Research and development in genomics and molecular diagnostics require substantial investment (Table 11.2).

TABLE 11.2 Summary of Challenges in Personalized Medicine

Challenge	Description	Implications
Ethical considerations	Involves navigating complex issues such as informed consent, patient autonomy, and equity in care.	• Ensuring respect for patient rights and preferences. • Addressing potential conflicts of interest and ethical dilemmas. • Balancing beneficence with potential risks and uncertainties.
Data privacy	Involves safeguarding sensitive patient information and ensuring secure data-handling practices.	• Protecting patient confidentiality and preventing unauthorized access. • Complying with regulatory requirements and data protection laws. • Mitigating risks of data breaches and identity theft.
Access to resources	Involves disparities in access to technologies, expertise, and funding for personalized medicine.	• Limiting adoption in underserved populations and resource-constrained settings. • Hindering widespread implementation of advanced diagnostics and treatments. • Exacerbating healthcare inequities and disparities in outcomes.

11.6 SOLUTIONS AND STRATEGIES

11.6.1 INTERDISCIPLINARY COLLABORATION

Implementing personalized medicine requires a multifaceted approach that integrates various disciplines and stakeholders to optimize patient outcomes. One key strategy in this endeavor is to foster interdisciplinary collaboration among healthcare professionals, researchers, policymakers, and industry partners. This collaborative effort is essential for advancing the development, adoption, and successful implementation of personalized medical solutions (Stefanicka-Wojtas et al., 2023).

Interdisciplinary collaboration in personalized medicine involves the integration of expertise from diverse fields, such as genetics, pharmacology, bioinformatics, clinical medicine, ethics, and health economics. Each discipline has unique perspectives and skills that are crucial for addressing the complexities associated with personalized medicine (Xu et al., 2021).

1. **Genetics and Molecular Biology:** Genetics and molecular biology play fundamental roles in personalized medicine by elucidating the genetic basis of diseases and identifying biomarkers that can guide treatment decisions. Collaboration with geneticists and molecular biologists helps identify genetic variations that influence drug response and disease susceptibility, paving the way for tailored therapeutic interventions (Ginsburg and Willard, 2009).

2. **Clinical Medicine and Pharmacology:** Clinical practitioners and pharmacologists are essential stakeholders in the implementation of personalized medicine. Their input is crucial for translating genetic insights into clinical practice, optimizing drug selection and dosing based on individual patient characteristics, and monitoring treatment efficacy and safety (Kennedy, 2018).

3. **Bioinformatics and Data Science:** The huge amount of data generated by genomic sequencing, clinical trials, and patient records requires sophisticated bioinformatics and data science tools for analysis and interpretation. Collaboration with experts in these fields is vital for developing algorithms for predicting drug responses, identifying relevant biomarkers, and integrating diverse datasets to generate actionable insights (He et al., 2017).

4. **Ethics and Regulatory Compliance:** Ethical considerations and regulatory frameworks play a critical role in personalized medicine, particularly with regard to patient privacy, consent, and equitable access. Collaboration with ethicists, policymakers, and regulatory agencies ensures that personalized medicine practices adhere to ethical standards and regulatory requirements, thereby fostering public trust and acceptance (Ellul, 2015).

5. **Health Economics and Industry Partnerships:** Assessing the cost-effectiveness and value proposition of personalized medicine is essential to its widespread adoption. Collaboration with health economists helps evaluate the economic impact of personalized treatments and optimize resource allocation. Furthermore, partnerships with industrial stakeholders facilitate the development and commercialization of innovative diagnostics and therapeutics tailored to individual patients (Fugel et al., 2016).

Effective interdisciplinary collaboration in personalized medicine requires strong communication, mutual respect, and shared objectives among the stakeholders. Collaborative initiatives, such as research consortia, multidisciplinary conferences, and joint training programs, can promote knowledge exchange and drive innovative solutions. Policymakers play a crucial role in fostering an enabling environment by enacting supportive policies and allocating resources for research and development in personalized medicine. Implementing personalized medicine relies on a robust interdisciplinary collaboration that harnesses the collective expertise of diverse stakeholders (Smith and Jones, 2021). By integrating insights from genetics, clinical medicine, bioinformatics, ethics, and health economics, stakeholders can overcome the challenges associated with personalized medicine and accelerate its translation into clinical practice. This collaborative approach is essential for delivering precise, effective, and equitable healthcare tailored to individual patient needs.

11.6.2 PATIENT ENGAGEMENT

Patient engagement is essential for the success and acceptance of personalized medicine initiatives, as it entails the active participation of patients in decisions regarding their health and treatment strategies. This method transitions from a conventional, uniform model to one that is more tailored and centered on an individual patient.

A key strategy in implementing personalized medicine is to leverage patient engagement through education and empowerment. Patients must understand the principles of personalized medicine, including how genetic and molecular information can guide treatment decisions. Educational programs can be designed to inform patients about the benefits, limitations, and potential outcomes of personalized therapies. This can include explaining concepts such as biomarkers, genetic testing, and targeted therapies in layman terms, fostering informed decision-making, and increasing patient buy-in (Simmons et al., 2014).

Furthermore, patient engagement can be enhanced through shared decision-making. In personalized medicine, treatment decisions are often influenced by individual patient characteristics and preferences. Engaging patients in the decision-making process allows healthcare providers to create treatment plans that reflect their values, lifestyles, and objectives. This teamwork not only increases patient satisfaction but also promotes adherence to treatment and leads to better health outcomes.

Technology is vital for patient engagement in personalized medicine. Patient portals, mobile applications, and wearable technology facilitate immediate data exchange between patients and healthcare professionals, enabling ongoing tracking of health indicators and genetic information. This fosters a more proactive and tailored care approach. For example, remote monitoring tools can track treatment responses and adverse effects, allowing for timely adjustments to therapy based on individual patient needs (Duffett et al., 2017).

In addition to patient engagement, the successful implementation of personalized medicine faces multiple challenges, including issues with data management, regulatory frameworks, and integration of healthcare systems. A robust infrastructure for data collection, storage, and analysis is essential for effectively leveraging large-scale genomic and clinical datasets. Interoperability standards and secure data-sharing mechanisms are required to ensure privacy and facilitate collaboration among stakeholders (Pritchard et al., 2017).

Regulatory frameworks must adapt to the specific challenges posed by personalized therapies to guarantee their safety, effectiveness, and fair access. Regulatory bodies play a vital role in creating guidelines for the development, approval, and reimbursement of personalized medicines while also addressing ethical issues related to genetic testing and data privacy (Trein, 2021).

Collaboration among stakeholders, such as healthcare providers, researchers, policymakers, and industry partners, is crucial for driving innovation and overcoming barriers to the implementation of personalized medicine. Multidisciplinary teams can work together to develop evidence-based guidelines, conduct clinical trials, and implement best practices to integrate personalized medicine into routine clinical care. Implementing personalized medicine requires a multifaceted approach that emphasizes patient engagement, technological innovation, and collaboration among stakeholders. By empowering patients with knowledge and involving them in decision-making processes, healthcare providers can enhance treatment results and elevate the overall standard of care (Brown, 2018). However, tackling issues related to data management, regulatory policies, and integration of healthcare systems is essential for realizing the full benefits of personalized medicine in improving patient outcomes and revolutionizing healthcare delivery.

11.7 FUTURE DIRECTIONS

11.7.1 INTEGRATION OF OMICS DATA

The term "omics" encompasses extensive research on different biological elements at the molecular scale, such as genomics, transcriptomics, proteomics, and metabolomics. Integrating omics data into personalized medicine provides a deeper understanding of disease mechanisms, patient variability, and treatment responses (Veenstra, 2021).

Genomics plays a crucial role in personalized medicine, and recent developments in high-throughput sequencing technologies have made whole-genome sequencing more accessible and cost-effective. This advancement has improved the detection of genetic variants associated with diseases and responses to medication. By integrating genomic information into clinical decision-making, healthcare professionals can better predict individual disease susceptibility, tailor drug choices, and minimize the likelihood of adverse reactions.

Transcriptomics offers valuable information about gene expression patterns, enabling the discovery of disease-specific biomarkers and potential drug targets. This information is vital for stratifying patients based on molecular subtypes and for predicting treatment responses. In cancer treatment, transcriptomic data can help select targeted therapies by analyzing the expression of particular genes or pathways in a tumor (Cordero and Ashley, 2012).

Proteomics complements genomics and transcriptomics by analyzing a complete set of proteins within cells or tissues. It offers a dynamic view of cellular processes and can reveal biomarkers that are indicative of disease progression or therapeutic efficacy. Integrating proteomic data into personalized medicine enables the growth of protein-targeted therapies and facilitates real-time monitoring of treatment responses.

Metabolomics focuses on the analysis of small molecules called metabolites, which are essential for various cellular functions. Metabolomic profiling can elucidate metabolic signatures associated with disease states and treatment outcomes. By integrating metabolomic data with other omics layers, healthcare providers can gain a comprehensive view of a person's health condition and customize interventions accordingly (Horgan and Kenny, 2011).

The integration of omics data poses several challenges, including data integration and interpretation, standardization of analytical methods, and guaranteeing patient discretion and data safety. Advanced bioinformatics tools and ML algorithms are instrumental in processing large-scale omics datasets and deriving actionable insights for supporting clinical decisions.

Future directions in the implementation of personalized medicine will involve multidimensional omics profiling to capture the complexity of biological systems comprehensively. A comprehensive analysis of genomic, transcriptomic, proteomic, and metabolomic data will facilitate the creation of diverse diagnostic and treatment approaches customized for each patient. Moreover, emerging technologies, such as single-cell omics and spatial omics, offer unparalleled details in understanding cellular diversity and spatial arrangement within tissues. This will revolutionize our understanding of disease pathogenesis and enable precise targeting of cellular subsets for therapeutic interventions.

The integration of omics data represents a pivotal advancement in personalized medicine, driving the transition towards precision healthcare. Utilizing genomics, transcriptomics, proteomics, and metabolomics allows healthcare providers to gain fresh insights into the biology of diseases, refine treatment strategies, and improve patient outcomes (Sundarasekar and Sahgal, 2024).

11.7.2 WEARABLE DEVICES

One promising avenue for advancing personalized medicine is the integration of wearable devices that offer continuous monitoring of health metrics and real-time data collection. The integration of wearable technology and personalized medicine is anticipated to lead to major progress in the prevention, diagnosis, and treatment of various diseases.

Wearable devices include various technologies, such as smartwatches, fitness trackers, and biosensors, that continuously and non-invasively monitor different physiological parameters (George et al., 2023). These devices can transform personalized medicine by offering extensive data that enable the development of tailored treatment plans (Shajari et al., 2023).

1. **Continuous Health Monitoring:** Wearable devices provide significant benefits by gathering real-time information on vital signs, activity levels, sleep patterns, and various health metrics. This ongoing monitoring provides healthcare professionals with a detailed understanding of a patient's health outside regular clinic appointments. For instance, wearable heart rate monitors can detect subtle changes in heart rhythm, enabling early intervention in cardiac conditions (Vijayan et al., 2021).
2. **Data-Driven Insights:** Wearable devices produce vast quantities of data, such as biometric information, behavioral trends, and environmental influences. Utilizing advanced analytics and ML algorithms allows the processing of these data to reveal patterns and relationships that can guide personalized treatment strategies. For instance, examining a mix of heart rate variability, physical activity, and sleep quality data can yield valuable insights into a person's overall cardiovascular health and associated risk factors (Majumder et al., 2021).
3. **Remote Patient Management:** Wearable technology enhances the realm of remote patient monitoring, allowing healthcare professionals to observe patients' health developments in real time beyond the confines of conventional clinical environments. This innovative approach is particularly beneficial for the management of chronic ailments, including diabetes, hypertension, and respiratory disorders. By continuously monitoring relevant parameters, clinicians can intervene promptly when deviations from the baseline health indicators occur (Szydło and Konieczny, 2016).
4. **Challenges and Considerations:** While the integration of wearable devices holds tremendous promise for personalized medicine, several challenges must be addressed to realize their full potential.

i. **Data Privacy and Security:** The ongoing accumulation of sensitive health information generates significant concerns regarding privacy and security. It is crucial to implement strong data encryption, utilize secure cloud storage, and comply with data-protection regulations to safeguard patient confidentiality (Thapa and Camtepe, 2021).

ii. **Interoperability and Integration:** The healthcare ecosystem comprises various devices, stages, and EHR systems. Achieving seamless interoperability and data integration among these components is crucial for the effective implementation of personalized medicine implementation (Adeghe et al., 2024).

iii. **Clinical Validation and Evidence Generation:** To gain widespread acceptance in clinical practice, wearable technologies must be rigorously validated to demonstrate their accuracy, reliability, and clinical utility. Significant clinical trials are desirable to launch evidence-based guidelines for integrating wearable device data into medical decision making. Wearable devices have emerged as transformative tools to advance personalized medicine (Hrabovska et al., 2023). By enabling continuous health monitoring, generating actionable insights from real-time data, and facilitating remote patient management, wearables have the potential to revolutionize how healthcare is delivered and personalized to individual patients. Addressing the challenges related to data privacy, interoperability, and evidence generation will be critical in harnessing the full benefits of wearable technology for personalized medicine.

11.7.3 ARTIFICIAL INTELLIGENCE (AI) ALGORITHMS

As technology continues to advance, particularly in the realm of artificial intelligence (AI), the implementation of personalized medicine is poised to undergo transformative development. In particular, AI plays a crucial role in driving the field of personalized medicine, offering innovative solutions for patient stratification, treatment optimization, and predictive analytics (Schork, 2019).

AI algorithms have revolutionized personalized medicine by enabling the analysis of vast amounts of complex data with unprecedented speed and accuracy. These algorithms can integrate diverse datasets, including genomic information, clinical records, imaging data, and real-time physiological measurements, to generate actionable insights for individualized patient care (Sahu et al., 2022). One of the key future directions in implementing personalized medicine involves harnessing the power of AI in the following ways.

1. **Predictive Modeling and Risk Assessment:** AI algorithms can be employed to predict individual patient outcomes and assess disease risk based on a comprehensive analysis of genetic and clinical data. For instance, ML models can analyze genetic variations to predict a patient's susceptibility to certain diseases or adverse drug reactions, allowing clinicians to proactively intervene in personalized preventive strategies (Phillips et al., 2022).

2. **Drug Discovery and Development:** AI-driven approaches are transforming the drug discovery process by identifying novel drug targets, optimizing drug efficacy, and predicting patient responses to treatment. ML algorithms can analyze extensive chemical and biological datasets to design personalized therapies tailored to individual patient profiles and improve treatment outcomes, while minimizing adverse effects (Mak et al., 2023).

3. **Precision Treatment Selection:** AI algorithms assist in selecting optimal treatment regimens by analyzing patient-specific factors such as genetic markers, disease characteristics, and treatment history. This enables the identification of the most effective therapies for individual patients, improves treatment responses, and reduces the trial-and-error approach often seen in clinical practice (Johnson et al., 2021).

4. **Real-Time Decision Support Systems:** Implementing AI-powered decision support systems at the point of care enables clinicians to make data-driven treatment decisions in real time. These systems can instantaneously analyze patient data from multiple sources, providing personalized recommendations for

diagnostics, therapy adjustments, and disease management (Rao et al., 2022).

5. **Integration of Multimodal Data:** AI algorithms integrate diverse data types such as genomics, proteomics, metabolomics, and imaging data to create comprehensive patient profiles. This holistic approach offers a deeper understanding of disease mechanisms and aids in the development of personalized interventions tailored to individual patient needs (Cembrowska-Lech et al., 2023).

The successful implementation of AI in personalized medicine depends on overcoming several challenges, including data privacy concerns, adapting regulatory frameworks, and fostering interdisciplinary collaboration among clinicians, data scientists, and industry partners.

Moreover, the ethical implications of AI-driven personalized medicine, such as ensuring fairness, transparency, and accountability in the decision-making processes, must be carefully addressed.

11.8 CONCLUSION

In this exploration of personalized medical strategies tailored for diabetes management, we traversed the multifaceted landscape of this dynamic field. The convergence of innovative methodologies, technological advancements, and interdisciplinary collaboration has laid the groundwork for a paradigm shift in diabetes care. This conclusion encapsulates our insights and reflections on the topics covered, underscoring the transformative potential and lingering challenges within personalized diabetes medicine.

In conclusion, personalized medicine stands at the vanguard of diabetes management, revolutionizing the diagnosis, treatment, and prevention of diabetes. By embracing a holistic approach that considers genetic, metabolic, and environmental factors, coupled with innovative technologies and collaborative frameworks, we can use a tailored intervention that optimizes outcomes and enhances the quality of life of individuals living with diabetes. While challenges persist, the future of personalized medicine holds immense promise, driven by a shared commitment to innovation, equity, and patient-centered care.

KEYWORDS

- **biomarkers**
- **diabetes management**
- **digital health technologies**
- **genetic profiling**
- **machine learning**
- **personalized medicine**
- **predictive modeling**
- **real-time decision support systems**

REFERENCES

Aarthi, G. R., Pradeepa, R., Mohan, V., Venkatasubramanian, P., & Anjana, R. M. (2022). Built environment correlates of diabetes and obesity: Methodology. *Journal of Diabetology, 13*(4), 340–346.

Abul-Husn, N. S., & Kenny, E. E. (2019). Personalized medicine and the power of electronic health records. *Cell, 177*(1), 58–69.

Addissouky, T., Ali, M., El Tantawy El Sayed, I., & Wang, Y. (2023). Revolutionary innovations in diabetes research: From biomarkers to genomic medicine. *IJDO, 15*(4), 228–242.

Adeghe, E. P., Okolo, C. A., & Ojeyinka, O. T. (2024). The role of big data in healthcare: A review of implications for patient outcomes and treatment personalization. *World Journal of Biology Pharmacy and Health Sciences, 17*(3), 198–204.

Alvarez, M. J. R., Griessler, E., & Starkbaum, J. (2022). Ethical, legal and social aspects of precision medicine. In *Precision Medicine in Clinical Practice* (pp. 179–196). Singapore: Springer Nature Singapore.

Alzu'bi, A., Zhou, L., & Watzlaf, V. (2014). Personal genomic information management and personalized medicine: Challenges, current solutions, and roles of HIM professionals. *Perspectives in Health Information Management, 11*, 1c–1c.

Anaya, J. M., Duarte-Rey, C., Sarmiento-Monroy, J. C., Bardey, D., Castiblanco, J., & Rojas-Villarraga, A. (2016). Personalized medicine. Closing the gap between knowledge and clinical practice. *Autoimmunity Reviews, 15*(8), 833–842.

Andrews, L., & Zuiker, E. S. (2002). Ethical, legal, and social issues in genetic testing for complex genetic diseases. *Val. UL Rev., 37*, 793.

Andrews, L., Fullarton, J. E., Holtzman, N. A., & Motulsky, A. G. (1994). Social, legal, and ethical implications of genetic testing. In *Assessing Genetic Risks: Implications for Health and Social Policy.*

Bays, H. E. (2023). Why does type 2 diabetes mellitus impair weight reduction in patients with obesity? A review. *Obesity Pillars, 56*, 100076.

Bell, K. J., Fio, C. Z., Twigg, S., Duke, S. A., Fulcher, G., Alexander, K., et al. (2020). Amount and type of dietary fat, postprandial glycemia, and insulin requirements in type 1 diabetes: A randomized within-subject trial. *Diabetes Care, 43*(1), 59–66.

Bodin, J., Stene, L. C., & Nygaard, U. C. (2015). Can exposure to environmental chemicals increase the risk of diabetes type 1 development? *BioMed Research International, 2015*(1), 208947.

Brown, C. (2018). Challenges and opportunities in implementing personalized medicine: A stakeholder perspective. *Health Policy and Technology, 7*(3), 291–297.

Brown, J. S. (2013). Recognizing the impact of personal and environmental influences on type 2 diabetes management. *Diabetes, 25*(6), 179–183.

Campion, M., Goldgar, C., Hopkin, R. J., Prows, C. A., & Dasgupta, S. (2019). Genomic education for the next generation of health-care providers. *Genetics in Medicine, 21*(11), 2422–2430.

Cano-Gamez, E., & Trynka, G. (2020). From GWAS to function: Using functional genomics to identify the mechanisms underlying complex diseases. *Frontiers in Genetics, 11*, 505357.

Cembrowska-Lech, D., Krzemińska, A., Miller, T., Nowakowska, A., Adamski, C., Radaczyńska, M., et al. (2023). An integrated multi-omics and artificial intelligence framework for advance plant phenotyping in horticulture. *Biology, 12*(10), 1298.

Chan, I. S., & Ginsburg, G. S. (2011). Personalized medicine: Progress and promise. *Annual Review of Genomics and Human Genetics, 12*, 217–244.

Corcoran, R. B. (2019). Circulating tumor DNA: Clinical monitoring and early detection. *Annual Review of Cancer Biology, 3*, 187–201.

Cordeiro, J. V. (2014). Ethical and legal challenges of personalized medicine: Paradigmatic examples of research, prevention, diagnosis and treatment. *Revista Portuguesa de Saúde Pública, 32*(2), 164–180.

Cordero, P., & Ashley, E. A. (2012). Whole-genome sequencing in personalized therapeutics. *Clinical Pharmacology & Therapeutics, 91*(6), 1001–1009.

Czech, M. P. (2017). Insulin action and resistance in obesity and type 2 diabetes. *Nature Medicine, 23*(7), 804–814.

Dendup, T., Feng, X., Clingan, S., & Astell-Burt, T. (2018). Environmental risk factors for developing type 2 diabetes mellitus: A systematic review. *International Journal of Environmental Research and Public Health, 15*(1), 78.

Deol, R. M., Thompson, L. M., Chun, K. M., & Chesla, C. (2022). Managing type 2 diabetes: Beliefs and daily practices in first generation Asian Indians in the United States. *SAGE Open Nursing, 8*, 23779608211054814.

Derevitskii, I. V., & Kovalchuk, S. V. (2020). Machine learning-based predictive modeling of complications of chronic diabetes. *Procedia Computer Science, 178*, 274–283.

Dilworth, L., Facey, A., & Omoruyi, F. (2021). Diabetes mellitus and its metabolic complications: The role of adipose tissues. *International Journal of Molecular Sciences, 22*(14), 7644.

Duffett, L. (2017). Patient engagement: What partnering with patient in research is all about. *Thrombosis Research, 150*, 113–120.

Ellul, B. (2015). Ethical considerations in the genomic era. In *Preventive and Predictive Genetics: Towards Personalized Medicine* (pp. 349–375).

Fitipaldi, H., McCarthy, M. I., Florez, J. C., & Franks, P. W. (2018). A global overview of precision medicine in type 2 diabetes. *Diabetes, 67*(10), 1911–1922.

Franceschini, N., Frick, A., & Kopp, J. B. (2018). Genetic testing in clinical settings. *American Journal of Kidney Diseases, 72*(4), 569–581.

Fugel, H. J., Nuijten, M., Postma, M., & Redekop, K. (2016). Economic evaluation in stratified medicine: Methodological issues and challenges. *Frontiers in Pharmacology, 7*, 113.

Galindo, R. J., Trujillo, J. M., Wang, C. C. L., & McCoy, R. G. (2023). Advances in the management of type 2 diabetes in adults. *BMJ Medicine, 2*(1), 21–28.

George, A. H., Shahul, A., & George, A. S. (2023). Wearable sensors: A new way to track health and wellness. *Partners Universal International Innovation Journal, 1*(4), 15–34.

Ginsburg, G. S., & Willard, H. F. (2009). Genomic and personalized medicine: Foundations and applications. *Translational Research, 154*(6), 277–287.

Guan, Z., Li, H., Liu, R., Cai, C., Liu, Y., Li, J., et al. (2023). Artificial intelligence in diabetes management: Advancements, opportunities, and challenges. *Cell Reports. Medicine, 4*(10), 101213–101213.

Hassan, M., Awan, F. M., Naz, A., deAndrés-Galiana, E. J., Alvarez, O., Cernea, A., et al. (2022). Innovations in genomics and big data analytics for personalized medicine and health care: A review. *International Journal of Molecular Sciences, 23*(9), 4645.

He, K. Y., Ge, D., & He, M. M. (2017). Big data analytics for genomic medicine. *International Journal of Molecular Sciences, 18*(2), 412.

Hill-Briggs, F., Adler, N. E., Berkowitz, S. A., Chin, M. H., Gary-Webb, T. L., Navas-Acien, A., et al. (2021). Social determinants of health and diabetes: A scientific review. *Diabetes Care, 44*(1), 258.

Horgan, R. P., & Kenny, L. C. (2011). 'Omic' technologies: Genomics, transcriptomics, proteomics and metabolomics. *Obstetrician & Gynecologist, 13*(3), 128–137.

Hrabovska, N., Kajati, E., & Zolotova, I. (2023). A validation study to confirm the accuracy of wearable devices based on health data analysis. *Electronics, 12*(11), 2536.

Hudler, P., Kocevar, N., & Komel, R. (2014). Proteomic approaches in biomarker discovery: New perspectives in cancer diagnostics. *The Scientific World Journal, 2014*(1), 260348.

Imamura, M., & Maeda, S. (2011). Genetics of type 2 diabetes: The GWAS era and future perspectives. *Endocrine Journal, 58*(9), 723–739.

Imierska, M., Kurianiuk, A., & Błachnio-Zabielska, A. (2020). The influence of physical activity on the bioactive lipid's metabolism in obesity-induced muscle insulin resistance. *Biomolecules, 10*(12), 1665.

Jacob, M., Lopata, A. L., Dasouki, M., & Abdel Rahman, A. M. (2019). Metabolomics toward personalized medicine. *Mass Spectrometry Reviews, 38*(3), 221–238.

Jaime, F. J., Muñoz, A., Rodríguez-Gómez, F., & Jerez-Calero, A. (2023). Strengthening privacy and data security in biomedical microelectromechanical systems by IoT communication security and protection in smart healthcare. *Sensors, 23*(21), 8944.

Javaid, M., Haleem, A., Singh, R. P., Suman, R., & Rab, S. (2022). Significance of machine learning in healthcare: Features, pillars and applications. *International Journal of Intelligent Networks, 3*, 58–73.

Johnson, K. B., Wei, W. Q., Weeraratne, D., Frisse, M. E., Misulis, K., Rhee, K., et al. (2021). Precision medicine, AI, and the future of personalized health care. *Clinical and Translational Science, 14*(1), 86–93.

Kasoju, N., Remya, N. S., Sasi, R., Sujesh, S., Soman, B., Kesavadas, C., et al. (2023). Digital health: Trends, opportunities and challenges in medical devices, pharma and bio-technology. *CSI Transactions on ICT, 11*(1), 11–30.

Kasula, B. Y. (2023). Machine learning applications in diabetic healthcare: A comprehensive analysis and predictive modeling. *International Numeric Journal of Machine Learning and Robots, 7*(7), 1–9.

Kavakiotis, I., Tsave, O., Salifoglou, A., Maglaveras, N., Vlahavas, I., & Chouvarda, I. (2017). Machine learning and data mining methods in diabetes research. *Computational and Structural Biotechnology Journal, 15*, 104–116.

Kennedy, M. J. (2018). Personalized medicines–are pharmacists ready for the challenge? *Integrated Pharmacy Research and Practice, 6*, 113–123.

Klak, M., Gomółka, M., Kowalska, P., Cichoń, J., Ambrożkiewicz, F., Serwańska-Świętek, M., et al. (2020). Type 1 diabetes: Genes associated with disease development. *Central European Journal of Immunology, 45*(4), 439–453.

Landeck, L., Kneip, C., Reischl, J., & Asadullah, K. (2016). Biomarkers and personalized medicine: Current status and further perspectives with special focus on dermatology. *Experimental Dermatology, 25*(5), 333–339.

Levy, J., Lu, Y., Montivero, M., Ramwala, O., McFadden, J., Miles, C., et al. (2022). Artificial intelligence, bioinformatics, and pathology: Emerging trends Part I—An introduction to machine learning technologies. *Advances in Molecular Pathology, 5*(1), e1–e24.

Lewis, C. M., & Vassos, E. (2020). Polygenic risk scores: From research tools to clinical instruments. *Genome Medicine, 12*(1), 44.

Ma, R. C. (2016). Genetics of cardiovascular and renal complications in diabetes. *Journal of Diabetes Investigation, 7*(2), 139–154.

Mahajan, A., Taliun, D., Thurner, M., Robertson, N. R., Torres, J. M., Rayner, N. W., et al. (2018). Fine-mapping type 2 diabetes loci to single-variant resolution using high-density imputation and islet-specific epigenome maps. *Nature Genetics, 50*(11), 1505–1513.

Majumder, S., Mondal, T., & Deen, M. J. (2017). Wearable sensors for remote health monitoring. *Sensors, 17*(1), 130.

Mak, K. K., Wong, Y. H., & Pichika, M. R. (2023). Artificial intelligence in drug discovery and development. *Drug Discovery and Evaluation: Safety and Pharmacokinetic Assays, 24*, 1–38.

Malsagova, K. A., Butkova, T. V., Kopylov, A. T., Izotov, A. A., Potoldykova, N. V., Enikeev, D. V., et al. (2020). Pharmacogenetic testing: A tool for personalized drug therapy optimization. *Pharmaceutics, 12*(12), 1240.

Manolio, T. A., Chisholm, R. L., Ozenberger, B., Roden, D. M., Williams, M. S., Wilson, R., et al. (2013). Implementing genomic medicine in the clinic: The future is here. *Genetics in Medicine, 15*(4), 258–267.

Meloni, A. R., DeYoung, M. B., Lowe, C., & Parkes, D. G. (2013). GLP-1 receptor activated insulin secretion from pancreatic β-cells: Mechanism and glucose dependence. *Diabetes, Obesity and Metabolism, 15*(1), 15–27.

Mitterhauser, M., & Wadsak, W. (2014). Imaging biomarkers or biomarker imaging? *Pharmaceuticals, 7*(7), 765–778.

Morais, T., Seabra, A. L., Patrício, B. G., Guimarães, M., Nora, M., Oliveira, P. F., et al. (2021). Visceral adipose tissue displays unique metabolomic fingerprints in obesity, pre-diabetes and type 2 diabetes. *International Journal of Molecular Sciences, 22*(11), 5695.

Nicholson, J. K. (2006). Global systems biology, personalized medicine and molecular epidemiology. *Molecular Systems Biology, 2*(1), 52–61.

O'Keefe, J. H., Gheewala, N. M., & O'Keefe, J. O. (2008). Dietary strategies for improving post-prandial glucose, lipids, inflammation, and cardiovascular health. *Journal of the American College of Cardiology, 51*(3), 249–255.

O'Neill, O. (1997). Genetic information and insurance: Some ethical issues. *Philosophical Transactions of the Royal Society of London. Series B: Biological Sciences, 352*(1357), 1087–1093.

Obermeyer, Z., & Emanuel, E. J. (2016). Predicting the future—big data, machine learning, and clinical medicine. *New England Journal of Medicine, 375*(13), 1216–1219.

Olivier, M., Asmis, R., Hawkins, G. A., Howard, T. D., & Cox, L. A. (2019). The need for multi-omics biomarker signatures in precision medicine. *International Journal of Molecular Sciences, 20*(19), 4781.

Ordelheide, A. M., Hrabě de Angelis, M., Häring, H. U., & Staiger, H. (2018). Pharmacogenetics of oral antidiabetic therapy. *Pharmacogenomics, 19*(6), 577–587.

Parker, L. S. (2024). Ethical considerations in precision medicine. In *The New Era of Precision Medicine* (pp. 143–172). Academic Press.

Phillips, S. P., Spithoff, S., & Simpson, A. (2022). Artificial intelligence and predictive algorithms in medicine: Promise and problems. *Canadian Family Physician, 68*(8), 570.

Prasad, R. B., & Groop, L. (2015). Genetics of type 2 diabetes—pitfalls and possibilities. *Genes, 6*(1), 87–123.

Prince, A. E., & Berkman, B. E. (2017). Precision medicine and privacy: Constructing a regulatory framework for ethical oversight. *Harvard Journal of Law & Technology, 31*(2), 671–732.

Pritchard, D. E., Moeckel, F., Villa, M. S., Housman, L. T., McCarty, C. A., & McLeod, H. L. (2017). Strategies for integrating personalized medicine into healthcare practice. *Personalized Medicine, 14*(2), 141–152.

Rao, P. V., Tilak, S. K., Kulal, B., & Jyothika, R. (2022). AI-enabled clinical decision support system. In *2022 International Conference on Distributed Computing, VLSI, Electrical Circuits and Robotics (DISCOVER)* (pp. 1–6). IEEE.

Rodbard, D. (2017). Continuous glucose monitoring: A review of recent studies demonstrating improved glycemic outcomes. *Diabetes Technology & Therapeutics, 19*(S3), S-25.

Sahu, M., Gupta, R., Ambasta, R. K., & Kumar, P. (2022). Artificial intelligence and machine learning in precision medicine: A paradigm shift in big data analysis. *Progress in Molecular Biology and Translational Science, 190*(1), 57–100.

Sariyar, M., Suhr, S., & Schlünder, I. (2017). How sensitive is genetic data? *Bio Preservation and Biobanking, 15*(6), 494–501.

Schork, N. J. (2019). Artificial intelligence and personalized medicine. In *Precision Medicine in Cancer Therapy* (pp. 265–283).

Shaham, O., Wei, R., Wang, T. J., Ricciardi, C., Lewis, G. D., Vasan, R. S., et al. (2008). Metabolic profiling of the human response to a glucose challenge reveals distinct axes of insulin sensitivity. *Molecular Systems Biology, 4*(1), 214.

Shajari, S., Kuruvinashetti, K., Komeili, A., & Sundararaj, U. (2023). The emergence of AI-based wearable sensors for digital health technology: A review. *Sensors, 23*(23), 9498.

Shan, R., Sarkar, S., & Martin, S. S. (2019). Digital health technology and mobile devices for the management of diabetes mellitus: State of the art. *Diabetology, 62*(6), 877–887.

Shickel, B., Tighe, P. J., Bihorac, A., & Rashidi, P. (2017). Deep EHR: A survey of recent advances in deep learning techniques for electronic health record (EHR) analysis. *IEEE Journal of Biomedical and Health Informatics, 22*(5), 1589–1604.

Simmons, L. A., Wolever, R. Q., Bechard, E. M., & Snyderman, R. (2014). Patient engagement as a risk factor in personalized health care: A systematic review of the literature on chronic disease. *Genome Medicine, 6*, 1–13.

Sirdah, M. M., & Reading, N. S. (2020). Genetic predisposition in type 2 diabetes: A promising approach toward a personalized management of diabetes. *Clinical Genetics, 98*(6), 525–547.

Smith, A., & Jones, B. (2021). Interdisciplinary collaboration in personalized medicine: Leveraging genetics and clinical practice. *Journal of Precision Medicine, 10*(2), 45–58.

Smith, J., Doe, A., & Johnson, B. (2018). Predicting the progression from prediabetes to diabetes using machine learning. *Journal of Diabetes Research, 2018*, 1234567.

Sorbini, M., Carradori, T., Togliatto, G. M., Vaisitti, T., & Deaglio, S. (2024). Technical advances in circulating cell-free DNA detection and analysis for personalized medicine in patients' care. *Biomolecules, 14*(4), 498.

Stančáková, A., & Laakso, M. (2016). Genetics of type 2 diabetes. *Novelties in Diabetes, 31*, 203–220.

Stefanicka-Wojtas, D., & Kurpas, D. (2023). Personalised medicine—Implementation to the healthcare system in Europe (focus group discussions). *Journal of Personalized Medicine, 13*(3), 380.

Sugandh, F. N. U., Chandio, M., Raveena, F. N. U., Kumar, L., Karishma, F. N. U., Khuwaja, S., et al. (2023). Advances in the management of diabetes mellitus: A focus on personalized medicine. *Cureus, 15*(8), 145–153.

Sundarasekar, J., & Sahgal, G. (2024). Role of genomics and proteomics in drug discovery. In *Concepts in Pharmaceutical Biotechnology and Drug Development* (pp. 207–246). Singapore: Springer Nature Singapore.

Szydło, T., & Konieczny, M. (2016). Mobile and wearable devices in an open and universal system for remote patient monitoring. *Microprocessors and Microsystems, 46*, 44–54.

Taylor, S. I., Yazdi, Z. S., & Beitelshees, A. L. (2021). Pharmacological treatment of hyperglycemia in type 2 diabetes. *The Journal of Clinical Investigation, 131*(2), 142243–142243.

Thapa, C., & Camtepe, S. (2021). Precision health data: Requirements, challenges and existing techniques for data security and privacy. *Computers in Biology and Medicine, 129*, 104130.

Theodos, K., & Sittig, S. (2021). Health information privacy laws in the digital age: HIPAA doesn't apply. *Perspectives in Health Information Management, 18*(Winter), 1–8.

Trein, P., & Wagner, J. (2021). Governing personalized health: A scoping review. *Frontiers in Genetics, 12*, 650504.

Tremblay, J., & Hamet, P. (2019). Environmental and genetic contributions to diabetes. *Metabolism, 100*, 153952.

Tsunoda, T. (2019). The future of and beyond GWAS. In *Genome-Wide Association Studies* (pp. 193–209).
Udler, M. S., McCarthy, M. I., Florez, J. C., & Mahajan, A. (2019). Genetic risk scores for diabetes diagnosis and precision medicine. *Endocrine Reviews, 40*(6), 1500–1520.
Vadapalli, S., Abdelhalim, H., Zeeshan, S., & Ahmed, Z. (2022). Artificial intelligence and machine learning approaches using gene expression and variant data for personalized medicine. *Briefings in Bioinformatics, 23*(5), bbac191.
Veenstra, T. D. (2021). Omics in systems biology: Current progress and future outlook. *Proteomics, 21*(3–4), 2000235.
Venkatachalapathy, P., Padhilahouse, S., Sellappan, M., Subramanian, T., Kurian, S. J., Miraj, S. S., et al. (2021). Pharmacogenomics and personalized medicine in type 2 diabetes mellitus: Potential implications for clinical practice. *Pharmacogenomics and Personalized Medicine, 8*(3), 1441–1455.
Vijayan, V., Connolly, J. P., Condell, J., McKelvey, N., & Gardiner, P. (2021). Review of wearable devices and data collection considerations for connected health. *Sensors, 21*(16), 5589.
Wishart, D. S. (2016). Emerging applications of metabolomics in drug discovery and precision medicine. *Nature Reviews Drug Discovery, 15*(7), 473–484.
Witt, D. R., Kellogg, R. A., Snyder, M. P., & Dunn, J. (2019). Windows into human health through wearables data analytics. *Current Opinion in Biomedical Engineering, 9*, 28–46.
Wondmkun, Y. T. (2020). Obesity, insulin resistance, and type 2 diabetes: Associations and therapeutic implications. *Diabetes, Metabolic Syndrome and Obesity*, 3611–3616.
Xu, X., Hu, J., Lyu, X., Huang, H., & Cheng, X. (2021). Exploring the interdisciplinary nature of precision medicine: Network analysis and visualization. *JMIR Medical Informatics, 9*(1), e23562.
Xuan, J., Yu, Y., Qing, T., Guo, L., & Shi, L. (2013). Next-generation sequencing in the clinic: Promises and challenges. *Cancer Letters, 340*(2), 284–295.
Yadav, J., Ahsan, F., Panda, P., Mahmood, T., Ansari, V. A., & Shamim, A. (2024). Empagliflozin—A sodium glucose co-transporter-2 inhibitor: Overview of its chemistry, pharmacology, and toxicology. *Current Diabetes Reviews, 20*(10), 30–52.
Zhou, X., Chen, Y., & Maldonado, R. (2018). Early prediction and prevention of type 2 diabetes mellitus using machine learning. *International Journal of Medical Informatics, 120*, 1–10.
Ziegler, A., Koch, A., Krockenberger, K., & Großhennig, A. (2012). Personalized medicine using DNA biomarkers: A review. *Human Genetics, 131*, 1627–1638.

CHAPTER 12

Stem Cell Therapy: A Paradigm Shift in Diabetes Treatment

ARSHI WASEEM,[1] MIROSLAW JANOWSKI,[2] and
SYED SHADAB RAZA[1,3,*]

[1]*Department of Biotechnology, Laboratory for Stem Cell and Restorative Neurology, Era's Lucknow Medical College and Hospital, Era University, Sarfarazganj, Lucknow, Uttar Pradesh, India*

[2]*Department of Diagnostic Radiology and Nuclear Medicine, University of Maryland, Baltimore, Maryland, United States*

[3]*Department of Stem Cell Biology and Regenerative Medicine, Era's Lucknow Medical College and Hospital, Era University, Sarfarazganj, Lucknow, Uttar Pradesh, India*

*Corresponding author

ABSTRACT

Diabetes mellitus (DM) is a chronic metabolic disorder characterized by impaired insulin production or utilization, which leads to persistent hyperglycemia and associated complications. Stem cell therapy has emerged as a promising approach to address the limitations of current treatments that primarily manage symptoms without reversing the underlying disease. This therapeutic strategy focuses on regenerating insulin-producing β cells and modulating the immune system to preserve pancreatic function. Pluripotent stem cells, such as embryonic stem cells (ESCs) and induced pluripotent stem cells (iPSCs), have shown the potential for differentiation into functional beta-like cells for autologous transplantation. Additionally, mesenchymal stem cells (MSCs) contribute to the reduction of

Diabetes: Novel Insights and Therapies. Anas Islam and Badruddeen (Eds)

DOI: 10.1201/9781779644596-17

inflammation and autoimmune responses, offering supportive roles in diabetes management. Despite the ongoing challenges in scaling production, achieving functional integration, and ensuring long-term safety, stem cell therapy represents a transformative avenue in diabetes research. This chapter examines the advancements, challenges, and future potential of stem cell therapy for delivering personalized and curative treatments for diabetes mellitus.

12.1 INTRODUCTION

A metabolic condition known as chronic hyperglycemia can be brought on by insufficient insulin secretion, compromised insulin action, or both. Insulin is a crucial anabolic hormone that influences the metabolism of proteins, fats, and carbohydrates (Poznyak et al., 2020). Because of insulin resistance, the metabolic abnormalities linked to diabetes primarily affect tissues such as skeletal muscles, adipose tissue, and the liver. The type and duration of diabetes can affect the severity of the symptoms. People with high blood sugar levels (BSLs), especially those who do not have any insulin, such as children, can experience symptoms such as weight loss, increased appetite, polydipsia, dysuria, and visual issues.

Access to reasonably priced insulin and other diabetes treatments is essential for the survival of patients with diabetes. By 2025, there will be a universally accepted goal to stop the increase in obesity and diabetes. Diabetes affects over 830 million people globally, most of whom reside in low-income and middle-income nations. More than 50% of individuals with diabetes do not receive treatment. Over the past few decades, there has been a steady increase in the number of people with diabetes and those who do not receive treatment for the disease.

12.2 STEM CELLS: AN OVERVIEW

All phases of life contain stem cells, a special type of cell population with the capacity to self-renew and specialize in several cell lineages. These cells are the source from which certain cell types within differentiated tissues and organs are produced, making them important mediators in the development of neonates, as well as in the restorative processes following injury or disease (Kolios et al., 2013). The main function of stem cells in adults is regenerative and restorative; however, in neonates, they differentiate and multiply into the various cell types and lineages needed for ongoing development (Dekoninck et al., 2019). Stem cells can perform specific physiological functions because of certain characteristics that distinguish them from terminally developed cells. Potency is the capacity of stem cells to differentiate into distinct cell types; stem cells can be categorized both by their origin and capacity to differentiate. Both totipotent and omnipotent stem cells can develop into all cell lineages required for adulthood and to build embryonic organs. Multipotent stem cells may only differentiate into one type of germline tissue, whereas pluripotent stem cells can differentiate into all three germ layers. Adult organ tissues contain oligopotent and unipotent stem cells that have committed to a certain cell lineage and are only capable of differentiating into cell types that belong to that lineage (Kolios et al., 2013). The inner cell mass of a blastocyst gives rise to potent ESCs. Legal and ethical considerations usually limit their spectrum of application, which is why mesenchymal stem cells (MSCs) are usually chosen. Without ethical concerns surrounding ESCs, MSCs can be extracted from a range of neonatal and adult tissues while retaining the capacity to develop into several cell types, enabling their use in therapeutic and research settings (Ding et al., 2011).

12.3 STEM CELLS CLASSIFICATION

The human body contains unspecialized stem cells. They can self-renew and differentiate into any type of cell. Both adult cells and embryos contain stem cells. The specialization process involves multiple steps. Unipotent stem cells cannot differentiate into as many different types of cells as pluripotent stem cells, because their developmental power decreases with each stage. This chapter will concentrate on stem cell classification (Hoang et al., 2022).

12.3.1 TOTIPOTENT STEM CELLS

Totipotent stem cells possess the ability to divide and develop into the cells of the entire organism. The ability of cells to differentiate into both embryonic and extra-embryonic tissues is known as totipotency (Malik et al., 2022). A zygote, which is created when a sperm fertilizes an egg, is an example of a totipotent cell. These cells have the potential to grow in the placenta or any one of the three germ layers. The inner cell mass of the blastocyst becomes pluripotent after approximately four days. The source of pluripotent cells is this structure (Ghazimoradi et al., 2022).

12.3.2 PLURIPOTENT STEM CELLS (PSCS)

All germ layer cells can be formed by pluripotent stem cells (PSCs), but extraembryonic tissues such as the placenta cannot. One such example is ESCs. The inner cell mass of preimplantation embryos is a source of ESCs (Liu et al., 2020; Sharkis et al., 2012). iPSCs obtained from the epiblast layer of implanted embryos provide an additional illustration. From fully pluripotent cells, such as ESCs and iPSCs, to representatives with less potency, multi-, oligo-, or unipotent cells, their pluripotency ranges. A teratoma development assay is one way to evaluate its spectrum and activity. iPSCs work similarly to PSCs and are intentionally produced from somatic cells (Aboul-Soud et al., 2021; Moradi et al., 2019). Their cultivation and application hold great promise for regenerative medicine, both now and in the future.

12.3.3 MULTIPOTENT STEM CELLS

Although multipotent stem cells can specialize in distinct cells of particular cell lineages, their range of differentiation is more limited than that of PSCs. One example is hematopoietic stem cells (HSCs), which may differentiate into many blood cell types (Worku et al., 2021). HSCs differentiate into oligopotent cells. They can only differentiate into related cells. It has been suggested that some multipotent cells are pluripotent cells because they can differentiate into unrelated cell types (Aprile et al., 2024).

12.3.4 UNIPOTENT STEM CELLS

Unipotent stem cells represent a highly specialized category of stem cells, characterized by their ability to self-renew and differentiate into a single, specific cell type within a defined lineage. This limited differentiation potential is complemented by their critical roles in tissue-specific maintenance and regeneration (Zakrzewski et al., 2019). For instance, epidermal stem cells in the basal layer of the skin are unipotent and contribute exclusively to the generation of keratinocytes, thereby ensuring continuous renewal of the epidermis. Similarly, spermatogonial stem cells in the testes are solely responsible for spermatozoa production and play a vital role in male fertility. Although their restricted potency minimizes the risk of undesired differentiation, it also limits their applicability in regenerative medicine, which requires diverse cell types. Nonetheless, their inherent self-renewal capacity and lineage-specific differentiation make them indispensable for sustaining tissue homeostasis and offer potential for targeted therapeutic interventions within specific domains (Mitalipov et al., 2009).

12.4 STEM CELL THERAPY IN DIABETES MELLITUS

Stem cell therapy is a promising treatment option for diabetes mellitus, particularly for addressing the underlying causes and consequences of the disease. With its potential advantages over conventional therapies, this novel strategy seeks to improve glycemic control and restore insulin production (Chen et al., 2020). The important facets of stem cell therapy in the treatment of diabetes are described in the following sections.

12.4.1 MESENCHYMAL STEM CELL (MSC) THERAPY IN DIABETES MELLITUS

Mesenchymal stem cells (MSCs) from various adult human tissues were used to differentiate them into cells that produce insulin. Several others include the endometrium, fibroblasts, liver cells, adipose tissue, bone marrow, and the umbilical cord or blood. However, bone marrow is the most abundant source of MSCs. Bone marrow MSCs offer several benefits (Ghoneim et al., 2020; Ullah et al., 2015). They are capable of self-replication and differentiation into cells that create bone, fat, and other tissues, both *in vitro* and *in vivo*. Both inside and outside lineage barriers retain the potential for multilineage differentiation. They grow and sustain their pluripotency, even under long-term culture conditions (Marques-Mari et al., 2009). Because MSCs are thought to be immunologically “inert” and have immunosuppressive properties, they are also favored for transplantation purposes. This makes them perfect candidates in situations where a properly matched donor is unavailable. In mouse models and human studies, MSCs promote HSC engraftment across lineage barriers when transplanted with other adult stem cells (Heris et al., 2022). Even though adult stem cells, including MSCs, have a higher differentiation capacity than ESCs and iPSCs, the latter are still preferred by transplantation scientists due to their "benign," nontumorigenic differentiation potential. MSCs have been used to effectively inhibit tumor growth *in vivo* (El-Badri et al., 2013).

12.4.2 INDUCED PLURIPOTENT STEM CELLS

Numerous *in vitro* and *in vivo* investigations have demonstrated how closely iPS and ES cells share their traits. Similar to ESCs, iPS cells have comparable morphological traits (Takahashi et al., 2007). *In vitro* research has demonstrated that iPS cells possess the ability to develop into cells of all three germ layers. Similar to human ESCs, iPS cells spontaneously group into a cluster of cells called embryoid bodies (EBs) when cultivated in suspension media used to cultivate and differentiate ESCs (Maehr et al., 2009).

12.4.3 EMBRYONIC STEM CELLS

The inner cell mass of blastocysts gives rise to pluripotent ESCs, which can differentiate into any type of cell in the human body. They are priceless tools for regenerative medicine because of their capacity to multiply endlessly while retaining pluripotency. As they provide a renewable reservoir of cells for therapeutic purposes, ESCs have been thoroughly investigated for their potential to replace or repair damaged tissues and organs. Because ESCs can produce β-cells that produce insulin, they have drawn much attention for their use in the treatment of diabetes mellitus. This offers a promising way to address the cellular deficiencies that underlie this disease (Docherty et al., 2007).

12.5 TREATMENT OF DIABETES MELLITUS WITH STEM CELLS

The first trial to assess the safety and effectiveness of autologous MSC therapy in individuals with newly diagnosed type 1 diabetes was published in 2015 by Swedish researchers (Nbib1068951). The median systemic single dose of stem cells isolated from the patient's iliac crest bone marrow was 2.75×10^6 cells/kg. They concluded that MSC injection produced encouraging C-peptide concentrations at the 1-year follow-up and did not cause any negative effects in any of the 10 patients. There were no functional differences in hemoglobin A1c (HbA1c) or insulin dosage between the control and MSC groups in this phase I trial. The safety, viability, and initial results of umbilical cord Wharton's jelly derived MSCs for newly diagnosed type 1 diabetes were investigated in a single-center, double-blind trial by Hu et al. (2013). The MSC-treated group had two intravenous infusions four weeks apart, with a mean cell count of 2.6×10^7. Between 9 and 24 months following MSC infusion, postprandial glucose and HbA1c levels were reduced in the experimental cohort. Additionally, the MSC group showed significant improvement in fasting C-peptide and insulin use. The authors concluded that umbilical cord MSC transplantation is safe and practical, based on their small trial, which was not powered to identify functional changes.

According to a Chinese pilot trial, placenta-derived MSCs were safe, simple, and may be effective when administered to individuals with type 2 diabetes who have had the disease for a long time (Jiang et al., 2011). 10 patients with poorly managed glucose, insulin dependence (≥0.7 U/kg/day) for at least a year, and type 2 diabetes for at least three years were included in this study. On average, the participants received three intravenous infusions of placental stem cells at intervals of one month, totaling 1.35×10^6/kg. All patients' HbA1c readings and insulin dosage showed a trend towards improvement six months after treatment. Additionally, following MSC treatment, there was an increase in the release of insulin and C-peptides. A group of people with other comorbidities, such as heart disease, kidney illness, and vascular problems, was also included in this trial, making them more representative of real-world clinical situations. Researchers have recently created MSCs that secrete insulin and administered them to patients with type 1 diabetes, together with HSCs (Thakkar et al., 2015). Compared to allogenic transplantation, autologous transplantation using the intrapancreatic route tended to have better postprandial glucose and C-peptide levels at 15–24 months. Further research is required to support the conclusions of both trials, which consider stem cell delivery to be a safe technique with prospective benefits.

Mouse-skin fibroblasts were used by Tateishi et al. (2008) and Park et al. (2008) to rewire iPS cells and induce their differentiation into cells that secrete insulin. When these insulin-secreting cells were injected into the portal vein of diabetic mice, the amount of insulin released dramatically increased. Furthermore, the findings showed that blood glucose levels (BGLs) dropped and that HbA1c levels returned to values that were comparable to those seen in people without diabetes. These findings demonstrate that islet cell damage in diabetic mice can be effectively treated with iPS cells. Zhang et al. (2009) and Maehr et al. (2011) effectively converted human iPS cells into cells that secrete insulin. Park et al. (2008) produced a range of iPS cell lines in 2008, including those generated from individuals with type 1 diabetes. These findings demonstrate that iPS cells could help diabetic patients with reduced islet cell counts overcome constraints related to donor tissue scarcity and immunological rejection after islet transplantation therapy, providing new hope for patients with diabetes.

When human pluripotent stem cells (hPSCs) were discovered, it became possible to create replacement cells and tissues for use in drug screening and diabetes treatment (Zhang et al., 2009). According to studies by Pagliuca et al. (2014), the *in vitro* production of insulin-producing pancreatic β cells from stem cells would offer a previously unheard-of cell source for diabetes medication discovery and cell transplantation therapy. They described a scalable differentiation strategy that can produce hundreds of millions of β-cells that respond to glucose *in vitro* from hPSC. These stem cell-derived β cells (SC-β) respond to glucose by fluxing Ca^{2+} and expressing the markers seen in mature β cells. Calcium signaling allows β cells to detect changes in glucose levels, and rising glucose levels cause membrane depolarization and an influx of calcium ions, which in turn causes insulin exocytosis (Mohammed et al., 2009; Pagliuca et al., 2014). Furthermore, these cells alleviated hyperglycemia in diabetic mice by secreting human insulin into the serum of mice in a glucose-regulated manner after transplantation. Without the use of transgenes or genetic modification, they produced glucose-responsive cells that exhibit important characteristics of β cells both *in vitro* and *in vivo* by sequentially modulating several signaling pathways in a three-dimensional cell culture system. It also demonstrated the potential of these cells in *in vivo* transplantation therapy for diabetes. iPS cells and other stem cell-based treatments may also help medicines come closer to a lasting solution for type 1 diabetes with further study (Godfrey et al., 2012; Lilly et al., 2016).

12.6 CLINICAL TRIALS BASED ON STEM CELL THERAPY TO TREAT DIABETES MELLITUS

Although preclinical research has not shown strong evidence, clinical trials have been conducted to test the theory that MSC-derived pancreatic progenitors produced *in vitro* develop into β-cells *in vivo*, either by themselves (Dave et al., 2015) or in combination with stem cells generated from the bone marrow (Thakkar et al., 2015). Currently, there is insufficient evidence to conclusively show the presence of mature functioning MSC-derived β-cells, even though both trials showed improvements in HbA1c, serum C-peptide, glutamic acid decarboxylase antibodies (GAD), and exogenous insulin requirement. The advantages of MSCs transplantation most likely stem from the ability of MSCs to modulate the immune system and/or protect indigenous islets. Compared to MSC-pancreatic progenitors alone, co-infusion of MSC-derived islet pancreatic progenitors with bone marrow-derived HSCs improved the long-term management of hyperglycemia (Dave et al., 2015; Thakkar et al., 2015).

Potential modes of action include the following: a paracrine effect through growth factor secretion (Salgado et al., 2010); extracellular matrix modulation, scavenging of reactive oxygen species (ROS), protection against hypoxia-induced apoptosis through exosome-derived microRNAs (miRNAs) (Najar et al., 2016); and modulation of the immune system (Carlsson et al., 2015; Najar et al., 2016) through the promotion of regulatory T cells and inhibition of T-cell proliferation, or interactions with other immune cell types, including macrophages, B cells, dendritic cells, and natural killer cells (Song et al., 2020).

Although the effect on T1D patients is still unclear, meta-analyses of data from finished clinical trials indicate that MSCs can protect islets in T2D patients. The small number of patients included in early MSC-based clinical studies for T1D, as well as the trial design that precludes suitable statistical analysis, have made it difficult to interpret these trials. Mesples et al. (2013) tested the effectiveness of autologous bone marrow stem cell transplantation (Mesples et al., 2020) and found improvements, particularly in the decrease of anti-pancreatic islet antibodies.

In the 12-month follow-up study, there was a drop in blood glucose and HbA1c, an increase in C-peptide, and negative values for islet cell antibodies (ICA), GAD, and insulin antibody levels. However, one available control patient had a similar decline in blood glucose and HbA1c levels, and one of the two recruited patients' C-peptide levels were not entirely maintained after a year. Interpretation of the data was equivocal because of the small number of treated patients and controls. 20 adult patients with recently diagnosed T1D participated in a similar trial (Carlsson et al., 2015) carried out in 2015 by Carlsson and his colleagues. 12 months after transplantation, C-peptide levels in treated patients responded to a mixed-meal tolerance test with preservation or even increase.

Although each of these trials indicated that MSC-based therapy supports β-cell health and function in patients with type 1 diabetes, the favorable results of controlled clinical trials are still being debated by systematic reviews and meta-analyses. The combined effect of HSC therapy, MSC-based therapy, and co-infusion of hematopoietic and multipotent MSCs led to increased C-peptide levels when compared with conventional insulin therapy, according to a 2018 meta-analysis (Gan et al., 2018), which included nine randomized controlled trials and 14 self-controlled trials. However, trials based on MSCs derived from umbilical cord blood have not reached a significant level. According to a meta-analysis of six controlled T1D trials published in 2019, there was no difference between the levels of fasting and stimulated C-peptide (Hwang et al., 2019). The only difference between the treatment and control groups was the decrease in HbA1c levels. To clarify the effectiveness of MSC therapy for T1D, results from current randomized controlled studies with a larger number of recruited patients and controls are required. MSC-based clinical trials for T2D have demonstrated consistent and strong efficacy in contrast to the dubious advantages of MSC-based treatments for T1D. Multipotent MSCs from various sources have been used in T2D MSC-based experiments. Improvements in C-pep levels, HbA1c values, and decreases in the necessary insulin dosage have been noted since the initial trial in 2009 (Bhansali et al., 2009) and in the most recent studies (Bhansali et al., 2017). Stimulated C-peptide and fasting C-peptide levels significantly increased according to a systematic evaluation of 10 T2D MSC-based trials (Hwang et al., 2019). Although several *in vitro* and *in vivo* pre-clinical studies have been conducted, the mechanism by which MSCs improve outcomes is still unknown. More research should be conducted to precisely determine this. Pluripotent human embryonic stem cells (hESCs) are extracted from the inner cell mass (Thomson et al., 1998). They can produce all three lineages (endoderm, mesoderm, and ectoderm) and can self-renew. They also exhibit genetic stability.

By ectopically overexpressing particular transcription factors, somatic cells can develop into induced pluripotent stem cells (iPSCs) (Takahashi et al., 2006). In addition to their potential for differentiation and self-renewal, the genetic stability of iPSCs remains unclear. Following growth, hESCs and iPSCs retain their pluripotency (Gerace et al., 2019), meeting the demand for the endless supply needed for therapeutic applications. Despite being a promising substitute for hESCs, iPSCs have not yet achieved the same level of differentiation into mature pancreatic endocrine cells as hESC methods (Kondo et al., 2018).

In Edmonton, an hESC-based pancreatic progenitor transplant was used to treat the first T1D patient in 2015. Using an encapsulation device called PEC-Encap (VC-01), the trial (NCT02239354, submitted in 2014) aimed to test a combination of hESC-derived pancreatic progenitor cells (PEC-01) (Kroon et al., 2008; Schulz et al., 2015) that, according to previous research using surrogate animals, should develop into functional insulin-producing cells (IPCs) upon transplantation. 40 million pancreatic progenitor cells were used in the initial transplant, including two encapsulation devices placed subcutaneously in the abdomen and six smaller encapsulation devices placed subcutaneously in the arm. These devices serve as sentinels that can be removed at various intervals to monitor cell survival and maturation.

An alternate encapsulation device (PEC-Direct, VC-02) with a modified membrane that permits vascularization but does not offer immune protection, necessitates the reintroduction of immunosuppressants. ViaCyte initiated the second 12-month trial (NCT03162926) in 2017. No modifications were made to the hESC-derived pancreatic progenitors. The current 2-year experiment (NCT03163511), which aims to investigate the safety and tolerability of VC-02 implanted subcutaneously in T1D participants with hypoglycemia unawareness, is ongoing as a result of successful outcomes. Furthermore, without triggering a foreign body reaction, the immunosuppressive regimen prevented the cells from being destroyed by allogeneic and autoimmune processes. There is no information on its effectiveness because the planned islet mass transplant was purposefully insufficient to return HbA1c levels to normal. Although only 30% of transplant recipients experience these benefits, future results could be enhanced by further refining the materials used in microencapsulation devices.

12.7 CHALLENGES IN STEM CELL-BASED THERAPY FOR DIABETES

Although cell-based treatments for diabetes have advanced considerably, numerous obstacles remain to be addressed. Although they have yielded important insights, clinical trials examining islet transplantation methods and encapsulation devices face several challenges, including oxygenation, host immunological responses, and inadequate long-term engraftment success. The goal of additive manufacturing and immunoengineering biomaterials to create 3D islet structures is to reduce inflammation and encourage graft revascularization. However, it is still difficult to consistently normalize BGLs in humans without the use of exogenous insulin. Research on genetically modified or progenitor-derived insulin-secreting β-like cells is being conducted in the fields of gene therapy and stem cell differentiation to optimize techniques that guarantee safety and functionality. Establishing stable and functional cells that can permanently restore normoglycemia without external assistance is a major challenge. Immunological response, which attacks both xenogeneic and allogeneic islet grafts, is a significant obstacle. Although local immunotherapy reduces systemic effects, it is still very difficult to avoid graft destruction using biomaterials that do not require immune suppression. To guarantee uniform function and long-term safety across batches, the translation of genetically reprogrammed cells into precise 3D islet construction also requires scalable manufacturing procedures. It is crucial to consider the safety, economic, ethical, and regulatory aspects that influence translational applications when evaluating advancements in cell-based diabetes therapies. Oversight organizations are essential for setting guidelines to protect patient welfare and promote therapeutic innovation at the regulatory level. In the US, the FDA is in charge of clinical trials and product approval; in Europe, the EMA offers complementary regulatory guidelines. Organ and cell allocation procedures in the United States are regulated by groups such as the Organ Procurement and Transplantation Network (OPTN) and the United Network for Organ Sharing (UNOS) (Parums et al., 2023; Witkowski et al., 2021). However, regulatory channels necessitate continual harmonization between agencies and jurisdictions when regenerative techniques deviate from conventional organ transplantation. To streamline guidelines in a patient-centric manner that balances safety, efficacy, and timely access to cutting-edge medications, it is essential that researchers, oversight bodies, and legislators have ongoing conversations. For example, the emergence of 3D bioprinted tissue constructions and β-cells produced from stem cells may make it difficult for existing drug and device frameworks to handle the manufacturing and product characterization challenges of these cutting-edge therapeutic solutions (Accolla et al., 2022). Upholding adherence to changing laws in clinics has an impact on research directives and patients' access to innovative treatments. From an ethical standpoint, it is critical to address clinical trial design, informed consent, and privacy protection for sensitive health data (Dezashibi et al., 2023; Joo et al., 2012). Prudence is necessary when it comes to the autonomy and agency of study participants in making decisions regarding experimental medicines. To prevent particular populations from encountering excessive obstacles, emphasis should also be placed on the equitable accessibility of new treatment choices. Depending on whether the cells are derived from adult, fetal, or embryonic tissues, there are ethical concerns regarding the cell source. Careful consideration must be given to logistical issues, such as the shipping and processing of stem cell-derived islets before transplantation. Thorough preclinical testing is necessary to maximize the carcinogenic potential of undifferentiated pluripotent stem cells. To transition medicines between animal and early human studies, it is necessary to have well-characterized cellular products that exhibit consistent safety and glucose-responsive insulin (GRI) secretion profiles similar to those of pancreatic islets. As treatments advance clinically, long-term animal model data demonstrating the absence of malignant transformation after transplantation help calm ethical safety concerns. In pursuit of curative objectives, researchers meticulously screened novel ideas to avoid participant side effects. Even though there are encouraging clinical signs, islet and stem cell transplantation procedures are still too costly for widespread use. To test methods, monitor long-term results, evaluate healthcare cost offsets from preventing the crippling consequences of diabetes, and calculate cost-benefit ratios for national reimbursement paradigms, the topic needs ongoing research. Large-scale interventional trials and longitudinal studies could be expedited by public-private collaborations to accurately measure the safety profiles and practical effectiveness of cellular treatments in comparison to intensive management and the expenses associated with intensive diabetes care. Catalytic manufacturing has the ability to completely recalibrate economics through ongoing advancements, such as 3D bioprinting, which can improve yields, standardize processes, and lower prices through scale. Researchers, oversight boards, and larger stakeholder networks can move cell-based therapies closer to providing transformative benefits for all communities by carefully and sensitively analyzing regulatory frameworks, informed consent procedures, risks and benefits, and financial considerations at both micro and macro levels. A diligent multidisciplinary approach strikes a balance between patient welfare and advancement. A variety of tactics can be used to overcome these restrictions. For example, sequencing treatments or gene-modified islets incorporated into vascularized biomaterial implants have shown promise in priming grafts in proregenerative settings prior to transplantation. Cross-disciplinary cooperation raises the possibility that in the long run, effective pancreatic cell or tissue engraftment may enable improved customized treatments for both diabetes and chronic pancreatitis to attain long-lasting insulin independence. In light of the continuous advancements in overcoming these obstacles, cell replacement techniques may enhance the treatment of diabetes.

12.8 FUTURE PERSPECTIVES AND THERAPEUTIC POTENTIAL

With the development of new treatment options for type 1 and type 2 diabetes, the prospects and therapeutic potential of stem cell research in diabetes mellitus are bright. By creating functioning insulin-producing β-cells, stem cell-based therapies seek to restore insulin production and glucose homeostasis, which are vital components of diabetes treatment. The ability of pluripotent stem cells, such as iPSCs and ESCs, to differentiate into β-like cells in the pancreas has made them promising candidates for autologous transplantation with a lower risk of immunological rejection. Owing to their immunomodulatory and anti-inflammatory properties, MSCs can maintain β-cell activity and reduce the inflammatory milieu, which is frequently linked to the advancement of diabetes. Additionally, bioengineering techniques, such as encapsulation technologies, are being developed, allowing β-cell transplants produced from stem cells to avoid immune attacks without requiring chronic immunosuppression. Organoid models of the pancreas offer novel platforms for drug discovery and disease modeling, while personalized medical approaches that make use of patient-specific iPSCs open the door to customized treatments. The intersection of precision medicine, bioengineering, and stem cell biology holds great promise for developing cures for diabetes mellitus, notwithstanding the difficulties in attaining exact functional integration, guaranteeing long-term safety, and scaling up the manufacturing process.

12.9 CONCLUSION

In conclusion, by addressing the underlying causes of diabetes mellitus, stem cell therapy has the potential to completely change the way the condition is treated. Restoring glycemic control may be possible with the capacity of stem cells to develop into insulin-producing β-cells, especially in individuals with severe β-cell loss. While MSCs have the potential to modulate inflammatory and autoimmune responses linked to the progression of diabetes, advances in pluripotent stem cell technology, including the use of embryos and iPSCs, have opened the door for the development of immunocompatible and customized therapies. By permitting precise genetic alterations and creating protective scaffolds for cell transplantation, emerging technologies, such as gene editing and bioengineering, significantly increase therapeutic potential. However, before broad clinical use, issues with transplanted cell integration, safety, scalability, and long-term viability must be resolved. The combination of stem cell biology, regenerative medicine, and cutting-edge therapeutic modalities is expected to revolutionize diabetes care as research advances, providing millions of patients worldwide with the prospect of long-lasting and possibly curative treatment.

KEYWORDS

- **3D bioprinting**
- **diabetes mellitus**
- **glucose homeostasis**
- **mesenchymal stem cells**
- **pluripotent stem cells**
- **regenerative medicine**
- **stem cell therapy**
- **β-cell regeneration**

REFERENCES

Aboul-Soud, M. A. M., Alzahrani, A. J., & Mahmoud, A. (2021). Induced pluripotent stem cells (iPSCs)—Roles in regenerative therapies, disease modelling and drug screening. *Cells, 10*(9), 2319. https://doi.org/10.3390/cells10092319 (accessed on 2nd February 2026).

Accolla, R. P., Simmons, A. M., & Stabler, C. L. (2022). Integrating additive manufacturing techniques to improve cell-based implants for the treatment of type 1 diabetes. *Advanced Healthcare Materials, 11*(13), e2200243. https://doi.org/10.1002/adhm.202200243 (accessed on 2nd February 2026).

Aprile, D., Patrone, D., Peluso, G., & Galderisi, U. (2024). Multipotent/pluripotent stem cell populations in stromal tissues and peripheral blood: Exploring diversity, potential, and therapeutic applications. *Stem Cell Research & Therapy, 15*(1), 139. https://doi.org/10.1186/s13287-024-03752-x (accessed on 2nd February 2026).

Bhansali, A., Upreti, V., Khandelwal, N., et al. (2009). Efficacy of autologous bone marrow-derived stem cell transplantation in patients with type 2 diabetes mellitus. *Stem Cells and Development, 18*(10), 1407–1416. https://doi.org/10.1089/scd.2009.0164 (accessed on 2nd February 2026).

Bhansali, S., Dutta, P., Kumar, V., et al. (2017). Efficacy of autologous bone marrow-derived mesenchymal stem cell and mononuclear cell transplantation in type 2 diabetes mellitus: A randomized, placebo-controlled comparative study. *Stem Cells and Development, 26*(7), 471–481. https://doi.org/10.1089/scd.2016.0275 (accessed on 2nd February 2026).

Carlsson, P. O., Schwarcz, E., Korsgren, O., & Le Blanc, K. (2015). Preserved β-cell function in type 1 diabetes by mesenchymal stromal cells. *Diabetes, 64*(2), 587–592. https://doi.org/10.2337/db14-0656 (accessed on 2nd February 2026).

Chen, S., Du, K., & Zou, C. (2020). Current progress in stem cell therapy for type 1 diabetes mellitus. *Stem Cell Research & Therapy, 11*(1), 275. https://doi.org/10.1186/s13287-020-01793-6 (accessed on 2nd February 2026).

Cito, M., Pellegrini, S., Piemonti, L., & Sordi, V. (2018). The potential and challenges of alternative sources of β cells for the cure of type 1 diabetes. *Endocrine Connections, 7*(3), R114–R125. https://doi.org/10.1530/EC-18-0012 (accessed on 2nd February 2026).

Dave, S. D., Vanikar, A. V., Trivedi, H. L., Thakkar, U. G., Gopal, S. C., & Chandra, T. (2015). Novel therapy for insulin-dependent diabetes mellitus: Infusion of *in vitro*-generated insulin-secreting cells. *Clinical and Experimental Medicine, 15*(1), 41–45. https://doi.org/10.1007/s10238-013-0266-1 (accessed on 2nd February 2026).

Dekoninck, S., & Blanpain, C. (2019). Stem cell dynamics, migration and plasticity during wound healing. *Nature Cell Biology, 21*(1), 18–24. https://doi.org/10.1038/s41556-018-0237-6 (accessed on 2nd February 2026).

Dezashibi, H. M., & Shabani, A. (2023). A mini-review of current treatment approaches and gene therapy as potential interventions for diabetes mellitus types 1. *Advanced Biomedical Research, 12*, 219. https://doi.org/10.4103/abr.abr_201_23 (accessed on 2nd February 2026).

Ding, D. C., Shyu, W. C., & Lin, S. Z. (2011). Mesenchymal stem cells. *Cell Transplantation, 20*(1), 5–14. https://doi.org/10.3727/096368910X (accessed on 2nd February 2026).

Docherty, K., Bernardo, A. S., & Vallier, L. (2007). Embryonic stem cell therapy for diabetes mellitus. *Seminars in Cell & Developmental Biology, 18*(6), 827–838. https://doi.org/10.1016/j.semcdb.2007.09.009 (accessed on 2nd February 2026).

El-Badri, N., & Ghoneim, M. A. (2013). Mesenchymal stem cell therapy in diabetes mellitus: Progress and challenges. *Journal of Nucleic Acids, 2013*, 194858. https://doi.org/10.1155/2013/194858 (accessed on 2nd February 2026).

Gan, J., Wang, Y., & Zhou, X. (2018). Stem cell transplantation for the treatment of patients with type 1 diabetes mellitus: A meta-analysis. *Experimental and Therapeutic Medicine, 16*(6), 4479–4492. https://doi.org/10.3892/etm.2018.6769 (accessed on 2nd February 2026).

Gerace, D., Martiniello-Wilks, R., Habib, R., et al. (2019). *Ex vivo* expansion of murine MSC impairs transcription factor-induced differentiation into pancreatic β-cells. *Stem*

Cells International, 2019, 1395301. https://doi.org/10.1155/2019/1395301 (accessed on 2nd February 2026).

Ghazimoradi, M. H., Khalafizadeh, A., & Babashah, S. (2022). A critical review on induced totipotent stem cells: Types and methods. *Stem Cell Research, 63*, 102857. https://doi.org/10.1016/j.scr.2022.102857 (accessed on 2nd February 2026).

Ghoneim, M. A., Refaie, A. F., Elbassiouny, B. L., Gabr, M. M., & Zakaria, M. M. (2020). From mesenchymal stromal/stem cells to insulin-producing cells: Progress and challenges. *Stem Cell Reviews and Reports, 16*(6), 1156–1172. https://doi.org/10.1007/s12015-020-10036-3 (accessed on 2nd February 2026).

Godfrey, K. J., Mathew, B., Bulman, J. C., Shah, O., Clement, S., & Gallicano, G. I. (2012). Stem cell-based treatments for type 1 diabetes mellitus: Bone marrow, embryonic, hepatic, pancreatic and induced pluripotent stem cells. *Diabetic Medicine, 29*(1), 14–23. https://doi.org/10.1111/j.1464-5491.2011.03433.x (accessed on 2nd February 2026).

Heris, R. M., Shirvaliloo, M., Abbaspour-Aghdam, S., et al. (2022). The potential use of mesenchymal stem cells and their exosomes in Parkinson's disease treatment. *Stem Cell Research & Therapy, 13*(1), 371. https://doi.org/10.1186/s13287-022-03050-4 (accessed on 2nd February 2026).

Hoang, D. M., Pham, P. T., Bach, T. Q., et al. (2022). Stem cell-based therapy for human diseases. *Signal Transduction and Targeted Therapy, 7*(1), 272. https://doi.org/10.1038/s41392-022-01134-4 (accessed on 2nd February 2026).

Hu, J., Yu, X., Wang, Z., et al. (2013). Long term effects of the implantation of Wharton's jelly-derived mesenchymal stem cells from the umbilical cord for newly-onset type 1 diabetes mellitus. *Endocrine Journal, 60*(3), 347–357. https://doi.org/10.1507/endocrj.ej12-0343 (accessed on 2nd February 2026).

Hwang, G., Jeong, H., Yang, H. K., et al. (2019). Efficacies of stem cell therapies for functional improvement of the β cell in patients with diabetes: A systematic review of controlled clinical trials. *International Journal of Stem Cells, 12*(2), 195–205. https://doi.org/10.15283/ijsc18076 (accessed on 2nd February 2026).

Jiang, R., Han, Z., Zhuo, G., et al. (2011). Transplantation of placenta-derived mesenchymal stem cells in type 2 diabetes: A pilot study. *Frontiers of Medicine, 5*(1), 94–100. https://doi.org/10.1007/s11684-011-0116-z (accessed on 2nd February 2026).

Joo, W. S., Jeong, J. H., Nam, K., Blevins, K. S., Salama, M. E., & Kim, S. W. (2012). Polymeric delivery of therapeutic RAE-1 plasmid to the pancreatic islets for the prevention of type 1 diabetes. *Journal of Controlled Release, 162*(3), 606–611. https://doi.org/10.1016/j.jconrel.2012.08.008 (accessed on 2nd February 2026).

Kaitsuka, T., Kobayashi, K., Otsuka, W., et al. (2017). Erythropoietin facilitates definitive endodermal differentiation of mouse embryonic stem cells via activation of ERK signaling. *American Journal of Physiology - Cell Physiology, 312*(5), C573–C582. https://doi.org/10.1152/ajpcell.00071.2016 (accessed on 2nd February 2026).

Kolios, G., & Moodley, Y. (2013). Introduction to stem cells and regenerative medicine. *Respiration, 85*(1), 3–10. https://doi.org/10.1159/000345615 (accessed on 2nd February 2026).

Kondo, Y., Toyoda, T., Inagaki, N., & Osafune, K. (2018). iPSC technology-based regenerative therapy for diabetes. *Journal of Diabetes Investigation, 9*(2), 234–243. https://doi.org/10.1111/jdi.12702 (accessed on 2nd February 2026).

Kroon, E., Martinson, L. A., Kadoya, K., et al. (2008). Pancreatic endoderm derived from human embryonic stem cells generates glucose-responsive insulin-secreting cells *in vivo*. *Nature Biotechnology, 26*(4), 443–452. https://doi.org/10.1038/nbt1393 (accessed on 2nd February 2026).

Lilly, M. A., Davis, M. F., Fabie, J. E., Terhune, E. B., & Gallicano, G. I. (2016). Current stem cell-based therapies in diabetes. *American Journal of Stem Cells, 5*(3), 87–98.

Liu, G., David, B. T., Trawczynski, M., & Fessler, R. G. (2020). Advances in pluripotent stem cells: History, mechanisms, technologies, and applications. *Stem Cell Reviews and Reports, 16*(1), 3–32. https://doi.org/10.1007/s12015-019-09935-x (accessed on 2nd February 2026).

Maehr, R. (2011). iPS cells in type 1 diabetes research and treatment. *Clinical Pharmacology & Therapeutics, 89*(5), 750–753. https://doi.org/10.1038/clpt.2011.1 (accessed on 2nd February 2026).

Maehr, R., Chen, S., Snitow, M., et al. (2009). Generation of pluripotent stem cells from patients with type 1 diabetes. *Proceedings of the National Academy of Sciences of the United States of America, 106*(37), 15768–15773. https://doi.org/10.1073/pnas.0906894106 (accessed on 2nd February 2026).

Malik, V., & Wang, J. (2022). Pursuing totipotency: Authentic totipotent stem cells in culture. *Trends in Genetics, 38*(7), 632–636. https://doi.org/10.1016/j.tig.2022.03.012 (accessed on 2nd February 2026).

Marques-Mari, A. I., Lacham-Kaplan, O., Medrano, J. V., Pellicer, A., & Simón, C. (2009). Differentiation of germ cells and gametes from stem cells. *Human Reproduction Update, 15*(3), 379–390. https://doi.org/10.1093/humupd/dmp001 (accessed on 2nd February 2026).

Matsuno, K., Mae, S. I., Okada, C., et al. (2016). Redefining definitive endoderm subtypes by robust induction of human induced pluripotent stem cells. *Differentiation, 92*(5), 281–290. https://doi.org/10.1016/j.diff.2016.04.002 (accessed on 2nd February 2026).

Mesples, A., Majeed, N., Zhang, Y., & Hu, X. (2013). Early immunotherapy using autologous adult stem cells reversed the effect of anti-pancreatic islets in recently diagnosed type 1 diabetes mellitus: Preliminary results. *Medical Science Monitor, 19*, 852–857. https://doi.org/10.12659/MSM.889525 (accessed on 2nd February 2026).

Mitalipov, S., & Wolf, D. (2009). Totipotency, pluripotency and nuclear reprogramming. *Advances in Biochemical Engineering/Biotechnology, 114*, 185–199. https://doi.org/10.1007/10_2008_45 (accessed on 2nd February 2026).

Mohammed, J. S., Wang, Y., Harvat, T. A., Oberholzer, J., & Eddington, D. T. (2009). Microfluidic device for multimodal characterization of pancreatic islets. *Lab on a Chip, 9*(1), 97–106. https://doi.org/10.1039/b809590f (accessed on 2nd February 2026).

Moradi, S., Mahdizadeh, H., Šarić, T., et al. (2019). Research and therapy with induced pluripotent stem cells (iPSCs): Social, legal, and ethical considerations. *Stem Cell Research & Therapy, 10*(1), 341. https://doi.org/10.1186/s13287-019-1455-y (accessed on 2nd February 2026).

Najar, M., Raicevic, G., Crompot, E., et al. (2016). The immunomodulatory potential of mesenchymal stromal cells: A story of a regulatory network. *Journal of Immunotherapy, 39*(2), 45–59. https://doi.org/10.1097/CJI.0000000000000108 (accessed on 2nd February 2026).

Pagliuca, F. W., Millman, J. R., Gürtler, M., et al. (2014). Generation of functional human pancreatic β cells *in vitro*. *Cell, 159*(2), 428–439. https://doi.org/10.1016/j.cell.2014.09.040 (accessed on 2nd February 2026).

Park, I. H., Arora, N., Huo, H., et al. (2008). Disease-specific induced pluripotent stem cells. *Cell, 134*(5), 877–886. https://doi.org/10.1016/j.cell.2008.07.041 (accessed on 2nd February 2026).

Parums, D. V. (2023). Editorial: First regulatory approval for allogeneic pancreatic islet beta cell infusion for adult patients with type 1 diabetes mellitus. *Medical Science Monitor, 29*, e941918. https://doi.org/10.12659/MSM.941918 (accessed on 2nd February 2026).

Poznyak, A., Grechko, A. V., Poggio, P., Myasoedova, V. A., Alfieri, V., & Orekhov, A. N. (2020). The diabetes mellitus-atherosclerosis connection: The role of lipid and glucose metabolism and chronic inflammation. *International Journal of Molecular Sciences, 21*(5), 1835. https://doi.org/10.3390/ijms21051835 (accessed on 2nd February 2026).

Salgado, A. J., Reis, R. L., Sousa, N. J., & Gimble, J. M. (2010). Adipose tissue derived stem cells secretome: Soluble factors and their roles in regenerative medicine. *Current Stem Cell Research & Therapy, 5*(2), 103–110. https://doi.org/10.2174/157488810791268564 (accessed on 2nd February 2026).

Schulz, T. C. (2015). Concise review: Manufacturing of pancreatic endoderm cells for clinical trials in type 1 diabetes. *Stem Cells Translational Medicine, 4*(8), 927–931. https://doi.org/10.5966/sctm.2015-0058 (accessed on 2nd February 2026).

Sharkis, S. J., Jones, R. J., Civin, C., & Jang, Y. Y. (2012). Pluripotent stem cell-based cancer therapy: Promise and challenges. *Science Translational Medicine, 4*(127), 127ps9. https://doi.org/10.1126/scitranslmed.3003920 (accessed on 2nd February 2026).

Song, N., Scholtemeijer, M., & Shah, K. (2020). Mesenchymal stem cell immunomodulation: Mechanisms and therapeutic potential. *Trends in Pharmacological Sciences, 41*(9), 653–664. https://doi.org/10.1016/j.tips.2020.06.009 (accessed on 2nd February 2026).

Takahashi, K., & Yamanaka, S. (2006). Induction of pluripotent stem cells from mouse embryonic and adult fibroblast cultures by defined factors. *Cell, 126*(4), 663–676. https://doi.org/10.1016/j.cell.2006.07.024 (accessed on 2nd February 2026).

Takahashi, K., Tanabe, K., Ohnuki, M., et al. (2007). Induction of pluripotent stem cells from adult human fibroblasts by defined factors. *Cell, 131*(5), 861–872. https://doi.org/10.1016/j.cell.2007.11.019 (accessed on 2nd February 2026).

Tateishi, K., He, J., Taranova, O., Liang, G., D'Alessio, A. C., & Zhang, Y. (2008). Generation of insulin-secreting islet-like clusters from human skin fibroblasts. *Journal of Biological Chemistry, 283*(46), 31601–31607. https://doi.org/10.1074/jbc.M806597200 (accessed on 2nd February 2026).

Thakkar, U. G., Trivedi, H. L., Vanikar, A. V., & Dave, S. D. (2015). Insulin-secreting adipose-derived mesenchymal stromal cells with bone marrow-derived hematopoietic stem cells from autologous and allogenic sources for type 1 diabetes mellitus. *Cryotherapy, 17*(7), 940–947. https://doi.org/10.1016/j.jcyt.2015.03.608 (accessed on 2nd February 2026).

Thomson, J. A., Itskovitz-Eldor, J., Shapiro, S. S., et al. (1998). Embryonic stem cell lines derived from human blastocysts [published correction appears in *Science*, 1998 Dec 4; *282*(5395), 1827]. *Science, 282*(5391), 1145–1147. https://doi.org/10.1126/science.282.5391.1145 (accessed on 2nd February 2026).

Ullah, I., Subbarao, R. B., & Rho, G. J. (2015). Human mesenchymal stem cells – Current trends and future prospective. *Bioscience Reports, 35*(2), e00191. https://doi.org/10.1042/BSR20150025 (accessed on 2nd February 2026).

Witkowski, P., Anteby, R., Olaitan, O. K., et al. (2021). Pancreatic islets quality and potency cannot be verified as required for drugs: Reflection on the FDA review of a biological license application for human islets. *Transplantation, 105*(12), e409–e410. https://doi.org/10.1097/TP.0000000000003880 (accessed on 2nd February 2026).

Worku, M. G. (2021). Pluripotent and multipotent stem cells and current therapeutic applications: Review. *Stem Cells and Cloning, 14*, 3–7. https://doi.org/10.2147/SCCAA.S304887 (accessed on 2nd February 2026).

Zakrzewski, W., Dobrzyński, M., Szymonowicz, M., & Rybak, Z. (2019). Stem cells: Past, present, and future. *Stem Cell Research & Therapy, 10*(1), 68. https://doi.org/10.1186/s13287-019-1165-5 (accessed on 2nd February 2026).

Zhang, D., Jiang, W., Liu, M., et al. (2009). Highly efficient differentiation of human ES cells and iPS cells into mature pancreatic insulin-producing cells. *Cell Research, 19*(4), 429–438. https://doi.org/10.1038/cr.2009.28 (accessed on 2nd February 2026).

Index

A

Abdominal
obesity, 40
pain, 8, 181, 182
Abnormal blood vessels, 15
Acromegaly, 10, 87, 100, 134
Actin cytoskeleton, 292
Acupuncture, 63, 66, 68
Adenosine monophosphate (AMP), 48, 141
activated protein kinase (AMPK), 141, 146, 169
Adenylate kinase, 299
Adipocyte, 48, 92, 282, 288, 298, 316, 321
hyperplasia, 316
lipolysis, 92
Adipokines, 282, 283, 298, 310, 315, 393
Adipose tissue (AT), 8, 103, 109, 135, 169, 256, 277, 282, 283, 297, 298, 311, 315, 316, 393, 394, 428, 431
Adiposity, 40, 42, 51, 279
Adrenocorticotropic hormone (ACTH), 100
Adult-onset diabetes, 4, 87
Advanced glycation end-product (AGE), 47, 84, 113
Aerobic exercise, 40
Aging population, 11, 64, 248, 315, 349
Air pollution, 13, 396
Aldosteronoma, 134
Allergens, 327
Allogenic transplantation, 433
American Diabetes Association (ADA), 6, 7, 9–11, 15, 93, 132, 207, 350
Amino acids, 46, 92, 101, 135, 285, 291, 293
Amphiphilic glycomacromolecules, 365
Amputations, 15, 72, 91, 147, 214
Amylin agonists, 143
Angioedema, 142
Antidiabetic, 130, 147–149, 151, 155, 164, 166–171, 173, 175, 179, 185, 186, 296, 362, 364, 370, 385, 391, 404
agents, 155, 164, 166, 171, 173, 175, 186
drugs, 171, 179, 296, 364, 391, 404
effects, 167–171, 173, 175
medications, 130, 179, 385
Antigen
presenting cells (APCs), 312, 326
specific immunotherapy (ASI), 330
Anti-inflammatory, 143, 146, 150, 167, 177, 228, 318–320, 325, 440
cytokine, 319, 320
Antioxidant
enzyme levels, 47
properties, 149, 151, 173, 175, 176
Anti-pancreatic islet antibodies, 435
Anxiety, 18
Apolipoprotein E (APOE), 297, 299
Aqueous solutions, 212, 219, 222
Arginine–insulin complexes (AINS), 218
Arterial walls, 15
Artificial
intelligence (AI), 16, 77–79, 205, 232, 233, 328, 358, 384, 386, 398, 402–405, 416–418
pancreas, 223, 231, 352–355
Asthma, 14
Atherosclerosis, 15, 16, 44, 104, 139, 281, 323
Atherosclerotic plaques, 16, 103, 105
Atypical antipsychotics, 10
Autoantigens, 327
Autoimmune
diabetes, 50, 72, 313, 324, 327
disease, 35, 88, 206, 309, 313, 333
disorders, 3, 275, 328, 390
response, 8, 51, 333, 390, 428, 441
Autoimmunity, 313, 317, 326, 335

Autologous transplantation, 427, 433, 440
Autonomic
nerve dysfunction, 15
nervous system (ANS), 226

B

B cells, 309, 313, 318, 326, 327, 331, 334, 435
Basophils, 311, 312
B-cell
activity, 313
compartment, 331
Bioactive
compounds, 148, 168, 169, 172, 175, 177, 178, 180, 182–184
molecules, 298
Bioavailability, 155, 184, 185, 211, 216, 217, 220, 231, 232, 368–370
Bio-breeding (BB), 37, 163, 164
Biocompatibility, 217, 220, 230, 365, 367, 368, 372
Biocompatible scaffolds, 362
Biodegradability, 217
Bioengineered tissues, 359, 360
Bioengineering, 347, 350, 352, 440, 441
Bioinformatics, 184–186, 287, 389, 399, 410, 411, 414
Biomarker, 99, 112, 183, 231, 248, 263–265, 313, 319, 332, 333, 400, 402–404, 408, 410, 412–414, 419
discovery, 301, 400, 401
Biomimetic system, 371
Bioprinting techniques, 361
Bioreactor, 375
Bisphenols, 19
Blood
flow, 72, 105, 106, 227
glucose
levels (BGLs), 3–7, 16, 18, 43, 44, 46, 63–68, 71–75, 85, 88, 109, 132, 145–148, 175–177, 179, 205, 210, 213, 214, 217–219, 221, 223, 226, 248, 276, 297, 310, 315, 346, 350, 352, 353, 357, 359, 362–365, 367, 369–372, 388, 390, 393, 394, 433, 438
measurement, 3, 7, 211, 251
meters, 86
monitoring, 69, 71, 90, 111, 212, 364
regulation, 353
pressure, 15, 16, 75, 102, 106–108, 111, 139, 177, 225, 227
sugar, 3, 5, 7, 15, 16, 41, 68, 86, 88, 90, 91, 105–110, 142, 143, 145, 147, 175, 205, 210, 211, 225, 284, 285, 350, 367, 384, 396, 428
level (BSL), 5, 14, 15, 41, 50, 68, 73, 86, 88, 90, 91, 104, 106, 108, 110, 112, 143, 145, 168, 169, 173, 175, 176, 210, 284, 350, 355, 357, 365, 384, 404, 428
vessels, 15, 103–108, 110, 208, 226, 315
Bloodstream, 46, 90, 222, 223, 316, 366, 387, 393
Blurred vision, 88, 107
Body
composition, 256
mass index (BMI), 40–42, 44, 97, 138, 226, 261, 283, 349
Bone marrow, 312, 316, 323, 431, 432, 435
Broad-spectrum immunosuppression, 334
Brown
adipose tissue (BAT), 298
seaweeds, 169
B-type natriuretic peptide (BNP), 401
Bulk metal electrodes, 215
Burning pain, 15

C

Calcium
ions, 434
phosphate, 222, 370
Calorie restriction (CR), 394
Canagliflozin, 142
Cancer
diagnosis, 401
treatment, 413
Capillary blood glucose (CBG), 145
Carbohydrates, 42, 47, 51, 85, 142, 147, 168, 210, 290, 310, 329, 394, 396, 428

Carbon nanotubes (CNTs), 210–212, 215
Cardiovascular
disease (CVD), 3, 8, 13, 16–18, 64, 67, 69, 99, 102–105, 112, 132, 137–139, 227, 281, 397
health, 16, 41, 106, 112, 178, 225, 264, 355, 394, 415
Catalase (CAT), 40, 47
Cell
biology, 280, 440, 441
death, 3, 309, 313, 318, 321, 325, 327
drug conjugates, 372
engineered pancreatic constructs (CEPCs), 362
lineages, 428–430
penetrating peptides (CPPs), 217
receptors, 35
transplantation, 347, 359, 434, 435, 439, 441
Cellular
architecture, 285
damage, 52, 103
dysfunction, 39
Centers for Disease Control and Prevention (CDC), 12, 18, 138, 139
Central
adiposity, 40, 51
nervous system (CNS), 43, 216
Ceruloplasmin, 297
Chemical-induced diabetes, 10
Chitosan (CS), 212, 217, 222, 223, 368–370
Chlorpropamide, 148
Cholesterol levels, 109, 111, 138, 146, 177
Chromatin
immunoprecipitation (ChIP), 99
remodeling, 253
structure, 50
Chromatography, 291
Chromium picolinate, 177
Chromosome 6, 8, 13, 35, 37, 209, 390
Chronic
hyperglycemia, 101, 130, 137, 393, 428
inflammation, 45, 49, 135, 280, 283, 315, 323, 334, 335, 393
kidney disease (CKD), 225
obstructive pulmonary disease (COPD), 14
Chylomicrons, 280
Cinnamon, 75, 172, 173, 179, 350
Circulating leukocytes, 322
Circulatory system, 43, 208
Clinical
decision
making (CDM), 20, 413
support (CDS), 402
manifestations, 38, 333
therapeutics, 260
trials, 130, 155, 178, 182, 232, 326, 330, 359, 361, 410, 413, 416, 434–438
Closed-loop systems, 90, 352, 354–356, 374, 375
Cognitive
behavioral therapy (CBT), 74
impairment, 43, 130
Coma, 43, 144
Combination therapy, 230, 331, 332
Comorbidities, 3, 14, 16, 17, 22, 84, 102, 104, 111, 112, 394, 433
Complementary and alternative medicine (CAM), 148
Computed
axial tomography (CAT), 40
tomography (CT), 73, 400
Congenital rubella syndrome (CRS), 134
Congestive heart failure (CHF), 141, 143
Continuous
glucose monitoring (CGM), 20, 21, 63, 65, 68, 71, 77, 79, 112, 113, 211, 231, 347, 353–356, 389, 405
positive airway pressure (CPAP), 113
Controlled insulin release, 365
Conventional
antidiabetic drugs, 171
pharmacotherapies, 178
Coronary
artery disease (CAD), 104, 105, 227, 260, 264
heart disease (CHD), 130
Cortisol, 9, 103
Coxsackie virus, 95, 96
C-peptide, 49, 72, 151, 280, 317, 325, 330, 385, 432, 433, 435, 436
C-reactive protein (CRP), 296

Cushing syndrome, 36
Cystic fibrosis (CF), 10, 87, 133
Cytokine, 43, 47, 94, 135–137, 274, 281, 283, 289, 309, 310, 313, 315, 316, 318, 319, 323–327, 334, 393
modulation, 334
production, 136
Cytomegalovirus (CMV), 134
Cytoplasmic antibodies, 314
Cytoskeleton, 292
Cytotoxic oligomers, 101

D

Dapagliflozin, 142
Data
analytics, 22, 386–388, 399, 402, 408
privacy, 78, 374, 384, 389, 399, 403, 407–409, 412, 416, 418
safety, 414
science, 410
Demographic
data, 10
transitions, 347
Dendrimers, 221, 369
Dendritic cells (DCs), 311, 316, 322, 323, 326, 327, 435
Deoxyribonucleic acid (DNA)
molecule, 94
technology, 13
Dephosphorylation, 135
Depolarization, 290, 434
Depression, 18, 74, 110
Depressive symptoms, 16, 41, 110
Dexamethasone, 275
Diabetes, 3–22, 33–44, 46, 48–52, 63–79, 83–88, 90–96, 98, 100–113, 129–134, 136–140, 142, 143, 145–151, 155, 163–168, 170–173, 176–179, 181, 183–186, 205–214, 216, 221–233, 247–266, 273–278, 282, 286, 289, 291–293, 295–299, 301, 309–372, 374, 375, 383–386, 389–398, 403–405, 415, 418, 419, 428, 431–434, 436–441
age-specific trends, 14
burden, 14, 64, 70, 185
chemical-induced diabetes, 10
classification, 7, 87
gestational diabetes mellitus (GDM), 9
type 1 diabetes mellitus (T1DM), 7
type 2 diabetes mellitus (T2DM), 8
comorbid conditions, 16
complications, 21, 67, 75, 138, 139, 208, 391, 397
data collection and analysis, 20
definition, 5
blood glucose levels, 6
HbA1c levels, 6
historical perspective, 5
modern definition, 5
oral glucose tolerance test (OGTT), 7
pathophysiological basis, 5
random blood sugar test, 7
dyslipidemia, 108
environmental contaminants, 19
epidemiology, 18, 19
etiology, 3, 34
genetics replication and meta-analysis (DIAGRAM), 253
global prevalence and incidence, 10
heritability, 247
immunomodulation, 310
insipidus, 346
machine learning applications, 20
macrovascular complications, 15
mellitus (DM), 3–5, 7–9, 16, 19, 22, 33–36, 38–40, 42–44, 48, 50–52, 63, 64, 66, 73, 79, 83–87, 108, 113, 129–134, 136–140, 143, 147, 148, 155, 163, 167, 173, 178, 186, 205–209, 233, 247, 248, 266, 274–276, 278, 279, 282, 285, 296, 300, 301, 310–313, 315, 320, 325, 330, 335, 346, 347, 349, 351, 362, 371, 375, 388–390, 427, 428, 431, 432, 440, 441
cultural aspects, 40
etiological factors, 36
gestational diabetes mellitus (GDM), 36
maturity-onset diabetes of the young (MODY), 36
type 1 diabetes mellitus (T1DM), 35
type 2 diabetes mellitus (T2DM), 35

type II (DMT2), 274–284, 286, 288, 289, 291, 293–299
metabolic syndrome, 19
microvascular complications, 14
monogenic diabetes syndromes, 9
morbidity burden, 17
mortality rate, 17
pathogenesis, 130, 137, 164–166, 184, 247, 293
pathophysiology, 5, 34, 39, 150, 166, 171, 185, 319, 326
prevalence, 10–12, 14, 18, 21, 22, 35, 38, 40, 64, 69, 70, 83, 207, 231, 248, 254, 349
prevention program (DPP), 254
real-world data utilization, 20
regional variations, 12
risk factors, 12
genetic predisposition, 12
lifestyle and behavioral factors, 13
secondary diabetes, 10
socioeconomic and environmental factors, 13
self-management education (DSME), 68
Diabetic
animal models, 171, 289, 320
cardiomyopathy, 371
dermopathy, 110
foot
disease, 21, 212, 227
infection (DFI), 228, 229
ulcer (DFU), 227–229
ketoacidosis (DKA), 8, 43
kidney disease, 17
nephropathy, 15, 36, 69, 72, 84, 91, 106, 107, 111
peripheral neuropathy (DPN), 226
retinal neurodegeneration (DRN), 225
retinopathy, 18, 69, 73, 91, 107, 108, 110, 111, 225
Diabetogenic immune cells, 318
Diagnostic
criteria, 6, 7
molecular biomarkers, 332
technologies, 65, 408
thresholds, 19
Digital
health, 232, 233, 402, 403, 419
PCR (dPCR), 401
Dipeptidyl peptidase-4 (DPP-4), 66, 68, 74, 140, 170, 254, 260, 394
Disease
mechanisms, 185, 254, 398, 400, 413, 418
pathophysiology, 273, 301
phenotype, 165, 166
progression, 4, 43, 111, 225, 263, 315, 328, 349, 384, 385, 387, 397, 401, 403, 404, 414
Disposition index (DI), 92
Distal sensory nerve fibers, 226
Dosage optimization, 398
Double vision, 107
Down syndrome, 134
Drug
delivery systems, 184, 185, 221, 374, 375
reactions, 387, 397, 417
Dyslipidemia, 44, 84, 104, 108, 109, 111, 138, 165, 225, 282, 329
Dyslipidemic profile, 108
Dysregulation, 19, 33, 150, 286, 315, 317
Dysuria, 428

E

Early
detection, 44, 72, 73, 106, 110, 111, 231, 401
diagnosis, 22, 66–68, 70, 109, 400
insulin response (EIR), 294, 295
stage cell death, 313
Economic burden, 4, 21, 69, 102, 129
Electrochemical enzymatic measurements, 214
Electron transport chain (ETC), 47, 290
Electronic health records (EHRs), 20, 264, 387, 389, 402, 407
Embryoid bodies (EBs), 432
Embryonic stem cells (ESCs), 360, 427, 429–432, 436, 440
Empagliflozin, 142
Encapsulated drugs, 364

Encapsulation techniques, 345
Encephalomyocarditis virus, 165
Endocrine
  disorders, 100, 134, 207
  disruptors, 19
Endogenous glucose, 364
Endoplasmic reticulum (ER), 44, 45, 136, 280, 287, 288, 292, 299, 313, 332
  kinase (PERK), 44, 136
Endothelial dysfunction, 103, 104
Endothelin-1 (ET-1), 135
Endothelium, 15
End-stage renal disease (ESRD), 18, 22, 106
Energy substrates, 43
Engineered
  biological systems, 345
  cells, 345, 353, 359
  cellular structures, 375
Environmental
  contaminants, 19, 22
  determinants, 262
  factors, 13, 35, 37, 38, 44, 50, 88, 94, 95, 97, 247, 256, 262, 263, 266, 276, 277, 384, 390, 392, 396, 418
  hazards, 322
  risks, 13
  stressors, 396
  toxins, 8, 396
Enzyme
  biofuel cell (EBFC), 212
  immobilization, 215
  nanoparticles, 371
Eosinophils, 311
Epidemiology, 18, 19
Epidermal growth factor (EGF), 228
Epigallocatechin gallate (EGCG), 167
Epigenetic, 50, 98, 99, 266
  factors, 94, 99, 248, 266
Epigenomics, 248, 266
Erectile dysfunction (ED), 107, 226
Ertugliflozin, 142
Ethnicity, 9, 39, 90, 96, 261
Ethnopharmacology, 149
Etiopathogenesis, 95
European Prospective Investigation into Cancer and Nutrition (EPIC), 255, 256
Evidence-based guidelines, 402, 413, 416
Exosomes, 282
Extracellular
  domain (ECD), 333
  matrix (ECM), 103, 225, 228, 362, 435
Eye damage, 91, 391

F

Family history of diabetes (FHD), 295, 296
Fasting
  glucose levels, 49, 66, 71, 93, 99, 131, 139, 142, 252
  plasma glucose (FPG), 43, 63, 65, 71, 93, 135, 141, 213
Fatigue, 9, 141
Fatty
  acid, 43, 45, 48, 49, 98, 103, 109, 113, 135, 137, 172, 177, 315, 316, 370
  mice, 292
Fecal transplants, 331
Feedback mechanisms, 285
Female sexual dysfunction (FSD), 226
Fibrinogen, 294, 299
Fibroblasts, 359
Fibrocalcific pancreatopathy, 133
Fibrous cap, 16
Fish oil supplements, 177
Flavin adenine dinucleotide (FAD), 47
Flavonoids, 148–150, 167, 173, 175
Fluorescein angiography, 107
Foam cells, 15, 16
Focused ultrasound system (FUS), 223
Foot ulcers, 15
Forecasting vascular complications, 247
Fractionation, 288, 294
Free fatty acids (FFAs), 45, 48, 103, 109, 113, 137, 138, 315
Functional antagonists, 46

G

Gastrointestinal (GI)
  mucosa, 49
  tract, 211, 368

Gene
environment interactions, 130, 186, 248, 266, 392
expression patterns, 401, 413
insulin secretion, 9
methylation, 137
Genetic, 18, 35, 38, 131, 253, 254, 257, 259, 261–263, 277, 333, 383, 384, 386, 387, 399, 410, 411
aberration, 87
mutations, 6, 397, 408
polymorphisms, 208, 265
predisposition, 12, 36–38, 45, 51, 52, 64, 148, 183, 254, 256, 262, 278, 383–385, 390, 391, 405, 407
profiling, 248, 265, 391, 419
testing, 261, 383, 385, 386, 388, 389, 392, 396–399, 403, 405, 406, 412
variants, 247, 249, 250, 252, 253, 258, 261, 265, 266, 278, 389–391, 397, 398, 413
Genome-wide association studies (GWAS), 9, 96, 208, 247, 250–253, 258, 260, 262, 266, 385, 397, 398
Genomic
markers, 400
medicine, 409
technologies, 385
Gestational diabetes mellitus (GDM), 3, 4, 6, 7, 9, 36, 39, 44, 51, 71, 87, 91, 132, 139, 206, 311
Global prevalence, 10, 11, 18, 130, 131, 254
Glomerular filtration rate (GFR), 141, 225
Glucagon, 33, 43, 45, 46, 51, 74, 99, 137, 141, 142, 144, 259, 274, 284–286, 331
glucagon-like peptide-1 (GLP-1), 51, 66, 68, 74, 99, 137, 140, 142, 143, 248, 260, 265, 331, 354, 356, 369, 393, 394
secretion, 33, 43, 137, 142, 144
Glucagonoma, 134
Glucocorticoid, 10, 41, 87, 134
Glucokinase (GCK), 36, 133, 143, 165
Glucolipotoxicity, 45
Gluconeogenesis, 85, 141, 146, 167, 168, 171, 297, 332
Glucose
concentrations, 41, 49, 146, 213, 214, 250–252, 351, 356, 365, 367, 369, 371
dehydrogenase (GDH), 213
fluctuations, 367, 368
glucose-6-phosphatase, 332
glucose-lowering therapies, 391
glucose-regulated protein (GRP), 288
glucose-responsive
insulin (GRI), 232, 347, 366, 369, 372, 374, 439
materials, 372
systems, 353, 364, 365, 375
technologies, 371
glucose-sensing components, 365
glucose-stimulated insulin secretion (GSIS), 146, 274, 286, 293
homeostasis, 33, 46, 52, 86, 150, 171, 176, 277, 285, 297, 299, 315, 320, 332, 363, 440, 441
intolerance, 9, 41, 164, 320
levels, 3, 4, 6, 7, 43–45, 49, 63–65, 68, 71, 76, 85, 132, 142, 143, 145–147, 171, 175–177, 205, 212, 213, 221, 248, 252, 259, 274, 279, 285, 290, 291, 310, 345, 346, 352, 355–357, 359, 360, 363–367, 370–372, 385, 386, 388, 389, 403, 404, 433, 434
metabolism, 6, 7, 19, 46, 52, 71, 73, 74, 92, 149, 165, 168–171, 175–178, 281, 283, 290, 325, 385, 393, 397
meter, 86, 212, 213, 223
monitoring, 21, 63, 65, 69, 71, 79, 90, 111–113, 205, 211, 212, 232, 233, 328, 351, 353–355, 364, 367, 389
monitors, 11, 78, 86, 347
oxidase (GOx), 213, 215, 371, 372
production, 5, 279
regulation, 5, 258, 345, 347, 350, 351, 353, 356, 360, 361, 364, 369, 371
tolerance, 3, 7, 9, 39, 44, 49, 63, 65, 91–93, 104, 131, 132, 136, 137, 139, 145, 146, 151, 176, 177, 251, 274, 294, 368, 385

toxicity, 45, 137, 139
transport, 48, 133, 143, 145, 149, 213, 221, 286, 321
Glucosidase enzymes, 369
Glutamic acid decarboxylase (GAD), 209, 314, 326, 332, 435
Glutathione peroxidase (GPx), 47, 292
Glycated hemoglobin, 72, 99, 132, 385
Glycemia, 6
Glycemic
control, 63, 66–68, 72–74, 77, 112, 129, 139, 170, 175–178, 208, 231, 252, 283, 329, 354–356, 363, 391–395, 397, 404, 405, 431, 440
dysregulation, 19
traits, 250–252, 260, 266
Glyceraldehyde-3-phosphate dehydrogenase (GAPDH), 299
Glycogenolysis, 85, 297, 332
Glycolytic flux, 84
GMP (good manufacturing practices), 180
Golgi apparatus (GA), 280
Good agricultural practices (GAP), 180
Gut
dysbiosis, 331
immune system, 50
microbiome, 8, 51, 98, 184
microbiota, 34, 48–50, 171, 178
Gymnemic acids, 175

H

Hazardous chemicals, 13
Healthcare
professionals, 70, 75, 78, 79, 112, 409, 410, 412, 413, 415
services, 17
systems, 18, 64, 67, 70, 149, 276, 328, 408, 412, 413
Health
inequities, 13
Insurance Portability and Accountability Act (HIPAA), 407
literacy, 76, 78
outcomes, 4, 13, 74, 76, 77, 79, 110, 130, 178, 186, 256, 259, 354, 358, 365, 367, 386, 392, 395, 396, 412
Heart
attack, 16, 18, 69, 108
disease, 84, 91, 103, 105, 129–131, 139, 212, 224, 226, 391, 398, 433
failure, 103, 105, 130, 141
rate, 106, 415
Heat shock proteins (HSPs), 290, 299
Hematopoietic stem cells (HSCs), 316, 430, 433, 435
Hemochromatosis, 10, 133
Hemoglobin A1c (HbA1c), 6, 63, 65, 72, 143, 213, 227, 250, 251, 432
levels, 3, 6, 88, 354, 355, 433, 435–437
values, 6
Hemopexin, 297
Hepatic glucose output (HGO), 135, 285
Hepatitis C enterovirus infection, 98
Hepatocellular lipids, 46
Hepatocyte nuclear factor 4α (HNF-4α), 36, 133
Hepatoma cells, 321
Herbal
formulations, 178
remedies, 148, 181, 346
supplements, 63, 66, 68, 74, 179, 182
Heritable epigenetic factors, 94
Heterogeneity, 4, 19, 38, 164, 265, 384, 389
Hexosamine pathway, 84, 225
High
blood pressure, 227
carbohydrate low-fat (HCLF), 328, 329
cholesterol, 105
content screening (HCS), 401
density
cholesterol, 138
lipoprotein (HDL), 49, 109, 138
fat diet, 165, 291, 298
glucose levels, 45, 367
risk populations, 254
Homeostasis, 33, 45, 46, 52, 86, 138, 150, 171, 176, 277, 285, 297, 299, 301, 315, 320, 322, 332, 334, 363, 431, 440, 441
Hormonal
disturbances, 10
regulation, 385

Hormone-sensitive lipase (HSL), 48, 103
Human
embryonic stem cells (hESCs), 436
islet, 47, 287, 288
amyloid polypeptide (hIAPP), 101
leukocyte antigen (HLA), 8, 13, 35, 51, 94, 95, 209, 313, 390, 391
placental lactogens (hPL), 9
pluripotent stem cells (hPSCs), 434
Hyaluronic acid, 371
Hydrogen peroxide (H_2O_2), 365
Hydroxyethyl methacrylate (HEMA), 219
Hyperglycemia, 8, 43–47, 52, 64, 67, 68, 71, 77, 83–86, 88, 92, 101, 105, 106, 111, 113, 130, 131, 135, 137, 141, 146, 147, 150, 163–165, 275, 277, 296, 311, 314, 315, 327, 351, 352, 354, 357, 363, 393, 405, 427, 428, 434, 435
Hyperglycemic crises, 47, 72, 85, 92, 98, 132, 228, 232, 330, 352, 365, 369, 371
Hyperinsulinemia, 283
Hyperlipidemia, 19, 45–47, 151, 227, 280
Hyperphosphorylation, 135
Hypertension, 19, 44, 84, 104, 105, 108, 111, 181, 225, 227, 251, 281, 415
Hyperthyroidism, 36, 134
Hypertriglyceridemia, 109
Hypertrophy, 144, 225, 292, 316
Hypoglycemia, 9, 43, 68, 77, 101, 109, 142, 144, 179, 180–182, 208, 231, 285, 351, 352, 354, 357, 360, 363, 364, 366, 369, 370, 372, 389, 405, 437
Hypoglycemic
agents, 4, 63, 74, 179, 180, 208, 347, 351, 397
episodes, 364, 369
Hypokalemia, 144

I

Imaging biomarkers, 402
Immature secretory vesicles, 280
Immune
cell, 274, 310, 318, 322, 323, 325, 326, 333, 334
checkpoint inhibitors, 327
function, 310
polarization, 310
dysregulation and polyendocrinopathy enteropathy X-linked (IPEX), 317
infiltrates, 313
regulation, 8, 333
system, 5, 49, 50, 88, 94, 151, 181, 209, 223, 309–312, 315, 321–323, 325–327, 334, 359, 390, 427, 435
tolerance induction (ITI), 334
Immunogenic vaccinations, 327
Immunoglobulin kappa-chain, 297
Immunoisolation techniques, 361
Immunological
checkpoints, 325, 326
microenvironments, 319
pathways, 334
rejection, 360, 361, 434, 440
synapse, 325
Immunometabolism, 310, 335
Immunomodulation, 309, 310, 333–335
Immunomodulatory
drugs, 330, 331
effects, 331
medications, 310, 331
Immunosuppressants, 10, 166, 437
Immunosuppression, 334, 359, 440
Immunotherapeutic approaches, 310
Immunotherapy, 309, 318, 328, 330, 332, 333, 438
Impaired
fasting glucose (IFG), 93, 131
glucose tolerance (IGT), 7, 44, 93, 131
Induced
pluripotent stem cells (iPSCs), 332, 360, 427, 436
Treg (iTreg), 327
Infectious diseases, 387
Inflammation, 15, 19, 43, 45, 46, 49, 50, 98, 99, 103–105, 109, 134, 135, 138, 145, 147, 168, 171, 177, 178, 210, 225, 228, 229, 279–281, 283, 295, 296, 298, 309, 310, 313–315, 319, 320, 322, 323, 327, 331, 334, 335, 393, 428, 438
Inflammatory
cytokines, 135–137, 274, 283, 316, 319, 325
disorders, 328

mediators, 319, 334
pathways, 33, 52, 103, 150, 277
response, 294, 319, 322, 325
Inhibitory receptors (IRs), 321, 325
Inositol
inositol-requiring enzyme 1 (IRE1), 44
trisphosphate (IP3), 45
Insulin (INS), 3–10, 16, 19–22, 33–37, 39, 41–43, 45–52, 63, 64, 66–68, 70–74, 77, 78, 83, 85–88, 90–92, 95, 96, 98–102, 104, 105, 109, 131–151, 164, 165, 167–171, 173, 175–179, 205–211, 217–224, 231–233, 248, 250–252, 259, 274, 276–283, 285, 286, 288–294, 296–299, 301, 309–311, 313–317, 319–321, 325, 326, 328, 329, 332–334, 345–347, 350–357, 359–361, 363–372, 374, 375, 384, 388–394, 396, 397, 403–405, 427, 428, 431–441
action, 5, 9, 10, 175, 205, 207, 220, 251, 278, 282, 370, 390, 428
administration, 90, 102, 211, 217, 231, 345, 352–354, 357, 363, 364, 367, 369
amyloidosis, 102
antigen, 332
autoantibody (IAA), 314, 326
deficiency, 8, 64, 132, 164, 207, 309, 390
delivery, 20, 21, 77, 102, 205, 211, 218–220, 222, 223, 231–233, 332, 351–357, 366, 368–372, 375
dosage, 353, 354, 403, 405, 432, 433, 436
injection, 4, 90, 208, 345, 352, 356, 357, 359, 370
insulin
promoter factor 1 (IPF-1), 36
dendrimer nanocomplexes, 370
dependent diabetes mellitus (IDDM), 4, 13, 35, 36, 86, 88, 132, 148, 207, 310, 359, 363
producing cells (IPCs), 353, 360, 361, 363, 437
responsive cells, 281
sensitizing agents, 292
production, 5, 8, 9, 35, 36, 43, 51, 52, 72–74, 95, 96, 109, 205, 209, 286, 310, 311, 316, 326, 347, 351, 352, 356, 360, 361, 364, 384, 388, 390, 393, 427, 431, 440
pump, 4, 64, 78, 86, 347, 353, 354
receptor substrate-1 (IRS-1), 48, 135, 136, 146, 209, 320, 321
resistance (IR), 3–9, 16, 19, 22, 33–36, 39, 42, 43, 45, 48, 49, 51, 52, 64, 73, 86, 87, 91, 92, 98, 99, 105, 109, 132, 134–138, 145–147, 164, 165, 207, 209, 210, 251, 252, 276–281, 283, 292, 294, 296, 298, 299, 301, 310, 311, 315, 316, 319–321, 325, 334, 388, 390, 393, 394, 396, 428
secretion, 4, 5, 8, 9, 36, 37, 41, 45–47, 63, 64, 68, 85, 86, 92, 96, 100, 109, 131, 134, 136, 137, 139, 141, 145–147, 149, 150, 164, 167, 168, 170, 175–177, 207, 250, 251, 274, 276, 277, 286, 291, 292, 310, 315, 350, 369, 370, 384, 390, 393, 428
secretory dysfunction, 46
sensitivity, 7, 37, 41, 48, 66, 67, 73, 74, 92, 104, 145, 146, 150, 167–171, 175–178, 259, 279–281, 283, 329, 334, 391, 393, 397
signaling, 48, 135, 145, 149, 165, 168, 169, 319, 320
therapy, 63, 66, 71, 72, 77, 91, 220, 221, 353, 354, 361, 364, 366, 369, 404, 405, 436
Interleukin (IL), 45, 47, 48, 136, 293, 313, 314, 316–322, 325, 327, 331
IL-6, 47, 48, 136, 293, 316, 318, 320–322
Intermediate-density lipoprotein (IDL), 108, 113
International Diabetes Federation (IDF), 10–12, 18, 64, 69, 130, 131, 147, 206, 248, 311
Islet
amyloid polypeptide (IAPP), 42, 45, 52, 101, 137
cell
antibody (ICA), 314, 326, 435

autoantibodies, 314, 326
communication, 285
infusion, 360
transplantation, 317, 361, 434, 437

J

Japanese population, 96
Jaundice, 9
Juvenile diabetes, 4, 88, 310

K

Kallikrein binding protein (KBP), 297
Ketoacidosis, 8, 35, 43
Kidney
damage, 15, 72, 225
failure, 15, 17, 69, 91, 106, 108
function, 111, 151
transplantation, 18
Klinefelter syndrome, 36, 134
Krebs cycle, 290, 291, 298

L

Laser photocoagulation, 15
Latent tuberculosis infection (LTBI), 320
Laurence–Moon–Biedl syndrome, 134
Leprechaunism, 134
Leptin resistance, 19
Lifelong immunosuppression, 359
Lifestyle
factors, 3, 18, 19, 21, 22, 44, 97, 138, 183, 254, 387, 392, 397, 403
interventions, 12, 17, 21, 63, 254, 385
modification, 18, 63, 65, 67–69, 72, 74, 79, 107, 349, 389
Lipid
levels, 16, 47, 151, 253, 397
metabolism, 108, 149, 169, 385
nanocarriers, 368
Lipodystrophy, 134, 144
syndromes, 134
Lipohypertrophy, 102
Lipoprotein, 108, 109, 280, 299, 301
lipase (LPL), 109, 281
Liposomes, 184, 217, 218, 231, 369, 372
Lipotoxicity, 45, 137
Lisofylline (LSF), 220
Liver insulin resistance, 299
LMICs (low- and middle-income countries), 12, 18, 70, 129
Logistic regression models, 11
Longitudinal data, 20
Long-lived cells, 318
Low-density
cholesterol, 138
lipoprotein (LDL), 15, 108, 109, 138, 280
Lymph nodes, 312, 323
Lymphatic circulation, 311
Lymphocyte, 16, 95, 311, 312, 314, 323, 324
activation genes (LAG), 325
homing receptors, 50
maturation, 326
Lymphocytic infiltration, 164
Lymphoid organs, 312, 323
Lysosomal proteins, 288

M

Machine learning (ML), 20, 22, 77, 79, 184, 186, 249, 384, 385, 398, 402–405, 414, 415, 417, 419
Macroangiopathy, 139
Macrophage, 15, 35, 135, 137, 219, 274, 311, 316, 322, 323, 334, 435
accumulation, 281, 316
infiltration, 47, 316
inflammatory protein (MIP), 316
polarization, 310
Macrosomia, 9, 91, 224
Macrovascular complications, 9, 15, 142, 150, 224
Magnetic resonance imaging (MRI), 73, 400
Major
depression, 110
histocompatibility complex (MHC), 37, 94
Marine
organisms, 148, 171
sponges, 169
Mass spectrometry (MS), 287, 288, 293, 294, 400, 401
Mast cells, 311

Matrix metalloproteinase 2 (MMP2), 47
Maturity-onset diabetes of the young (MODY), 36, 51, 87, 132, 251
Mesenchymal stem cell (MSCs), 427, 429, 431–435, 436, 440, 441
Metabolic
 abnormalities, 35, 310, 428
 biomarkers, 313
 diseases, 254
 disorders, 7, 85, 130, 253
 disturbances, 166, 182
 markers, 18
 profile, 183, 383, 384, 392, 394, 395
 profiling, 386
 syndrome, 3, 19, 22, 177, 209, 276, 315
Metabolism, 6, 7, 19, 41, 46, 52, 71, 73, 74, 85, 92, 96, 100, 108, 134, 143, 149, 163, 165, 168–171, 175–178, 184, 185, 216, 221, 279, 281, 283, 286, 290, 310, 325, 327, 346, 369, 371, 385, 393, 397, 428
Metabolomics, 183, 248, 266, 386, 387, 400, 401, 413, 414, 418
 clusters (MGCs), 49
Metagenomics, 248, 266
Methylation, 50, 94, 99, 100, 137
Mexican population, 42
Microalbuminuria, 15, 72, 151
Microaneurysms, 15, 73
Microangiopathy, 139
Microbiota-host interaction, 34
Micro-electromechanical systems (MEMS), 223
Microneedle (MN), 372
Microorganisms, 169, 311
Microvascular, 9, 14, 142, 150, 224, 247, 276
 problems, 224
Mild hyperglycemia, 44
Minor allele frequency (MAF), 250–252
Mitochondria, 101, 136, 139, 287, 288
Mitochondrial
 dysfunction, 138
 genes, 289
 pathways, 47
 proteins, 298, 299
 stress, 19
Mitogen-activated protein (MAP), 136, 321
Mobile applications, 77, 412
Monoclonal antibodies (mAbs), 331
Monocytes, 15, 45, 316, 323
Monogenic diabetes, 9, 132, 251, 265
Monozygotic twins, 37, 96
Mulberry leaf alkaloids, 175
Multidimensional omics profiling, 414
Multi-omics data, 184, 248, 249, 266
Multi-organ autoimmunity, 317
Multiple genetic factors, 13
Mumps virus, 95, 96
Muscle IGF receptor (MKR ML), 292
Myeloid cells, 316, 323
Myotonic dystrophy (DM), 134

N

Nanoelectromechanical systems (NEMS), 223
Nanomaterials, 211, 214, 215, 223
Nanomedicine, 211, 232, 368, 375
Nanoparticles (NPs), 48, 184, 211, 212, 215, 216, 218, 219, 222, 223, 228, 230, 231, 333, 368, 370–372
Nanosensors, 211, 214
Nanotechnology, 186, 205, 210, 211, 214, 222, 230–233, 368, 372
National
 Center for Biotechnology Information (NCBI), 94
 Diabetes Data Group (NDDG), 86
Natural
 killer (NK), 322–324, 331, 435
 products, 129, 130, 133, 148, 150, 167, 171, 173, 177–186
 Treg (nTreg), 327
Nausea, 8, 141, 144
Necrobiosis lipoidica diabeticorum, 111
Neonatal diabetes, 9, 87, 132, 251, 261
Nephropathy, 3, 8, 15, 36, 67, 69, 72, 84, 105, 106, 110, 111, 131, 139, 225, 281, 391
Nerve damage, 15, 90, 107, 111, 226
Nervous system, 43, 83, 103, 106, 216, 226
Neurodegenerative diseases, 101

Neuroendocrine dysfunction, 210
Neurological disorders, 84
Neuropathy, 3, 8, 15, 17, 18, 21, 64, 67, 69, 84, 91, 105–107, 111, 129–131, 139, 147, 151, 281, 397
Neutral protamine Hagedorn (NPH), 144
Neutrophils, 227, 311, 322
Newborn hypoglycemia, 9
Next-generation sequencing (NGS), 247, 397, 400, 401
Nicotinamide adenine dinucleotide (NAD), 47
Nicotinic acid, 134
Niosomes, 218
Nonalcoholic fatty liver disease (NAFLD), 48, 131
Non-coding
  DNA, 99
  RNA (ncRNA), 50
Non-healing ulcers, 72
Non-insulin-dependent diabetes mellitus (NIDDM), 86, 87, 132, 148, 207
Non-obese diabetic (NOD), 37, 163, 164, 312, 324, 331
Non-proliferative diabetic retinopathy (NPDR), 107, 108, 225, 226
Non-viral cell transfection, 216
Normal glucose tolerance (NGT), 49, 93, 294–296, 320
Normoglycemia, 208, 211, 438
Novel
  drug targets, 417
  immunomodulatory therapies, 334
  therapies, 360
Nuclear magnetic resonance (NMR), 400
Nutraceuticals, 177
Nutritional polysaccharides, 49

O

Obesity, 9–12, 14, 18, 21, 22, 35, 40, 42, 45, 48, 49, 51, 52, 64, 69, 70, 84, 86, 87, 90, 96–99, 104, 109, 112, 131, 134, 137, 138, 164, 165, 206, 208, 209, 248, 251, 253, 277, 278, 280, 283, 284, 291, 292, 298, 299, 315, 321, 347, 349, 390, 392–394, 403, 428
Observational cohort studies, 254
Obstructive sleep apnea (OSA), 98
Omics
  data, 184, 248, 249, 266, 384, 386, 413, 414
  technologies, 18, 183, 358
Optical coherence tomography (OCT), 72, 73
Oral
  administration, 208, 370, 371
  antihyperglycemic agents, 43
  glucose tolerance test (OGTT), 3, 7, 9, 63, 65, 71, 91, 93, 132, 251
  hypoglycemic agents, 4, 63, 179, 347, 397
Organ
  damage, 182
  Procurement and Transplantation Network (OPTN), 438
  rejection, 359
  transplantation, 438
Organic acids, 149
Osteoporosis, 329
Oxidative
  damage, 138
  phosphorylation, 47, 135
  stress, 16, 33, 45, 47, 52, 98, 99, 103, 104, 136, 145, 147, 150, 151, 167, 168, 175–178, 208, 216, 226, 279–281, 283, 292

P

Pacific Islanders, 39, 40, 278
Pancreas, 4, 5, 10, 36, 64, 85, 86, 90, 98, 101, 132, 147, 166, 221, 223, 231, 274, 277, 284, 285, 287, 288, 293, 297, 310, 313, 332, 346, 350, 352–356, 359, 360, 364, 365, 388, 390, 393, 440
Pancreatectomy, 133, 163, 164, 293
Pancreatic
  beta cells, 5, 7–9, 35, 43, 46, 52, 74, 87, 88, 92, 95, 96, 137, 147, 149, 164, 166–168, 175, 206, 211, 221, 223, 231, 290, 309, 311, 318, 325, 326, 332, 333, 345, 359, 360, 362, 364, 434

cells, 42, 96, 175, 209, 274–276, 293, 313, 319
dysfunction, 87
hormones, 285
islet, 45, 85, 99–101, 137, 164, 285, 439
microenvironment, 361
organoids, 360
pathology, 42
polypeptide, 285
progenitors, 434, 435, 437
tissue, 50, 52, 359–362, 369
Pancreatitis, 10, 36, 87, 133, 440
Pathogenesis, 8, 19, 34, 36, 39, 42, 43, 130, 134, 136, 137, 147, 164–166, 183, 184, 247, 254, 256, 266, 274, 276, 289, 293, 296, 299, 321, 414
Pathophysiology, 5, 34, 38, 39, 50, 150, 164, 166, 171, 185, 252, 273, 274, 280, 300, 301, 312, 316, 319, 326, 327, 386
Peptides, 140, 169–171, 215, 217, 313, 368, 433
Perfluorinated compounds (PFCs), 19
Peripheral
artery disease (PAD), 72, 103, 104
neuropathy, 107, 130, 147
vascular disease (PVD), 130, 131, 224, 281
Permanent neonatal diabetes mellitus (PNDM), 132
Personal health information (PHI), 407, 408
Personalized
medicine, 183, 185, 231, 233, 265, 266, 334, 351, 365, 384, 386–389, 396, 398–403, 405–419
therapies, 412, 417
Pesticides, 10, 182
P-glycoprotein (P-gp), 299
Pharmaceutical, 52, 149, 150, 259, 366, 367
compounds, 52
drugs, 180
Pharmacogenomics, 184–186, 265, 266, 400
Pharmacological
activities, 167, 169, 170
properties, 167, 186
treatments, 11, 112, 393, 394
Pharmacology, 73, 410
Pharmacotherapy, 63, 65, 66, 68, 79, 385
Phenolic acids, 175
Phenylboronic acid (PBA), 365, 367, 372
Pheochromocytoma, 134
Phosphorylation, 47, 135, 146, 286, 317, 320, 321
pH
responsive cationic polymeric micelles (PCPMs), 220
sensitive biodegradable polymers, 222
Physical
activity, 11, 19, 41, 52, 63, 73, 76, 90, 91, 96, 109, 254, 277, 279, 328, 330, 349, 354, 385, 390, 392–397, 404, 405, 415
exercise, 66, 265, 283, 395
inactivity, 37, 41, 70, 90, 104, 138, 209, 349
Physiological
parameters, 392, 415
processes, 5, 183, 264, 350
Phytochemicals, 175, 176, 178
Phytotherapy, 186
Placenta, 9, 36, 323, 429, 430, 433
Placental stem cells, 433
Plant-based medicines, 350
Plasma
glucose (PG), 37, 41, 43, 49, 63, 65, 71, 93, 132, 135, 145, 213, 366
triglyceride (TG) levels, 49, 108, 109
Plasminogen activator inhibitor-1 (PAI-1), 16, 48
Platelet aggregation, 16
Pluripotent stem cells (PSCs), 332, 360, 427, 429, 430, 434, 436, 439–441
Poly(lactic-co-glycolic acid) (PLGA), 217, 368
Poly(styrene-co-maleic acid), 220
Polyacrylamide (PAM), 222
Polyacrylic acid (PAA), 222
Polyanhydrides, 222
Polyaniline nanoparticles (PAni-NPs), 212
Polycystic ovary syndrome (PCOS), 9, 139

Polydipsia, 8, 9, 44, 92, 428
Polyendocrinopathy enteropathy, 317
Polyethylene glycol (PEG), 210, 222
Polygenic risk scores (PRS), 398
Polyinosinic-polycytidylic acid, 324
Polymer degradation, 372
Polymeric nanocarrier systems, 368
Polymersomes, 366
Polynuclear phagocytes, 312
Polyol pathway activation, 47
Polyphagia, 8
Polyphenols, 149, 168, 173
Polysaccharides, 49, 167–170, 216, 296
Polyurethanes (PU), 222
Polyuria, 8, 9, 34, 85, 92, 151, 346
Porphyria, 134
Positron emission tomography (PET), 400
Postprandial
    glucose levels, 6, 142
    hyperglycemia, 135, 141
Post-receptor insulin resistance, 35
Potassium ATP (KATP), 261, 290
Prader–Willi syndrome (PWS), 134
Prebiotic/postbiotic therapies, 331
Precision medicine, 4, 18, 112, 113, 205, 230, 358, 364, 384, 386, 387, 404, 408, 440
Prediabetes, 6, 93, 98, 282, 319, 403
Predictive modeling, 384, 404, 405, 419
Preeclampsia, 9, 36, 91
Preventive strategies, 34, 257, 398, 417
Pro-apoptotic signals, 45
Probiotics, 171
Pro-coagulant state, 16
Progesterone, 9
Prognosis, 38, 400, 401
Pro-inflammatory
    cytokines, 135–137, 274, 283
    mediators, 319
Proinsulin processing, 45, 46, 250, 252, 279, 313
Proliferative diabetic retinopathy (PDR), 107, 108, 225
Proliferator-activated receptor-gamma coactivator alpha-1 (PGCα-1), 99
Protein
    disulfide isomerase (PDI), 288, 299
    expression, 275, 289, 293, 300, 301
    folding, 45
    kinase C (PKC), 47, 135, 225, 226, 321
    protein interactions, 301
    tyrosine phosphatase (PTPN2), 169, 209, 314, 317, 321, 325, 326, 333
Proteinuria, 15, 106, 225
Proteomic techniques, 248, 264, 266, 273–275, 287–289, 291, 293, 294, 298–301, 332, 386, 387, 400–402, 413, 414, 418
Psychological distress, 18, 69
Psychosocial support, 21, 71
Public health, 11, 14, 21, 22, 69, 70, 347, 396
    interventions, 22
    policies, 22
    strategies, 14, 21
Pyridoxal phosphate (PLP), 332

Q

Quality control (QC), 180, 182, 183, 186
Quality of life (QoL), 3, 18, 63–69, 71, 73, 77, 79, 106, 107, 110, 112, 211, 226, 232, 247, 249, 265, 346, 347, 353, 365, 369, 375, 384, 395, 418

R

Racial disparities, 38
Radiation, 97
Random
    blood sugar assessment, 3
    glucose test, 93
Reactive oxygen species (ROS), 45–47, 136, 164, 228, 280, 290, 435
Real-time
    decision support systems (RT-DSS), 419
    glucose measurements, 354
    monitoring, 20, 367, 414
Real-world data (RWD), 20, 22
Red blood cell membranes (RBCMs), 212
Regenerative medicine, 232, 333, 430–432, 441
Regulatory
    mechanisms, 137, 331, 357

standards, 365
T cells, 316, 435
Renal
failure, 17, 64, 212, 247
impairment, 142
Respiratory distress syndrome (RDS), 9
Resveratrol, 172, 175
Retinopathy, 3, 6, 8, 15, 17, 18, 64, 69, 73, 91, 103, 105, 107, 108, 110, 111, 131, 139, 151, 225, 281, 391, 405
Revascularization, 229, 438
Rheumatoid arthritis (RA), 325
Risk
assessment, 137, 262, 263, 392, 398
factors, 9, 12–14, 18, 19, 22, 40, 52, 70, 73, 90, 95–97, 100, 104, 109, 112, 138, 139, 147, 208, 225–227, 247, 248, 261, 277, 279, 295, 315, 391, 403, 415
Rubella virus, 95, 96

S

Sarco/endoplasmic Reticulum Ca2+ ATPase (SERCA), 45
Saturated fatty acid (SFA), 135
Screen-printed electrodes (SPEs), 214
Secretory granules, 286, 288, 290, 292, 333
Sedentary behavior, 9, 11, 44
Seizures, 43
Self
management, 68, 69, 71, 74, 76, 111, 112, 231, 350, 385, 386, 403
renewal capacity, 431
reported data, 255
Sepsis, 17
Serine/threonine phosphorylation, 135, 321
Serum insulin, 221
Short-chain fatty acid (SCFA), 49, 171, 331
Silicon-on-insulator (SOI), 223
Silk fibroin, 365
Single nucleotide polymorphisms (SNPs), 48, 317, 400
Skeletal muscle, 41, 92, 99, 146, 169, 279, 292, 299, 311, 321, 428
Skin
transplantation, 228
ulcers, 227
Sleep apnea, 98, 109, 110
Slow-healing wounds, 91
Smart therapeutic system, 364
Smooth muscle cells, 16
Social determinants of health (SDOH), 22
Socioeconomic
factors, 64, 76, 349
status, 13, 14, 76, 97, 396
Sodium-glucose cotransporter 2 (SGLT2), 51, 66, 68, 74, 142, 143, 248, 265, 354, 356, 394
Solid lipid nanoparticles (SLNs), 218, 219, 368
Somatic cells, 95, 430, 436
Somatostatinoma, 134
Spectrometry, 291
Spermatogonial stem cells (SSCs), 430
Standard therapies, 183
Standardized
criteria, 19
mortality rate (SMR), 17
Statistical models, 11
Steady-state ROS, 280
Stem cell, 359
therapy, 359, 428, 431, 440, 441
β cells (SC-β), 434
Streptozotocin (STZ), 151, 163–165, 295–297
Stroke, 16, 18, 43, 69, 91, 104, 105, 108, 130, 212, 224, 226, 281
Sulfonylureas, 66, 68, 74, 91, 140, 142, 259, 261, 391, 394
Superoxide dismutase 1 (SOD1), 47
Surface
alterations, 232
enhanced laser desorption/ionization time-of-flight spectrometry (SELDI TOF-MS), 294
Survival rates, 11
Susceptibility molecules, 13
Sympathetic nervous system (SNS), 103
Sympathoadrenal symptoms, 43
Synthetic
biology, 345, 347, 350, 352, 353, 355, 358, 364, 372, 374, 375
insulins, 347
molecules, 351, 374

Systemic inflammation, 99, 134, 310

T

Telemedicine platforms, 385
Teplizumab, 333
Teratogenic effects, 36
Terpenoids, 148, 150, 168, 170
Therapeutic
 drugs, 363, 366
 efficacy, 232, 366, 367, 374, 414
 molecules, 365
 strategies, 167, 183, 260, 261, 350, 354
Thiazide diuretics, 10
Thiazolidinediones (TZDs), 140, 259
Thioredoxin (TXN), 47
Three-dimensional (3D), 360–363, 434, 438, 439, 441
 bioprinting, 360, 361, 439, 441
 culture systems, 362, 363
Threonine phosphorylation, 135, 321
Thrombosis, 16, 103, 105
Tissue
 engineering, 359, 361–363, 368
 regeneration, 205, 228, 232, 233, 369
 scaffolds, 362
Titanium dioxide (TiO_2), 215
T-lymphocytes (T-cells), 8, 16, 35, 95, 309, 312, 314–316, 322, 324–326, 331, 334, 435
Traditional
 Chinese medicine (TCM), 176
 medicinal plants, 155, 173, 178
Transcription factors, 50, 253, 363, 436
Transcriptomic data, 248, 266, 386, 387, 413, 414
Transferrin, 297
Transient neonatal diabetes mellitus (TNDM), 132
Transition metals, 47
Transmembrane, 333
Transmucosal adhesive (TLA), 149
Transplantation, 18, 87, 90, 228, 229, 317, 347, 359–362, 427, 431, 433–435, 437–441
Transthyretin (TTR) tetramer, 297
Triglycerides, 103, 280
Tuberculosis (TB), 132, 320
Tumor necrosis factor-α (TNF-α), 48, 136, 138, 313, 316, 318, 320–322
Two-dimensional (2D), 207, 288, 362
Type 1 diabetes (T1D), 3, 5, 7, 12, 17, 35, 38, 43, 64, 66, 67, 69, 71, 72, 74, 87, 88, 95, 96, 109, 147, 164–166, 206, 207, 209, 310, 312–319, 323–334, 349, 360, 362, 363, 390, 391, 393, 432–437
 mellitus (T1DM), 3, 4, 7–10, 35–39, 42–44, 50, 51, 87, 88, 90, 94–96, 99–102, 208, 209, 310, 312–314, 319, 321, 324, 329, 332, 349, 350, 362
Type 2 diabetes (T2D), 3–5, 8, 11–13, 16, 17, 21, 22, 35, 37, 39, 40, 42–44, 46, 48, 51, 52, 64, 66–70, 72–74, 87, 90, 91, 109, 133, 136–140, 143, 164–166, 206–209, 221, 223, 224, 226, 227, 250–259, 262–266, 310, 315, 316, 319, 320, 323, 325–327, 329, 333, 334, 347, 349, 351, 353, 390, 391, 393, 394, 433, 435, 436, 440
 mellitus (T2DM), 3, 4, 7–10, 12, 35, 37–45, 48, 49, 51, 52, 87, 92, 93, 96–101, 133, 134, 137, 139, 140, 147, 208–210, 226, 260, 281, 282, 310, 311, 315, 319, 321, 332, 349–351
Tyrosine kinase, 321

U

Uncontrolled diabetes, 67
Unfolded protein response (UPR), 45, 136
United
 Kingdom Prospective Diabetes Study (UKPDS), 6, 16
 Network for Organ Sharing (UNOS), 438
Universal stem cells, 361
Urbanization, 10–12, 34, 64, 69, 349
Urinary
 excretion, 296
 glucose levels, 212
Urticaria, 142

V

Vascular
- endothelial growth factor (VEGF), 228
- inflammation, 19
- insufficiency, 227

Very-low-density lipoprotein (VLDL), 108, 109, 138, 280
Viral infections, 88, 95, 209
Visceral fat, 9, 40, 98, 393
Vision loss, 18, 73, 226
Visual impairment, 9
Vitamin D
- deficiency, 8
- insufficiency, 88

W

Waist circumference (WC), 40, 256
Waist-to-hip ratio (WHR), 40, 41
Wearable
- devices, 20, 211, 231, 357, 385, 386, 414, 415
- sensing technologies, 210
- technologies, 367, 384, 386, 416

Weight
- gain, 98, 102, 143, 144, 147, 208, 394
- loss, 8, 44, 71, 88, 91, 141, 178, 283, 329, 428
- management, 63, 349

Wolfram syndrome, 134
World Health Organization (WHO), 6, 41, 83, 84, 86, 131, 132, 208, 276, 315, 347
Wound
- dressing, 228, 229
- healing, 111, 217, 228, 229

X

Xenogeneic islet grafts, 438
Xenografts, 229

Y

Yoga, 63, 66, 68, 74, 75
Young adults, 132, 280

Z

Zinc (Zn) supplements, 177
Zucker diabetic fatty (ZDF), 172, 291
Zucker fatty (ZF), 291